WHAT YOU MAY NOT KNOW ABOUT BARTONELLA, BABESIA, LYME DISEASE AND OTHER TICK & FLEA-BORNE INFECTIONS

IMPROVING TREATMENT SPEED, RECOVERY & PATIENT SATISFACTION

James Schaller, MD, MAR

and

Kimberly Mountjoy, MS

International University Infectious Disease Press
Bank Towers • Newgate Center (305)
5150 Tamiami Trail North [Highway 41]
Naples, Florida 34103

Cover Art: Nick Botner

Lead Research and Research Study Acquisitions: Randal Blackwell

Copy Editing by Kimberly Mountjoy, Lindsay Gibson,
Jeremy Schaller and anonymous patients from all over the world

Wholesale discount requires purchase of at least twenty copies and can be in five book units. Fax request to (239) 304-1987 and (239) 263-6760.

Library of Congress Cataloging Data

Schaller, J.L; Mountjoy, K.

ISBN: 978098408895942

What you may not know about bartonella, babesia, lyme disease and other tick & flea-borne infections: improving treatment speed, recovery & patient satisfaction

by J.L. Schaller and K. Mountjoy

1.Tick infections 2. Flea infections 3. Bartonella 4. Babesia 5. Lyme disease

Manufactured in the United States of America

First Edition

To my beloved friends in USA prisons,
with a hope we will end our leadership as the PRISON NATION,
and lead in liberty and not inmate numbers.

Let our nation return to timely trials,
end cruel and unusual excessive sentences,
allow the poor to have a good defense,
and may our peace officers never exceed the facts.

Let our prisons never have any element of torture—
the time is already a torture.

Contents

Tick and Flea Infection Emerging Medicine

Politics and Powers

I will simply be very clear and frank about the current debate over tick infections and what I see as a full-time reader and researcher. I do not mean to be disrespectful, but I do mean to start ending nonsense.

First, when you get a doctorate in medicine, you take an oath that allows you to wrestle with the complexity of medicine. Samples include dealing with emerging infections like HIV/AIDS, the new versions of Hepatitis, Stem cell technology explosions, nutritional science (which only exists outside of the pharmaceutical and medical device control of treatment options), drug resistant strains of tuberculosis, and *over a thousand complex medical issues, so you get some room to wiggle.*

Simply, it is naive to assume the USA has all the answers when we are not even in the top 50 nations in terms of physician numbers per population, and many physicians in the United States are leaving medicine. So my comments are not meant to control over 800,000 physicians of which over 80% are not in the AMA and who care for over 300 million Americans.

I do not have all the answers in the area of tick and flea infections. And while working on my fifth book on Babesia, I found that books on parasites by smart authors have only one to three pages on Babesia; perhaps no one has all the answers.

Confusingly, the real debate or hate seems to center around the four letter word, "Lyme," referring to "Lyme disease." And the hatred this topic generates is similar to race hatred as seen in the Civil War or other periods of race hatred. Simply, this is an error, and also shows a lack of insight in how we all think.

If you trust a patient report more than an evidence based study or vice versa, I will support you. I trust both and neither.

And so in legal situations, I will defend a healer who wants to treat a patient for one infection for a short time, yet I will also support a healer who wants to treat a number of infections for a longer time. I recall a wonderful history professor, who allowed me to speak very bluntly once. I am not proud of this, but I told him he was far too hard on grading and was too confusing. He was actually a very good teacher. He simply smiled and said, "That may all be true, but when you have a doctorate, you get to present the information in a way you feel is best, and no teacher is the same, and I also get to set the line you have to cross for each grade." He was patient. I was clueless.

And the training of the average physician is far in excess of a regular doctoral student and far more brutal, not to mention my extra college time and graduate degree. But this time allowed me to learn something pure pre-meds never learned.

IT IS IMPOSSIBLE TO HAVE COMPLETELY OBJECTIVE SCIENCE. THE SCIENTIST OR PHYSICIAN BRINGS TO THE TABLE MANY ASSUMPTIONS AND APPROACHES THAT ARE NOT SCIENCE, BUT SOCIOLOGY, PHILOSOPHIES, PREJUDICES AND MANY BIASES.

Since most pre-medicine educations are very weak on the philosophy of knowledge and of self-examination, this all sounds like fluff—but it is not fluff. Physicians must know what they bring to the table, and what guides their non-objective science and medicine. Even untrained patients are aware that physicians are biased in many ways, thus increasingly seek care outside synthetic patented pharmaceutical options and medical devices.

Those added years in humanities studies taught me to learn how to think critically and introspectively. Most physicians do not know how to weigh the assumptions and biases in every study. Simply, as

Kuhn has said in *The Structure of Scientific Revolutions,* here are some profound cliff notes about medicine. It is time for all of us to grow up and identify our religious or ultimate beliefs. For example, many years ago, anything from Harvard or the ten top journals was considered fact. This is nonsense, and I am not happy admitting to this belief, which is a type of early adolescent intellectual crush.

Some key elements on the philosophy of science are required for any basic college level understanding of science and medicine, or one is really not educated or aware of the forces creating "certainty in medicine."

Thomas S. Kuhn reminds us of what many other philosophers of science and bias have written.

A. Medical students, residents and physicians are given massive amounts of information which is a type of brain washing that may be correct in many parts, but it is a guild position. These beliefs about "facts" are required to get a medical degree and license to practice medicine. As a physician, I can assure you the volume of information is massive, uncreative, and must be deeply learned mentally to pass tests. So it has a deep hold on your mind.

B. Leaders of the medical guild can be unaware that what they hold as sacred "facts" do not fit some patients or some realities. The human body and its pathology are infinitely complex, and mastery of all aspects is impossible. Top medical sages can suppress or devalue new ideas because they undermine strongly held medical science beliefs.

C. The idea that research is unbiased is false. In fact, "research" is a strong attempt to make patients and disease fit into the positions supplied by an extremely regimented medical school and residency education. In this education you are not asked what you think, you are told what to think. Even with relentless revisions of "facts," many miss the obvious—if medical facts need to be revised routinely, perhaps "current positions" is a more accurate description for them than "facts."

D. If you present information that challenges the positions of the core medical community, you are treated like an anarchist, hated and degraded when new, possibly contradictory information emerges. It is threatening the core beliefs of the medical community "guild"—since they believe the current position is just fine. The nucleus members of the guild holding to these principles use their journals, professional societies, continuing education classes and mentoring to preserve the past core beliefs.

I am currently writing an updated tick and flea infection text to help the many fine healers and patients seeking the most up to date knowledge and the best tailored care. It contains over 400 pages of references alone. Below is a small sample of the points from this textbook. When one studies emerging infections, it is impossible to finish learning. I continually update my positions every season.

I stand on the shoulders of at least 500 authors and medical professionals, and while I might not always agree with their positions, they push you to find critical new information.

It should be noted that a negative finding, such as the discovery that a certain type of treatment fails, is always very useful. A poor treatment leads to increased illness over time, even if in the initial months it appears to be useful.

Please consider these points below. My goal is not to have you agree 100%, but to have you simply ponder these issues.

What do we do with people who still feel ill after a treatment with doxycycline at the approved dose?

When a person has "Lyme disease," is there ever a reason to treat longer than a few weeks? If the treatment is helping the patient more each week, do you still stop treatment at a set time? In other words, if Jane is better in her function, or some sign or symptom each week, do you still stop at a set day?

As a Former Director of a Research Center in Infectious Disease has said, "No one is saying that they're not suffering from something. It's just that it doesn't have anything to do with chronic Lyme disease."

Let us start with what is fairly obvious in some unknown percentage of patients. Simply, they do not feel well, and while they may have some psychiatric or cognitive complaints, they do not meet criteria of somatization or hypochondriasis, because *when I do testing for things like inflammation markers, and anti-inflammation hormones or peptides, nutrient deficits, hormone status, etc., I see pathology that is medical, not PRIMARY psychiatric disorders.*

It is important that we accept that some percentage of patients remain ill regardless of the approach. And I do not think at this stage it matters if it is 5% or 95%. If it is you or your loved ones, 5% is worth serious discussion, meaning, are you going to stop care if your relative is getting better on any treatment?

Few physicians always use probiotics with antibiotics. And those that do prescribe them do not understand 99% of probiotics are very poor.

Fifteen years ago I clung to a few preferred probiotics, due to the usual seduction—many strains at high colony numbers. I had health care workers take high doses of these probiotics, after which they stopped for 5 days and I did a stool culture. Every stool sample yielded the same result: a total lack of the good bacteria required for health. These brands would not prevent a C. difficile bacterial infection of the intestines—a real problem. No one should ever be given an antibiotic for any duration, 2 weeks or 2 months, without top probiotics. I mention this in more detail in my first Babesia textbook, *The Diagnosis and Treatment of Babesia*. Simply, if no number or other further designation follows the name of the bacteria, it is a strain with no proof it can bind and proliferate in the 30 feet of intestine. Also, having only one strain of good bacteria is like having one finger. Some of this information was available in the 1980's.

Some probiotics with no specified strains have been used in research to decrease intestinal disease. For example, they merely refer to an "acidophilus." I would see these as possibly of use since in a study of patients in the real world they appear to offer a benefit, even though they may have sub-optimal strains. Only about a dozen international probiotics are known to bind to the gut wall, reproduce rapidly and work together like a piano player's fingers. Two good ones are Theralac and Dr. Ohirra probiotics.

In summary, I would suggest ***antibiotics never be used without top quality carefully selected probiotics***—the duration of antibiotic use does not matter. There is always some unknown risk.

If physicians are sincerely concerned about C. difficile and resistant strains, they should start by reading *Probiotics: A Clinical Guide*, by Floch and Kim, who are both physicians.

Always start one treatment at a time, and do not add or increase two things in the same day.

Years ago the chairman of a famous Ivy League medical department and the editor of the top pediatric journal asked me to write on dosing medication to decrease side effects. All treatment of any kind needs to be isolated. You should typically add only one new treatment at a time, and no more than one new thing in a day. Further, if you increase a dose, it is regarded as a **new** treatment. Therefore, if you start three things and do not feel right, get a rash or cannot work because of the treatment, you have no idea how to tailor it. Why? You have three possible causes for your problem. Being told to "grin and bear it" is not very caring and it is not tailored care. If we can tailor a suit, we can tailor biochemical interventions.

The suggested testing using only a direct Lyme ELISA test is confusing.

The ELISA test is respected lab testing, but while it is very good in some situations, tick and flea infection medicine may not be one of them. For example, patients can have a marked change in results by simply being 35,000 feet high in a plane, having a surgery or for many other reasons. But even if 90% are correct, that means 1 in 10 will be missed. Since the infections carried by the Ixodes tick may be serious if untreated, this is a risk, assuming even a 90% sensitive ELISA test result.

What do you do when the ELISA changes from positive to negative (or vice versa) without any medical intervention? As I said, diagnosis is messy in emerging infections, and that is reality. In order for physicians to keep their insurance contract, they have to order the least number of tests possible—it is like a source of pride and skill. Amusingly, medical board members, appointed as a reward for involvement in political medicine, are acting for insurance companies by an excessive dependence on one lab test to diagnose, and by often calling more complete lab testing which shows positive findings "wasted labs" and "bad medicine."

If it is good enough for MAYO, HOPKINS, and the CLEVELAND CLINIC, it is surely good enough for any passionate clinician who wants to do a good and thorough job. No one would dare attack an Ivy League physician for ordering extra labs.

Let me make this simple. You have a parent, spouse, sibling or child who is ill. Seven smart physicians are unable to find the cause of their sickness. So you go to see a specialist in diagnostic medicine.

This doctor wants to order ten tests that have never been ordered before. Indeed, the lab staff and your primary care doctor have no idea what these tests are meant to show. Do you do these unfamiliar labs or ignore the consult? Your loved one's health is hanging in the balance.

Do not be more "moral" than the DEA if you need controlled drugs to function.

Some patients need strong treatments to keep their job or function in school. These may include medicines for sleep, anxiety, focus, pain or depression. Some options are traditional medications that are controlled substances. These can all be made into transdermal treatments, or treatments that go through the skin. Some may reject these as "unnatural" perhaps because they have not been used carefully since some healers do not understand that in *an infected or inflamed brain these medications cannot be dosed in "routine suggested ways."*

If a patient has depression, restlessness and trouble with concentration, do you know which of these should be handled first? I strongly suggest depression is always treated before anxiety, and anxiety before focus defects. If you do not do this carefully and with close communication between the patient and the healer, you can commit chemical battery.

Other options for depression, anxiety, focus or pain may be called "functional, integrative or alternative medicine." Some of these are very effective, but can fail with neurological infection or brain inflammation. For example, SAM-e is an exceptional anti-depressant, but St. Johns Wort is normally ineffective in serious depression. No single school of medicine has all the answers. Therefore, my appeal is to be open to what works. "Natural" options are often profoundly useful. However, in some areas we have very limited natural options, and I am not going to lie to a patient and oversell an alternative medicine option that usually is ineffective. Some health care workers are excited about one type of treatment. I am excited when Mrs. Jones or Mr. Smith experience help from a wide range of possible treatments, and the labs show the treatment is actually working. Each patient comes before any type of pet treatment.

Medicine is dead without both the freedom of thought and the ability to treat patients individually.

Much medical care is reduced to being a bank teller or lawn mower repairman. Further, the ability to see uniqueness in each patient, and not merely trends, makes medicine both human and advanced. Why? Because the biochemistry of infections and unique human bodies create the possibility of profound variety in treatments.

Freedom of Thought in the French Tradition is useful here. I am the son of a genius physician father who served with both the American Army and Navy. This meant I was born in my beloved France while he served, and I mention this only because **the French can teach us a lesson on intellectual freedom.**

Watch two men in passionate and sober debate in a French café. Minutes later they are eating and enjoying that special treasure of friendship exemplified by the second US President John Adams and his best friend and wife, Abigail Adams, or as depicted in the Hebrew Bible between Jonathan and David.

My point?

Many French people *do not fuse an idea with the person holding to that opinion, and once discussed, it is shelved.* In other countries, you *are* your opinion. Amazingly, you can be the sports team you praise. This needs to be very clear when one is dealing with beliefs in the area of emerging flea and tick infections with new species found monthly. We need to make our point passionately and reasonably but without reaching the point of hatred. When people reach that place, they do unethical, unnecessary and destructive things to the physicians who disagree with them. As an MD, I can offer an opinion and feel that it is as good as yours, unless you are--by actual study and actual experience--better than me. Infectious disease experts are typically not experts on tick and flea infections, since they do not have the time to read 7,000 journal articles while working full-time with HIV, Herpes, MRSA, Hepatitis and the other top ten infections. In the same way, I will never do surgical work because that requires supervised cutting skills that I have never learned.

Further, patients and researchers filter. Those who are of the Lyme only infection model go to those who hold to that approach. And if they get very ill later, they never go back. Others see physicians who are very IV centered and use the HIV or TB model. They believe the long-term IV Lyme centered model is the best approach..

Each of them sees the annoyed patients of the other, but not the successes. I know patients that have gone to IDSA physicians who were treated 30 days or less and have been fine for at least five years. I have seen patients who were treated exactly according to IDSA guidelines yet were still very ill. And they are becoming disabled. The issue is not why they are worse, since it is not always an IV antibiotic deficit, but simply the reality that the patient is not functioning after "curative care." And let us not mention they need psychiatric medicines for their residual body troubles. All tick borne infections can cause neurologic and psychiatric troubles.

In this book I will discuss things definitely not known by most specialists in infectious disease or those with a serious interest in Flea and Tick infections.

Further, even I do not agree with my positions after six months, because so much is changing and new in every aspect of these bacteria, protozoa and viruses. Emerging infections and a set "guideline" kept over five years may be a functional contradiction. "Emerging" and a single type of treatment does not make sense logically or practically.

If you do not agree with what I write on a topic, fine. I might agree I was wrong next year.

Some feel "correctness" is based on location of the physician's office or what staff they have joined. Having rejected prestigious places repeatedly, I do not get this medical Mecca or Vatican type of thinking.

My father went to a highly respected Ivy League Medical school. I rejected invitations to the same school, in order to avoid being mugged and shot, and because he was not pleased with his experience. Sites that rate schools are silly, because faculty can change in a year, and very few in the USA have the advanced wisdom and time to know each aspect of a training program.

So I do not weigh the expertise of any physician based on the name of an institution. Some with my temperament are adverse to required "meetings" because they can waste time. Some select physicians are as passionate about study as any person running a large grant study. Yet some reading oriented physicians also want to actually see patients, get to know them, and offer advanced personal tailored medical care based on both published materials and consults with many solid state, national, and international clinicians.

Indeed, one of my close friends, who spent much time at the National Institutes of Health and was part of many large studies, is now a strong clinical research practitioner, and the pearls he has found from treating patients he shares with me one to ten years before a study confirms his experience with hundreds. This type of physician is a legitimate practitioner, and saying one has to do either pure "research" or pure "clinical" care is too polarized.

Indeed, a functional cancer cure and other discoveries I have made occurred after patients went to the top respected medical centers in America, and were not helped. In my training in medicine and metaphysics, we were taught how to think, weight the studies, and that clinical medicine often had no study to use or available studies had so many exclusion criteria that generalized use was difficult. "Pure patients" with one issue really do not exist, and likely never in those with one or more tick bites over years.

I have a strong belief that a doctorate in medicine allows one some freedom to seek out options to heal. These treatment proposals should not be limited by large insurance companies or pharmaceutical companies defining the options in our tool box. Simply, if a physician and a competent patient want to pursue a particular treatment, as long as it is not a profound and clear danger to the patient, they should be allowed to make that choice.

Therefore, I do not regard doctors as children, so I will defend, by all ethical and aggressive means, any attack on any position regarding the treatment of tick and flea-borne infections. I will defend any sincere practitioner regardless of their style of treatment. Since I have yet to meet someone who has been reading research papers full-time on these infections for eight years, I have no one that I feel fully shares my identical opinion. So I would support those who reject some of my beliefs on these emerging infections.

Why? Thankfully, we do not have Stalins or Hitlers in medicine. We have patients, and more new and emerging information on these infections than any human can read. Deferring to a small number of "top studies" or to "patient experiences" is not definitive medicine. It is an assumption about knowledge showing a lack of philosophical maturity common in those who have had rigorous science training divorced from advanced modern philosophy. It is perfectly fine if you do not agree with each new very specific clinical real world medical point that I make. I do not even agree with many of my own practices nine months ago in this area of tick and flea infections.

I believe very strongly in liberty, therefore, I do not believe that doctors who have soberly reflected on their treatment approach should ever be sued or reported to medical boards. States are coming to the same conclusion.

The lesson of the debates in New York State, in which a widely known MD asserted that the duration of one infection--Lyme--can be flexible, is that making every doctor treat every patient for a short time or for a long time is outside the law of medicine.

When a physician studies intensely, and for many years, in one area of medicine they slowly develop a strong advanced set of research based beliefs. While this approach can drop their yearly income markedly, if they read over 15 hours a week, it will profoundly lift their wisdom in any topic. Reading 40-50 hours a week has allowed me to offer a very small number of patients very thorough care.

Bartonella is no footnote and is more common than Lyme.

Many years ago when I first got involved in the **super specialty** of tick and flea infection medicine, no one took Bartonella seriously. It was presented as an easy to kill infection, and of no real concern. It was rarely discussed at infection medicine meetings, in guidelines or infection textbooks. (I noticed the same thing after publishing four books on Babesia--the parasite books I purchased only had two pages on this serious infection).

When I published the most recent book on Bartonella, it showed that Bartonella did not have two or three skin patterns, but vast numbers. This was a fully new and massively expanded diagnostic tool based on reading the world literature and examining heavily infected patients. I was also surprised that no one was looking for the chemicals altered by the presence of Bartonella and the dynamic of these chemicals when both Babesia and Bartonella are present. You can read this in the latter sections of my textbook, *Babesia 2009 Update*.

This year a new human Bartonella species was added to the over thirty-five Bartonella species publically published in Genetic Data banks. It was discovered and highlighted by the talented veterinarian researcher Edward Breitschwerdt. He has said things more clearly than the ideas I was pondering in 2005, while doing most of my Bartonella book reading. He has said simply, but with devastating and highly useful clarity that **Bartonella testing is terrible, the treatments are poor,** it is typically found on the outside of red blood cells, and the current research on Bartonella is pathetic—one study at NIH. If this was not enough, he said in 2011, **"Bartonella is carried by more vectors than any infection on the earth."** So it is hardly a backdoor "co-infection." Indeed, this month Bartonella was literally shown to alter human DNA. The implications of this possibility are staggering, and may support what I reported six years ago—Bartonella is not killed simply or easily. My appeal is simple: treating it like a footnote infection is outdated and harmful.

Finally, based on the position above that Bartonella has the largest number of vectors in nature, perhaps Lyme is the "co-infection."

The treatments for Bartonella are based on terribly outdated testing or are very experimental without real proof by *indirect* and advanced direct testing.

I am embarrassed to admit that six years ago I felt you could rule out Bartonella by a simple antibody test—an IgM and an IgG. When only one species was being tested for in North America, it was also easy to ignore that other Bartonella species infect humans. Further, in 2005 I was amazed to learn how much Bartonella suppresses immunity. It lowers fevers and at times drops antibodies for many common tick and flea-borne infections. Further, we found that most proposed treatments in traditional and integrative medicine at best stun Bartonella, and do not cure or even drop body load much. Treatments that are promoted because patients "feel better" are not clear proof. Patients feel better for a hundred reasons, and that is not science, it is psychotherapy. Many healers treating Bartonella are using good treatment options, but they do not know how to use indirect and direct testing to confirm effectiveness. This means treatment variables are chaotic, and at times treatments are mixed up like a stew. This approach is very dangerous because Bartonella can cause literal death, in addition to injuring every organ twenty different ways (based on a review of the world literature).

If someone has a Western Blot with a "band" or antibody highly specific against Lyme, how can that be ignored?

The interpretation of the Lyme Western Blot test is very faith based, and is not like pure math. Indeed, in one recent study from China, they take the position that one band or antibody against an infection shows the infection is present. They even consider the non-specific spirochete antibody to be useful if you prove it is not caused by other spirochetes.

Let us talk about how to interpret a Western Blot Test. Some say these tests are either "negative" or "positive." This does not sound like medicine, but an arbitrary religious-type faith position.

If a person has one "fingerprint band," some feel this is proof of Lyme disease. These highly specific bands, widely accepted in the world literature, are 13, 14, 17, 21, 23, 24, 25, 28, 31, 34, 35, 37, 39, 47, 50, 54, 83, 84, 93 and 94. The lab can be a junk lab that invests nothing to optimize their testing kit, but if one of these bands is positive—Lyme is present. In the last six years IGeneX has been attacked for their Western Blot despite the fact that five samples every four months from New York State have been correct 98% of the time for over a decade. What lab is that correct on negative and positive blind controls?

Has any other lab invested so much for so long, to create the best test? If your clinician wants to use an ELISA first, this is a gamble. To put it bluntly, many patients and physicians report that the ELISA test as a screening tool is useless, missing even the most obvious PCR positive patients with clear past histories of massive Bull's Eye rashes, which, while not the norm, provide evidence of spirochetes. Do we assume all patients reporting a clear tick bite and many tick infection symptoms are 100% liars or inept?

The best treatment for you is not merely one intervention type or school of healing.

You should never be treated by only one school or philosophy of healing or only one type of intervention. Too many healers are only using the options that are rooted in their highly specific training.

The treatment of tick infections involves many types of medicine and affects many body systems. Therefore healers need to know many types of medicine. Many types of healing can be of use. But I also believe in each school of healing some parts are not of use in treating tick and flea-borne infections. One reason I have had to learn so many types of medicine over the last two decades is that my education was obviously only a starting point as a healer. I have had to try so many credible treatments of different types because that offered the best help to patients. No one type of treatment works for all the facets of tick and flea-borne infections. One has to have a broad range of options.

Treatment given season after season and year after year with poor monitoring might be cheap, but it is very inadequate care.

Currently I drive the cheapest car I could find. If a huge SUV hits me, I am toast. What is the point of the illustration? You get what you pay for. If someone is seeing 20 or more patients a day, that is hardly going to allow them to adjust and tune many facets of your treatment. Tick infections hit virtually every part of the body. So a healer has to know many systems of the body—hormones, inflammation, nutrients, improving functionality quickly, compounding medicine, preventing cancer and preventing clots. Further, they must also understand that these infections can impact any organ or human body chemical system.

The bite you see is rarely the first bite.

While it is well known that the more common stages of biting ticks are very hard to see, what is not appreciated is that, **based on animal studies, any rash may be a sign of a past bite** that occurred 1, 5, or 20 years earlier. Further, more advanced and informed lab tests, showing the biochemical domino effect of tick infections over years, are often very abnormal in people reporting symptoms from a "first bite." If you are a physician or nurse practitioner and do not know the 15-20 indirect labs altered by tick and flea infections, that is a concern.

The diagnosis of tick and flea infections is dirty, confusing and hardly easy.

For example, what do you think when the Lyme ELISA is negative, only the IgG 23 "fingerprint" Lyme infection band on the Western Blot is positive, and a PCR for Lyme is positive?

That does not fit some formulas proposed in emerging infection medicine. Further, in traditional medicine, a diagnosis is made by an excellent history and interview of the patient followed by a physical exam—labs merely support the diagnosis. That is one reason I noted the dermatology differences in vast numbers of highly infected Bartonella patients compared to uninfected normal patients. Bartonella alters blood vessels and skin tissue in perhaps over eighty skin markings. When I started my investigation of vast numbers of published and unpublished skin signs, only two or three patterns were discussed. Now, slowly, people are mentioning and posting images of Bartonella that have never existed as "Bartonella images" in the 100 years since its discovery.

The new wave of Lyme disease or Babesia infection mockery is both naive and unkind to patients.

Tick infections are emerging infections. Emerging means no one has the foundation to be cocky. Some believe physicians are only useful when they "reassure" patients they do not have any of the hundred possible species and variants of the infectious agents carried in an Ixodes tick. Since more and more of the population is moving away from traditional allopathic (MD) medicine, perhaps this is not a good issue to mock. One can suggest a course of action for any infection if they wish. But the notion of utter mastery shows a lack of insight into the many complex ways these infection clusters exist after a few bites by the Ixodes tick over a few years. Amusingly, one researcher mentioned to me she found tapeworm DNA in an Ixodes tick. I do not think she or I feel you can get a tapeworm from a tick bite, but if you can find tapeworm DNA inside the gut of a tick, you can find virtually anything.

The loss of insight and an increase in rigidity is sometimes the first symptom of infection with brain and body inflammation.

One danger in some people is they have no idea they are losing productivity or insight, because that awareness comes from the higher and more advanced areas of the brain. Self-reflection is an advanced type of brain function, and it can be impaired if more than a small area of the brain is infected and inflamed. Once someone has this problem they may never be willing to be examined.

Chronic tick infections over years drop anti-inflammation chemicals and increase inflammation chemicals with serious results.

When one's body is chronically inflamed, some other things start to happen. One's vulnerability to autoimmunity increases and depending on which type of autoimmunity, one can become disabled or die. Further, one can have an increase in allergies. These can be allergies to foods, synthetic medicines, and at times even herbs. Finally, one can also become highly sensitive to volatile chemicals, and it requires immense work to maintain a work, school or living location free of synthetic chemicals.

Routine treatments to reverse systemic and deeply entrenched inflammation are generally trivial and ineffective.

If you read a book on lowering inflammation, you will see the same twenty options that are listed in other books or journal articles. Unfortunately these do not work when dealing with immense long term chronic inflammation secondary to a series of missed tick and flea-borne infections. We have some options for this problem, but they are outside the realm of this short article.

The dose that causes misery is not required for effective killing.

Some healers feel you should never feel an effective antibiotic, and others feel you are not getting any benefit unless you feel terrible. As the Greeks and Calvin said, perhaps the best position is the middle way. If a medication seems to be having an effect that causes discomfort which is not a side effect, what is wrong with lowering it to a dose just below the level of discomfort? I am almost embarrassed to raise this issue, but do so because it is a common issue.

Very advanced pharmacology is needed to address physical, neurologic, hormonal, nutritional and psychiatric problems in tick infection medicine.

Sometimes the most important first treatments are not things that kill infections. Sometimes people need care for their extremely low vitamin D level, depression, irritability, anxiety, rage, fatigue, insomnia, cognitive deficits and agitation which are hardly rare with tick and flea infections left untreated for a significant period of time.

This is very important and few physicians are familiar with the dosing for these infections and the common presence of inflammation in the brain which causes these problems. For example, we suggest all capsules and tablets should never be started over the quarter mark of the smallest option. But the end effective dose may be profoundly high. These are not primary psychiatric disorders, but disorders secondary to infections, infection debris and inflammation of the brain.

The notion that an Ixodes tick carries only "Lyme Disease" is a 1990's notion.

If a clinician uses advanced, direct and highly important indirect testing to look for the increasing number of infections carried by tiny Ixodes ticks (deer ticks), it is clear that organisms besides Lyme are present routinely in Ixodes ticks. The idea that Ixodes ticks only carry one infection is a disaster. Ixodes ticks carry multiple bacteria, parasites, and viruses. For example, Bartonella is far more common than Lyme disease.

There is no correct starting dose for virtually any medication.

I was asked years ago by two top editors to write an article on "sensitive and careful dosing in clinical practice." They noticed within my various papers we were pointing out the need for tailored dosing instead of chemical battery. For example, all medications should begin with a first dose that is below a full tablet or capsule, because sometimes it is 20 times more effective than normal. Always start with a fraction of the lowest dose pill and this can be increased over a mere 24 hours.

One should never increase or start two treatments on the same day.

This is chaos, and causes confusion if you have a reaction to the medications. You do not know if one of the treatments is creating a side effect or is working well. Also, if a patient develops uncomfortable feelings, either from the die off of an organism or from medication side effects, they become demoralized, and the cause is unclear with many treatments. Simply, no two people have even been treated by me the same from start to finish, and this is why a cure book on all major tick-borne infections cannot be published.

Further, if you increase one treatment and add another, you have implemented two new treatments on the same day. I would not do this if it can be avoided.

Is the new explosion of "Lyme Literate" or "LLMD experts" really trained to do more than basic screening?

Generally when I am trying to pursue an expertise in any aspect of tick and flea-borne infections, I spend years engaged in full-time reading on the topic and try to talk with the leaders around the world who know the most on the topic. Unfortunately, as of 2010, "Lyme Literate" really means that you have gone to a couple conferences, learned the basics from the last five to ten years, and some also shadowed one or two physicians for days to a week while they see patients.

This is a good starting place, but does not make one "tick-infection literate" in any serious manner. Finding someone that knows how to use a wide range of labs which will check for a direct and indirect presence of the infections from ticks, who has read thousands of articles, and consults with physicians and scientists regularly for success and failures along with finding new solutions is extremely rare in the world. Yet we do need every screening healer we can get.

Routine speed I.V. treatment of most new patients is an error.

Some individuals treating Lyme disease do a fairly rapid assessment and quickly put all of their patients on an I.V. like they are running a mill. It is almost as if they say "It is nice to meet you, let's get you started on your I.V. quickly." There are many problems with this approach and far too many to discuss here. The first problem is that the volume of spirochetes that can die with an invasive I.V. could be too much and release Lyme debris and/or Lyme biotoxins, such as BbTox1, which can increase inflammation.

I.V. and all other types of Lyme treatment work profoundly better if one or more new Bartonella treatments are used. We find these new treatments every few seasons. As previously stated in my first Townsend article on the "Reasons for Lyme Treatment Failure," the most common treatments for Bartonella come from a mere 25 basic Bartonella treatment articles or infection handbooks. They lead to relapse even when they appear to work for variable periods of time.

I.V. gall bladder emergencies are too frequent. One reason some insurance companies do not want to do prolonged I.V. treatment is because of gallbladder emergencies. I am fairly stunned that the only thing given to protect the gall bladder and liver with the use of I.V. medications is Actigall, and some do not prescribe anything when giving I.V. treatment. Many have little knowledge of advanced ways to protect the liver, and yet use liver stressing treatments. For example, any dose of azithromycin, Mepron, Malarone, Diflucan or I.V. or injected muscle antibiotics can stress the liver, and low doses that do not stress the liver may lead to residual infections.

Following the guidelines of practitioners with famous names, university titles or organization leadership positions might be unwise.

If a healer is famous or has a title or "chair" or is high in an organization, the more brutally busy the healer can be, sometimes working 12 hours virtually every day. So this healer can never read high volumes of new material published this season. Therefore, no organization, government agency, web site or person has the definitive, updated information on tick-infection medicine in the USA or the world. No single organization or group of organizations can provide people with authoritative instruction in how to treat each individual profoundly unique patient.

All guidelines for medicine are flawed and outdated within one month of publication.

The explosion of new published material and non-published discoveries by hundreds of international healers makes guidelines mere suggestions.

Hundreds of thousands of articles are published every few months. In our practice, we have only published five percent of what we have found. Similarly, many fellow researchers I know also have limited time to publish their discoveries.

Further, as mentioned before, the great philosopher of science, Kuhn, has shown that there are so many variables that impact all scientists, that the notion that any group of physicians can give unbiased purely scientific recommendations is impossible. Obvious guideline errors are present in all current tick and flea-borne infection guidelines.

Different guidelines have unusually specific treatment plans which are not even appropriate for cars from the 1950s, let alone current automobiles which have different types of oil and different amounts of recommended oil, and electrical and computer systems that are stunning in complexity.

The human body, when it is infected with a cluster of tick infections, is a billion times more complex than any automobile. Some guidelines use highly dated doses from studies that are fifteen years old. Other guidelines do not even mention infections such as persistent human atypical Bartonella, which has vastly more vectors than Lyme disease, or Babesia which suppresses the immune system in highly specific ways that some guideline agencies and groups seem to totally ignore.

In conclusion, one example that months matter in research relates to the CDC Morgellons' study which admits it intentionally ignored critical indirect Bartonella tests TNF-a and IL-6, and used highly insensitive markers for inflammation (sedimentation rate). They opted for a "skin-primary" approach, which I have said repeatedly over five years is a waste of time. They also seemed to limit the importance of fatigue and cognitive deficits which are not associated with delusions.

What is not mentioned in the CDC paper is a new paper by Middelveen and Stricker, showing spirochetes cause colored fibers in bovines as part of their full-body disease--my Morgellons' patients always have full-body issues. Clearly, this paper was not read in the months before the CDC paper hit the world news. So months matter in clinical real-world medicine.

Sample References

Pearson ML, Selby JV, Katz KA, Cantrell V, Braden CR, et al. (2012) Clinical, Epidemiologic, Histopathologic and Molecular Features of an Unexplained Dermopathy. PLoS ONE 7(1): e29908. doi:10.1371/journal.pone.0029908

Middelveen, M., & Stricker, R. (2011). Clinical,Cosmetic and Investigational Dermatology,4,167-177

Savely, V., Stricker, R. (2010). Morgellons disease: Analysis of a population with clinically confirmed microscopic subcutaneous fibers of unknown etiology. Clinical, Cosmetic and Investigational Dermatology 3, 67–78.

Evans NJ, Blowey RW, Timofte D, et al. Association between bovine digital dermatitis treponemes and a range of 'non-healing' bovine hoof disorders. Vet Rec. 2011 Feb 26;168(8):214. Epub 2011 Feb 15.

A complete lack of meaningful knowledge of the immense magnitude and danger of Bartonella is very dangerous.

This stealth bacterium has over ten different ways to infect you, and not merely a few types of ticks. It kills, harms every organ, decreases fevers and immune defenses, and does not fully respond to the top ten "published" traditional or alternative treatments. In one case report it appears that Bartonella turned off all the antibodies to five tick-borne infections, including its own antibody titer levels. In this medical family they self-treated with a new Bartonella agent and this resulted in an explosion of western blot Lyme disease bands and all major deer tick infection antibody titers suddenly rose to profound levels because the immune system was no longer suppressed against them by Bartonella. Therefore, merely by the use of this newly uncovered Bartonella treatment, all of these patients' negative labs at a large national lab turned positive after being repeatedly negative.

The use of fetish, "favorite" medications, herbs or newly "discovered" causes of prolonged illness can waste time for patients.

Of course, any healer studying traditional or progressive medications is serving all. My appeal in this criticism is not to reject the fine work done by at least two hundred people internationally on traditional antibiotics, protozoa medications, anti-viral drugs, herbs used for a wide range of infections, essential oils, and at least fifty progressive alternative treatments.

However, like the experience of falling in love, when one love becomes all you think about, this is not optimal medicine when you fall in love with a few treatments.

For example, minocycline, tetracycline, clarithromycin, rifampin, azithromycin, HBOT, Rife, special saunas, ozone, I.V. nutrients to "boost immunity," chelation, confused detox formulas, Artemisia derivatives, essential oil combinations, I.V. medications, various weak alcohol based herbal programs, various energy machines, and a hundred other options found in chat rooms and Lyme disease "information" sites, are not meant to be the sole or primary style of all patient treatment.

Carpenters use select tools at select times for select needs. Nevertheless, with my thanks for the above passion of those that promote these and hundreds of others of treatments, they have to pass blind rigorous simple direct and indirect testing to show they work, and very few know how to do such testing. I feel it is an error to only use an antibiotic which has limited mechanisms for killing bacteria.

I have published the most current textbook on Artemisia derivatives, including artemisinin (qinghaosu) and many other toxic forms that should be avoided. And yet, despite being the most recent practical clinical book on the topic, based on a year of full-time study with Chinese consultants and WHO consultants, it has been ignored, and instead of artesunate being used, inferior artemisinin is used. Why?

The final approach that is worthy of mention is the "I only do natural treatments" approach.

Unfortunately when I interview some of these individuals, many of whom are quite smart and well read, they are aware of allopathic medication side effects, but not the toxic components of the herbs they are using. Individuals using essential oils, including those that prescribe them, usually have never read a book on the various toxicities and safety concerns of essential oils. Some of them have excellent effects and others can provide help, but also have side effect risks and others should never be used internally at all in anything more than a minimal dose.

The "new" yearly or bi-yearly cause of Lyme disease treatment failures is possibly wrong.

A few years ago, the existence of a Lyme biofilm was proposed. Many spirochetes make biofilms so this was not really a surprise, but not addressing these may undermine treatment outcomes.

Indeed, many types of spirochetes in the mouth are known to cause biofilms, and they are believed to limit antibiotic effectiveness. Organizations with millions in grants and research money have never addressed this issue.

I am currently working on a textbook that addresses the many treatment options for attacking biofilms. No article or book exists that explores the twenty-plus ways that I would propose to beat a Lyme biofilm. It is believed by some professionals that highly specific enzymes, drugs, or one mineral can undermine a Lyme biofilm. Yet enzymes are like highly specific keys, and no single enzyme has been a proven "key" to undermining a Lyme biofilm.

I was appreciative that a few brilliant researchers found that the Bb Lyme spirochete had a biofilm in recent years. But I was actually stunned this was felt to be new, since spirochetes routinely have biofilms, and there is immense research on dental spirochetes going back many years on biofilm promoting dental disease. A review of the major world literature shows about 25 treatment options to handle biofilms. No one has offered more than a small number of basic options to beat this problem. Perhaps it increases treatment relapses and failures, but that is not what I usually see.

If biofilms slow treatment, here are a few sample options from the 25 in the literature. NAC is a liver health supplement given for acetaminophen overdose (Tylenol) and it undermines some biofilms.

Another approach is to give a constant select antibiotic, such as azithromycin (Zithromax), and over time if the blood level is constant, it will connect to the surface of the biofilms and work its way into the biofilm, and ultimately into contact with the bacteria. Finally, digestive enzymes such as proteases are sometimes able to hinder many biofilms. Some promote a single enzyme as the magic cure to every biofilm type and variation made by tick and flea based infections. My strong opinion is these are never the reason for relapse alone, and one enzyme is never a sure thing against the many types of biofilms in humans.

Is it wise to reject a consult with a top thought leader due to cost?

When I think back over the hundreds of physicians, PhDs, herbal experts, nurses, alternative healing practitioners and even poorly educated addicts whom I treated decades ago, it is clear to me that, while none of them was perfect, all have helped me immeasurably. Currently, at least 50 physicians are defamed for their fees when treating tick-borne infections and this can end their entire career. Many physicians who are associated with the Infectious Diseases Society of America (IDSA) have said that patients with tick infections are harder to deal with than those with other very serious infections. Some physicians stop their treatment of any patients with tick or flea infections because of the way they are treated.

The same applies to bonding with a healer. I often seek the wisdom of people that may be annoying, irritable, tired, simplistic, insulting, or confusing. But the fact of the matter is that virtually every healer I have known, regardless of specialty, philosophy and ideology, has taught me a lesson that helps patients. I have literally seen patients decide to go with physicians who have virtually no knowledge of tick-borne disease, because they were "caring and friendly."

Further some want a "local" physician, as if geography is the same as expertise and knowledge.

So how do you pick someone to examine the possibility you have a tick or flea-borne infection?

1) It may take a number of appointments to get better.

2) There is no better use of any income than improving your health and the health of your loved ones.

3) However, are you wasting it on healer after healer who is sincere, but does not have a complete passion to master these illnesses, and a good track record of improving lives, including the lives of very ill patients? I will not debate how

long it takes to kill Bartonella, Babesia and Lyme when they have been missed for twenty years. But it may be that one session will not cure all **your ills.**

The use of herbal treatments without solid follow-up by direct and indirect means needs careful study.

Currently, one finds herbs that are mixed in grain alcohol with a fiftieth of the potency of a capsule, that are supposedly cures to tick-borne disease. In our examination of these inherited treatment failures, we have not found that these low potency alcohol based herbs cure. Others offer high priced herbs and "know" they are successful, and often recommend one size for all adults living on the earth. Often their understanding of advanced herbal processing, standardization and the multiple chemicals in any herb is limited. In any event, in our outcome studies we have found that these herbs at best may limit body infection volume slightly. It is profoundly important to use effective herbs with a tailored, specialized dosage for each individual or you are merely experiencing "mill medicine." If you are self-treating with herbs or if your healer promotes "one-size-fits-all," you are accepting health care inferior to dog medicine.

Advice from web sites and chat rooms usually does not apply to you. No two people are ever to be treated exactly the same.

To seek advice on the Internet is a concern of most physicians and healers. Sometimes you can find mature balanced support from those who are healthy, but not new, advanced and solidly credible information for your medical care. Many leaders in tick infection medicine report they are quoted incorrectly, and that the information is often wrong, sometimes dangerous and wastes time and money.

Practitioners are not aware of current treatment approaches.

Practitioners who follow a year-after-year I.V. treatment approach are not "up-to-date" in their knowledge of Lyme. Ten years of Lyme disease treatment is not acceptable. These so called "cure" treatments often merely lower the body's pathogen load or decrease symptoms without fully eradicating all the different types of infectious agents.

If someone never examines indirect testing for Bartonella, or assumes Bartonella can only make a few skin alterations, they are sadly very dated.

Any proposed treatments that ignore Bartonella means the treatments proposed are not applicable to this decade. It has been very well established that Bartonella is both a highly common vector infection, and is carried in both ticks and many other vectors like fleas. Bartonella is in the ticks that carry Lyme and Babesia.

Further, since we are on the topic of Bartonella, it is stunning to see the immense certainty published in some studies about the complete and perfect effectiveness of azithromycin (Zithromax), rifampin, mycobutin, Levaquin, Cipro, doxycycline or minocycline. When I read these studies I am thankful people are looking to treat this infection that can kill at an unknown frequency, and harm most organs 15-20 ways, but it is a concern that the studies seem to be reasonable, yet the conclusion is simply wrong.

When you read full-time two years, not two months, on this infection, you learn all the new publically defined species, and the new species that infect humans, as well as the immune suppression abilities and realize that brilliant researchers have to understand more about the infections' ability to hide, and suppress each other as well as the limits to test kits before they do a study.

One is reminded of the lovely and compelling studies about Epstein-Barr virus (EBV) as a cause of fatigue and other ills, and how this position as a reported cause of fatigue is simply not true. And any infection or inflammation disorder, in my opinion, can cause EBV to show abnormal results.

So my only point here is to discuss another angle on Bartonella in tick and flea infection troubles.

Routine Bartonella treatments are not effective. So why is the research that shows I was right six years ago ignored?

Right now the infection with more vectors than any infection on earth has one study being done at the National Institutes of Health—it is Bartonella. So we should be stunned if any study is done on the treatments of Bartonella that contradict that Bartonella is very easy to kill. Most clinicians feel Bartonella is trivial and very easy to kill and also easy to remove. I have read these unusually designed and confident papers—often five to ten times.

Let me briefly mention some materials that no one seems to read that undermines the simplistic approaches common in treating Bartonella.

Research shows the common "best treatments" for Bartonella agree with what I published six years ago--they are ineffective. Why? Possibly in part due to Bartonella resistance to the treatment.

The chief mechanisms by which antibiotics work are now found to be undermined by Bartonella. So the treatments published in the past about perfect effectiveness may not have any use now. My study and opinion in 2005 was these were rarely effective in people in 2004.

In new research, antibiotic resistant mutations have been found in *B. henselae, B. quintana and B. bacilliformis*.

In one study 20 new *Bartonella* isolates to fluoroquinolones were examined, and resistance to some quinolones was found. Another author reports: fluoroquinolones alone should not be used for the treatment of bartonellosis since there is an intrinsic low level of resistance due to the gyrA mutation. Moreover, high level of resistance to fluoroquinolones is easily obtained. It is surprising that so many physicians prescribe Levaquin, ciprofloxacin (Cipro) and moxifloxacin (Avelox). These are supposed to have restricted use, including the 4th generation class Avelox. These all have clear tendon damage risks, and a profoundly high risk of C. difficile and MRSA infections. I only see perhaps 1 in 100 patients who are treated with quinolone antibiotics who are also on any probiotic, and only 1 in 500 who are on good probiotics that bind to the wall of the intestines, proliferate and work in synergy.

The facts are that quinolones increase the risk of developing tendonitis and tendon rupture in patients of all ages taking fluoroquinolones. Many quinolones are no longer available due to severe toxicity issues.

Further, azithromycin was effective only until the second passage for *B. henselae* isolates obtained from cats. Other studies show azithromycin, rifampin and quinolone resistance in various Bartonella variants.

Finally, some feel aminoglycosides are the best treatment, but some research tells physicians not to count on an effective use.

Why do guidelines and physicians suggest treatments that may be worthless?

In summary, cat scratch disease does not typically respond well to the cliche options in fair papers. That these troubled treatments are not obvious to very smart MD's, DO's or PhD's shows the terribly poor knowledge they have about Bartonella.

Sample Supporting References

Angelakis E, Biswas S, Taylor C, Raoult D, Rolain JM. Heterogeneity of susceptibility to fluoroquinolones in Bartonella isolates from Australia reveals a natural mutation in gyrA. J Antimicrob Chemother. 2008 Jun;61(6):1252-5. Epub 2008 Mar 10.

Angelakis E, Raoult D, Rolain JM. Molecular characterization of resistance to fluoroquinolones in Bartonella henselae and Bartonella quintana. J Antimicrob Chemother. 2009 Jun;63(6):1288-9. Epub 2009 Apr 15. PMID:19369272

Barbian KD, Minnick MF. A bacteriophage-like particle from Bartonella bacilliformis. Microbiology. 2000 Mar;146 (Pt 3):599-609.

Battisti JM, Smitherman LS, Samuels DS, Minnick MF. Mutations in Bartonella bacilliformis gyrB confer resistance to coumermycin A1. Antimicrob Agents Chemother. 1998 Nov;42(11):2906-13.

Biswas S, Maggi RG, Papich MG, Breitschwerdt EB. Molecular mechanisms of Bartonella henselae resistance to azithromycin, pradofloxacin and enrofloxacin. J Antimicrob Chemother. 2010 Mar;65(3):581-2. Epub 2009 Dec 18.

Biswas S, Raoult D, Rolain JM. Molecular characterization of resistance to macrolides in Bartonella henselae. Antimicrob Agents Chemother. 2006 Sep;50(9):3192–3.

Biswas S, Raoult D, Rolain JM. Molecular mechanisms of resistance to antibiotics in Bartonella bacilliformis. J Antimicrob Chemother. 2007 Jun;59(6):1065-70. Epub 2007 Apr 21.

Biswas S, Raoult D, Rolain JM. A bioinformatic approach to understanding antibiotic resistance in intracellular bacteria through whole genome analysis. Int J Antimicrob Agents. 2008 Sep;32(3):207-20. Epub 2008 Jul 10.

Biswas S, Raoult D, Rolain JM. Molecular mechanism of gentamicin resistance in Bartonella henselae. Clin Microbiol Infect. 2009 Dec;15 Suppl 2:98-9. PMID:20584166

Biswas S, Raoult D, Rolain JM. Molecular characterisation of resistance to rifampin in Bartonella quintana. Clin Microbiol Infect. 2009 Dec;15 Suppl 2:100-1. Epub 2009 Dec 24. PMID:19929979

del Valle LJ, Flores L, Vargas M, García-de-la-Guarda R, Quispe RL, Ibañez ZB, Alvarado D, Ramírez P, Ruiz J. Bartonella bacilliformis, endemic pathogen of the Andean region, is intrinsically resistant to quinolones. Int J Infect Dis. 2010 Jun;14(6):e506-10. Epub 2009 Dec 6.

Meghari S, Rolain JM, Grau GE, Platt E, Barrassi L, Mege JL, Raoult D. Antiangiogenic effect of erythromycin: an in vitro model of Bartonella quintana infection. J Infect Dis. 2006 Feb 1;193(3):380-6. Epub 2005 Dec 27.

Minnick MF, Wilson ZR, Smitherman LS, Samuels DS. gyrA mutations in ciprofloxacin-resistant Bartonella bacilliformis strains obtained in vitro. Antimicrob Agents Chemother. 2003 Jan;47(1):383-6.

Some treatments that cost a good deal of money and time may be ineffective.

For example, the use of hyperbaric oxygen (HBOT) for the treatment of tick-borne infections fails. Results from studies of the use of HBOT in mice are not applicable to humans. To prove that HBOT is useless for the treatment of tick-borne infections, I decided to perform a self-funded study to examine its benefits for the treatment of Lyme (Borrelia), Babesia, Ehrlichia and Bartonella. The family strongly wanted this care but could not afford it, so I paid for them to receive these treatments from David Perlmutter, MD, who believed this would be a successful treatment. After approximately 120 treatments at 2.4 atmospheres for 90 minutes each, administered by very accomplished HBOT techs, the results were not what any expected. Even though the treatments were three times per week at a great facility, the treatment failed.

All participants, after these treatments, still had clear positive findings for all four infections. Therefore, there is no validity to the claim that HBOT "kills" Babesia, Bartonella, Ehrlichia or Lyme disease. I have talked to the late Dr. Fife in detail about his HBOT study and carefully evaluated the HBOT research of Dr. Robert Lombard, who accepted patients on routine antibiotic and antimalarial *treatments while getting HBOT,* which has further confirmed this finding, because people did not return to baseline quickly in four weeks, as expected with double treatment.

I love HBOT treatment for many medical problems, and we know it does kill surgical and some other infections, but it does not cure common tick and flea-borne infections. It may help other aspects of patients' suffering, but I defer that to other physicians and healers.

Many medicines, healing machines and top retail herbal options are of limited help, or are sold at very inflated prices by healers.

Ignoring new data leads to treatment failures.

All medical groups have founders who represent the core beliefs of their organization. These founders are closed-minded about receiving new information. This is simply human nature. For example, different friends who are researchers have performed new surgical techniques or found newer, more useful treatments in many areas of medicine, as have I, and the first response is inertia and a lack of interest. It is so bad, that I discuss new discoveries with patients before physicians.

For example, around 2000, I found a functional "cancer" cure. I found it only because my co-author with a full-time top orthodontry practice asked me firmly to research it along with five other topics. And once I proved it was a solid winner, he shared my paper over and over with oncologists and other cancer experts to get it noticed. If he had not been so driven on this finding, many more would have died from HES or Idiopathic Hypereosinophilia Syndrome. Few exist in the healing professions like my co-author, Dr. Glenn Burkland, who was not only willing to study outside his field, and help find the new serious finding, but also willing to nag people to read and accept this very new information. It is no wonder he is a peerless top clinician and researcher. But we see that excellence often comes from outside clique locations. For example, the only current hospital wing dedicated to tick infection research is at Columbia run by psychiatrist B. Fallon, MD. Indeed, most of those who designed the Infectious Diseases Society of America guidelines on Lyme disease were not infection specialists. They were not afraid to use people with other specialties. Any organization willing to admit that doctors outside their specialization can add information to their guidelines is acting wisely. If neurologists use psychiatrists and psychiatrists use neurologists, in position papers, I feel the papers will be better.

In the same way, I have interests in many specialties, and not mere infection medicine. And yet now I have published eight books on advanced tick-borne infections, all showing new types of information, without an infection fellowship. For some "Lyme-literate" physicians, it took educated patients "throwing a copy" of one of my books at them before they read this new information, and by then **many years had already passed.** Some health care workers believe in a Lyme literate Pope or President, but no such expert exists. Sure, some offer useful information from past investigations. However, no one has mastered modern tick-borne medicine and all the newest co-infection information. And we know from the history of medicine that in every generation that positions from medical "elite" are most often limited and flawed.

Right now I am working on a *Babesia Treatment Update* and a *Three Volume Tick Infections* series, and they are so difficult and involve over 500 pages of references, that I will likely wait until 2013. New data usually comes from those working and reflecting full-time on a topic, and we are quite open to error if we mock such people. I know some have mocked my research and study. I end up treating too many of their patients. I take no delight in saying this alienating statement, but I care more about patients than looking or sounding "professional."

Sick physicians, sick nurses, sick chiropractors or sick herbal physicians (NDs) are trying to treat sick patients.

I have been asked by a number of physicians to share my various impressions of literature reviews of thousands of articles, and they are obviously asking primarily for themselves. They do not want to be patients but want thirty to sixty minute summaries of things that require forty to eight hundred pages to begin to answer.

They are ill themselves and need treatment help. I have asked them to stop treating themselves, and to do an hour consultation with very extensive labs. Most have refused. Tragically, what they could have learned by fixing themselves would have translated into real help for their patients.

My position on these infections fits no one protocol or approach, so I can help any professional regardless of their orientation. In the treatment of tick-borne infections we have limited tools, but enough to offer options other types of healers can accept.

Current treatment recommendations are profoundly flawed or too simplistic.

*   I.V. treatments are often used without herbal or synthetic antibiotic cyst busters. Surprisingly, some even mock the notion of spirochete cyst forms.

*   The most common treatment for Babesia is 750 mg per teaspoon of Mepron, taken twice a day. This treatment fails in some patients and is too high a starting dose for some people.

*   The most commonly used herbal Babesia cures are artemisinin, dihydroartemisinin, or artesunate (for example, Zhang Artemisia from Heprapro.com uses artesunate). The latter involves a "standard" dose of one capsule three times a day. Artemisinin is poor at killing Babesia and three artesunate do not cure most patients. Further, in patients with high systemic inflammation, three artesunate per day may be too uncomfortable. The patient may need some new approaches we have designed to help this very serious problem of chronic high inflammation.

*   Azithromycin (Zithromax) is **not** effective at killing Babesia at a mere 500 mg a day. It does kill Babesia at 2,000 mg which was published years ago. All of the approaches listed in infection books and articles can fail at published and recommended doses, even after long trials of treatment.

A lack of two-year blind studies leads to treatment failures for Bartonella. For example, I have found that high doses of Levaquin, rifampin, Zithromax, doxycycline, Mycobutin, acupuncture, Ceftin, Cipro, Axelox, gentamicin, Omnicef, Cumanda and Banderol all fail to cure Bartonella. These antibiotics, along with Rife machines that are used at various optimal frequencies and powers, may lower the body's pathogen load and lead to initial and convincing feelings of improvement, but none of these treatments leads to a cure for Bartonella.

The current tests for Babesia, Bartonella and Ehrlichia are limited.

Some DNA or PCR tests that are processed by a popular East Coast lab often miss a positive infection up to ten times. If a lab needs ten urine or blood samples to show a positive result, it is not functional. Some labs are only fair at tissue PCR testing, when the tissue has clear Lyme, Babesia and Bartonella that can be observed microscopically. This is a diagnostic disaster.

Amazingly, some rely upon large national labs to do manual examinations of red blood cells to look for Babesia and Bartonella. I have never seen a large national lab detect Babesia or Bartonella in over 600 manual smears. No national lab has been able to capture these infections in patients with certain strains of Babesia and Bartonella. I have repeatedly offered to assist them in improving their technology by linking them with hematology experts in tick-borne infections. They did not care that their manual smears were worthless, and I was repeatedly ignored.

The knowledge base about both Bartonella testing and treatment is so poor it borders on the catastrophic.

Bartonella is one of the most common infections in the world. Calling it a "co-infection" may be an error. If anything, Lyme (Borrelia) might be the "co-infection." Bartonella is found in vast numbers of common vectors including dust mites, fleas, flea feces, pet saliva, ticks, etc. Amazingly, it can turn off or lower antibodies to Lyme disease, Babesia, Ehrlichia, Anaplasma and even itself. Bartonella floats in blood and also enters all blood vessel walls without causing a fatal fever, and indeed, actually lowers fevers. It is the ultimate stealth infection. It turns off antibodies, fevers and immune function defense chemicals as it damages organs in anywhere from 15-60 different ways. Many organs can be harmed 15-20 ways and the brain at least 60 ways.

The use of fixed "protocols" or "procedures" in the treatment of tick-borne infections is "machine mill" medicine.

Why? It treats each ill human person as a machine that is built the same and has the exact same problems, which in turn objectifies the patient and flirts with the sociopathic. We see this mindset in serious criminals, who mold people into objects in an effort to fit their skewed perceptions of the world. It is junk medicine to apply a blanket protocol to a unique human body, with a complex and multi-faceted infection cluster and unique biochemical response. Treating in this manner is poor "mill medicine," plain and simple.

Bartonella turns off the production of antibodies to infections like Babesia, Lyme disease and Ehrlichia; it must always be considered in tick and flea medicine.

I would suggest that practitioners learn the 60 different skin patterns that can be created by Bartonella or a mix of Bartonella/Lyme infections. It would also be useful for them to become familiar with the indirect lab markers that are associated with Bartonella infections, as well as those that are associated with mixed Bartonella/Babesia infections, such as IL-6, IL-1B, TNF-alpha, ECP, and VEGF. We discuss clinical patterns that are seen as a result of these lab results in the *Babesia 2009 Update* book and *The Diagnosis and Treatment of Bartonella* book.

Some patients have very few Babesia protozoa parasites, but they are causing serious trouble in their bodies. Practitioners don't recognize them to be a problem, however. Their small numbers cause them to be missed in visual "FISH" exams, PCR and antibody tests. But indirect testing can allow them to be detected.

Most labs don't test for new species of Babesia and Bartonella. Yet there are special ways to detect these infections. Most international labs are unable to test for Babesia duncani or the many other documented species of Babesia (15) or Bartonella (10) that infect humans.

Practitioners cannot rule out the presence of these infection species just because patients test negative for them. One way to reduce treatment failures is to use new medical techniques to detect stealth Babesia. (Babesia can cause symptoms of ongoing fatigue, headaches and weight gain, as well as others, while hindering the treatment of Lyme disease).

The "trick" is simple: a patient is given at least two Babesia killing medications such as Mepron, artesunate or Malarone (given for the proguanil). These medications are used for four days at a dose that both patient and physician feel is worth the risk. Usually, at least one of the medications will kill a few Babesia parasites. Approximately ten to fourteen days later, a follow up lab test is performed, in which blood is drawn and VEGF, TNF-alpha, IL-6, IL-1B, and ECP levels are assayed. ECP is used to kill parasites. The new ECP level is compared to the baseline. If the ECP or TNF-alpha levels rise and VEGF falls, it can be a sign of Babesia "die-off." (Eosinophils release ECP and possibly react to the single-celled parasite Babesia or Babesia debris as if a larger parasite, which is the primary role of Eosinophils—killing large parasites). An increase in either IL-6 or IL-1B is not routine, but an increase after these trials is a sign that suspicions exist for the presence of Babesia.

An added option is to wait six weeks after using this lab technique and have the patient tested for antibodies to Babesia microti or duncani. One juvenile patient with profound illness, who was increasingly disabled after being seen by approximately fifteen physicians, was finally diagnosed in this manner, and after three weeks of triple Babesia treatment, had significant clinical improvement for the first time in six years.

Not being able to detect stealthy, low-volume Babesia is a common problem when treating tick and flea-borne infections. Talented health care workers commonly miss these red blood cell parasites, but this trick usually causes these singled-celled parasites to show up and can save patients from years of failed treatment.

First, look at these five labs below. Alone, they can each be low, normal or high for many reasons. But in tick and flea infection medicine, reading patterns of them can be helpful.

TNF-a represents Tumor Necrosis Factor-alpha

IL-6 represents Interleukin 6

IL-1b represents Interleukin 1b

VEGF represents Vasoendothelial Growth Factor

ECP means Eosinophil Cationic Protein

I will not go too deeply into the function of these common labs, except to say that VEGF makes and opens blood vessels. **Bartonella makes VEGF (and so do mold toxins such as those measured reliably by Real Time Labs). If your skin or labs show Bartonella findings and the VEGF is not well above normal, something is likely going on. What could it be? It could be that Babesia is present and suppressing full body blood VEGF levels,** but it does not stop the production in some patients of Bartonella skin markings consistent with the 40 **different** skin markings illustrated in my two-volume color Bartonella book. These markings appear less often in children under nine years old, because they have had less time to develop.

Bartonella suppresses other labs such as the TNF-a, IL-6 and IL-1b. So in the presence of only Bartonella and Lyme, these labs are **typically low and often *below* normal.**

Bartonella and Lyme Infection

TNF-a	low
IL-6	low
IL-1b	low
VEGF	high

Babesia and Lyme without Bartonella

First, since I believe Bartonella is one of the most common bacterial infections on earth, the notion that Babesia and Lyme would exist without at least one species variant of Bartonella would be unusual. But since Bartonella medicine and lab testing surrounding this powerful stealth infection is 20 years behind the times, the belief that some people have just these two infections is common. So let's discuss what it would look like in this theoretical situation. (This assumes no 15/16-6/5-51 HLA).

TNF-a	high
IL-6	normal-high
IL-1b	normal-high
VEGF	low-normal

Babesia and Bartonella Together

TNF-a	high

Bartonella lowers the value of this lab, so if it is high, is something driving it high, such as Babesia? It should be low with Bartonella alone.

IL-6	low-normal-high

While Bartonella lowers this, in the presence of Babesia, it may or may not become increased. If it is in the 40th percentile or higher, this is suspicious for Babesia.

IL-1b	low-normal-high

While Bartonella lowers this, in the presence of Babesia, it may or may not become increased. If it is in the 30th percentile or higher, this is suspicious for Babesia.

Please do not assume **both** IL-6 and IL-1b will both go up in the presence of Babesia. **In fact, sometimes only TNF-a or IL-6 or IL-1b increases, while the other two remain low.**

VEGF	**low-normal**

Generally even **very low numbers of Babesia will bring high levels of VEGF down.** At times Babesia will reduce VEGF significantly to moderate or low "normal" blood levels in the accepted range of the test.

On occasion Babesia makes VEGF so low it is actually unable to be measured. One new problem with some laboratories is that they have had a new flood of thousands of VEGF tests being done on very ill patients. Some of these have very low VEGF blood levels. So at least one large lab, LabCorp, has revised its normal range markedly downward based on very ill patients. Therefore their new normal range is based on an ill patient population and not healthy and normal patients. The outcome then, if a lab alters the lowest "normal" range to zero, is that they have created a statistical and clinical flaw, much like saying the normal range for human eyes is zero—two. In the same way, some Labs actually say a VEGF of **zero** is part of the normal range. Wrong. A VEGF of 31-85 is fine for our purposes here.

The critical point is that Bartonella manufactures VEGF directly or indirectly, creating a *high level of VEGF* in the blood and also in tissues. (Sometimes the skin shows evidence of VEGF). It is the chemical that sometimes causes various red, burgundy and blue blood vessel findings all over the body. If a person has Bartonella alone with Lyme, VEGF is almost always going to be above the normal range. If VEGF is low or normal, one common cause in a person with Lyme disease or ixodes tick exposure risk is a Babesia infection.

Finally, let me merely mention the meaning of ECP or Eosinophil Cationic Protein. It is used by eosinophil cells to kill parasites, but not single-celled parasites as a rule. Sometimes the ECP is in the top 15%. In the presence of effective Babesia killing in about 60 percent of Babesia positive patients, ECP is over the top normal level.

Sample Bartonella Laboratory References

1. Cerimele F, Brown LF, Bravo F, Ihler GM, Kouadio P, Arbiser JL. Infectious angiogenesis: Bartonella bacilliformis infection results in endothelial production of angiopoetin-2 and epidermal production of vascular endothelial growth factor. *Am J Pathol.* 2003;163(4):1321-1327.

2. Dehio C. Recent progress in understanding bartonella-induced vascular proliferation. *Curr Opin Microbiol.* 2003;6(1):61-65.

3. Herremans M, Bakker J, Vermeulen MJ, Schellekens JF, Koopmans MP. Evaluation of an in-house cat scratch disease IgM ELISA to detect bartonella henselae in a routine laboratory setting. *Eur J Clin Microbiol Infect Dis.* 2008. 10.1007/s10096-008-0601-8.

4. Kempf VA, Schairer A, Neumann D, et al. Bartonella henselae inhibits apoptosis in mono mac 6 cells. *Cell Microbiol.* 2005;7(1):91-104. 10.1111/j.1462-5822.2004.00440.x.

5. Lappin MR, Breitschwerdt E, Brewer M, Hawley J, Hegarty B, Radecki S. Prevalence of bartonella species antibodies and bartonella species DNA in the blood of cats with and without fever. *J Feline Med Surg*. 2008. 10.1016/j.jfms.2008.06.005.

6. Mathieu S, Vellin JF, Poujol D, Ristori JM, Soubrier M. Cat scratch disease during etanercept therapy. *Joint Bone Spine*. 2007;74(2):184-186. 10.1016/j.jbspin.2006.05.017.

7. Popa C, Abdollahi-Roodsaz S, Joosten LA, et al. Bartonella quintana lipopolysaccharide is a natural antagonist of toll-like receptor 4. *Infect Immun*. 2007;75(10):4831-4837. 10.1128/ IAI.00237-07.

8. Raoult D, Dutour O, Houhamdi L, et al. Evidence for louse-transmitted diseases in soldiers of napoleon's grand army in vilnius. *J Infect Dis*. 2006;193(1):112-120. 10.1086/498534.

9. Resto-Ruiz SI, Schmiederer M, Sweger D, et al. Induction of a potential paracrine angiogenic loop between human THP-1 macrophages and human microvascular endothelial cells during bartonella henselae infection. *Infect Immun*. 2002;70(8):4564-4570.

10. Vermeulen MJ, Diederen BM, Verbakel H, Peeters MF. Low sensitivity of bartonella henselae PCR in serum samples of patients with cat-scratch disease lymphadenitis. *J Med Microbiol*. 2008;57(Pt 8):1049-1050. 10.1099/ jmm.0.2008/001024-0.

The Bartonella testing of most national labs is surprisingly poor.

It is stunning to read about so-called "sages" who report that patients don't have Bartonella just because a large lab didn't find antibodies to the infection in their blood.

First, these "sages" do not understand that Bartonella turns off its own antibodies, and that the large labs only check for one (or two) species that infect humans, and their cut-off titers are unrealistically high.

Bartonella FISH testing is now available (except in New York State) from IGeneX and is useful but should never be the only test. Fry Clinical Laboratories has a very sensitive smear that shows Bartonella. We have found that when they report Bartonella, we see indirect labs that are consistent with the presence of Bartonella. These indirect labs are mentioned in a full and complete review of the international PubMed articles on the topic which I have read over many years.

Infections and inflammation decrease insight.

Tick-borne infections routinely destroy patients' ability to have insight into treatments and lead to personality changes and/or rigid resistance to testing. This is largely due to an impaired frontal lobe (the part of the brain involved in self-awareness). Examples of decreased insight are demonstrated by the following situations:

a. Patients feeling like they are cured when they have only experienced partial improvement in their symptoms.

b. Patients intentionally going to practitioners who use inferior labs.

c. Patients refusing, with eccentric resistance, to be tested for tick-borne infections.

d. Patients dismissing positive test results with a wave of their hand.

Some patients insist that their problem is mold alone and not tick-borne infections.

They cannot believe **both** indoor mold and tick-borne infections are important. The idea that one could be causing 80 percent of their symptoms and the other was "the straw that broke the camel's back" is a concept they reject.

Some patients get ill after a flood, large leak or some other water intrusion problem. They feel they are ill only because of mold mycotoxins in their home that have formed 36-48 hours after water intrusion into drywall, insulation, carpeting and other dust or cellulose-filled materials. The EPA reports that 30 percent of US structures have indoor mold. Some of these indoor molds have war-grade chemicals on their surfaces. When the tomb room of the last King of Poland, Casimir IV was opened in Paris in 1973, ten of the twelve scientists who were present died. One survivor had expertise in mold and subsequently found specific toxic mold species. I must confess that as a certified mold investigator and certified mold remediator, I am utterly stunned that many physicians actually dismiss the notion of indoor mold being related to illness.

Here is one example why that is a scientific error.

Mold chemicals from mummies kill tomb researchers

In recent years, some "mold experts" ignoring almost 100% of the 33,000 mycotoxin references in PubMed, and who are also weak on remediation, have received public attention. Others seem to know nothing about the illnesses caused by mold other than 1970's leaky gut issues or spore illness found in severely immune suppressed people who are very rare. We have known for at least 30 years illness can be caused by the chemicals from indoor mold. In medical schools, no one is really taught this information.

Most of us have heard the term "Beware the Mummy's Curse." Many individuals working in archeology or tomb robbery have died soon after opening and entering tombs or handling their contents.

Perhaps the caution began when Lord Carnarvon, an elderly and medically frail expert in Egyptian archeology, was involved in the excavation of King Tut's tomb in 1922. After 5 years, 11 who had entered the tomb were dead.

Since such tombs typically had fruits, vegetables, meats, clothing and furniture, molds would naturally form in these dark places and form spores and their surface toxins that could last thousands of years. The first to enter these tombs, before they were aired out, would get a huge dose of mold toxins.

This seems to be the general belief of scholars from all over the Middle East, Europe and America.

This was further supported by the examination of the mummy of Ramesses II of ancient Egypt, which was examined in a research Museum in Paris in 1976, and over 89 different species of molds were found in or on the mummy. The researchers were fortunately careful enough to be wearing special masks.

One of the most serious recent mold toxin Archeology disasters occurred when the tomb of a famous 15th century Polish leader, King Casimir, was opened in 1973 by 12 researchers. The wooden coffin was heavily rotted inside the tomb. In a few days, four of the 12 were dead. Soon six more died. One of the two survivors was Dr. Smyk who was an expert microbiologist and suffered 5 years with new neurological balance trouble. He studied some tomb artifacts in great detail and found clear Aspergillus and Penicillin species that make dangerous mycotoxins, such as aflatoxins…

Is it any wonder that experts on this topic, like Dr. Barbara Janinka from the Polish Institute of Engineering and Dr.'s Poirier and Feder, in their book *Dangerous Places: Health, Safety, and Archaeology,* remind us of an old observation about archaeology—when you go home after a hard day in the field and blow your nose, you blow out dirt." Feder said, "Clearly you have been breathing it in, and if you have been exposed to molds, spores, or fungi that lay dormant in the earth, there is at least a possibility of being exposed to some nasty stuff."

However, if the reader does not follow the required home, school, office, church or synagogue mold prevention hygiene steps, the same molds that have killed archeologists in the past can become part of your world. And in many cases, in ways much more than a runny nose or red eyes!

Examples of scholars who believe toxic molds like Aspergillus and Penicillium species make poisons like Ochratoxins, and have been responsible for Archeologist deaths include: Dr. Ezzeddin Taha of Cairo University, the Italian physician Dr. Nicola Di Paolo, French physician Dr. Caroline Stenger-Phillip, physician Dr. Hans Merk and microbiologist Dr. G. Kramer—both from Germany.

Sample Supporting References

- news.nationalgeographic.com

- www.quaktestusa.com

- www.catchpenny.org

- B. Janinska. Historical buildings and mould fungi. Not only vaults are menacing with "Tutankhamen's Curse." *Foundations of Civil and Environmental Engineering*. (2002): 43-54. www.unmuseum.org

- meta-religion.com/Archaeology/Africa/Egypt/tut_curse.htm

Residing in a moldy location prevents people from being cured from tick and flea-borne infections.

This significant factor was the catalyst for my decision to co-author two mold remediation books. We have also known since the 1880's that the combination of dust and high humidity leads to mold and bacteria growth indoors. Their presence makes Lyme disease much more difficult to cure.

Only 1 in 1000 physicians has read 500 articles on indoor water intrusion's impact on health. One fascinating article includes possible mold chemicals used in the Vietnam War (Wannamaker, *Military Medicine*, Ch. 24).

Further, we can measure three top dangerous mycotoxins in your body. Specifically, in an ELISA test done by Dr. Hooper at his Real Time Laboratory, he routinely finds aflatoxins, ochratoxins and trichothenes in the urine of my mold exposed patients. So for example, the Collier county sheriff building and jail here in Naples is filled with mold, rat urine and rats, and the "remediation" is inept, so many staff are retiring, or going out on disability. No one really cares or has a clue the illness this is causing—they simply are ignorant or do not listen.

This sheriff building and jail had ERMI testing done that was positive. ERMI is a research tool developed by the EPA and the results are serious, but no administrator understands that these employees in Naples, Florida are better when away from the sheriff building because it is apparently a "sick building." So here are the possible causes of illness from our example, the sheriff building and jail of Naples.

A. Mold toxins—there are 33,000 articles on these in PubMed. Anyone who questions the sicknesses caused by mycotoxins is illiterate, a sadistic boss, or an insurance company prostitute. I have seen toxicologists, who have not read a full book or 40 articles on mold water illness, report a sick building is safe. Amusingly, every military field of battle medical book I own has a section on the treatment of mycotoxin poison. The military are not fools.

B. Mold inflammation chemicals—when molds eat, they produce a flurry of substances, and some of these increase inflammation in mammals like humans.

C. Bacteria—water inside any structure is really a disaster. If it is dried very fast, in 36 hours or less, generally no health risks exist. Of course this means in all the locations where the water reached. I was recently an expert in a New Jersey utilities case, and the utilities visitor never realized the water was inside the walls, the kitchen ceiling and around the window structure. Why? Because he could care less. We see the same inept ignorance or sadistic bosses running the Naples Florida jail and sheriff building, which has massive mold found in past inspections and a current EPA designed ERMI test. In the past, visible mold was handled by renovators or "remediators" of which 95 percent in Florida and probably other states are vastly under trained. The jail/sheriff offices also have rat urine which has biologically active water. Over twenty bacteria species create toxins when water is present indoors. For example, you have probably heard that the famous Legionnaires' infections in our treasured veterans were due to water in the hotel's AC ducts. I recall very vividly the outbreak of Legionnaires' in the hotel where I attended meetings monthly. One would think from reading infection books that we know everything about all infections. Such hubris is absurd and quickly dispatched by merely refraining from excess alcoholic beverages.

Indeed, the mortality at the original American Legion convention in 1976 was high despite the closeness of the University of Pennsylvania's elite infectious disease department, who are gifted at telling people they are not ill when they feel ill. Thirty-four died and approximately one hundred-eighty were infected.

Despite the obvious infectious symptoms, the infectious agents were not identified for some time as was the case with HIV. Legionnaires' disease was simply caused by a bacterium that takes advantage of standing water. And it is hardly the only killing bacterium that is present in standing water associated with leaks in a home, school or work structure. Legionnaires' disease is still fatal, but the percentage of people surviving is better in recent outbreaks and single infections. We know that standing water in almost any location has some risk if nothing is present to kill the organisms. So as mentioned, prisons and structures with poor ventilation due to building defects, terribly clogged or cheap filters, or a ventilation system with bends in the ducts, allow for condensation of water in the ducts of the air conditioner system, which will allow the infected invisible vapor to infect people very far away, infecting anyone not immune to the strain of bacteria.

Finally, please understand, this is a sample dangerous bacterium associated with still water. It is hardly the only one that can cause illness and death.

D. Bacteria biotoxins—in the section above we focused on the infection of water related bacteria. But these bacteria also make biotoxins. These bacteria toxins are dangerous. One you have heard of is related to food poisoning. It is why some food makes people vomit. However, if a location with these biotoxins is fully dried, the bacteria biotoxins should decay. In contrast, mold biotoxins do not easily decay.

It is a medical error to ignore patients sleeping over 9 hours a day or under 7 hours a day.

Some patients with tick or flea infections need over 9 hours of sleep, or cannot sleep 7 hours. Their complaints of fatigue must be taken very seriously, and one must not assume it is the vague "fibromyalgia" which can also be associated with a wide range of things mentioned in this book.

Papers that accept a Fibromyalgia diagnosis quickly are not advanced 2012 medicine nor do they show full-time study in these areas.

If a patient has significant troubles with fatigue, it is possible the infections or other sicknesses mentioned in this book might apply.

For example, if someone is excessively fatigued, here would be some basic labs to order and the result that might fit with the topics in this book.

- [ ] Low free DHT

- [ ] Low FreeT3

- [ ] High Reverse T3

- [ ] One of the many thyroid system auto-immunity labs

- [ ] ECP is over 2010 top range or unable to be measured

- [ ] Babesia lab that has at least a 5% positive reporting range is indeterminate or positive.

- [ ] Urine Real Time mycotoxins are positive

- [ ] The Western Blot is interpreted in a manner similar to some Chinese physicians—if a band is specific for Lyme, it is Lyme positive.

- [ ] Low free testosterone

- ☐ IL-6 is very low

- ☐ IL-1B is very low

- ☐ Vitamin D is under 39 or very low normal

- ☐ WBC count is under 5.0

- ☐ Platelets are under 190.

- ☐ MSH is in lower 20th percentile. Any range that starts at zero is absurd. Five years ago a zero level was never normal, so the norm was changed due to sick patients. If LabCorp is used, the range of normal is 40-85.

- ☐ VIP is in the low 25th percentile

- ☐ C4a is in excess of normal

- ☐ MMPI is over 300 (a top range of over 300 is an error)

One could add dozens of other tests but these are a start.

If any patient reports that any of these are problems, Babesia, Bartonella and Lyme disease should be considered. But Babesia causes the worst fatigue, and using a massive mill lab to test for Babesia is naive. Patients with positive DNA or PCR testing and visualized Babesia inside cells are usually called negative when their blood is sent to large volume labs.

Lyme has at least one surface biotoxin, the patented BbTox1, and some people cannot detoxify this biotoxin.

Patients with 15/16--6/5--51 HLA patterns and possibly others, are possibly unable to remove Lyme biotoxins (R. Shoemaker) and must take a binder like Cholestyramine, which has been used to bind biotoxins since the 1970's. Other HLA patterns have been identified in 2009 that may be responsible for the body slowly releasing Lyme biotoxins. It is not clear how much of this toxin and other inflammatory chemicals are removed by USP purity clay, activated charcoal, top probiotics, cholestyramine, NAC, Cal-D-Glucarate, Milk Thistle or glutathione.

The research in PubMed over many years shows that one binder will always fail to remove some mycotoxins. So an informed and well-read position is the use of multiple agents.

Many patients who have had tick-borne infections have very high levels of inflammation.

High starting doses of antibiotics exacerbate this problem and complicate healing. Therefore, all starting doses of medications or herbs should be very low and gradually raised to higher levels. Additionally, liver-protecting substances should be given in conjunction with these remedies. Starting at full dosing in a "medically sensitive" patient is akin to committing chemical battery. Reactions to massive die-off of infectious organisms may be confused with allergic reactions and can cause panic attacks, shortness of breath, chest pain and severe migraines. This sloppy, one-size-fits-all approach is common in large practices in which a few major "protocols" are routine.

Medical "Band-Aids" are often required to save a job, a marriage and to care for children, but practitioners don't always prescribe these.

They are often a highly useful component of care, however. Pain, fatigue, severe insomnia, depression and anxiety often increase with die-off reactions or as a result of the presence of the infections. Band-Aid treatments are therefore often useful and helpful for patients. I treat people who run companies, schools, very large families and professional teams. They want to sleep 13 hours per day. They need stimulants for a period of time. The use of natural or synthetic stimulant options is discussed in *The Diagnosis and Treatment of Babesia* (available from Amazon.com or www.LymeBook. com). Patients do not benefit from sleep in excess of 8.5 hours. It may just serve to get them fired!

Health care workers have a huge inability to see the core flaw in all "Lyme," "Babesia" and Human "Bartonella" testing research.

Many physicians are no longer comfortable thinking about tick and flea infections for a wide range of reasons. And if they are very busy, they may only have time to open a book and try what was suggested the year before the book was written. They may also fear using a dose below or above what is listed. Some patients can only handle a lower dose or they get side effects; others do not feel better without a higher dose.

First, I have looked over many sincere and well intentioned studies. The common massive error in these studies is the limited reading and experience that promotes the quasi-religious belief that a lab test can be 100 percent accurate and the researcher can find patients that have pure Babesia, Bartonella, Ehrlichia, or Lyme disease. The reality is that it is absolutely impossible as of 2011 to use simplistic *direct labs,* which look for species established by approximately the year 2000 and not after, to determine what infections I just mentioned are present. And we are not even talking about the flood of viruses and other newly discovered different types of infections routinely carried by Ixodes ticks that we know about in 2012 if one is aggressively reading and attending conferences.

Of course some exceptions exist. If a person lives in New York City and has a cat, and never is exposed to anything but concrete and tar, they may just get Bartonella from their pet. And roughly 100 years ago, all southern cattle were destroyed by Babesia, and I believe that was Babesia alone. But these are exceptions.

In summary, studies that *rule out other infections with the wave of simple PCR or titer lab tests are throwbacks to 1995 medicine.* Any finding is markedly suspect, first, because tick and flea infections are not spread as mono-infections among humans, and second, since single infections do not exist as a rule, lab results may be skewed by the presence of more than one infectious agent.

Reading and researching the ***indirect labs changed by one or many of these infections*** make it clear you are missing infections if you assume the study population has "a single infection." But this requires years of full-time reading to dent this topic, and not merely a few hours at an infection conference.

Look at some sample ways Bartonella hides and alters immunity to understand how serious it can be to you.

Bartonella can:

☐ lower your temperature

☐ suppress antibodies

☐ make new tissue

☐ make new blood vessels or new cavities for blood. This is ***not rare*** if you know how and where to look. Increased VEGF is routine, and if VEGF is not high, one should consider the presence of Babesia immediately.

☐ use bacteriophages—small virus outer shells that carry genetic information to defeat host defense mechanisms and allow survival in a host.

☐ invade the critically important endothelial cells as targets

☐ undermine many cell functions

☐ invade cells

☐ increase inflammation

☐ suppress apoptosis (cell death)

☐ stimulate cell reproduction

☐ create tumor-like growths

☐ impair monocytes so that they no longer devour bacteria properly

☐ persistently decrease CD8+ lymphocytes (cancer fighting cells)

☐   change adhesion molecule expression (downregulation of
      L-selectin, VLA-4, and LFA-1)

☐   harm some CD8+ T lymphocytes

☐   limit antigen presentation in human lymph nodes

This is a highly limited set of examples. Why is this new to people?
Why is it unknown to most smart physicians?

Sample Supporting References

Harms A, Dehio C. Intruders below the Radar: Molecular Pathogenesis of Bartonella spp. Clin Microbiol Rev. 2012 Jan;25(1):42-78.

Maggi RG, Breitschwerdt EB. Isolation of bacteriophages from Bartonella vinsonii subsp. berkhoffii and the characterization of Pap31 gene sequences from bacterial and phage DNA. J Mol Microbiol Biotechnol. 2005;9(1):44-51. PMID:16254445

Andersen-Nissen E, Smith KD, Strobe KL, Barrett SL, Cookson BT, Logan SM, Aderem A. Evasion of Toll-like receptor 5 by flagellated bacteria. Proc Natl Acad Sci U S A. 2005 Jun 28;102(26):9247-52. Epub 2005 Jun 13.

Ahsan N, Holman MJ, Riley TR, Abendroth CS, Langhoff EG, Yang HC. Peloisis hepatis due to Bartonella henselae in transplantation: a hemato-hepato-renal syndrome. Transplantation. 1998 Apr 15;65(7):1000-3.

Dehio C. Molecular and cellular basis of bartonella pathogenesis. Annu Rev Microbiol. 2004;58:365-90.

Pappalardo BL, Brown TT, Tompkins M, Breitschwerdt EB. Immunopathology of Bartonella vinsonii (berkhoffii) in experimentally infected dogs. Vet Immunol Immunopathol. 2001 Dec;83(3-4):125-47.

Pulliainen AT, Dehio C. Persistence of Bartonella spp. stealth pathogens: from sub-clinical infections to vasoproliferative tumour formation. FEMS Microbiol Rev. 2012 Jan 9. [Epub ahead of print]

Smith KJ, Skelton HG, Tuur S, Larson PL, Angritt P. Bacillary angiomatosis in an immunocompetent child. Am J Dermatopathol. 1996 Dec;18(6):597-600.

Bartonella has psychiatric and neurology effects in excess of current awareness.

In my TV interview and paper on brain effects, I show Bartonella can cause ADHD, ADD, depression, manic symptoms and severe insomnia.

Here are some other findings summarized. Bartonella can cause:

- ☐ trouble speaking

- ☐ acute neurological disease

- ☐ stroke

- ☐ granulomas or other tissue changes of the brain

- ☐ bacteremia

- ☐ retinitis

- ☐ musculoskeletal disorders

- ☐ liver disease

- ☐ spleen disease

- ☐ muscle myocarditis

- ☐ fever of unknown cause

- ☐ new illness after a blood transfusion

- ☐ Encephalitis lethargica with a possible statue-like, speechless and motionless state. It often creates high fever, sore throat, headache, double vision, delayed physical and mental response, sleep inversion, catatonia and lethargy. In acute cases, patients may enter a coma-like state (akinetic mutism). Patients may also experience abnormal eye movements ("oculogyric crises"), Parkinsonism, upper body weakness, muscular pains, tremors, neck rigidity, and behavioral changes including psychosis. A vocal tic is sometimes present.

☐ Fully normal lymph nodes or enlarged nodes—large nodes are not a routine finding

☐ malaise

☐ dementia

Sample Supporting References

Becker JL. Vector-borne illnesses and the safety of the blood supply. Curr Hematol Rep. 2003 Nov;2(6):511-7.

Ben-Ami R, Ephros M, Avidor B, Katchman E, Varon M, Leibowitz C, Comaneshter D, Giladi M. Cat-scratch disease in elderly patients. Clin Infect Dis. 2005 Oct 1;41(7):969-74. Epub 2005 Aug 30.

Bloch KC, Glaser C. Diagnostic approaches for patients with suspected encephalitis. Curr Infect Dis Rep. 2007 Jul;9(4):315-22.

Brenneis C, Scherfler C, Engelhardt K, Helbok R, Brössner G, Beer R, Lackner P, Walder G, Pfausler B, Schmutzhard E. Encephalitis lethargica following Bartonella henselae infection. J Neurol. 2007 Apr;254(4):546-7. Epub 2007 Mar 12.

Chan L, Reilly KM, Snyder HS. An unusual presentation of cat scratch encephalitis. J Emerg Med. 1995 Nov-Dec;13(6):769-72.

Centers for Disease Control and Prevention (CDC). Encephalitis associated with cat scratch disease--Broward and Palm Beach Counties, Florida, 1994. MMWR Morb Mortal Wkly Rep. 1994 Dec 16;43(49):909, 915-6.

Cherinet Y, Tomlinson R. Cat scratch disease presenting as acute encephalopathy. Emerg Med J. 2008 Oct;25(10):703-4.

Dreher A, Grevers G. [Cat scratch disease. An overview for the ENT physician].[Article in German]. Laryngorhinootologie. 1996 Jul;75(7):403-7.

Edouard S, Raoult D. [Bartonella henselae, an ubiquitous agent of proteiform zoonotic disease].[Article in French]. Med Mal Infect. 2010 Jun;40(6):319-30. Epub 2009 Dec 29.

Fouch B, Coventry S. A case of fatal disseminated Bartonella henselae infection (cat-scratch disease) with encephalitis. Arch Pathol Lab Med. 2007 Oct;131(10):1591-4.

Genizi J, Kasis I, Schif A, Shahar E. Effect of high-dose methyl-prednisolone on brainstem encephalopathy and basal ganglia impairment complicating cat scratch disease. Brain Dev. 2007 Jul;29(6):377-9. Epub 2006 Dec 15.

Gerber JE, Johnson JE, Scott MA, Madhusudhan KT. Fatal meningitis and encephalitis due to Bartonella henselae bacteria. J Forensic Sci. 2002 May;47(3):640-4.

Glaser CA, Gilliam S, Schnurr D, Forghani B, Honarmand S, Khetsuriani N, Fischer M, Cossen CK, Anderson LJ; California Encephalitis Project, 1998-2000. In search of encephalitis etiologies: diagnostic challenges in the California Encephalitis Project, 1998-2000. Clin Infect Dis. 2003 Mar 15;36(6):731-42. Epub 2003 Mar 3.

Grzeszczuk A, Ziarko S, Kovalchuk O, Stańczak J. Etiology of tick-borne febrile illnesses in adult residents of North-Eastern Poland: report from a prospective clinical study. Int J Med Microbiol. 2006 May;296 Suppl 40:242-9. Epub 2006 Mar 10.

Kusumanto YH, Veenhoven RH, Bokma JA, Schellekens JF. [2 patients with atypical manifestations of cat-scratch disease].[Article in Dutch]. Ned Tijdschr Geneeskd. 1997 Feb 22;141(8):385-7.

Marienfeld CB, Dicapua DB, Sze GK, Goldstein JM. Expressive aphasia as a presentation of encephalitis withBartonella henselae infection in an immunocompetent adult. Yale J Biol Med. 2010 Jun;83(2):67-71.

Marra CM. Neurologic complications of Bartonella henselae infection. Curr Opin Neurol. 1995 Jun;8(3):164-9.

McGrath N, Wallis W. Cat-scratch encephalopathy. Neurology. 1998 Oct;51(4):1239. PMID:9781592

McGrath N, Wallis W, Ellis-Pegler R, Morris AJ, Taylor W. Neuroretinitis and encephalopathy due to Bartonella henselae infection. Aust N Z J Med. 1997 Aug;27(4):454. PMID:9448896

Nishio N, Kubota T, Nakao Y, Hidaka H. Cat scratch disease with encephalopathy in a 9-year-old girl. Pediatr Int. 2008 Dec;50(6):823-4.

[No authors listed]. From the Centers for Disease Control and Prevention. Encephalitis associated with cat scratch disease--Broward and Palm Beach counties, Florida, 1994. JAMA. 1995 Feb 22;273(8):614. PMID:7531250

Noah DL, Bresee JS, Gorensek MJ, Rooney JA, Cresanta JL, Regnery RL, Wong J, del Toro J, Olson JG, Childs JE. Cluster of five children with acute encephalopathy associated with cat-scratch disease in south Florida. Pediatr Infect Dis J. 1995 Oct;14(10):866-9.

Ogura K, Hara Y, Tsukahara H, Maeda M, Tsukahara M, Mayumi M. MR signal changes in a child with cat scratch disease encephalopathy and status epilepticus. Eur Neurol. 2004;51(2):109-10. Epub 2004 Feb 11.

Rombaux P, M'Bilo T, Badr-el-Din A, Theate I, Bigaignon G, Hamoir M. Cervical lymphadenitis and cat scratch disease (CSD): an overlooked disease? Acta Otorhinolaryngol Belg. 2000;54(4):491-6.

Singhal AB, Newstein MC, Budzik R, Cha JH, Rordorf G, Buonanno FS, Panzara MA. Diffusion-weighted magnetic resonance imaging abnormalities in Bartonella encephalopathy. J Neuroimaging. 2003 Jan;13(1):79-82.

Skarphédinsson S, Jensen PM, Kristiansen K. Survey of tickborne infections in Denmark. Emerg Infect Dis. 2005 Jul;11(7):1055-61.

Tattevin P, Lellouche F, Bruneel F, Régnier B, De Broucker T. [Bartonella henselae meningoencephalitis].[Article in French]. Rev Neurol (Paris). 2001 Jul;157(6-7):698-700.

Trelles JO, Palomino L, Trelles L. [Neurologic form of Carrion's disease. Clinical-anatomical study of 9 cases].[Article in Spanish]. Rev Neuropsiquiatr. 1969 Dec;32(4):245-306. PMID:5384732

Weston KD, Tran T, Kimmel KN, Maria BL. Possible role of high-dose corticosteroids in the treatment of cat-scratch disease encephalopathy. J Child Neurol. 2001 Oct;16(10):762-3.

Tick and flea infection medicine is not simple if you study each infection in ticks and fleas thoroughly.

Let me share my bias since, unlike some who had no training in the foundations of their thinking due to their overloaded science trainings, I have some sense of my biases. The first is I do not see tick and flea infection medicine as being as simple as a cold or a strep throat. I see it like HIV, a very large non-fatal third degree burn, or a massive car accident.

First, in keeping with one of my beloved Master's professors Harvie Conn at Westminster, who taught me Kuhn's *The Structure of Scientific Revolutions,* I used hyperbole to allow you to hear me. HIV is worse than tick infections, even if you have not been treated for your insect bite in thirty years. But you get the larger point that these complexes of injected infectious agents are not as simple as a strep throat.

With each passing year of full-time reading, I feel that this is a super-specialization. So a course, a week of lectures, or following an infection specialist on rounds for two weeks is not training, it is merely learning some basic ideas. But my appeal is the tick infection complex of infections is not basic.

This is a problem. If healthcare practitioners haven't spent 3,000 hours learning about this complex, emerging area of medicine, one that requires a great deal of study in years, then their patients need to find practitioners that are serious about it, instead of someone who is just "doing them a favor" by simply running a few tests.

If I had HIV, I would fly into Washington DC to see a top expert in this infection. I would not want someone who is "somewhat interested" in this disease.

Some patients relapse due to "treatment fatigue," meaning, they are taking too many pills each day even if some are just supplements.

I respect those that try to offer hope and encourage people by telling them that all tick and flea infections are easy to cure. But I also respect those that keep treating in one of many ways when the patient is not back to normal. However, this latter group is often on so many supplements that the patient feels exhausted from simply swallowing all the pills.

I have treated people who have seen all types of doctors with an interest in these infections. Some treated them for a month and others treated them longer.

My appeal to all healers is that asking someone to take 30 pills a day for longer than 2 months is a turn off, so be sure they really need it *or they will get fed up*. For example, some very ill patients may be on I.V. antibiotics or I.V. nutrients for an extended time, and any improvement clinically appears to be over, but some keep treating— I.V.

Others have various healers such as NDs, Chiropractors and integrative physicians, who feel that various supplements can be of use, and have Ms. Levin and Mr. Donaldson taking 40 pills per day. Others waste money on testing that we already know. For example, when I did a toxic water study, I realized every one of my patients had at least three metals above the "healthy" range. So I stopped testing for heavy metals after this was found in about eighty people—they are in all our bodies, and no test is needed to show what is true of all in industrialized nations.

So just give them what prevents clots, strokes, heart attacks, and cancer and lowers inflammation and also give them something for depression, agitation, panic, insomnia, and focus defects. It is a serious problem if they lose their job due to an inability to function.

Many natural and synthetic stimulants are available and should be discussed with your physicians or other health care workers.

So only give what is needed and what the labs show is low in terms of nutrients and hormones so as to keep people from getting fed up and putting them at the end of their treatment rope. This is what happens when practitioners do not treat them fully and effectively at the beginning of their treatment. They get treatment fatigue. Patients should consider a short treatment break, and discuss this option frankly with their health care providers. They should not confuse cure with improvement.

If you are opting for short tick infection care, this is not an issue. However, we all know some patients feel your standard approach helped partly, and want to continue care. It is your presuppositions and your bias for finding truth that will determine what you do. And I will defend you whatever you decide.

The treatment dose that "stuns organisms" is not the same dose that leads to a cure.

Sandy read a book on Babesia I wrote, and could not get anyone to give her a trial of an anti-malarial drug. So because she felt her signs and symptoms fit Babesia [See my Bartonella, Babesia and Lyme disease checklist book on Amazon.com], she purchased some artesunate and tried it herself. It was a modest dose, but *far too high as a starting dose* based on my Chinese connections and my own Artemesia and artesunate book research.

Sandy had new severe fatigue, a new severe headache, and chills and sweats. She strongly felt this was consistent with an effective dose, and a top Chinese MD agreed with her. In two days, all her symptoms were gone, and she "felt the best" in her life. She then stopped her herbal malaria medication.

One way to understand Sandy's report is to understand what she did. She took an herbal Chinese drug called "sweet wormwood" [it is **not** wormwood] and she had many symptoms that were new and these started 90 minutes after her artesunate self-trial—a semi-synthetic derivative of the Artemesia grown all over the world, such as in Wisconsin for our troops. And so I believe she felt poorly not from the medication, but from its ability to kill a protozoa or a single-celled parasite like Babesia. But why would she feel so much better and feel ill for a full 48 hours after taking the artesunate?

I believe the reason is simple.

A cure is not a mere reduction in bacterial load or stunning the infection. For example, using Bicillin LA 1.2 million units once a week, without a cyst buster may make someone feel better, but are you sure Lyme cysts do not exist? Are you willing to bet your family's health that it is unlike syphilis which has clear cysts? My bias is frank and open: cysts seem very likely from a review of other spirochetes and some Lyme disease research. And this has not been an area of primary research, so dismissing the idea seems confusing. So my appeal is the possibility of leaving some "Lyme seeds" might be unwise. And people may relapse not merely due to repeat infections, or inflammation residue, but due to active cysts.

It you are leaving cysts you will probably not fully cure patients of Lyme disease. So months or years after receiving "appropriate treatment," the levels of the body's cancer-fighting cells, marked by some as the CD 8/57, may still be under 90. Further, Vitamin D levels can fall into the lower 15th percentile due to active infection and cause an increase in cancer risk and thinning bones. These latter two indirect tests might be associated with Lyme disease and possibly other tick-borne infections. (The C4a test is definitely **not** specific for Lyme, since the presence of many infections or inflammation increases it, but it should probably not be in the top 95 percent or never above normal range).

Cynical relatives, friends or other health care workers defame some healing experts who are actually helping the patient.

You are getting better, or you relate to a physician, but others use the following types of put downs.

The doctor costs too much according to some relatives or strangers. I have insurance—the best in my state. And non-surgeons have never spent over 20 minutes with me, including "intakes" in many years. The real use of my insurance has been paying for covered very expensive surgeries and hospital costs.

Perhaps in your experience you had other healers who took your insurance. But too often I hear that the physicians seem to have "no real interest" in your problems and "did not help or listen fully," or simply passed you on to a "nice" physician extender such as a physician assistant or a nurse.

Having someone listen is very serious. Having a sub-specialist physician listen for over 30 minutes is very rare. They might not be the smartest and may not figure out all your troubles, but being heard matters. I am ashamed to say, at times, I feel I "know what people are thinking," and respond too fast, and it turns out I did not hear them accurately. It really takes time to hear a patient fully.

Others in your life or total strangers insult the healer because you are not getting better. It is true many healers do not know what they are doing, or do not know more than how to do simple screening. But sometimes your family and friends forget you were sick a very long time when you came for care. And extensive labs--not just a few tubes of blood--showed you had multi-body system defects. So if someone is disabled, I do not see anyone from any camp, group or tradition raising the functionally dead patient in a wheelchair in a single season. Any physician who is even willing to try to help someone who is a possible walking malpractice case should get a parade, because if the person continues to do poorly, you often see two undertakers—one for the ill patient and one for the attacked

MD. It is one reason my Canadian patients tell me the sick are often rejected as patients during intakes by family physicians.

Self-treatment rarely leads to your cure.

We all know you should not be your own lawyer. And medicine is 500 times more complex than one state's law. Being a top physician is not merely about the physician's cognitive abilities, but it is about the broadness of that physician's academic research in medicine and medical biochemistry. Due to the explosion of information about tick borne diseases, I read 50 hours a week, and feel I am falling behind.

Some reject "experts" due to cost even when they use physician extenders--their level of expertise is much less. Others search the land of all answers--the Internet. But the internet also has every answer, including utter nonsense. And no group has the corner on false medicine. It is so easy to say this ultra-conservative group with only 100 percent synthetic drug options is the right thinkers, but you would be markedly wrong. Others feel only "rebels" offer effective treatment options, but their proof is "Ms. Jones felt better on treatment F."

So if you are going to treat yourself, who will play the pipe to lead you? Some health care practitioners seem too narrow in their approach to treatment, while others are open to virtually everything. So patients get into a medical boat and push themselves out to sea. They read like crazy. They try treatments A through T. They read testimonials of hundreds of patients. They try a wide range of non-prescription options. Some days, weeks or months, they feel better. Other weeks, they don't feel so good. They are upset. They ask themselves, "Why do I have to do all the work and learning?" This is not a good place for them to be. People exist who have already explored 98 percent of the things that those with Lyme are going to explore over the next ten years. They need mentors.

In many of my books and many Internet sites, patients can read about preventing flea and tick bites.

I believe it was Nadelman who proposed that longer term illness was the result of repeated bites. He is quite correct in pointing out that repeated bites happen far too much.

Robert is a hunter. Susan is a hiker. They both love the outdoors passionately. Both were diagnosed with a tick or flea infection of some type. They were given treatment. And they went back to the outdoor living they love. But they only changed their behavior a little bit.

If they use protection it is "spotty."

a. Both own a dog, but neither makes sure the tick and flea killing protection is up to date. They may miss the application date by 2 or 3 weeks at times. When asked, they blame the "busyness" of life.

b. Both are fine having their dog in their bedroom, and when asked to be "honest," both admit to "occasionally" allowing the dog into the foot of the bed and allowing the dog to "kiss" their face or fingers with saliva.

c. Robert reports using permethrin on his hunting clothes last season. He has washed these clothes, but has no idea the permethrin potency he applied to his hunting clothes, and does not know how many times they have been washed. So he has no idea if a tick can crawl onto his skin or if the clothing will kill it in a second.

d. Susan does apply permethrin to her "running shoes and socks" but does **not** realize it must be fully dry to work. She also does **not apply any type of protection above her ankles** due to fear of "cancer causing chemicals."

e. Neither looks over their dogs for fleas or ticks for more than 45 seconds after time outside.

f.   Neither looks over their body other than a quick look at their naked body just before getting into the shower or the bathtub. When asked if they "inspected" their body after walking, running or hunting, they actually both smiled. The concept seemed amusing.

g.   Both have used DEET but primarily for mosquito contact and "occasionally" to prevent tick bites.

h.   Both really did not understand the simple basics about permethrin. For example, permethrin is an insecticide derived from the chrysanthemum family of plants. You do not put it on your skin, but apply it to clothing and allow it to dry before use—skin chemicals denature it so skin contact is not advised. It will not "spook" animals for viewing pleasure or during hunting, since it is odorless. It can survive washing, but the number of washings allowed is related to the concentration. It can stun or kill ticks based on the percentage on clothing and contact duration. Some feel it may have side effects, such as those experienced by those who used it in the Gulf War, but these soldiers were exposed to many other things as well.

i.   Susan has used an herbal mix of cedar, geranium, cilantro and another essential oil. She was unsure if it was of any use. What would you say to her? It matters because if you do not understand prevention of tick, flea or insect bites, depending on the location, she could become very ill.

Therefore let me propose some tentative thoughts from the research. I do not claim it is perfect or complete.

First, many feel we need to look at mosquito and tick products differently, meaning, a substance that repels a mosquito may not repel a tick. I hope this is obvious. Many well intentioned people confuse these very different insects. Simply, it is much harder to repel ticks.

Second, we have some research that suggests some organic substances and new substances are as good as DEET or better.

Here are just a few summary findings:

a. The oil of J. communis was nearly as potent as DEET according to top researcher John Carroll writing in 2011 (J Vector Ecol. 2011 Dec;36(2):258-68).

b. Many authors and studies report that DEET needs very high potency to have any meaningful repelling effects against ticks—at dosing far above what is effective against mosquitoes. Some suggest, for example, that high concentrations at 35% may not work to repel ticks, at least not after an hour, and also complain that it melts synthetic clothing, packaging and may have health risks.

c. Semmler reports in Parasitology Research (2011) that saltidin, p-menthan-diol and IR 3535 showed long-lasting effects, and the combination of saltidin and Vitex extracts was very good. [Saltidin is icaridin which is also called, "picaridine or KBR 3023" and is also sold as "Bayrepel." Vitex is an herb with many names, many proposed uses over many centuries and a full discussion would be tangential].

d. Zhang and Klun report that Isolongifolenone is easily synthesized from inexpensive turpentine oil and is cheaper and safer, and is at least as effective as DEET. If this were true, a higher concentration might be worth researching. (2009)

e. Dr. Bissinger published that the EPA approved an extract from wild tomatoes, 2-undecanone, now called, "BioUD," which is 200 to 400 percent more powerful at repelling ticks than DEET (*Exp Appl Acarol.* 2009).

In summary, many herbal derivatives, particularly in the oil or liquid forms which "off-gas" as their means of repelling ticks, include these sample substances mentioned above. The most pronounced effects were observed for the oils of citronella, cloves and lily of the valley. These three at specific concentrations or doses were reported as repelling ticks as effectively as DEET. Further, these substances are not single oils, and some parts were significantly more effective at repelling. For example, parts of citronellol, geraniol (oil of citronella and lily of the valley) and eugenol (oil of cloves) showed pronounced repelling effects along with phenethyl alcohol which is found in small amounts in the oil from lily of the valley. This was reported by Swedish professors, Thorsell, Mikiver and Tunon in 2006 in *Phytomedicine*.

What these three Swedish researchers report reflects a thread in other papers, specifically, if essential oils or other types of oils that can become vapors to make contact with ticks, and are effective at repelling or killing ticks, they can replace DEET. Using these oils, either alone or in combinations, and perhaps with higher dosing, individuals can successfully repel ticks from their skin with greater safety than DEET.

In conclusion, some individuals who are infected with Bartonella, Lyme, Babesia or any other tick infections become fair at protecting themselves. Learning how to prevent repeated bites merely takes thirty minutes of Internet study. It is worth the time. But the first lesson is realizing that the most common infectious tick is very small and requires close attention — not merely a ten second glance as you rush into the shower or bathtub.

Here is a sample case of how sometimes a tick infection cluster is highly complex in body effects.

Thomas Nolan is an FBI worker. He has been struggling with some fatigue, headaches and fair quality sleep for six months.

He has seen about two dozen physicians.

He has some red papules and skin tags on his physical. Further, he is unable to do a heel to toe walking test or one leg raise test well enough to pass a field sobriety test. So if a sheriff or police officer with a High School education did a medical exam on him to determine if he was on drugs or alcohol, he would fail and go to jail. He also has some very slight nystagmus or horizontal jerking of the eye that is borderline positive, which could also result in a DUI arrest. He does not drink or use illegal drugs.

Mr. Nolan's labs showed:

- ☐ a WBC of 4.6 – a low normal

- ☐ A free testosterone below abnormally low

- ☐ A DHT or dihydrotestosterone level abnormally low

- ☐ Anticardiolipin is positive

- ☐ ANA is high normal

- ☐ DHEA is within the normal range but very low

- ☐ VIP is undetectable

- ☐ C4a is 5780 or above normal

- ☐ Vitamin D level of 28 or low

- ☐ CD 57/8 is in the low normal range

- ☐ TNF alpha is 1.4

- ☐ IL-6 is zero

- ☐ IL-1B is unmeasurable

- ☐ ECP is borderline high

- ☐ VEGF is 120

- ☐ LYME ELISA is negative

- ☐ LYME WESTERN BLOT is "negative" with a positive 31 and 39 band

- ☐ Antibody testing for Bartonella, Babesia, Anaplasma is negative

- ☐ Ehrlichia titer is positive in one test

- ☐ MMP-9 of 437 which is too high, but called normal in the reference range

- ☐ EBV positive

- ☐ C-peptide high

- ☐ C-reactive protein high

- ☐ HLA DR/DQ of 16-5 and 4-3 according to QUEST laboratory. (Quest requires two codes for all five HLA results. These results are identical to LabCorp results)

- ☐ CMV positive

- ☐ HHP-6 positive

I am not going to tell you some of the many possible reasons for these results. It is likely fair to say that it is rare to find a physician who understands the meaning or possible meanings of this information from Mr. Nolan. Anyone who mocks them by saying they are "nonsense" and that each of these labs has "many possible reasons" is half correct. None are nonsense but **each has many possible**

causes. However, such comments reveal an inability to see meta-patterns in patients who are not getting better. My only point here is to show in a simple example that systemic infections over time have very dynamic effects, and that tick and flea infections might be a super specialization in medicine. If some of these labs and issues are foreign, it may be a sign of a very complex biochemical domino effect of tick and flea infections that is not appreciated by busy clinicians only trying to keep up with insurance codes and a 50-hour per week full-time practice.

The creative ways to decrease the numbers of Ixodes ticks and to decrease infections in humans from them are markedly flawed.

An important book of medicine in 2011 was R. Ostfeld's *Lyme Disease: The Ecology of a Complex System.* In this book he mentions many strong insights for Lyme disease prevention that includes comments that Lyme diagnosis, prevention and treatment is primitive in each area, and is unimpressed with treatments that are fifty years old. He considers the knowledge of Babesia transmission very primitive without even a good list of reservior hosts. Frankly, he feels the ecological science surrounding Ixodes ticks and Lyme is filled with blind faith convictions which rejected superior science over past decades and made Lyme disease a deer and mouse disease, which is false.

He reminds us that part of the cause of the Black Death or Plague was close proximity of fleas and rats to humans, and the increase of defragmented forests and brush increases contact between humans and ticks and lowers species diversity, with the immense loss of predators like wolves and cougars who would remove large numbers of tick-carrying small mammals. Effective carriers of infected ticks like chipmunks, shrews and rodents thrive in fragmented locations such as homes and schools with small strips of woods or brush near structures with people. Birds which can carry Ixodes ticks effectively are also more common in fragmented areas with construction and wild brush being mixed in small areas.

Ostfeld strongly opposes the idea of deer being at the center of tick infections, and mentions that research exists in which *over 70 percent of the deer are removed from islands so the deer cannot be replaced easily as on the mainland, and the infectious rodents actually carried more ticks. Deer removal solutions, such as expensive deer fences or aggressive hunting,* give very "inconsistent" results, and initially may increase infections. The notion of Lyme and other diseases as "deer infections" is wrong and too simplistic. It is also false that white footed mice are critical for transmission of tick infections. They are immensely easy to catch and due to hairless ears the ticks are vividly clear to researchers. Ostfeld expresses, repeatedly, that faith-like "science" claims regarding carriers and ticks were false. For example, according to various beliefs about North-East USA coastal limits, weather and optimal tick locations it was initially felt that the cold Midwest and Texas and California would **not** be states with high number of infections, yet they are states with many infectious Ixodes ticks.

Solutions to decrease infections, such as 4 pillar posts with tick killers next to "deer" food are not merely "deer devices," because many animals eat from them. Also cotton ball devices with miscellaneous insecticides to kill ticks in rodent nests fail according to high quality studies (Daniels 1991, Stafford 1992). Further, these products along with "bait boxes" are used by many other mammals and not merely mice. My impression of Ostfeld is that he supports an "all of the above" approach, with a full rejection of any notion that this is a deer and white footed mouse disease as immensely simplistic and refuted. He seems troubled by the time wasted by the focus on these two core animals.

Some animals are useful at lowering Ixodes ticks such as opossums, who can eat 5,300 larval ticks a week (pg 127), and some types of birds which kill ticks based on their grooming. Gray squirrels are also poor vectors for tick infection in humans. But he is not suggesting we drop thousands of opossums as a tick control solution.

He reports that burning of wild areas is not effective at reducing infections from ticks.

Using Guinea hens as an approach to reducing tick infections is not an informed option since they only eat adult Ixodes ticks in thin growth areas like lawns--younger forms such as nymphal forms are not reduced in lawns that have these hens compared to lawns without them. Adult Ixodes ticks are not the primary cause of human infections. The use of a Nematode parasite is also an approach recommended to reduce Ixodes ticks, since Ostfeld reports they are also only effective against adult ticks.

He reports that while predators may play a role in control, rodent food profoundly promotes Ixodes tick population growth. So for example, acorns on the forest floor may matter more than raptors like owls and hawks. Some trees may be less supportive of rodents such as birches and most conifers which have seeds too small for rodent food.

Vaccines against tick bites include the same chemicals that make tick bites painless and invisible. He proposes vaccines against tick antihistamines, anti-coagulants, pain killing chemicals and anti-inflammatory chemicals in tick saliva.

While some focus on deer control approaches, at times the number of acorns eaten by mice was a better predictor of Lyme disease than deer numbers.

Ostfeld does feel that having diversity in every aspect of forests may be helpful in some locations. He believes that having many animal varieties likely decreases infection rates rather than having the limited varieties of animals and birds that can survive in small, fragmented green areas between homes or other structures. Further, many ticks escape being killed by some proposed tick control approaches by living deeper in the floor of a wild vegetation area. Ostfeld also suggests that the fungal species Metarhizium anisopliae and Beauveria bassiana can kill ticks and may offer promise. (pp. 179-80).

Tick and flea-borne infections cause isolation.

They ruin relationships due to the sick person's fogginess, poor insight, depression, various addictions, rage, anxiety, extreme hostility, or because the individual refuses to get treatment. These infections can even sometimes provoke violence in those infected. This hinders recovery.

I believe Bartonella is likely the worst cause of these problems, but Lyme and Babesia and the die-off reactions that they cause can also increase them.

Isolation leads to decreased treatment options because wisdom and financial support often comes from communities. A mobile society, such as is found in the USA as compared to the Czech Republic, can decrease supports for solid medical wisdom and financial options.

Slow physical decay and the slow alteration of a personality can ultimately lead to unemployment, jail for impulsive actions, divorce and the loss of family relationships and friendships. This, in turn, leads to profound isolation in sickness. Isolated humans, as Mother Teresa often said, are the poorest beings on earth.

Checklists for Bartonella, Babesia and Lyme Disease

The Bartonella Checklist
Increasing Suspicion of an Emerging Stealth Infection
James L. Schaller, M.D., M.A.R.

Introduction

In 2011 a new human Bartonella species was added to the over thirty-five Bartonella species currently publically published in Genetic Data banks. It was discovered and highlighted by the talented veterinarian researcher Edward Breitschwerdt. He has said things more clearly than the ideas I was pondering in 2005, while doing most of the research for my Bartonella book. He said simply, but with devastating and highly useful clarity, that **Bartonella testing is terrible, the treatments are poor,** it is typically found on the outside of red blood cells, and the current research on Bartonella is pathetic—one study at NIH. If this was not enough, he said in 2011, **"Bartonella is carried by more vectors than any infection on the earth."** So it is hardly a backdoor "co-infection." Perhaps Lyme is the "co-infection."

Recently, the German researchers Kaiser and Riess summarized Bartonella research in this manner: after 2 decades of Bartonella research, knowledge on transmission and pathology of these bacteria is still limited. Bartonella species have emerged to be important pathogens in human and veterinary medicine.

Why create a check list when a physician can just order an antibody test? First, I have found at times, Bartonella can turn off its own antibodies, and those caused by other tick and flea-borne infections in humans. In a study of sixty-one Bartonella infected dogs, Perez and Maggi reported recently that most Bartonella infected dogs **did not have detectable Bartonella antibodies.**

The criteria listed below may have causes unrelated to Bartonella. For example, each year more studies show the presence of poly infections, and this raises the problem of which infection is causing what symptom, sign or lab test change. For example, most tick infections can cause headache or fatigue. Knowing which infection is the cause does become clear if you are doing very advanced treatments that are designed to kill only one infection. The limitation of these poly infection studies is that typically the testing detection rate for each tick or flea-borne infection is not over 95% for all possible species and strains possibly infecting humans.

However, since Bartonella can disable and kill healthy people, the **checklist below is set to catch virtually every infected patient.** This is neither right nor wrong. Philosophy, sociology, presuppositions, medical fashion and psychology usually all play a role in setting cut offs for a diagnosis. All science is guided by presuppositions, and that is why even math research is guided by a wide range of variables. **In medicine, psychology, philosophical assumptions and sociology control all of medicine** but are unappreciated due to a lack of training. **See Kuhn's *The Structure of Scientific Revolutions* exceptionally summarized at the following link: http://des.emory.edu/mfp/Kuhn.html**

THE BARTONELLA CHECKLIST
James Schaller, M.D., M.A.R.
(Please Check Any Symptoms That Apply)

PSYCHIATRIC AND NEUROLOGICAL

☐ Current anxiety that was not present at age ten

☐ Current depression not present at age sixteen

☐ Knee-jerk emotional responses worse than past decades and worsening

☐ Brain fog

☐ Depression

☐ Depression that is not **fully** controlled on **routine anti-depressant doses,** or high dose antidepressants are required to control mood [**Improvement of mood** or being "less depressed" is not successful depression treatment.]

☐ Anxiety is poorly controlled with average dosing

☐ Depression is poorly controlled by reasonable treatment trials.

☐ Suicidal feelings or routine thoughts of death

☐ Crying

☐ Obsessive thoughts or fear in excess of event

☐ Obsessive thoughts that intrude into the mind which are in excess of normal

☐ A decrease in pleasure

☐ Rage worse with time

☐ Irritability worse with time

☐ Impatience is greater when compared to ten years ago [in a child--any irritability in excess of what is common for most children with an identical age].

☐ Cursing or hostile speech that is worse over time

☐ Increased addictions that are very resistant to typical recovery ranges

☐ Increased impulsivity in contrast to past years or past decades

☐ Severe neurological disorders without a clear cause

☐ Severe psychiatric troubles that do not seem to fit with the diagnostic criteria or there is trouble controlling symptoms with treatment

☐ New physical, emotional or verbal abuse in the home which was not present in the past

☐ Panic attacks that were not present at ten years of age

☐ Anxiety medication has to be increased to **very high levels** to continue past benefit

☐ Diagnosed as having bipolar disorder, but do not fit the criteria well

☐ Any psychiatric disorder that also shows **medical pathology in laboratory tests**

☐ Restlessness

☐ Combative behavior

☐ A parent, grandparent, child or sibling with suicide attempts

☐ A parent, grandparent, child or sibling who has started physical or extreme verbal fights

☐ Intermittent confusion

☐ Seizures

☐ Brain lesions seen on a brain scan such as an MRI or CT of the head

☐ Short term memory deficits

☐ Difficulty in learning new information

DERMATOLOGY OR SKIN

☐ Persistent rashes that last over 3 weeks

☐ Nodules under the skin

☐ Hyper-pigmentation or dark areas of skin which were not present at birth

☐ Hypo-pigmentation or obvious light areas of skin

☐ Unexplained hair loss

☐ Spontaneous breaks or holes in the skin as small as a millimeter

☐ Skin ulcerations

☐ Stretch marks in eccentric locations, e.g., arms, upper side under armpit, around armpit or on the back

☐ Stretch marks filled with red, pink, purple or dark blue color which are not caused by pregnancy or weight loss [remember, many with many pregnancies or weight loss do not have 20 stretch marks]

☐ Any skin markings or growths **greater** than most people

☐ Blood vessels or color on skin **greater** than most people

☐ Red papules of **any** size

- ☐ Skin tags including ones removed by a dermatologist or shaved off

- ☐ Unusual blood vessels of any kind including inside organs such as bladder or intestinal walls

- ☐ Any skin finding in excess of 95% of most humans

- ☐ Skin findings showing increased blood vessels of any size

- ☐ Skin findings showing increased tissue formation that is increased over the flatness of surface skin [This may be due to Bartonella, untreated Lyme disease, or both infections and systemic inflammation]

- ☐ Skin showing blood vessels that are too large or too many for **the location of the blood vessels**, e.g., surface thigh and calf skin with very thick surface blood vessels or legs, upper arms or shoulders have explosions of many fine blood vessels

- ☐ Burning skin sensations [this may have many causes].

- ☐ Itching without a clear cause and which is hard to control and remove

- ☐ Skin erosion without a clear cause such as a fire, fall or chemical burn

- ☐ Minor cuts or scratches which heal slowly

- ☐ Very slow healing after a surgery

- ☐ "Granulomas" or balls of tissue

- ☐ Formication or feelings of being bitten by bugs or bug sensations on skin with no bugs on the skin

EYE

☐ Retina infection

☐ Retina infarct or dead tissue in the back of the eye

☐ Neuroretinitis or inflammation of the retina and optic nerve in the back of the eye

☐ Uveitis or inflammation of the middle layer of the eye or the interior eye

☐ Papilledema or swelling of the optic nerve as it enters the back of the eye due to raised intracranial pressure

☐ Stellate maculopathy

☐ Acute blurred vision

☐ Sudden and/or significant change in vision

HEART

☐ Endocarditis or inflammation of the heart

☐ Heart valve pathology

☐ Enlargement of the heart

☐ Any amount of dead cardiac tissue

☐ Arrhythmias of the heart

☐ Palpitations unrelated to panic attacks

GENERAL MEDICAL

☐ Sleep medications take 90-120 minute to take effect instead of 30 minutes

☐ Insomnia [If profound fatigue is present, this might not apply]

☐ A temperature under 98.3 in a sick person.   A temperature under 99.0 if Lyme disease or Babesia is also present

☐ An uncomfortable infection in the body with no discernible cause

☐ Gastroesophageal reflux disease (GERD)

☐ Diarrhea

☐ Colitis or an inflammation of the colon

☐ Liver enlargement with no clear cause

☐ Blood vessel proliferation or increased numbers in any internal organs

☐ Lesions or wounds with no clear cause

☐ A sore throat with no other clear reason

☐ A persistent sore throat in humidity in excess of 45% [low humidity dries out throat tissue]

☐ Gingivitis or bleeding during flossing

☐ Unusual discomfort on the soles of the feet especially in the morning

☐ Puffy tissue on insole or any part of ankles

☐ Ankle "edema" or expanded tissue that does not pit when pressed [because it is expanded tissue and not merely fluid]

☐ Bone pain

☐ Inflammation of the outer bone surface or osteomyelitis

☐ Joint pain [this can be also due to Lyme disease and many other medical problems]

- ☐ Muscle pain [this can be also due to Lyme disease and many other medical problems]

- ☐ Medical problems described as "idiopathic" (of unknown or unclear cause)

- ☐ Presence of two tick or flea infections with two positive tick or flea-borne viruses, bacteria or protozoa.

As previously mentioned, Bartonella has more than 30 published species in public genetic databases and has more vectors than possibly any infection in the world. Therefore, the presence of other infections such as tick-borne viruses, bacteria or protozoa, should raise suspicion. Some of these include Babesia, STARI (Masterson's Disease), Neoehrlichia, Anaplasma, Lyme disease, Mycoplasmas, Q Fever, Rocky Mountain spotted fever (Rickettsia), tick-borne relapsing fever, Tularemia (bacteria), Ehrlichia, Protozoa FL1953, and viruses such as CMV, HHV-6, Coxsackie B Types 1, 2, 3, 4, 5, 6, Parvo B-19 or Powassan.

POSSIBLE LABORATORY FINDINGS

- ☐ IL-6 is very low.

- ☐ IL-1B is very low.

- ☐ TNF-alpha is in lower 10% of normal range.

- ☐ VEGF is above the normal range [however, if Babesia is present or being treated the VEGF will fall into normal or abnormal low levels].

- ☐ X-ray of the bone may show areas of bone loss.

- ☐ Biopsies of lymph nodes are negative for Mycoplasma and no clear evidence of other infections or illnesses are found

- ☐ Biopsies of lymph nodes appearing similar to sarcoidosis

☐ Tissue biopsies which are abnormal but with no clear cause of tissue problems

☐ A swab of a fresh scratch or bite skin lesion is positive for Bartonella.

ENVIRONMENT

☐ Exposure to cats and dogs in excess of very incidental rare contact

☐ **Exposure to cats and dogs** that have been strays or go outside [reviews of hundreds of professional journal articles make this a risk in an unknown percentage]

☐ Ticks or fleas are found on any pet you contact

☐ The patient's **mother** is suspected of having Bartonella based on newer direct and **indirect testing.**

☐ A **sibling, father, spouse or child** with any tick or flea-borne infection who shared with the patient a residence or vacation location with proximity to brush

☐ Outdoor exposure to outdoor environments such as brush, wild grasses, wild streams or woods which happened **without** the use of DEET on skin and Permethrin on all clothing **(It only takes one exposure to get a bite**.   If you used protection "most of the time," you were still exposed.)

☐ Exposure to lice

☐ Flea bites or flea exposure

☐ Exposure to pets that are exposed to ticks or fleas

☐ A scratch from a cat

☐ A bite from a cat or dog

☐ Exposure to biting flies

☐ Hunting, living or vacationing near deer or small mammals

☐ Clear exposure to any type of tick. [Bartonella is carried by a huge number of carriers, but for now, the percent that carry Bartonella is not known. Further, the capacity to detect all new species in the vectors or in humans infected does not exist or is not routinely available in direct testing of all human infectious Bartonella organisms in both large or specialty labs].

☐ Ticks found on your clothing

☐ Ticks found on your skin

☐ Ticks found in your home or car, vacation spot or recreation area

If one reads the majority of Bartonella journal articles, it seems clear Bartonella harms the body in hundreds of ways. But for our purposes in diagnosis, the above criteria should be enough to prevent a missed diagnosis. More criteria exist. Certainty claims or criticism about Bartonella positions without reading at least of 1,000 articles is confusing. How is this possible with new Bartonella findings and understandings each month? There are also new species whose genetic sequences show their uniqueness almost every month in public databases. In this spirit, this scale is meant merely to increase suspicion of Bartonella, which is a super stealth infection that takes perhaps fifty days to grow out on some bacteria growth plates, and floats in the blood as it lowers fevers. It also clearly suppresses some key immune system fighting chemicals. Cure claims made without the use of **indirect** testing, markedly documented in superior journals, should be examined further to prove effectiveness.

Dr. Schaller is the author of 30 books and 27 top journal articles. His publications address issues in at least twelve fields of medicine.   He has the most recent textbook on Bartonella. He has published on Bartonella under the supervision of the former editor of the *Journal of the American Medical Association (JAMA)*, and his entries on multiple tick and flea borne infections, including Bartonella [along with Babesia and Lyme disease] were published in a respected infection textbook endorsed by the NIH Director of Infectious Disease.   He has seven texts on tick and flea-borne infections based on his markedly unique full-time research and study practice, which is not limited to either finite traditional or integrative progressive medicine. Dr. Schaller has read on these emerging problems for many years.

Bibliography (Bartonella)

Aberer E. Lyme borreliosis--an update. J Dtsch Dermatol Ges. 2007 May;5(5):406-14. [Article in English, German]. J Dtsch Dermatol Ges. 2007 May;5(5):406-14. PMID:17451386

Abuzeid WM, Ruckenstein MJ. Spirochetes in otology: are we testing for the right pathogens?   Otolaryngol Head Neck Surg. 2008 Jan;138(1):107-9. PMID:18165003

Accorinti M. Ocular bartonellosis. Int J Med Sci. 2009;6(3):131-2. Epub 2009 Mar 19. PMID:19319232

Adamska M. [Bartonella spp. as a zoonotic pathogens transmitting by blood-feeding arthropods].[Article in Polish]. Wiad Parazytol. 2010;56(1):1-9. PMID:20450002

Aguero-Rosenfeld ME, Wang G, Schwartz I, Wormser GP. Diagnosis of lyme borreliosis. Clin Microbiol Rev. 2005 Jul;18(3):484-509. PMID:16020686

Al-Attar N, Ruimy R, Baron F, Hvass U. Bartonella endocarditis complicating congenital heart disease. BMJ Case Rep. 2009;2009. pii: bcr06.2008.0092. Epub 2009 Mar 17. PMID:21686936

Alves AS, Milhano N, Santos-Silva M, Santos AS, Vilhena M, de Sousa R. Evidence of Bartonella spp., Rickettsia spp. and Anaplasma phagocytophilum in domestic, shelter and stray cat blood and fleas, Portugal. Clin Microbiol Infect. 2009 Dec;15 Suppl 2:1-3. Epub 2009 Mar 26. PMID:19416279

Anan'eva LP, Studentsov EE, Levin E. [Detection of anti-Borrelia antibodies by immunoblotting in Lyme borreliosis].[Article in Russian]. Klin Lab Diagn. 2002 Jun;(6):45-7. PMID:12132378

Ang CW, Notermans DW, Hommes M, Simoons-Smit AM, Herremans T. Large differences between test strategies for the detection of anti-Borrelia antibodies are revealed by comparing eight ELISAs and five immunoblots. Eur J Clin Microbiol Infect Dis. 2011 Aug;30(8):1027-32. Epub 2011 Jan 27. PMID:21271270

Angelakis E, Edouard S, La Scola B, Raoult D. Bartonella henselae in skin biopsy specimens of patients with cat-scratch disease. Emerg Infect Dis. 2010 Dec;16(12):1963-5. PMID:21122232

Angelakis E, Lepidi H, Canel A, Rispal P, Perraudeau F, Barre I, Rolain JM, Raoult D. Human case of Bartonella alsatica lymphadenitis. Emerg Infect Dis. 2008 Dec;14(12):1951-3. PMID:19046532

Angelakis E, Pulcini C, Waton J, Imbert P, Socolovschi C, Edouard S, Dellamonica P, Raoult D. Scalp eschar and neck lymphadenopathy caused by Bartonella henselae after Tick Bite. Clin Infect Dis. 2010 Feb 15;50(4):549-51. PMID:20070235

Angelakis E, Roux V, Raoult D, Rolain JM. Real-time PCR strategy and detection of bacterial agents of lymphadenitis. Eur J Clin Microbiol Infect Dis. 2009 Nov;28(11):1363-8. Epub 2009 Aug 14. PMID:19685089

Arav-Boger R, Crawford T, Steere AC, Halsey NA. Cerebellar ataxia as the presenting manifestation of Lyme disease. Pediatr Infect Dis J. 2002 Apr;21(4):353-6. PMID:12075773

Arvand M, Raoult D, Feil EJ. Multi-locus sequence typing of a geographically and temporally diverse sample of the highly clonal human pathogen Bartonella quintana. PLoS One. 2010 Mar 19;5(3):e9765. PMID:20333257

Assi MA, Yao JD, Walker RC. Lyme disease followed by human granulocytic anaplasmosis in a kidney transplant recipient. Transpl Infect Dis. 2007 Mar;9(1):66-72. PMID:17313478

Atamanyuk I, Raja SG, Kostolny M. Bartonella henselae endocarditis of percutaneously implanted pulmonary valve: a case report. J Heart Valve Dis. 2011 Jan;20(1):94-7. PMID:21396492

Bacon RM, Biggerstaff BJ, Schriefer ME, Gilmore RD Jr, Philipp MT, Steere AC, Wormser GP, Marques AR, Johnson BJ. Serodiagnosis of Lyme disease by kinetic enzyme-linked immunosorbent assay using recombinant VlsE1 or peptide antigens of Borrelia burgdorferi compared with 2-tiered testing using whole-cell lysates. J Infect Dis. 2003 Apr 15;187(8):1187-99. Epub 2003 Apr 2. PMID:12695997

Bakken JS, Dumler JS. Clinical diagnosis and treatment of human granulocytotropic anaplasmosis. Ann N Y Acad Sci. 2006 Oct;1078:236-47. PMID:17114714

Ball R, Shadomy SV, Meyer A, Huber BT, Leffell MS, Zachary A, Belotto M, Hilton E, Bryant-Genevier M, Schriefer ME, Miller FW, Braun MM. HLA type and immune response to Borrelia burgdorferi outer surface protein a in people in whom arthritis developed after Lyme disease vaccination. Arthritis Rheum. 2009 Apr;60(4):1179-86. PMID:19333928

Barbier F, Fournier PE, Dauge MC, Gallien S, Raoult D, Andremont A, Ruimy R. Bartonella quintana coinfection in Staphylococcus aureus endocarditis: usefulness of screening in high-risk patients? Clin Infect Dis. 2009 May 1;48(9):1332-3. PMID:19344260

Baty G, Lanotte P, Hocqueloux L, Prazuck T, Bret L, Romano M, Mereghetti L. [PCR rDNA 16S used for the etiological diagnosis of blood culture negative endocarditis].[Article in French]. Med Mal Infect. 2010 Jun;40(6):358-62. Epub 2009 Sep 30. PMID:19796889

Bayliss DB, Steiner JM, Sucholdolski JS, Radecki SV, Brewer MM, Morris AK, Lappin MR. Serum feline pancreatic lipase immunoreactivity concentration and seroprevalences of antibodies against Toxoplasma gondii and Bartonella species in client-owned cats. J Feline Med Surg. 2009 Aug;11(8):663-7. Epub 2009 Jun 26. PMID:19560385

Beall MJ, Chandrashekar R, Eberts MD, Cyr KE, Diniz PP, Mainville C, Hegarty BC, Crawford JM, Breitschwerdt EB. Serological and molecular prevalence of Borrelia burgdorferi, Anaplasma phagocytophilum, and Ehrlichia species in dogs from Minnesota. Vector Borne Zoonotic Dis. 2008 Aug;8(4):455-64. PMID:18302532

Becker JL. Vector-borne illnesses and the safety of the blood supply. Curr Hematol Rep. 2003 Nov;2(6):511-7. PMID:14561396

Belgard S, Truyen U, Thibault JC, Sauter-Louis C, Hartmann K. Relevance of feline calicivirus, feline immunodeficiency virus, feline leukemia virus, feline herpesvirus and Bartonella henselae in cats with chronic gingivostomatitis. Berl Munch Tierarztl Wochenschr. 2010 Sep-Oct;123(9-10):369-76. PMID:21038808

Bellissimo-Rodrigues F, da Fonseca BA, Martinez R. Bacillary angiomatosis in a pregnant woman. Int J Gynaecol Obstet. 2010 Oct;111(1):85-6. Epub 2010 Jul 21. PMID:20650456

Bernabeu-Wittel J, Luque R, Corbi R, Mantrana-Bermejo M, Navarrete M, Vallejo A, Bernabeu-Wittel M. Bacillary angiomatosis with atypical clinical presentation in an immunocompetent patient. Indian J Dermatol Venereol Leprol. 2010 Nov-Dec;76(6):682-5. PMID:21079313

Bhengsri S, Baggett HC, Peruski LF Jr, Morway C, Bai Y, Fisk TL, Sitdhirasdr A, Maloney SA, Dowell SF, Kosoy M. Bartonella spp. infections, Thailand. Emerg Infect Dis. 2010 Apr;16(4):743-5. PMID:20350414

Bhengsri S, Baggett HC, Peruski LF, Morway C, Bai Y, Fisk TL, Sitdhirasdr A, Maloney SA, Dowell SF, Kosoy M. Bartonella seroprevalence in rural Thailand. Southeast Asian J Trop Med Public Health. 2011 May;42(3):687-92. PMID:21706948

Bhide M, Yilmaz Z, Golcu E, Torun S, Mikula I. Seroprevalence of anti-Borrelia burgdorferi antibodies in dogs and horses in Turkey. Ann Agric Environ Med. 2008 Jun;15(1):85-90. PMID:18581984

Bianda JC, Dedes W. [Positive polymerase chain reaction for Bartonella henselae in conjunctival granuloma].[Article in German]. Klin Monbl Augenheilkd. 2009 Apr;226(4):347. Epub 2009 Apr 21. PMID:19384797

Binnicker MJ, Jespersen DJ, Harring JA, Rollins LO, Bryant SC, Beito EM. Evaluation of two commercial systems for automated processing, reading, and interpretation of Lyme borreliosis Western blots. J Clin Microbiol. 2008 Jul;46(7):2216-21. Epub 2008 May 7. PMID:18463211

Bitam I, Dittmar K, Parola P, Whiting MF, Raoult D. Fleas and flea-borne diseases. Int J Infect Dis. 2010 Aug;14(8):e667-76. Epub 2010 Mar 1. PMID:20189862

Blanco JR, Jado I, Marín M, Sanfeliu I, Portillo A, Anda P, Pons I, Oteo JA. [Microbiological diagnosis of emerging bacterial pathogens: Anaplasma, Bartonella, Rickettsia, and Tropheryma whipplei].[Article in Spanish]. Enferm Infecc Microbiol Clin. 2008 Nov;26(9):573-80. PMID:19100178

Bodaghi B. [New etiological concepts in uveitis].[Article in French]. J Fr Ophtalmol. 2005 May;28(5):547-55. PMID:15976725

Bodaghi B. [Ocular manifestations of Lyme disease].[Article in French]. Med Mal Infect. 2007 Jul-Aug;37(7-8):518-22. Epub 2007 Mar 21. PMID:17376626

Boggs SR, Fisher RG. Bone pain and fever in an adolescent and his sibling. Cat scratch disease (CSD). Pediatr Infect Dis J. 2011 Jan;30(1):89, 93-4. PMID:21513084

Bolton JG, Galeckas KJ, Satter EK. Inoculation bartonellosis in an adult: a case report. Cutis. 2010 Jan;85(1):37-42. PMID:20184210

Boltri JM, Hash RB, Vogel RL. Patterns of Lyme disease diagnosis and treatment by family physicians in a southeastern state. J Community Health. 2002 Dec;27(6):395-402. PMID:12458782

Branda JA, Aguero-Rosenfeld ME, Ferraro MJ, Johnson BJ, Wormser GP, Steere AC. 2-tiered antibody testing for early and late Lyme disease using only an immunoglobulin G blot with the addition of a VlsE band as the second-tier test. Clin Infect Dis. 2010 Jan 1;50(1):20-6. PMID:19947857

Branda JA, Linskey K, Kim YA, Steere AC, Ferraro MJ. Two-tiered antibody testing for Lyme disease with use of 2 enzyme immunoassays, a whole-cell sonicate enzyme immunoassay followed by a VlsE C6 peptide enzyme immunoassay. Clin Infect Dis. 2011 Sep;53(6):541-7. PMID:21865190

Breitschwerdt EB, Maggi RG. A confusing case of canine vector-borne disease: clinical signs and progression in a dog co-infected with Ehrlichia canis and Bartonella vinsonii ssp. berkhoffii. Parasit Vectors. 2009 Mar 26;2 Suppl 1:S3. PMID:19426442

Breitschwerdt EB, Maggi RG. Comparative medical features of canine and human bartonellosis. Clin Microbiol Infect. 2009 Dec;15 Suppl 2:106-7. Epub 2009 Apr 30. PMID:19438635

Breitschwerdt EB, Maggi RG, Varanat M, Linder KE, Weinberg G. Isolation of Bartonella vinsonii subsp. berkhoffii genotype II from a boy with epithelioid hemangioendothelioma and a dog with hemangiopericytoma. J Clin Microbiol. 2009 Jun;47(6):1957-60. Epub 2009 Apr 15. PMID:19369441

Brewer NT, Weinstein ND, Cuite CL, Herrington JE. Risk perceptions and their relation to risk behavior. Ann Behav Med. 2004 Apr;27(2):125-30. PMID:15026296

Brinar VV, Habek M. Rare infections mimicking MS. Clin Neurol Neurosurg. 2010 Sep;112(7):625-8. Epub 2010 May 2. PMID:20439131

Brook I. The bacteriology of salivary gland infections. Oral Maxillofac Surg Clin North Am. 2009 Aug;21(3):269-74. PMID:19608044

Brown DB, Huang YC, Kannenberg EL, Sherrier DJ, Carlson RW. An acpXL mutant of Rhizobium leguminosarum bv. phaseoli lacks 27-hydroxyoctacosanoic acid in its lipid A and is developmentally delayed during symbiotic infection of the determinate nodulating host plant Phaseolus vulgaris. J Bacteriol. 2011 Sep;193(18):4766-78. Epub 2011 Jul 15. PMID:21764936

Brown EL, Kim JH, Reisenbichler ES, Höök M. Multicomponent Lyme vaccine: three is not a crowd. Vaccine. 2005 May 25;23(28):3687-96. PMID:15882529

Buchmann AU, Kempf VA, Kershaw O, Gruber AD. Peliosis hepatis in cats is not associated with Bartonella henselae infections. Vet Pathol. 2010 Jan;47(1):163-6. PMID:20080497

Bunikis J, Barbour AG. Laboratory testing for suspected Lyme disease. Med Clin North Am. 2002 Mar;86(2):311-40. PMID:11982304

Burbelo PD, Bren KE, Ching KH, Coleman A, Yang X, Kariu T, Iadarola MJ, Pal U. Antibody profiling of Borrelia burgdorferi infection in horses. Clin Vaccine Immunol. 2011 Sep;18(9):1562-7. Epub 2011 Jul 20. PMID:21775514

Capitta P, Zobba R, Masala G, Cocco R, Tola S, Parpaglia ML. Isolation and characterization of Bartonella strains in cats in Italy. Transbound Emerg Dis. 2010 Jun;57(3):201-4. Epub 2010 Mar 14. PMID:20345572

Caponetti GC, Pantanowitz L, Marconi S, Havens JM, Lamps LW, Otis CN. Evaluation of immunohistochemistry in identifying Bartonella henselae in cat-scratch disease. Am J Clin Pathol. 2009 Feb;131(2):250-6. PMID:19141385

Carvounis PE, Mehta AP, Geist CE. Orbital myositis associated with Borrelia burgdorferi (Lyme disease) infection. Ophthalmology. 2004 May;111(5):1023-8. PMID:15121383

Casalta JP, Gouriet F, Richet H, Thuny F, Habib G, Raoult D. Prevalence of Coxiella burnetii and Bartonella species as cases of infective endocarditis in Marseilles (1994-2007). Clin Microbiol Infect. 2009 Dec;15 Suppl 2:152-3. Epub 2009 Sep 28. PMID:19793124

Cermakova Z, Ryskova O, Honegr K, Cermakova E, Hanovcova I. Diagnosis of Lyme borreliosis using enzyme immunoanalysis. Med Sci Monit. 2005 Apr;11(4):BR121-5. Epub 2005 Mar 24. PMID:15795690

Cetin E, Sotoudeh M, Auer H, Stanek G. Paradigm Burgenland: risk of Borrelia burgdorferi sensu lato infection indicated by variable seroprevalence rates in hunters. Wien Klin Wochenschr. 2006 Nov;118(21-22):677-81. PMID:17160606

Chang CC, Chen YJ, Tseng CS, Lai WL, Hsu KY, Chang CL, Lu CC, Hsu YM. A comparative study of the interaction of Bartonella henselae strains with human endothelial cells. Vet Microbiol. 2011 Apr 21;149(1-2):147-56. Epub 2010 Oct 7. PMID:21035278

Cherry NA, Maggi RG, Cannedy AL, Breitschwerdt EB. PCR detection of Bartonella bovis and Bartonella henselae in the blood of beef cattle. Vet Microbiol. 2009 Mar 30;135(3-4):308-12. Epub 2008 Sep 21. PMID:19019574

Cheung VW, Moxham JP. Cat scratch disease presenting as acute mastoiditis. Laryngoscope. 2010;120 Suppl 4:S222. PMID:21225820

Chiaraviglio L, Duong S, Brown DA, Birtles RJ, Kirby JE. An immunocompromised murine model of chronic Bartonella infection. Am J Pathol. 2010 Jun;176(6):2753-63. Epub 2010 Apr 15. PMID:20395436

Chmielewski T, Fiett J, Gniadkowski M, Tylewska-Wierzbanowska S. Improvement in the laboratory recognition of lyme borreliosis with the combination of culture and PCR methods. Mol Diagn. 2003;7(3-4):155-62. PMID:15068385

Choi P, Qin X, Chen EY, Inglis AF Jr, Ou HC, Perkins JA, Sie KC, Patterson K, Berry S, Manning SC. Polymerase chain reaction for pathogen identification in persistent pediatric cervical lymphadenitis. Arch Otolaryngol Head Neck Surg. 2009 Mar;135(3):243-8. PMID:19289701

Chomel BB, Kasten RW, Williams C, Wey AC, Henn JB, Maggi R, Carrasco S, Mazet J, Boulouis HJ, Maillard R, Breitschwerdt EB. Bartonella endocarditis: a pathology shared by animal reservoirs and patients. Ann N Y Acad Sci. 2009 May;1166:120-6. PMID:19538271

Chu BC, Tam VT. A serologically proven case of cat-scratch disease presenting with neuroretinitis. Hong Kong Med J. 2009 Oct;15(5):391-3. PMID:19801700

Colton L, Zeidner N, Lynch T, Kosoy MY. Human isolates of Bartonella tamiae induce pathology in experimentally inoculated immunocompetent mice. BMC Infect Dis. 2010 Jul 30;10:229. PMID:20673363

Coulter P, Lema C, Flayhart D, Linhardt AS, Aucott JN, Auwaerter PG, Dumler JS. Two-year evaluation of Borrelia burgdorferi culture and supplemental tests for definitive diagnosis of Lyme disease. J Clin Microbiol. 2005 Oct;43(10):5080-4. PMID:16207966

Costa V, Sommese L, Casamassimi A, Colicchio R, Angelini C, Marchesano V, Milone L, Farzati B, Giovane A, Fiorito C, Rienzo M, Picardi M, Avallone B, Marco Corsi M, Sarubbi B, Calabrò R, Salvatore P, Ciccodicola A, Napoli C. Impairment of circulating endothelial progenitors in Down syndrome. BMC Med Genomics. 2010 Sep 13;3:40. PMID:20836844

Coyle PK. Lyme disease. Curr Neurol Neurosci Rep. 2002 Nov;2(6):479-87. PMID:12359100

Cunha BA, Cohen YZ, McDermott B. Fever of unknown origin (FUO) due to babesiosis in a immunocompetent host. Heart Lung. 2008 Nov-Dec;37(6):481-4. Epub 2008 Sep 30. PMID:18992633

Curi AL, Machado D, Heringer G, Campos WR, Lamas C, Rozental T, Gutierres A, Orefice F, Lemos E. Cat-scratch disease: ocular manifestations and visual outcome. Int Ophthalmol. 2010 Oct;30(5):553-8. Epub 2010 Jul 30. PMID:20668914

Da Silva K, Chussid S. Cat scratch disease: clinical considerations for the pediatric dentist. Pediatr Dent. 2009 Jan-Feb;31(1):58-62. PMID:19320261

Dabrowska-Bień J, Pietniczka-Załeska M, Rowicki T. [Cat scratch disease--a diagnostic problem, case report].[Article in Polish]. Otolaryngol Pol. 2009 Mar-Apr;63(2):154-7. PMID:19681487

Das BB, Wasser E, Bryant KA, Woods CR, Yang SG, Zahn M. Culture negative endocarditis caused by Bartonella henselae in a child with congenital heart disease. Pediatr Infect Dis J. 2009 Oct;28(10):922-5. PMID:19738506

Dautović-Krkić S, Cavaljuga S, Ferhatović M, Mostarac N, Gojak R, Hadzović M, Hadzić A. [Lyme borreliosis in Bosnia and Herzegovina--clinical, laboratory and epidemiological research].[Article in Bosnian]. Med Arh. 2008;62(2):107-10. PMID:18669233

de Caprariis D, Dantas-Torres F, Capelli G, Mencke N, Stanneck D, Breitschwerdt EB, Otranto D. Evolution of clinical, haematological and biochemical findings in young dogs naturally infected by vector-borne pathogens. Vet Microbiol. 2011 Apr 21;149(1-2):206-12. Epub 2010 Oct 16. PMID:21106311

de La Blanchardière A, Fournier PE, Haustraete E, du Cheyron D, Lepage O, Verdon R. [Infective endocarditis due to Bartonella henselae following a rupture of a cerebral aneurysm].[Article in French]. Med Mal Infect. 2009 Jun;39(6):394-6. Epub 2008 Dec 18. PMID:19097835

De Martino SJ. [Role of biological assays in the diagnosis of Lyme borreliosis presentations. What are the techniques and which are currently available?].[Article in French]. Med Mal Infect. 2007 Jul-Aug;37(7-8):496-506. Epub 2007 May 23. PMID:17512148

De Martino S, Jaulhac B. [Lyme borreliosis].[Article in French]. Rev Prat. 2005 Mar 15;55(5):471-7. PMID:15895947

de Paz HD, Larrea D, Zunzunegui S, Dehio C, de la Cruz F, Llosa M. Functional dissection of the conjugative coupling protein TrwB. J Bacteriol. 2010 Jun;192(11):2655-69. Epub 2010 Apr 2. PMID:20363945

Dekkers MJ, Dees A, Weidema WF, Bartelsman M, Veeken H, Hart W. [Clinical thinking and decision making in practice. A man with abdominal pain, weight loss and fever].[Article in Dutch]. Ned Tijdschr Geneeskd. 2009 Jan 31;153(5):174-80. PMID:19256242

Delforge ML. [On the usefulness of serology testing in infectious diseases: selected topics].[Article in French]. Rev Med Brux. 2011 Sep;32(4):285-8. PMID:22034758

DePietropaolo DL, Powers JH, Gill JM, Foy AJ. Diagnosis of lyme disease. Am Fam Physician. 2005 Jul 15;72(2):297-304. PMID:16050454

DePietropaolo DL, Powers JH, Gill JM, Foy AJ. Diagnosis of Lyme disease. Del Med J. 2006 Jan;78(1):11-8. PMID:16548394

Desenclos JC, Laporte A, Brouqui P. [Louse-borne infections in humans].[Article in French]. Med Mal Infect. 2011 Jun;41(6):295-300. Epub 2011 Mar 30. PMID:21450425

Dessau RB, Bangsborg JM, Ejlertsen T, Skarphedinsson S, Schønheyder HC. Utilization of serology for the diagnosis of suspected Lyme borreliosis in Denmark: survey of patients seen in general practice. BMC Infect Dis. 2010 Nov 1;10:317. PMID:21040576

Dessau RB, Bangsborg JM, Jensen TP, Hansen K, Lebech AM, Andersen CØ. [Laboratory diagnosis of infection caused by Borrelia burgdorferi].[Article in Danish]. Ugeskr Laeger. 2006 Aug 21;168(34):2805-7. PMID:16942701

Diniz PP, Wood M, Maggi RG, Sontakke S, Stepnik M, Breitschwerdt EB. Co-isolation of Bartonella henselae and Bartonella vinsonii subsp. Berkhoffii from blood, joint and subcutaneous seroma fluids from two naturally infected dogs. Vet Microbiol. 2009 Sep 18;138(3-4):368-72. Epub 2009 Feb 4. PMID:19560291

Donnelly EF. Preview: Lyme disease vaccines. Med Health R I. 1998 Nov;81(11):373-5. PMID:15580796

dos Santos AP, dos Santos RP, Biondo AW, Dora JM, Goldani LZ, de Oliveira ST, de Sá Guimarães AM, Timenetsky J, de Morais HA, González FH, Messick JB. Hemoplasma infection in HIV-positive patient, Brazil. Emerg Infect Dis. 2008 Dec;14(12):1922-4. PMID:19046522

Douglas TA, Tamburro D, Fredolini C, Espina BH, Lepene BS, Ilag L, Espina V, Petricoin EF 3rd, Liotta LA, Luchini A. The use of hydrogel microparticles to sequester and concentrate bacterial antigens in a urine test for Lyme disease. Biomaterials. 2011 Feb;32(4):1157-66. Epub 2010 Oct 28. PMID:21035184

Dowers KL, Hawley JR, Brewer MM, Morris AK, Radecki SV, Lappin MR. Association of Bartonella species, feline calicivirus, and feline herpesvirus 1 infection with gingivostomatitis in cats. J Feline Med Surg. 2010 Apr;12(4):314-21. Epub 2009 Dec 2. PMID:19959386

Drummond MR, Gilioli R, Velho PE. Bartonellosis diagnosis requires careful evaluation. Braz J Infect Dis. 2010 May-Jun;14(3):217. PMID:20835501

Dubey JP, Bhatia CR, Lappin MR, Ferreira LR, Thorn A, Kwok OC. Seroprevalence of Toxoplasma gondii and Bartonella spp. antibodies in cats from Pennsylvania. J Parasitol. 2009 Jun;95(3):578-80. PMID:19061304

Dubey JP, Lappin MR, Kwok OC, Mofya S, Chikweto A, Baffa A, Doherty D, Shakeri J, Macpherson CN, Sharma RN. Seroprevalence of Toxoplasma gondii and concurrent Bartonella spp., feline immunodeficiency virus, and feline leukemia virus infections in cats from Grenada, West Indies. J Parasitol. 2009 Oct;95(5):1129-33. Epub 2009 Apr 22. PMID:19385716

Durá-Travé T, Yoldi-Petri ME, Gallinas-Victoriano F, Lavilla-Oiz A, Bove-Guri M. Neuroretinitis Caused by Bartonella henselae (Cat-Scratch Disease) in a 13-Year-Old Girl. Int J Pediatr. 2010;2010:763105. Epub 2010 Jun 15. PMID:20628521

Dutta A, Schwarzwald HL, Edwards MS. Disseminated bartonellosis presenting as neuroretinitis in a young adult with human immunodeficiency virus infection. Pediatr Infect Dis J. 2010 Jul;29(7):675-7. PMID:20216243

Edlow JA. Erythema migrans. Med Clin North Am. 2002 Mar;86(2):239-60. PMID:11982300

Edouard S, Gonin K, Turc Y, Angelakis E, Socolovschi C, Raoult D. Eschar and neck lymphadenopathy caused by Francisella tularensis after a tick bite: a case report. J Med Case Reports. 2011 Mar 19;5:108. PMID:21418587

Edouard S, Raoult D. [Bartonella henselae, an ubiquitous agent of proteiform zoonotic disease].[Article in French]. Med Mal Infect. 2010 Jun;40(6):319-30. Epub 2009 Dec 29. PMID:20042306

Eisen L, Eisen RJ, Chang CC, Mun J, Lane RS. Acarologic risk of exposure to Borrelia burgdorferi spirochaetes: long-term evaluations in north-western California, with implications for Lyme borreliosis risk-assessment models. Med Vet Entomol. 2004 Mar;18(1):38-49. PMID:15009444

Eldøen G, Vik IS, Vik E, Midgard R. [Lyme neuroborreliosis in More and Romsdal].[Article in Norwegian]. Tidsskr Nor Laegeforen. 2001 Jun 30;121(17):2008-11. PMID:11875896

Elston DM, Do H. What's eating you? Cat flea (Ctenocephalides felis), Part 1: Clinical features and role as a disease vector. Cutis. 2010 May;85(5):231-6. PMID:20540412

Eppes SC, Childs JA. Comparative study of cefuroxime axetil versus amoxicillin in children with early Lyme disease. Pediatrics. 2002 Jun;109(6):1173-7. PMID:12042561

Ergin C, Akkaya Y, Kiriş Satılmış O, Yılmaz C. [Comparison of the indirect immunofluorescence assay performance of bartonella henselae antigens obtained by co-cultivation in vero and HeLa cells].[Article in Turkish]. Mikrobiyol Bul. 2011 Jul;45(3):461-7. PMID:21935779

Eschner AK. Effect of passive immunoglobulin transfer on results of diagnostic tests for antibodies against Borrelia burgdorferi in pups born to a seropositive dam. Vet Ther. 2008 Fall;9(3):184-91. PMID:19003779

Exner MM, Lewinski MA. Isolation and detection of Borrelia burgdorferi DNA from cerebral spinal fluid, synovial fluid, blood, urine, and ticks using the Roche MagNA Pure system and real-time PCR. Diagn Microbiol Infect Dis. 2003 Aug;46(4):235-40. PMID:12944012

Feder HM Jr, Abeles M, Bernstein M, Whitaker-Worth D, Grant-Kels JM. Diagnosis, treatment, and prognosis of erythema migrans and Lyme arthritis. Clin Dermatol. 2006 Nov-Dec;24(6):509-20. PMID:17113969

Feng S, Kasten RW, Werner JA, Hodzic E, Barthold SW, Chomel BB. Immunogenicity of Bartonella henselae P26 in cats. Vet Immunol Immunopathol. 2009 Dec 15;132(2-4):251-6. Epub 2009 May 18. PMID:19500857

Fenimore A, Varanat M, Maggi R, Schultheiss P, Breitschwerdt E, Lappin MR. Bartonella spp. DNA in cardiac tissues from dogs in Colorado and Wyoming. J Vet Intern Med. 2011 May-Jun;25(3):613-6. PMID:21539606

Fonollosa A, Galdos M, Artaraz J, Perez-Irezabal J, Martinez-Alday N. Occlusive vasculitis and optic disk neovascularization associated with neuroretinitis. Ocul Immunol Inflamm. 2011 Feb;19(1):62-4. Epub 2010 Oct 31. PMID:21034304

Font RL, Del Valle M, Mitchell BM, Boniuk M. Cat-scratch uveitis confirmed by histological, serological, and molecular diagnoses. Cornea. 2011 Apr;30(4):468-71. PMID:21099401

Fournier PE, Thuny F, Richet H, Lepidi H, Casalta JP, Arzouni JP, Maurin M, Célard M, Mainardi JL, Caus T, Collart F, Habib G, Raoult D. Comprehensive diagnostic strategy for blood culture-negative endocarditis: a prospective study of 819 new cases. Clin Infect Dis. 2010 Jul 15;51(2):131-40. PMID:20540619

Gan JJ, Mandell AM, Otis JA, Holmuhamedova M, Perloff MD. Suspecting optic neuritis, diagnosing Bartonella cat scratch disease. Arch Neurol. 2011 Jan;68(1):122-6. PMID:21220684

Gardner GC, Kadel NJ. Ordering and interpreting rheumatologic laboratory tests. J Am Acad Orthop Surg. 2003 Jan-Feb;11(1):60-7. PMID:12699372

Garro AC, Rutman M, Simonsen K, Jaeger JL, Chapin K, Lockhart G. Prospective validation of a clinical prediction model for Lyme meningitis in children. Pediatrics. 2009 May;123(5):e829-34. PMID:19403476

Gaumond G, Tyropolis A, Grodzicki S, Bushmich S. Comparison of direct fluorescent antibody staining and real-time polymerase chain reaction for the detection of Borrelia burgdorferi in Ixodes scapularis ticks. J Vet Diagn Invest. 2006 Nov;18(6):583-6. PMID:17121087

Geng Z, Hou XX, Wan KL, Hao Q. [Isolation and identification of Borrelia burgdorferi sensu lato from ticks in six provinces in China].[Article in Chinese]. Zhonghua Liu Xing Bing Xue Za Zhi. 2010 Dec;31(12):1346-1348. PMID:21223661

Girard YA, Fedorova N, Lane RS. Genetic diversity of Borrelia burgdorferi and detection of B. bissettii-like DNA in serum of north-coastal California residents. J Clin Microbiol. 2011 Mar;49(3):945-54. Epub 2010 Dec 22. PMID:21177909

Glatz M, Fingerle V, Wilske B, Ambros-Rudolph C, Kerl H, Müllegger RR. Immunoblot analysis of the seroreactivity to recombinant Borrelia burgdorferi sensu lato antigens, including VlsE, in the long-term course of treated patients with erythema migrans. Dermatology. 2008;216(2):93-103. Epub 2008 Jan 23. PMID:18216470

Glatz M, Golestani M, Kerl H, Müllegger RR. Clinical relevance of different IgG and IgM serum antibody responses to Borrelia burgdorferi after antibiotic therapy for erythema migrans: long-term follow-up study of 113 patients. Arch Dermatol. 2006 Jul;142(7):862-8. PMID:16847202

Godfroid E, Min Hu C, Humair PF, Bollen A, Gern L. PCR-reverse line blot typing method underscores the genomic heterogeneity of Borrelia valaisiana species and suggests its potential involvement in Lyme disease. J Clin Microbiol. 2003 Aug;41(8):3690-8. PMID:12904377

Goldstein RE, Cordner AP, Sandler JL, Bellohusen BA, Erb HN. Microalbuminuria and comparison of serologic testing for exposure to Borrelia burgdorferi in nonclinical Labrador and Golden Retrievers. J Vet Diagn Invest. 2007 May;19(3):294-7. PMID:17459861

Gooskens J, Templeton KE, Claas EC, van Dam AP. Evaluation of an internally controlled real-time PCR targeting the ospA gene for detection of Borrelia burgdorferi sensu lato DNA in cerebrospinal fluid. Clin Microbiol Infect. 2006 Sep;12(9):894-900. PMID:16882295

Gouriet F, Samson L, Delaage M, Mainardi JL, Meconi S, Drancourt M, Raoult D. Multiplexed whole bacterial antigen microarray, a new format for the automation of serodiagnosis: the culture-negative endocarditis paradigm. Clin Microbiol Infect. 2008 Dec;14(12):1112-8. PMID:19076842

Greco T Jr, Conti-Kelly A, Greco T. Antiphospholipid antibodies in patients with purported 'chronic Lyme disease'. Lupus. 2011;20(13):1372-7. Epub 2011 Jul 5. PMID:21729977

Grumbkow PV, Zipp A, Seidenberg V, Fehren-Schmitz L, Kempf VA, Groß U, Hummel S. Brief communication: Evidence of Bartonella quintana infections in skeletons of a historical mass grave in Kassel, Germany. Am J Phys Anthropol. 2011 Sep;146(1):134-137. PMID:21710687

Gulati A, Yalamanchili S, Golnik KC, Lee AG. Cat Scratch Neuroretinitis: The Role of Acute and Convalescent Titers for Diagnosis. J Neuroophthalmol. 2011 Sep 21. [Epub ahead of print]. PMID:21941214

Guptill L. Bartonellosis. Vet Microbiol. 2010 Jan 27;140(3-4):347-59. Epub 2009 Nov 18. PMID:20018462

Guptill L. Feline bartonellosis. Vet Clin North Am Small Anim Pract. 2010 Nov;40(6):1073-90. PMID:20933137

Haddad FA, Nadelman RB. Lyme disease and the heart. Front Biosci. 2003 Sep 1;8:s769-82. PMID:12957829

Halperin JJ. Nervous system Lyme disease. Vector Borne Zoonotic Dis. 2002 Winter;2(4):241-7. PMID:12804165

Hamer SA, Tsao JI, Walker ED, Mansfield LS, Foster ES, Hickling GJ. Use of tick surveys and serosurveys to evaluate pet dogs as a sentinel species for emerging Lyme disease. Am J Vet Res. 2009 Jan;70(1):49-56. PMID:19119948

Hassler D, Schnauffer M, Ehrfeld H, Müller E. Disappearance of specific immune response after successful therapy of chronic Lyme borreliosis. Int J Med Microbiol. 2004 Apr;293 Suppl 37:161-4. PMID:15147000

Hengge UR, Tannapfel A, Tyring SK, Erbel R, Arendt G, Ruzicka T. Lyme borreliosis. Lancet Infect Dis. 2003 Aug;3(8):489-500. PMID:12901891

Hernandez-Da-Mota S, Escalante-Razo F. Bartonellosis causing bilateral Leber neuroretinitis: a case report. Eur J Ophthalmol. 2009 Mar-Apr;19(2):307-9. PMID:19253255

Heyman P, Cochez C, Bigaignon G, Guillaume B, Zizi M, Vandenvelde C. Human Granulocytic Ehrlichiosis in Belgium: an underestimated cause of disease. J Infect. 2003 Aug;47(2):129-32. PMID:12860146

Hoey JG, Valois-Cruz F, Goldenberg H, Voskoboynik Y, Pfiffner J, Tilton RC, Mordechai E, Adelson ME. Development of an immunoglobulin M capture-based enzyme-linked immunosorbent assay for diagnosis of acute infections with Bartonella henselae. Clin Vaccine Immunol. 2009 Feb;16(2):282-4. Epub 2008 Dec 3. PMID:19052161

Holmes NE, Opat S, Kelman A, Korman TM. Refractory Bartonella quintana bacillary angiomatosis following chemotherapy for chronic lymphocytic leukaemia. J Med Microbiol. 2011 Jan;60(Pt 1):142-6. Epub 2010 Oct 14. PMID:20947664

Holmgren AR, Matteson EL. Lyme myositis. Arthritis Rheum. 2006 Aug;54(8):2697-700. PMID:16871548

Houck JA, Hojgaard A, Piesman J, Kuchta RD. Low-density microarrays for the detection of Borrelia burgdorferi s.s. (the Lyme disease spirochete) in nymphal Ixodes scapularis.   Ticks Tick Borne Dis. 2011 Mar;2(1):27-36. Epub 2010 Nov 27. PMID:21771534

Hristea A, Hristescu S, Ciufecu C, Vasile A. Seroprevalence of Borrelia burgdorferi in Romania. Eur J Epidemiol. 2001;17(9):891-6. PMID:12081110

Hsieh JW, Tung KC, Chen WC, Lin JW, Chien LJ, Hsu YM, Wang HC, Chomel BB, Chang CC. Epidemiology of Bartonella infection in rodents and shrews in Taiwan. Zoonoses Public Health. 2010 Sep;57(6):439-46. PMID:19538457

Huang J, Dai L, Lei S, Liao DY, Wang XQ, Luo TY, Chen Y, Hang ZB, Li GD, Dong DD, Xu G, Gu ZC, Hao JL, Hua P, He L, Duan FL. [Application of Warthin-Starry stain, immunohistochemistry and transmission electron microscopy in diagnosis of cat scratch disease].[Article in Chinese]. Zhonghua Bing Li Xue Za Zhi. 2010 Apr;39(4):225-9. PMID:20654119

Hufschmidt A, Müller-Felber W, Tzitiridou M, Fietzek UM, Haberl C, Heinen F. Canalicular magnetic stimulation lacks specificity to differentiate idiopathic facial palsy from borreliosis in children. Eur J Paediatr Neurol. 2008 Sep;12(5):366-70. Epub 2008 Feb 21. PMID:18206409

Hunfeld KP, Ernst M, Zachary P, Jaulhac B, Sonneborn HH, Brade V. Development and laboratory evaluation of a new recombinant ELISA for the serodiagnosis of Lyme disease. Wien Klin Wochenschr. 2002 Jul 31;114(13-14):580-5. PMID:12422605

Hunfeld KP, Kraiczy P, Kekoukh E, Schäfer V, Brade V. Standardised in vitro susceptibility testing of Borrelia burgdorferi against well-known and newly developed antimicrobial agents--possible implications for new therapeutic approaches to Lyme disease. Int J Med Microbiol. 2002 Jun;291 Suppl 33:125-37. PMID:12141737

Hunfeld KP, Ruzic-Sabljic E, Norris DE, Kraiczy P, Strle F. In vitro susceptibility testing of Borrelia burgdorferi sensu lato isolates cultured from patients with erythema migrans before and after antimicrobial chemotherapy. Antimicrob Agents Chemother. 2005 Apr;49(4):1294-301. PMID:15793100

Hunfeld KP, Stanek G, Straube E, Hagedorn HJ, Schörner C, Mühlschlegel F, Brade V. Quality of Lyme disease serology. Lessons from the German Proficiency Testing Program 1999-2001. A preliminary report. Wien Klin Wochenschr. 2002 Jul 31;114(13-14):591-600. PMID:12422607

Hunt PW. Molecular diagnosis of infections and resistance in veterinary and human parasites. Vet Parasitol. 2011 Aug 4;180(1-2):12-46. Epub 2011 May 27. PMID:21700392

Irshad FA, Gordon RA. Bartonella henselae neuroretinitis in a 15-year-old girl with chronic myelogenous leukemia. J AAPOS. 2009 Dec;13(6):602-4. PMID:20006827

Ivacic L, Reed KD, Mitchell PD, Ghebranious N. A LightCycler TaqMan assay for detection of Borrelia burgdorferi sensu lato in clinical samples. Diagn Microbiol Infect Dis. 2007 Feb;57(2):137-43. Epub 2006 Sep 20. PMID:16989975

Jacobs DJ, Scott ML, Slusher MM. Localised retinal vasculitis in cat scratch disease. BMJ Case Rep. 2009;2009. pii: bcr09.2008.0904. Epub 2009 Mar 17. PMID:21686569

Jäderlund KH, Egenvall A, Bergström K, Hedhammar A. Seroprevalence of Borrelia burgdorferi sensu lato and Anaplasma phagocytophilum in dogs with neurological signs. Vet Rec. 2007 Jun 16;160(24):825-31. PMID:17575245

James FM, Engiles JB, Beech J. Meningitis, cranial neuritis, and radiculoneuritis associated with Borrelia burgdorferi infection in a horse. J Am Vet Med Assoc. 2010 Nov 15;237(10):1180-5. PMID:21073390

Jeanclaude D, Godmer P, Leveiller D, Pouedras P, Fournier PE, Raoult D, Rolain JM. Bartonella alsatica endocarditis in a French patient in close contact with rabbits. Clin Microbiol Infect. 2009 Dec;15 Suppl 2:110-1. Epub 2009 Apr 30. PMID:19438633

Jennings F, Lambert E, Fredericson M. Rheumatic diseases presenting as sports-related injuries. Sports Med. 2008;38(11):917-30. PMID:18937522

Jobe DA, Lovrich SD, Asp KE, Mathiason MA, Albrecht SE, Schell RF, Callister SM. Significantly improved accuracy of diagnosis of early Lyme disease by peptide enzyme-linked immunosorbent assay based on the borreliacidal antibody epitope of Borrelia burgdorferi OspC. Clin Vaccine Immunol. 2008 Jun;15(6):981-5. Epub 2008 Apr 16. PMID:18329555

Johnson JL, Ginsberg HS, Zhioua E, Whitworth UG Jr, Markowski D, Hyland KE, Hu R. Passive tick surveillance, dog seropositivity, and incidence of human lyme disease. Vector Borne Zoonotic Dis. 2004 Summer;4(2):137-42. PMID:15228814

Johnson L, Aylward A, Stricker RB. Healthcare access and burden of care for patients with Lyme disease: a large United States survey. Health Policy. 2011 Sep;102(1):64-71. Epub 2011 Jun 14. PMID:21676482

Johnson L, Stricker RB. Treatment of Lyme disease: a medicolegal assessment. Expert Rev Anti Infect Ther. 2004 Aug;2(4):533-57. PMID:15482219

Juchnowicz D, Rudnik I, Czernikiewicz A, Zajkowska J, Pancewicz SA. [Mental disorders in the course of lyme borreliosis and tick borne encephalitis].[Article in Polish]. Przegl Epidemiol. 2002;56 Suppl 1:37-50. PMID:12194228

Kaçar N, Taşli L, Demirkan N, Ergin C, Ergin S. HIV-negative case of bacillary angiomatosis with chronic hepatitis B. J Dermatol. 2010 Aug;37(8):722-5. PMID:20649715

Kaiser PO, Riess T, O'Rourke F, Linke D, Kempf VA. Bartonella spp.: throwing light on uncommon human infections. Int J Med Microbiol. 2011 Jan;301(1):7-15. Epub 2010 Sep 15. PMID:20833105

Kalogeropoulos C, Koumpoulis I, Mentis A, Pappa C, Zafeiropoulos P, Aspiotis M. Bartonella and intraocular inflammation: a series of cases and review of literature. Clin Ophthalmol. 2011;5:817-29. Epub 2011 Jun 16. PMID:21750616

Kamoi K, Yoshida T, Takase H, Yokota M, Kawaguchi T, Mochizuki M. Seroprevalence of Bartonella henselae in patients with uveitis and healthy individuals in Tokyo. Jpn J Ophthalmol. 2009 Sep;53(5):490-3. Epub 2009 Oct 22. PMID:19847604

Kanjwal K, Karabin B, Kanjwal Y, Grubb BP. Postural orthostatic tachycardia syndrome following Lyme disease. Cardiol J. 2011;18(1):63-6. PMID:21305487

Kantas I, Katotomichelakis M, Vafiadis M, Kaloutsa ZV, Papadakis CE. Serous labyrinthitis as a manifestation of cat scratch disease: a case report. J Med Case Reports. 2009 Sep 15;3:7405. PMID:20519021

Karan' LS, Koliasnikova NM, Toporkova MG, Makhneva MA, Nadezhdina MV, Esaulkova AIu, Romanenko VV, Arumova EA, Platonov AE, Maleev VV. [Usage of real time polymerase chain reaction for diagnostics of different tick-borne infections].[Article in Russian]. Zh Mikrobiol Epidemiol Immunobiol. 2010 May-Jun;(3):72-7. PMID:20734723

Karolak J, Gotz-Wipckowska A. [Neuroretinitis in cat scratch disease].[Article in Polish]. Klin Oczna. 2010;112(4-6):131-4. PMID:20825068

Karosi T, Rácz T, Szekanecz E, Tóth A, Sziklai I. Recurrent laryngeal nerve paralysis due to subclinical Lyme borreliosis. J Laryngol Otol. 2010 Mar;124(3):336-8. Epub 2009 Sep 10. PMID:19740453

Karris MY, Litwin CM, Dong HS, Vinetz J. Bartonella henselae Infection of Prosthetic Aortic Valve Associated with Colitis. Vector Borne Zoonotic Dis. 2011 Nov;11(11):1503-5. Epub 2011 Jun 24. PMID:21702667

Kaufmann J, Buccola JM, Stead W, Rowley C, Wong M, Bates CK. Secondary symptomatic parvovirus B19 infection in a healthy adult. J Gen Intern Med. 2007 Jun;22(6):877-8. Epub 2007 Mar 24. PMID:17384979

Kaya AD, Parlak AH, Ozturk CE, Behcet M. Seroprevalence of Borrelia burgdorferi infection among forestry workers and farmers in Duzce, north-western Turkey. New Microbiol. 2008 Apr;31(2):203-9. PMID:18623985

Kelly JJ. Evaluation of peripheral neuropathy. Part III: vasculitic, infectious, inherited, and idiopathic neuropathies. Rev Neurol Dis. 2005 Spring;2(2):70-9. PMID:19813300

Khoudri I, Frémont G, Flageul B, Brière J, Dubertret L, Viguier M. [Bilateral inguinal lymphadenopathy and erythema nodosum: an uncommon presentation of cat scratch disease].[Article in French]. Rev Med Interne. 2011 Mar;32(3):e34-6. Epub 2010 Jun 19. PMID:20646798

Kim D, Kordick D, Divers T, Chang YF. In vitro susceptibilities of Leptospira spp. and Borrelia burgdorferi isolates to amoxicillin, tilmicosin, and enrofloxacin. J Vet Sci. 2006 Dec;7(4):355-9. PMID:17106227

Klotz SA, Ianas V, Elliott SP. Cat-scratch Disease. Am Fam Physician. 2011 Jan 15;83(2):152-5. PMID:21243990

Koga T, Taguchi J, Suzuki M, Higa Y, Kamimura T, Nishimura M, Arakawa M. Cat scratch disease presenting with a retroperitoneal abscess in a patient without animal contacts. J Infect Chemother. 2009 Dec;15(6):414-6. PMID:20012734

Koneva OA, Anan'eva LP, Shtannikov AV, Evsegneev SI, Baranova EV. [Comparative analysis of use of two strains of various genotypes of Borrelia burgdorferi sensu lato as antigens for antibody identification in Ixodes tick borreliosis by indirect immunofluorescence].[Article in Russian]. Klin Lab Diagn. 2003 May;(5):41-3. PMID:12822309

Koo M, Manalili S, Bankowski MJ, Sampath R, Hofstadler SA, Koo J. A "silent culture-negative" abdominal aortic mycotic aneurysm: Rapid detection of Bartonella species using PCR and high-throughput mass spectrometry. Hawaii Med J. 2010 Mar;69(3):68-9. PMID:20397506

Kornreich BG, Craven M, McDonough SP, Nydam DV, Scorza V, Assarasakorn S, Lappin M, Simpson KW. Fluorescence In-situ Hybridization for the Identification of Bacterial Species in Archival Heart Valve Sections of Canine Bacterial Endocarditis. J Comp Pathol. 2011 Oct 24. [Epub ahead of print]. PMID:22030263

Krause PJ, McKay K, Thompson CA, Sikand VK, Lentz R, Lepore T, Closter L, Christianson D, Telford SR, Persing D, Radolf JD, Spielman A; Deer-Associated Infection Study Group. Disease-specific diagnosis of coinfecting tickborne zoonoses: babesiosis, human granulocytic ehrlichiosis, and Lyme disease. Clin Infect Dis. 2002 May 1;34(9):1184-91. Epub 2002 Apr 4. PMID:11941544

Krupka I, Knauer J, Lorentzen L, O'Connor TP, Saucier J, Straubinger RK. Borrelia burgdorferi sensu lato species in Europe induce diverse immune responses against C6 peptides in infected mice. Clin Vaccine Immunol. 2009 Nov;16(11):1546-62. Epub 2009 Sep 2. PMID:19726618

Krupka I, Straubinger RK. Lyme borreliosis in dogs and cats: background, diagnosis, treatment and prevention of infections with Borrelia burgdorferi sensu stricto. Vet Clin North Am Small Anim Pract. 2010 Nov;40(6):1103-19. PMID:20933139

Kubicka-Trzaska A, Oleksy P, Karska-Basta I, Romanowska-Dixon B. [Acute posterior multifocal placoid pigment epitheliopathy (APMPPE)—a therapeutic dilemma].[Article in Polish]. Klin Oczna. 2010;112(4-6):127-30. PMID:20825067

Kubová Z, Szanyi J, Langrová J, Kremlácek J, Kuba M, Honegr K. Motion-onset and pattern-reversal visual evoked potentials in diagnostics of neuroborreliosis. J Clin Neurophysiol. 2006 Oct;23(5):416-20. PMID:17016151

Kvasnicka HM, Thiele J. [Differentiation of granulomatous lesions in the bone marrow].[Article in German]. Pathologe. 2002 Nov;23(6):465-71. Epub 2002 Oct 8. PMID:12436300

Lagal V, Postic D, Ruzic-Sabljic E, Baranton G. Genetic diversity among Borrelia strains determined by single-strand conformation polymorphism analysis of the ospC gene and its association with invasiveness. J Clin Microbiol. 2003 Nov;41(11):5059-65. PMID:14605139

Lakos A, Reiczigel J, Solymosi N. The positive predictive value of Borrelia burgdorferi serology in the light of symptoms of patients sent to an outpatient service for tick-borne diseases. Inflamm Res. 2010 Nov;59(11):959-64. Epub 2010 May 13. PMID:20461540

Lange D, Oeder C, Waltermann K, Mueller A, Oehme A, Rohrberg R, Marsch W, Fischer M. Bacillary angiomatosis. [Article in English, German]. J Dtsch Dermatol Ges. 2009 Sep;7(9):767-69. PMID:19298547

Ledue TB, Collins MF, Young J, Schriefer ME. Evaluation of the recombinant VlsE-based liaison chemiluminescence immunoassay for detection of Borrelia burgdorferi and diagnosis of Lyme disease. Clin Vaccine Immunol. 2008 Dec;15(12):1796-804. Epub 2008 Oct 22. PMID:18945880

Lemos ER, Mares-Guia MA, Almeida DN, Silva RG, Silva CM, Britto C, Lamas CC. [Traveler's fever associated with cervical adenomegaly and antibodies for Bartonella sp in a Brazilian patient returning from South Africa].[Article in Portuguese]. Rev Soc Bras Med Trop. 2010 Jul-Aug;43(4):472-3. PMID:20802956

Lencáková D, Fingerle V, Stefancíková A, Schulte-Spechtel U, Petko B, Schréter I, Wilske B. Evaluation of recombinant line immunoblot for detection of Lyme disease in Slovakia: comparison with two other immunoassays. Vector Borne Zoonotic Dis. 2008 Jun;8(3):381-90. PMID:18279004

Lesseva M, Christova I, Miloshev G. Cloning and expression of recombinant flagellar protein flaB from Borrelia burgdorferi. Folia Med (Plovdiv). 2007;49(3-4):58-62. PMID:18504936

Levy S, O'Connor TP, Hanscom JL, Shields P. Utility of an in-office C6 ELISA test kit for determination of infection status of dogs naturally exposed to Borrelia burgdorferi. Vet Ther. 2002 Fall;3(3):308-15. PMID:12447839

Lienhardt B, Irani S, Gaspert A, Weishaupt D, Boehler A. Disseminated infection with Bartonella henselae in a lung transplant recipient. J Heart Lung Transplant. 2009 Jul;28(7):736-9. PMID:19560704

Lin EY, Tsigrelis C, Baddour LM, Lepidi H, Rolain JM, Patel R, Raoult D. Candidatus Bartonella mayotimonensis and endocarditis. Emerg Infect Dis. 2010 Mar;16(3):500-3. PMID:20202430

Littman MP. Canine borreliosis. Vet Clin North Am Small Anim Pract. 2003 Jul;33(4):827-62. PMID:12910746

Ljøstad U, Skarpaas T, Mygland A. Clinical usefulness of intrathecal antibody testing in acute Lyme neuroborreliosis. Eur J Neurol. 2007 Aug;14(8):873-6. PMID:17662007

Loeckx I, Tuerlinckx D, Jespers S, Marchant AS, Bodart E. [A clinical case of spontaneous involution of systemic cat scratch disease].[Article in French]. Rev Med Liege. 2010 Feb;65(2):78-80. PMID:20344917

López-Alberola RF. Neuroborreliosis and the pediatric population: a review. Rev Neurol. 2006 Apr 10;42 Suppl 3:S91-6. PMID:16642458

Lünemann JD, Gelderblom H, Sospedra M, Quandt JA, Pinilla C, Marques A, Martin R. Cerebrospinal fluid-infiltrating CD4+ T cells recognize Borrelia burgdorferi lysine-enriched protein domains and central nervous system autoantigens in early lyme encephalitis. Infect Immun. 2007 Jan;75(1):243-51. Epub 2006 Oct 23. PMID:17060473

Lynch T, Iverson J, Kosoy M. Combining culture techniques for Bartonella: the best of both worlds. J Clin Microbiol. 2011 Apr;49(4):1363-8. Epub 2011 Feb 2. PMID:21289156

Macarez R, Bazin S, Lagauche D, Soullié B, Giordano P, May F, Guigon B. [Onset of Leber's hereditary optic neuropathy in association with borreliosis].[Article in French]. J Fr Ophtalmol. 2005 Dec;28(10):1095-100. PMID:16395203

Macdonald K. Infective endocarditis in dogs: diagnosis and therapy. Vet Clin North Am Small Anim Pract. 2010 Jul;40(4):665-84. PMID:20610018

Magalhães RF, Cintra ML, Barjas-Castro ML, Del Negro GM, Okay TS, Velho PE. Blood donor infected with Bartonella henselae. Transfus Med. 2010 Aug 1;20(4):280-2. Epub 2010 Mar 24. PMID:20345384

Magalhães RF, Urso Pitassi LH, Lania BG, Barjas-Castro ML, Neves Ferreira Velho PE. Bartonellosis as cause of death after red blood cell unit transfusion. Ultrastruct Pathol. 2009 Jul-Aug;33(4):151-4. PMID:19728230

Maggi RG, Mascarelli PE, Pultorak EL, Hegarty BC, Bradley JM, Mozayeni BR, Breitschwerdt EB. Bartonella spp. bacteremia in high-risk immunocompetent patients. Diagn Microbiol Infect Dis. 2011 Dec;71(4):430-7. Epub 2011 Oct 13. PMID:21996096

Maggi RG, Reichelt S, Toliver M, Engber B. Borrelia species in Ixodes affinis and Ixodes scapularis ticks collected from the coastal plain of North Carolina. Ticks Tick Borne Dis. 2010 Dec;1(4):168-71. Epub 2010 Oct 20. PMID:21771524

Magnarelli LA, Bushmich SL, IJdo JW, Fikrig E. Seroprevalence of antibodies against Borrelia burgdorferi and Anaplasma phagocytophilum in cats. Am J Vet Res. 2005 Nov;66(11):1895-9. PMID:16334946

Magnarelli LA, Lawrenz M, Norris SJ, Fikrig E. Comparative reactivity of human sera to recombinant VlsE and other Borrelia burgdorferi antigens in class-specific enzyme-linked immunosorbent assays for Lyme borreliosis. J Med Microbiol. 2002 Aug;51(8):649-55. PMID:12171295

Magnarelli LA, Stafford KC 3rd, Ijdo JW, Fikrig E. Antibodies to whole-cell or recombinant antigens of Borrelia burgdorferi, Anaplasma phagocytophilum, and Babesia microti in white-footed mice. J Wildl Dis. 2006 Oct;42(4):732-8. PMID:17255439

Magri JM, Johnson MT, Herring TA, Greenblatt JF. Lyme disease knowledge, beliefs, and practices of New Hampshire primary care physicians. J Am Board Fam Pract. 2002 Jul-Aug;15(4):277-84. PMID:12150460

Maguiña C, Guerra H, Ventosilla P. Bartonellosis. Clin Dermatol. 2009 May-Jun;27(3):271-80. PMID:19362689

Manalai P, Bhalavat RM, Dobbs MR, Lippmann S. Coma falsely attributed to Lyme disease. J Ky Med Assoc. 2008 Jul;106(7):317-9. PMID:18777697

Marangoni A, Moroni A, Accardo S, Cevenini R. Borrelia burgdorferi VlsE antigen for the serological diagnosis of Lyme borreliosis. Eur J Clin Microbiol Infect Dis. 2008 May;27(5):349-54. Epub 2008 Jan 16. PMID:18197445

Marienfeld CB, Dicapua DB, Sze GK, Goldstein JM. Expressive aphasia as a presentation of encephalitis with Bartonella henselae infection in an immunocompetent adult. Yale J Biol Med. 2010 Jun;83(2):67-71. PMID:20589186

Martín L, Vidal L, Campins A, Salvá F, Riera M, Carrillo A, Sáez de Ibarra JI. Bartonella as a cause of blood culture-negative endocarditis. Description of five cases. [Article in English, Spanish]. Rev Esp Cardiol. 2009 Jun;62(6):694-7. PMID:19480767

Martinez-Diaz GJ, Kim J, Bruckner AL. A toddler with facial nodules: a case of idiopathic facial aseptic granuloma. Dermatol Online J. 2010 Jan 15;16(1):9. PMID:20137751

Marques AR, Hornung RL, Dally L, Philipp MT. Detection of immune complexes is not independent of detection of antibodies in Lyme disease patients and does not confirm active infection with Borrelia burgdorferi. Clin Diagn Lab Immunol. 2005 Sep;12(9):1036-40. PMID:16148168

Maruyama S. [Cat-scratch disease].[Article in Japanese]. Nihon Rinsho. 2010 Jun;68 Suppl 6:244-7. PMID:20942049

Mastrandrea S, Simonetta Taras M, Capitta P, Tola S, Marras V, Strusi G, Masala G. Detection of Bartonella henselae--DNA in macronodular hepatic lesions of an immunocompetent woman. Clin Microbiol Infect. 2009 Dec;15 Suppl 2:116-7. Epub 2009 Sep 28. PMID:19793123

Mavin S, Evans R, Milner RM, Chatterton JM, Ho-Yen DO. Local Borrelia burgdorferi sensu stricto and Borrelia afzelii strains in a single mixed antigen improves western blot sensitivity. J Clin Pathol. 2009 Jun;62(6):552-4. Epub 2009 Feb 23. PMID:19240047

Mavin S, Hopkins PC, MacLennan A, Joss AW, Ho-Yen DO. Urban and rural risks of Lyme disease in the Scottish Highlands. Scott Med J. 2009 May;54(2):24-6. PMID:19530498

Mavin S, McDonagh S, Evans R, Milner RM, Chatterton JM, Ho-Yen DO. Interpretation criteria in Western blot diagnosis of Lyme borreliosis. Br J Biomed Sci. 2011;68(1):5-10. PMID:21473255

Mazepa AW, Kidd LB, Young KM, Trepanier LA. Clinical presentation of 26 anaplasma phagocytophilum-seropositive dogs residing in an endemic area. J Am Anim Hosp Assoc. 2010 Nov-Dec;46(6):405-12. PMID:21041333

McGinnis J, Bohnker BK, Malakooti M, Mann M, Sack DM. Lyme disease reporting for Navy and Marine Corps (1997-2000). Mil Med. 2003 Dec;168(12):1011-4. PMID:14719627

Mead P. Lyme disease testing. Lancet Infect Dis. 2006 Mar;6(3):122-3. PMID:16500589

Metz CH, Buer J, Bornfeld N, Lipski A. Bilateral Bartonella henselae neuroretinitis with stellate maculopathy in a 6-year-old boy. Infection. 2011 Aug 9. [Epub ahead of print]. PMID:21826435

Meyniel C, Wiertlewski S. [Optic neuritis].[Article in French]. Rev Med Interne. 2010 Jul;31(7):481-5. PMID:20434241

Michos A, Dessypris N, Pourtsidis A, Moschovi M, Polychronopoulou S, Athanasiadou-Piperopoulou F, Kalmanti M, Syriopoulou VP, Mavrouli MD, Petridou ET. Delayed exposure to infections and childhood lymphomas: a case-control study. Cancer Causes Control. 2009 Jul;20(5):795-802. Epub 2009 Jan 25. PMID:19169895

Mietze A, Morick D, Köhler H, Harrus S, Dehio C, Nolte I, Goethe R. Combined MLST and AFLP typing of Bartonella henselae isolated from cats reveals new sequence types and suggests clonal evolution. Vet Microbiol. 2011 Mar 24;148(2-4):238-45. Epub 2010 Sep 21. PMID:20863631

Misić-Majerus L, Bujić N, Madarić V, Avsic-Zupanc T. [An abortive type of tick-borne meningoencephalitis].[Article in Croatian]. Acta Med Croatica. 2003;57(2):111-6. PMID:12879690

Mitchell BM, Font RL. Molecular detection of Bartonella henselae for the diagnosis of cat scratch disease and bacillary angiomatosis of the conjunctiva. Cornea. 2011 Jul;30(7):807-14. PMID:21282991

Mofenson LM, Brady MT, Danner SP, Dominguez KL, Hazra R, Handelsman E, Havens P, Nesheim S, Read JS, Serchuck L, Van Dyke R; Centers for Disease Control and Prevention; National Institutes of Health; HIV Medicine Association of the Infectious Diseases Society of America; Pediatric Infectious Diseases Society; American Academy of Pediatrics. Guidelines for the Prevention and Treatment of Opportunistic Infections among HIV-exposed and HIV-infected children: recommendations from CDC, the National Institutes of Health, the HIV Medicine Association of the Infectious Diseases Society of America, the Pediatric Infectious Diseases Society, and the American Academy of Pediatrics. MMWR Recomm Rep. 2009 Sep 4;58(RR-11):1-166. PMID:19730409

Montcriol A, Benard F, Fenollar F, Ribeiri A, Bonnet M, Collart F, Guidon C. Fatal myocarditis-associated Bartonella quintana endocarditis: a case report. J Med Case Reports. 2009 Jul 17;3:7325. PMID:19830188

Morrison C, Seifter A, Aucott JN. Unusual presentation of Lyme disease: Horner syndrome with negative serology. J Am Board Fam Med. 2009 Mar-Apr;22(2):219-22. PMID:19264948

Morway C, Kosoy M, Eisen R, Montenieri J, Sheff K, Reynolds PJ, Powers N. A longitudinal study of Bartonella infection in populations of woodrats and their fleas. J Vector Ecol. 2008 Dec;33(2):353-64. PMID:19263856

Mrázek V, Bartůněk P, Varejka P, Janovská D, Bína R, Hulínská D. [Prevalence of antiborrelia antibodies in two populations: various interpretations of the same data].[Article in Czech]. Epidemiol Mikrobiol Imunol. 2002 Feb;51(1):19-22. PMID:11881295

Muenzel D, Duetsch S, Fauser C, Slotta-Huspenina J, Gaa J, Rummeny EJ, Holzapfel K. Diffusion-weighted magnetic resonance imaging in cervical lymphadenopathy: report of three cases of patients with Bartonella henselae infection mimicking malignant disease. Acta Radiol. 2009 Oct;50(8):914-6. PMID:19636985

Mullegger RR, Glatz M. Is serological follow-up useful for patients with cutaneous Lyme borreliosis? Curr Probl Dermatol. 2009;37:178-82. Epub 2009 Apr 8. PMID:19367102

Müller NF, Kaiser PO, Linke D, Schwarz H, Riess T, Schäfer A, Eble JA, Kempf VA. Trimeric autotransporter adhesin-dependent adherence of Bartonella henselae, Bartonella quintana, and Yersinia enterocolitica to matrix components and endothelial cells under static and dynamic flow conditions. Infect Immun. 2011 Jul;79(7):2544-53. Epub 2011 May 2. PMID:21536788

Murdoch W, Rosin FC. One presentation, two continents: left wrist myositis of distinct etiology in genetically similar individuals. J Am Board Fam Med. 2009 Jul-Aug;22(4):408-11. PMID:19587255

Murray MA, Zamecki KJ, Paskowski J, Lelli GJ Jr. Ocular bacillary angiomatosis in an immunocompromised man. Ophthal Plast Reconstr Surg. 2010 Sep-Oct;26(5):371-2. PMID:20683276

Murray TS, Shapiro ED. Lyme disease. Clin Lab Med. 2010 Mar;30(1):311-28. PMID:20513553

Myint KS, Gibbons RV, Iverson J, Shrestha SK, Pavlin JA, Mongkolsirichaikul D, Kosoy MY. Serological response to Bartonella species in febrile patients from Nepal. Trans R Soc Trop Med Hyg. 2011 Dec;105(12):740-2. Epub 2011 Sep 28. PMID:21955739

Naesens R, Vermeiren S, Van Schaeren J, Jeurissen A. False positive Lyme serology due to syphilis: report of 6 cases and review of the literature. Acta Clin Belg. 2011 Jan-Feb;66(1):58-9. PMID:21485767

Namekata MS, Clifford DL, Kasten RW, Henn JB, Garcelon DK, Coonan TJ, Chomel BB. Seroprevalence of Bartonella spp. in the endangered island fox (Urocyon littoralis). Vet Microbiol. 2009 Apr 14;136(1-2):184-7. Epub 2008 Oct 28. PMID:19058928

Nghiem PP, Schatzberg SJ. Conventional and molecular diagnostic testing for the acute neurologic patient. J Vet Emerg Crit Care (San Antonio). 2010 Feb;20(1):46-61. PMID:20230434

Nigrovic LE, Thompson AD, Fine AM, Kimia A. Clinical predictors of Lyme disease among children with a peripheral facial palsy at an emergency department in a Lyme disease-endemic area. Pediatrics. 2008 Nov;122(5):e1080-5. Epub 2008 Oct 17. PMID:18931349

Nijssen E, Cescau S, Vayssier-Taussat M, Wang J, Biville F. Identification of mechanisms involved in iron and haem uptake in Bartonella birtlesii: in silico and in vivo approaches. Clin Microbiol Infect. 2009 Dec;15 Suppl 2:118-9. Epub 2009 Apr 30. PMID:19438629

Nishio N, Kubota T, Nakao Y, Hidaka H. Cat scratch disease with encephalopathy in a 9-year-old girl. Pediatr Int. 2008 Dec;50(6):823-4. PMID:19067901

Nunes Rosado FG, Stratton CW, Mosse CA. Clinicopathologic correlation of epidemiologic and histopathologic features of pediatric bacterial lymphadenitis. Arch Pathol Lab Med. 2011 Nov;135(11):1490-3. PMID:22032579

Occorsio P, Orso G, di Martino L. [Ticks and the pediatrician]. [Article in Italian]. Parassitologia. 2004 Jun;46(1-2):115-8. PMID:15305698

O'Connor TP, Esty KJ, Hanscom JL, Shields P, Philipp MT. Dogs vaccinated with common Lyme disease vaccines do not respond to IR6, the conserved immunodominant region of the VlsE surface protein of Borrelia burgdorferi. Clin Diagn Lab Immunol. 2004 May;11(3):458-62. PMID:15138170

Oliver J, Means RG, Kogut S, Prusinski M, Howard JJ, Layne LJ, Chu FK, Reddy A, Lee L, White DJ. Prevalence of Borrelia burgdorferi in small mammals in New York state. J Med Entomol. 2006 Sep;43(5):924-35. PMID:17017230

Owen DC. Is Gulf War Syndrome actually chronic Lyme disease? Med Hypotheses. 2005;64(4):717-20. PMID:15694687

Pachner AR, Dail D, Li L, Gurey L, Feng S, Hodzic E, Barthold S. Humoral immune response associated with lyme borreliosis in nonhuman primates: analysis by immunoblotting and enzyme-linked immunosorbent assay with sonicates or recombinant proteins. Clin Diagn Lab Immunol. 2002 Nov;9(6):1348-55. PMID:12414773

Palecek T, Kuchynka P, Hulinska D, Schramlova J, Hrbackova H, Vitkova I, Simek S, Horak J, Louch WE, Linhart A. Presence of Borrelia burgdorferi in endomyocardial biopsies in patients with new-onset unexplained dilated cardiomyopathy. Med Microbiol Immunol. 2010 May;199(2):139-43. Epub 2010 Jan 6. PMID:20052487

Panic G, Stanulovic V, Popov T. Atrio-ventricular block as the first presentation of disseminated Lyme disease. Int J Cardiol. 2011 Aug 4;150(3):e104-6. Epub 2010 Mar 11. PMID:20226549

Papadopouli E, Michailidi E, Papadopoulou E, Paspalaki P, Vlahakis I, Kalmanti M. Cervical lymphadenopathy in childhood epidemiology and management. Pediatr Hematol Oncol. 2009 Sep;26(6):454-60. PMID:19657996

Pape M, Mandraveli K, Alexiou-Daniel S. Clinical aspects of Bartonella infection in northern Greece. Clin Microbiol Infect. 2009 Dec;15 Suppl 2:91-2. Epub 2009 May 18. PMID:19456804

Patil N, Bariola JR, Saccente M, Vyas KS, Bradsher RW Jr. A clinical review of Lyme disease in Arkansas. J Ark Med Soc. 2010 Feb;106(8):186-8. PMID:20218039

Pennisi MG, La Camera E, Giacobbe L, Orlandella BM, Lentini V, Zummo S, Fera MT. Molecular detection of Bartonella henselae and Bartonella clarridgeiae in clinical samples of pet cats from Southern Italy. Res Vet Sci. 2010 Jun;88(3):379-84. Epub 2009 Dec 5. PMID:19963231

Perez C, Hummel JB, Keene BW, Maggi RG, Diniz PP, Breitschwerdt EB. Successful treatment of Bartonella henselae endocarditis in a cat. J Feline Med Surg. 2010 Jun;12(6):483-6. Epub 2010 Feb 6. PMID:20138559

Pérez C, Maggi RG, Diniz PP, Breitschwerdt EB. Molecular and serological diagnosis of Bartonella infection in 61 dogs from the United States. J Vet Intern Med. 2011 Jul-Aug;25(4):805-10. Epub 2011 May 25. PMID:21615498

Pérez GJ, Munita SJ, Araos BR, López GJ, Stevenson AR, González AP, Pérez CD, Noriega RL. [Cat scratch disease associated neuroretinitis: clinical report and review of the literature].[Article in Spanish]. Rev Chilena Infectol. 2010 Oct;27(5):417-22. PMID:21186508

Peters GB 3rd, Bakri SJ, Krohel GB. Cause and prognosis of nontraumatic sixth nerve palsies in young adults. Ophthalmology. 2002 Oct;109(10):1925-8. PMID:12359616

Pfrommer S, Maier M, Mayer C, Erben A, Engelmann V, Lohmann CP. [Vasoproliferative retinal tumours].[Article in German]. Ophthalmologe. 2011 Mar;108(3):265-8. PMID:21153829

Phillips SE, Burrascano JJ, Horowitz R, Savely VR, Stricker RB. Lyme disease testing. Lancet Infect Dis. 2006 Mar;6(3):122. PMID:16500590

Piérard-Franchimont C, Quatresooz P, Piérard GE. Skin diseases associated with Bartonella infection: facts and controversies. Clin Dermatol. 2010 Sep-Oct;28(5):483-8. PMID:20797506

Pinna A, Puglia E, Dore S. Unusual retinal manifestations of cat scratch disease. Int Ophthalmol. 2011 Apr;31(2):125-8. Epub 2011 Jan 26. PMID:21267628

Pitassi LH, Cintra ML, Ferreira MR, Magalhães RF, Velho PE. Blood cell findings resembling Bartonella spp. Ultrastruct Pathol. 2010 Feb;34(1):2-6. PMID:20070147

Podsiadły E, Sapiejka E, Dabrowska-Bień J, Majkowski J, Tylewska-Wierzbanowska S. [Diagnostics of cat scratch disease and present methods of bartonellosis recognition--a case report]. [Article in Polish]. Pol Merkur Lekarski. 2009 Feb;26(152):131-5. PMID:19388519

Polat E, Turhan V, Aslan M, Müsellim B, Onem Y, Ertuğrul B. [First report of three culture confirmed human Lyme cases in Turkey].[Article in Turkish]. Mikrobiyol Bul. 2010 Jan;44(1):133-9. PMID:20455410

Pomelova VG, Kharitonenkov IG, Sadykbekova RK, Bychenkova TA, Anan'eva LP, Sokolova MV, Osin NS. [Designing and clinical testing of immune-enzyme and immunofluorescence test systems for serodiagnosis of ixodes borreliosis].[Article in Russian]. Vestn Ross Akad Med Nauk. 2004;(1):3-7. PMID:15022545

Pourel J. [Clinical diagnosis of Lyme borreliosis in case of joint and muscular presentations].[Article in French]. Med Mal Infect. 2007 Jul-Aug;37(7-8):523-31. Epub 2007 Mar 26. PMID:17368783

Probert W, Louie JK, Tucker JR, Longoria R, Hogue R, Moler S, Graves M, Palmer HJ, Cassady J, Fritz CL. Meningitis due to a "Bartonella washoensis"-like human pathogen. J Clin Microbiol. 2009 Jul;47(7):2332-5. Epub 2009 May 13. PMID:19439538

Przytuła L, Gińdzieńska-Sieśkiewicz E, Sierakowski S. [Diagnosis and treatment of Lyme arthritis].[Article in Polish]. Przegl Epidemiol. 2006;60 Suppl 1:125-30. PMID:16909789

Pulliainen AT, Dehio C. Bartonella henselae: subversion of vascular endothelial cell functions by translocated bacterial effector proteins. Int J Biochem Cell Biol. 2009 Mar;41(3):507-10. Epub 2008 Oct 25. PMID:18992392

Que YA, Moreillon P. Infective endocarditis. Nat Rev Cardiol. 2011 Jun;8(6):322-36. Epub 2011 Apr 12. PMID:21487430

Quebatte M, Dehio M, Tropel D, Basler A, Toller I, Raddatz G, Engel P, Huser S, Schein H, Lindroos HL, Andersson SG, Dehio C. The BatR/BatS two-component regulatory system controls the adaptive response of Bartonella henselae during human endothelial cell infection. J Bacteriol. 2010 Jul;192(13):3352-67. Epub 2010 Apr 23. PMID:20418395

Qureshi M, Bedlack RS, Cudkowicz ME. Lyme disease serology in amyotrophic lateral sclerosis. Muscle Nerve. 2009 Oct;40(4):626-8. PMID:19697382

Ramsey AH, Belongia EA, Chyou PH, Davis JP. Appropriateness of Lyme disease serologic testing. Ann Fam Med. 2004 Jul-Aug;2(4):341-4. PMID:15335133

Reis C, Cote M, Le Rhun D, Lecuelle B, Levin ML, Vayssier-Taussat M, Bonnet SI. Vector competence of the tick Ixodes ricinus for transmission of Bartonella birtlesii. PLoS Negl Trop Dis. 2011;5(5):e1186. Epub 2011 May 31. PMID:21655306

Reis C, Cote M, Paul RE, Bonnet S. Questing ticks in suburban forest are infected by at least six tick-borne pathogens. Vector Borne Zoonotic Dis. 2011 Jul;11(7):907-16. Epub 2010 Dec 15. PMID:21158500

Renou F, Raffray L, Gerber A, Moiton MP, Ferrandiz D, Yvin JL. [Hepatic localization of cat scratch disease in an immunocompetent patient].[Article in French]. Med Mal Infect. 2010 Mar;40(3):172-4. Epub 2009 Jul 17. PMID:19616394

Ricart JJ. [Infective endocarditis due to Bartonella quintana]. [Article in Spanish]. Medicina (B Aires). 2008;68(6):478. PMID:19147434

Roberts DM, Caimano M, McDowell J, Theisen M, Holm A, Orff E, Nelson D, Wikel S, Radolf J, Marconi RT. Environmental regulation and differential production of members of the Bdr protein family of Borrelia burgdorferi. Infect Immun. 2002 Dec;70(12):7033-41. PMID:12438383

Rodríguez C M, Giachetto L G, Cuneo E A, Gutiérrez B Mdel C, Shimchack R M, Pírez G MC. [Cat-scratch disease with bone compromise: atypical manifestation].[Article in Spanish]. Rev Chilena Infectol. 2009 Aug;26(4):363-9. Epub 2009 Sep 23. PMID:19802407

Rolain JM, Boureau-Voultoury A, Raoult D. Serological evidence of Bartonella vinsonii lymphadenopathies in a child bitten by a dog. Clin Microbiol Infect. 2009 Dec;15 Suppl 2:122-3. Epub 2009 Apr 3. PMID:19374641

Rooks YL, Corwell B. Common urgent musculoskeletal injuries in primary care. Prim Care. 2006 Sep;33(3):751-77, viii. PMID:17088159

Rostoff P, Konduracka E, El Massri N, Gackowski A, Kruszec P, Zmudka K, Piwowarska W. [Lyme carditis presenting as acute coronary syndrome: a case report].[Article in Polish]. Kardiol Pol. 2008 Apr;66(4):420-5. PMID:18473271

Roubaud-Baudron C, Fortineau N, Goujard C, Le Bras P, Lambotte O. [Cat scratch disease with bone involvement: a case report and literature review].[Article in French]. Rev Med Interne. 2009 Jul;30(7):602-8. Epub 2009 Mar 19. PMID:19303175

Roux F, Boyer E, Jaulhac B, Dernis E, Closs-Prophette F, Puéchal X. Lyme meningoradiculitis: prospective evaluation of biological diagnosis methods. Eur J Clin Microbiol Infect Dis. 2007 Oct;26(10):685-93. PMID:17629757

Ruckenstein MJ, Prasthoffer A, Bigelow DC, Von Feldt JM, Kolasinski SL. Immunologic and serologic testing in patients with Ménière's disease. Otol Neurotol. 2002 Jul;23(4):517-20; discussion 520-1. PMID:12170155

Rudnik I, Konarzewska B, Zajkowska J, Juchnowicz D, Markowski T, Pancewicz SA. [The organic disorders in the course of Lyme disease].[Article in Polish]. Pol Merkur Lekarski. 2004 Apr;16(94):328-31. PMID:15517926

Ruzić-Sabljić E, Maraspin V, Lotric-Furlan S, Jurca T, Logar M, Pikelj-Pecnik A, Strle F. Characterization of Borrelia burgdorferi sensu lato strains isolated from human material in Slovenia. Wien Klin Wochenschr. 2002 Jul 31;114(13-14):544-50. PMID:12422599

Saisongkorh W, Kowalczewska M, Azza S, Decloquement P, Rolain JM, Raoult D. Identification of candidate proteins for the diagnosis of Bartonella henselae infections using an immunoproteomic approach. FEMS Microbiol Lett. 2010 Sep 1;310(2):158-67. Epub 2010 Jul 9. PMID:20695898

Salehi N, Custodio H, Rathore MH. Renal microabscesses due to Bartonella infection. Pediatr Infect Dis J. 2010 May;29(5):472-3. PMID:20072078

Sanfeliu I, Antón E, Pineda V, Pons I, Perez J, Font B, Segura F. Description of Bartonella spp. infections in a general hospital of Catalonia, Spain. Clin Microbiol Infect. 2009 Dec;15 Suppl 2:130-1. Epub 2009 May 18. PMID:19456816

Sanguinetti-Morelli D, Angelakis E, Richet H, Davoust B, Rolain JM, Raoult D. Seasonality of cat-scratch disease, France, 1999-2009. Emerg Infect Dis. 2011 Apr;17(4):705-7. PMID:21470466

Sankatsing SU, Kolader ME, Bouma BJ, Bennink RJ, Verberne HJ, Ansink TM, Visser CE, van der Meer JT. 18F-fluoro-2-deoxyglucose positron emission tomography-negative endocarditis lenta caused by Bartonella henselae. J Heart Valve Dis. 2011 Jan;20(1):100-2. PMID:21404906

Sasseigne G, Herbert A, Larvol L, Damade R, Cartry O. [Fever and abdominal pain in a 56-year-old woman].[Article in French]. Rev Med Interne. 2009 Dec;30(12):1049-53. Epub 2009 Oct 7. PMID:19815317

Sauer A, Hansmann Y, Jaulhac B, Bourcier T, Speeg-Schatz C. [Ocular Lyme disease occurring during childhood: Five case reports.][Article in French]. J Fr Ophtalmol. 2011 Jun 20. [Epub ahead of print]. PMID:21696850

Scheidegger F, Quebatte M, Mistl C, Dehio C. The Bartonella henselae VirB/Bep system interferes with vascular endothelial growth factor (VEGF) signalling in human vascular endothelial cells. Cell Microbiol. 2011 Mar;13(3):419-31. Epub 2010 Dec 3. PMID:21044238

Schoen RT. A case revealing the natural history of untreated Lyme disease. Nat Rev Rheumatol. 2011 Mar;7(3):179-84. Epub 2010 Dec 21. PMID:21173795

Scott C, Azwa A, Cohen C, McIntyre M, Desmond N. Cat scratch disease: a diagnostic conundrum. Int J STD AIDS. 2009 Aug;20(8):585-6. PMID:19625597

Shah SS, Zaoutis TE, Turnquist J, Hodinka RL, Coffin SE. Early differentiation of Lyme from enteroviral meningitis. Pediatr Infect Dis J. 2005 Jun;24(6):542-5. PMID:15933566

Sherr VT. Panic attacks may reveal previously unsuspected chronic disseminated lyme disease. J Psychiatr Pract. 2000 Nov;6(6):352-6. PMID:15990495

Smajlovic F, Ibralic M. Color Doppler pseudolymphomatous manifestations of the cat scratch disease. Med Arh. 2009;63(5):297-9. PMID:20380135

Smismans A, Goossens VJ, Nulens E, Bruggeman CA. Comparison of five different immunoassays for the detection of Borrelia burgdorferi IgM and IgG antibodies. Clin Microbiol Infect. 2006 Jul;12(7):648-55. PMID:16774561

Steere AC, McHugh G, Damle N, Sikand VK. Prospective study of serologic tests for lyme disease. Clin Infect Dis. 2008 Jul 15;47(2):188-95. PMID:18532885

Stek CJ, van Eijk JJ, Jacobs BC, Enting RH, Sprenger HG, van Alfen N, van Assen S. Neuralgic amyotrophy associated with Bartonella henselae infection. J Neurol Neurosurg Psychiatry. 2011 Jun;82(6):707-8. Epub 2010 Aug 14. PMID:20710009

Stiles J. Bartonellosis in cats: a role in uveitis? Vet Ophthalmol. 2011 Sep;14 Suppl 1:9-14. PMID:21923819

Stone EG, Lacombe EH, Rand PW. Antibody testing and Lyme disease risk. Emerg Infect Dis. 2005 May;11(5):722-4. PMID:15890128

Stricker RB. Counterpoint: long-term antibiotic therapy improves persistent symptoms associated with lyme disease. Clin Infect Dis. 2007 Jul 15;45(2):149-57. Epub 2007 Jun 5. PMID:17578772

Stricker RB, Delong AK, Green CL, Savely VR, Chamallas SN, Johnson L. Benefit of intravenous antibiotic therapy in patients referred for treatment of neurologic Lyme disease. Int J Gen Med. 2011;4:639-46. Epub 2011 Sep 6. PMID:21941449

Stricker RB, Green CL, Savely VR, Chamallas SN, Johnson L. Safety of intravenous antibiotic therapy in patients referred for treatment of neurologic Lyme disease. Minerva Med. 2010 Feb;101(1):1-7. PMID:20228716

Stricker RB, Johnson L. Lyme wars: let's tackle the testing. BMJ. 2007 Nov 17;335(7628):1008. PMID:18006976

Stricker RB, Johnson L. Chronic Lyme disease and the 'Axis of Evil'. Future Microbiol. 2008 Dec;3(6):621-4. PMID:19072179

Stricker RB, Johnson L. Lyme disease: the next decade. Infect Drug Resist. 2011;4:1-9. Epub 2011 Jan 7. PMID:21694904

Strle F, Videcnik J, Zorman P, Cimperman J, Lotric-Furlan S, Maraspin V. Clinical and epidemiological findings for patients with erythema migrans. Comparison of cohorts from the years 1993 and 2000. Wien Klin Wochenschr. 2002 Jul 31;114(13-14):493-7. PMID:12422589

Stübs G, Fingerle V, Wilske B, Göbel UB, Zähringer U, Schumann RR, Schröder NW. Acylated cholesteryl galactosides are specific antigens of Borrelia causing lyme disease and frequently induce antibodies in late stages of disease. J Biol Chem. 2009 May 15;284(20):13326-34. Epub 2009 Mar 23. PMID:19307181

Sugiyama H, Sahara M, Imai Y, Ono M, Okamoto K, Kikuchi K, Nagai R. Infective endocarditis by Bartonella quintana masquerading as antineutrophil cytoplasmic antibody-associated small vessel vasculitis. Cardiology. 2009;114(3):208-11. Epub 2009 Jul 15. PMID:19602882

Suh B, Chun JK, Yong D, Lee YS, Jeong SH, Yang WI, Kim DS. A report of cat scratch disease in Korea confirmed by PCR amplification of the 16S-23S rRNA intergenic region of Bartonella henselae. Korean J Lab Med. 2010 Feb;30(1):34-7. PMID:20197720

Sun J, Fu G, Lin J, Song X, Lu L, Liu Q. Seroprevalence of Bartonella in Eastern China and analysis of risk factors. BMC Infect Dis. 2010 May 20;10:121. PMID:20482887

Sureda A, García D, Loma-Osorio P. [Embolic stroke as the first manifestation of Bartonella henselae endocarditis in an immunocompetent patient].[Article in Spanish]. Enferm Infecc Microbiol Clin. 2010 Jan;28(1):64-5. Epub 2009 May 1. PMID:19409676

Susta L, Uhl EW, Grosenbaugh DA, Krimer PM. Synovial Lesions in Experimental Canine Lyme Borreliosis. Vet Pathol. 2011 Nov 10. [Epub ahead of print]. PMID:22075774

Swanson SJ, Neitzel D, Reed KD, Belongia EA. Coinfections acquired from ixodes ticks. Clin Microbiol Rev. 2006 Oct;19(4):708-27. PMID:17041141

Sykes JE. Feline hemotropic mycoplasmas. J Vet Emerg Crit Care (San Antonio). 2010 Feb;20(1):62-9. PMID:20230435

Sykes JE, Lindsay LL, Maggi RG, Breitschwerdt EB. Human coinfection with Bartonella henselae and two hemotropic mycoplasma variants resembling Mycoplasma ovis. J Clin Microbiol. 2010 Oct;48(10):3782-5. Epub 2010 Aug 11. PMID:20702675

Sykes JE, Westropp JL, Kasten RW, Chomel BB. Association between Bartonella species infection and disease in pet cats as determined using serology and culture. J Feline Med Surg. 2010 Aug;12(8):631-6. Epub 2010 May 31. PMID:20570199

Szaleniec J, Oleś K, Składzień J, Strek P. [Cat scratch disease--an underestimated diagnosis].[Article in Polish]. Otolaryngol Pol. 2009 May-Jun;63(3):271-3. PMID:19886535

Talarek E, Duszczyk E, Zarnowska H. [Diagnostic difficulties in neuroborreliosis in children].[Article in Polish]/ Przegl Epidemiol. 2007;61(1):73-8. PMID:17702442

Tang YW. Duplex PCR assay simultaneously detecting and differentiating Bartonella quintana, B. henselae, and Coxiella burnetii in surgical heart valve specimens. J Clin Microbiol. 2009 Aug;47(8):2647-50. Epub 2009 Jun 24. PMID:19553582

Tarasów E, Ustymowicz A, Zajkowska J, Hermanowska-Szpakowicz T. [Neuroborreliosis: CT and MRI findings in 14 cases. Preliminary communication].[Article in Polish]. Neurol Neurochir Pol. 2001 Sep-Oct;35(5):803-13. PMID:11873593

Tasher D, Armarnik E, Mizrahi A, Liat BS, Constantini S, Grisaru-Soen G. Cat scratch disease with cervical vertebral osteomyelitis and spinal epidural abscess. Pediatr Infect Dis J. 2009 Sep;28(9):848-50. PMID:19654566

Tavora F, Burke A, Li L, Franks TJ, Virmani R. Postmortem confirmation of Lyme carditis with polymerase chain reaction. Cardiovasc Pathol. 2008 Mar-Apr;17(2):103-7. Epub 2007 May 11. PMID:18329555

Tay ST, Kamalanathan M, Rohani MY. Borrelia burgdorferi (strain B. afzelii) antibodies among Malaysian blood donors and patients. Southeast Asian J Trop Med Public Health. 2002 Dec;33(4):787-93. PMID:12757227

ten Hove CH, Gubler FM, Kiezebrink-Lindenhovius HH. Back pain in a child caused by cat scratch disease. Pediatr Infect Dis J. 2009 Mar;28(3):258. PMID:19209087

Teng JL, Yeung MY, Yue G, Au-Yeung RK, Yeung EY, Fung AM, Tse H, Yuen KY, Lau SK, Woo PC. In silico analysis of 16S rRNA gene sequencing based methods for identification of medically important aerobic Gram-negative bacteria. J Med Microbiol. 2011 Sep;60(Pt 9):1281-6. Epub 2011 Apr 15. PMID:21498652

Terekhova D, Sartakova ML, Wormser GP, Schwartz I, Cabello FC. Erythromycin resistance in Borrelia burgdorferi. Antimicrob Agents Chemother. 2002 Nov;46(11):3637-40. PMID:12384380

Terrada C, Bodaghi B, Conrath J, Raoult D, Drancourt M. Uveitis: an emerging clinical form of Bartonella infection. Clin Microbiol Infect. 2009 Dec;15 Suppl 2:132-3. Epub 2009 Jun 22. PMID:19548998

Thompson A, Mannix R, Bachur R. Acute pediatric monoarticular arthritis: distinguishing lyme arthritis from other etiologies. Pediatrics. 2009 Mar;123(3):959-65. PMID:19255026

Thompson GR 3rd, Lunetta JM, Johnson SM, Taylor S, Bays D, Cohen SH, Pappagianis D. Early treatment with fluconazole may abrogate the development of IgG antibodies in coccidioidomycosis. Clin Infect Dis. 2011 Sep;53(6):e20-4. PMID:21865185

Ticona E, Huaroto L, Garcia Y, Vargas L, Madariaga MG. The pathophysiology of the acute phase of human bartonellosis resembles AIDS. Med Hypotheses. 2010 Jan;74(1):45-9. Epub 2009 Aug 7. PMID:19665314

Tiemstra JD, Khatkhate N. Bell's palsy: diagnosis and management. Am Fam Physician. 2007 Oct 1;76(7):997-1002. PMID:17956069

Topolovec J, Puntarić D, Antolović-Pozgain A, Vuković D, Topolovec Z, Milas J, Drusko-Barisić V, Venus M. Serologically detected "new" tick-borne zoonoses in eastern Croatia. Croat Med J. 2003 Oct;44(5):626-9. PMID:14515426

Trafny DJ, Oyama MA, Wormser C, Reynolds CA, Singletary GE, Peddle GD. Cardiac troponin-I concentrations in dogs with bradyarrhythmias before and after artificial pacing. J Vet Cardiol. 2010 Dec;12(3):183-90. Epub 2010 Oct 28. PMID:21030328

Tsai YL, Chomel BB, Chang CC, Kass PH, Conrad PA, Chuang ST. Bartonella and Babesia infections in cattle and their ticks in Taiwan. Comp Immunol Microbiol Infect Dis. 2011 Mar;34(2):179-87. Epub 2010 Dec 30. PMID:21194750

Tsuneoka H, Yanagihara M, Otani S, Katayama Y, Fujinami H, Nagafuji H, Asari S, Nojima J, Ichihara K. A first Japanese case of Bartonella henselae-induced endocarditis diagnosed by prolonged culture of a specimen from the excised valve. Diagn Microbiol Infect Dis. 2010 Oct;68(2):174-6. PMID:20846591

Tuerlinckx D, Bodart E, Garrino MG, de Bilderling G. Clinical data and cerebrospinal fluid findings in Lyme meningitis versus aseptic meningitis. Eur J Pediatr. 2003 Mar;162(3):150-3. Epub 2003 Jan 21. PMID:12655417

Tuháčková J, Běláková J, Krupka M, Neperený J, Chumela J, Weigl E, Vrzal V. Testing of the Biocan B inj. ad us. vet. vaccine and development of the new recombinant vaccine against canine borreliosis. Biomed Pap Med Fac Univ Palacky Olomouc Czech Repub. 2005 Dec;149(2):297-302. PMID:16601776

Tylewska-Wierzbanowska S, Chmielewski T. Limitation of serological testing for Lyme borreliosis: evaluation of ELISA and western blot in comparison with PCR and culture methods. Wien Klin Wochenschr. 2002 Jul 31;114(13-14):601-5. PMID:12422608

Ullmann AJ, Gabitzsch ES, Schulze TL, Zeidner NS, Piesman J. Three multiplex assays for detection of Borrelia burgdorferi sensu lato and Borrelia miyamotoi sensu lato in field-collected Ixodes nymphs in North America. J Med Entomol. 2005 Nov;42(6):1057-62. PMID:16465748

Umekoji A, Fukai K, Yanagihara S, Ono E, Sowa J, Ishii M. Rapid detection of Bartonella henselae heat shock protein DNA by nested polymerase chain reaction from swollen lymph nodes of a patient with cat-scratch disease. J Dermatol. 2009 Oct;36(10):548-50. PMID:19785710

Valverde-Gubianas M, Ramos-López JF, López-Torres JA, Toribio-García M, Milla-Peñalver C, Gálvez Torres-Puchol J, Medialdea-Marcos S. [Neuroretinitis. Clinical cases].[Article in Spanish]. Arch Soc Esp Oftalmol. 2009 Aug;84(8):389-94. PMID:19728239

Varela AS, Luttrell MP, Howerth EW, Moore VA, Davidson WR, Stallknecht DE, Little SE. First culture isolation of Borrelia lonestari, putative agent of southern tick-associated rash illness. J Clin Microbiol. 2004 Mar;42(3):1163-9. PMID:15004069

Vayssier-Taussat M, Le Rhun D, Deng HK, Biville F, Cescau S, Danchin A, Marignac G, Lenaour E, Boulouis HJ, Mavris M, Arnaud L, Yang H, Wang J, Quebatte M, Engel P, Saenz H, Dehio C. The Trw type IV secretion system of Bartonella mediates host-specific adhesion to erythrocytes. PLoS Pathog. 2010 Jun 10;6(6):e1000946. PMID:20548954

Vázquez M, Sparrow SS, Shapiro ED. Long-term neuropsychologic and health outcomes of children with facial nerve palsy attributable to Lyme disease. Pediatrics. 2003 Aug;112(2):e93-7. PMID:12897313

Vermeulen MJ, Verbakel H, Notermans DW, Reimerink JH, Peeters MF. Evaluation of sensitivity, specificity and cross-reactivity in Bartonella henselae serology. J Med Microbiol. 2010 Jun;59(Pt 6):743-5. Epub 2010 Mar 11. PMID:20223899

Vianello M, Marchiori G, Giometto B. Multiple cranial nerve involvement in Bannwarth's syndrome. Neurol Sci. 2008 Apr;29(2):109-12. Epub 2008 May 16. PMID:18483708

Vitale G, Incandela S, Incandela C, Micalizzi A, Mansueto P. Isolation and characterization of Bartonella quintana from the parotid gland of an immunocompetent man. J Clin Microbiol. 2009 Mar;47(3):862-4. Epub 2009 Jan 7. PMID:19129406

Vorstman JA, Kuiper H. [Peripheral facial palsy in children: test for lyme borreliosis only in the presence of other clinical signs].[Article in Dutch]. Ned Tijdschr Geneeskd. 2004 Apr 3;148(14):655-8. PMID:15106315

Vostal K, Zakovska A. Two-year study of examination of blood from wild rodents for the presence of antiborrelian antibodies. Ann Agric Environ Med. 2003;10(2):203-6. PMID:14677912

Wagner B, Freer H, Rollins A, Erb HN. A fluorescent bead-based multiplex assay for the simultaneous detection of antibodies to B. burgdorferi outer surface proteins in canine serum. Vet Immunol Immunopathol. 2011 Apr 15;140(3-4):190-8. Epub 2010 Dec 10. PMID:21208663

Wagner B, Freer H, Rollins A, Erb HN, Lu Z, Gröhn Y. Development of a multiplex assay for the detection of antibodies to Borrelia burgdorferi in horses and its validation using Bayesian and conventional statistical methods. Vet Immunol Immunopathol. 2011 Dec 15;144(3-4):374-81. Epub 2011 Aug 17. PMID:21890217

Wang CW, Chang WC, Chao TK, Liu CC, Huang GS. Computed tomography and magnetic resonance imaging of cat-scratch disease: a report of two cases. Clin Imaging. 2009 Jul-Aug;33(4):318-21. PMID:19559357

Webster JD, Miller MA, DuSold D, Ramos-Vara J. Effects of prolonged formalin fixation on the immunohistochemical detection of infectious agents in formalin-fixed, paraffin-embedded tissues. Vet Pathol. 2010 May;47(3):529-35. Epub 2010 Mar 23. PMID:20332424

Weinspach S, Tenenbaum T, Schönberger S, Schaper J, Engers R, Rueggeberg J, Mackenzie CR, Wolf A, Mayatepek E, Schroten H. Cat scratch disease--heterogeneous in clinical presentation: five unusual cases of an infection caused by Bartonella henselae. Klin Padiatr. 2010 Mar;222(2):73-8. Epub 2009 Sep 29. PMID:19790029

Weinstein A. Editorial commentary: laboratory testing for Lyme disease: time for a change? Clin Infect Dis. 2008 Jul 15;47(2):196-7. PMID:18532894

Welc-Faleciak R. [Current state of the knowledge of Bartonella infections].[Article in Polish]. Przegl Epidemiol. 2009;63(1):11-7. PMID:19522219

Welc-Faleciak R, Rodo A, Siński E, Bajer A. Babesia canis and other tick-borne infections in dogs in Central Poland. Vet Parasitol. 2009 Dec 23;166(3-4):191-8. Epub 2009 Sep 26. PMID:19837515

Wendling D, Sevrin P, Bouchaud-Chabot A, Chabroux A, Toussirot E, Bardin T, Michel F. Parsonage-Turner syndrome revealing Lyme borreliosis. Joint Bone Spine. 2009 Mar;76(2):202-4. Epub 2009 Jan 14. PMID:19147387

Woodcock S. Lyme disease testing. Lancet Infect Dis. 2006 Mar;6(3):122. PMID:16500588

Wormser GP, Liveris D, Hanincová K, Brisson D, Ludin S, Stracuzzi VJ, Embers ME, Philipp MT, Levin A, Aguero-Rosenfeld M, Schwartz I. Effect of Borrelia burgdorferi genotype on the sensitivity of C6 and 2-tier testing in North American patients with culture-confirmed Lyme disease. Clin Infect Dis. 2008 Oct 1;47(7):910-4. PMID:18724824

Wormser GP, Nowakowski J, Nadelman RB, Visintainer P, Levin A, Aguero-Rosenfeld E. Impact of clinical variables on Borrelia burgdorferi-specific antibody seropositivity in acute-phase sera from patients in North America with culture-confirmed early Lyme disease. Clin Vaccine Immunol. 2008 Oct;15(10):1519-22. Epub 2008 Aug 20. PMID:18716009

Wormser GP, Ramanathan R, Nowakowski J, McKenna D, Holmgren D, Visintainer P, Dornbush R, Singh B, Nadelman RB. Duration of antibiotic therapy for early Lyme disease. A randomized, double-blind, placebo-controlled trial. Ann Intern Med. 2003 May 6;138(9):697-704. PMID:12729423

Wright SA, Tucker JR, Donohue AM, Castro MB, Kelley KL, Novak MG, Macedo PA. Avian hosts of Ixodes pacificus (Acari: Ixodidae) and the detection of Borrelia burgdorferi in larvae feeding on the Oregon junco. J Med Entomol. 2011 Jul;48(4):852-9. PMID:21845945

Yamada Y, Ohkusu K, Yanagihara M, Tsuneoka H, Ezaki T, Tsuboi J, Okabayashi H, Suwabe A. Prosthetic valve endocarditis caused by Bartonella quintana in a patient during immunosuppressive therapies for collagen vascular diseases. Diagn Microbiol Infect Dis. 2011 Jul;70(3):395-8. Epub 2011 May 10. PMID:21558050

Yilmaz C, Ergin C, Kaleli I. [Investigation of Bartonella henselae seroprevalence and related risk factors in blood donors admitted to Pamukkale University Blood Center].[Article in Turkish]. Mikrobiyol Bul. 2009 Jul;43(3):391-401. PMID:19795614

Yoon HJ, Lee WC, Choi YS, Cho S, Song YG, Choi JY, Kim CO, Kim EJ, Kim JM. Cervical lymphadenitis in a patient coinfected with Toxoplasma gondii and Bartonella henselae. Vector Borne Zoonotic Dis. 2010 May;10(4):415-9. PMID:19874186

Youssef D, Shams WE, El Abbassi A, Moorman JP, Al-Abbadi MA. Combining cytomorphology and serology for the diagnosis of cat scratch disease. Diagn Cytopathol. 2011 Mar;39(3):210-3. PMID:21319324

Zajkowska JM, Hermanowska-Szpakowicz T, Wysocka J, Pancewicz S, Lipska A, Kasprzycka E. [Estimation of platelet counts and their morphological parameters in patients infected by borrelia burgdorferi].[Article in Polish]. Wiad Lek. 2001;54(11-12):668-73. PMID:11928555

Zapater Latorre E, Castillo Ruiz A, Alba García JR, Armengot Carceller M, Sancho Rieger J, Basterra Alegría J. [Bilateral peripheral facial paralysis secondary to Lyme disease].[Article in Spanish]. An Otorrinolaringol Ibero Am. 2004;31(5):447-58. PMID:15566265

Zarraga M, Rosen L, Herschthal D. Bacillary angiomatosis in an immunocompetent child: a case report and review of the literature. Am J Dermatopathol. 2011 Jul;33(5):513-5. PMID:21285862

Zarzycka B, Pieczara A, Skowron-Kobos J, Krzemiński Z. [Prevalence IgG antibodies against Bartonella henselae in children with lymphadenopathy].[Article in Polish]. Przegl Epidemiol. 2008;62(4):759-65. PMID:19209738

Zeidner NS, Schneider BS, Dolan MC, Piesman J. An analysis of spirochete load, strain, and pathology in a model of tick-transmitted Lyme borreliosis. Vector Borne Zoonotic Dis. 2001 Spring;1(1):35-44. PMID:12653134

Zenone T. Systemic Bartonella henselae Infection in Immunocompetent Adult Presenting as Fever of Unknown Origin. Case Report Med. 2011;2011:183937. Epub 2011 May 5. PMID:21629850

Zekraoui Y, Megzari A, El Alloussi T, Berraho A. [Unilateral neuroretinitis revealing cat-scratch disease].[Article in French]. Rev Med Interne. 2011 Apr;32(4):e46-8. Epub 2010 Jun 19. PMID:20646795

Zhang L, Cui F, Wang L, Zhang L, Zhang J, Wang S, Yang S. Investigation of anaplasmosis in Yiyuan County, Shandong Province, China. Asian Pac J Trop Med. 2011 Jul;4(7):568-72. PMID:21803311

Zhong J, Skouloubris S, Dai Q, Myllykallio H, Barbour AG. Function and evolution of plasmid-borne genes for pyrimidine biosynthesis in Borrelia spp. J Bacteriol. 2006 Feb;188(3):909-18. PMID:16428394

Zobba R, Chessa G, Mastrandrea S, Pinna Parpaglia ML, Patta C, Masala G. Serological and molecular detection of Bartonella spp. in humans, cats and dogs from northern Sardinia, Italy. Clin Microbiol Infect. 2009 Dec;15 Suppl 2:134-5. Epub 2009 May 18. PMID:19456814

The Babesia Checklist

Improving Detection of A Common, Emerging Stealth Infection

James L. Schaller, M.D., M.A.R.

Introduction

Below are examples of signs, symptoms and indirect ways to help increase the diagnosis of Babesia. An examination of public genetic databases shows that well over thirty-five species exist, many of which have variants.

Please note that an unknown percentage of people infected with this single celled parasite have no symptoms, at least for many years.

This checklist is not meant to be used as a definitive tool to diagnose Babesia. It is my expert opinion that no definitive 100% or even 98% accurate tool exists.

My goal is merely to decrease illness in those people who are positive but do not show up as positive on a basic direct test (false negative).

Indeed, it is not uncommon for a patient with Babesia to present with a negative test result over ten times, regardless of the laboratory, and then to show up with a positive on DNA testing when exposed to two or three treatments against protozoa for three days, or to have new conversion from negative to positive antibody testing six weeks after a similar provocation trial.

I do not oppose or endorse such approaches, but feel it necessary to mention that the same outcome has occurred with "Malaria-prevention" treatment. Additionally, there have been instances in which the use of herbs, such as artesunate, for cancer prevention, has resulted in an unintended outcome: the conversion of a Babesia antibody titer from negative to positive.

Having authored four books on the topic of Babesia, I have created this scale based on years of full-time reading and a passion to advance detection. This checklist is meant to prevent false negatives: some patients who appear to be negative may not actually be negative. I have done this because my years of full-time reading and research have shown me that missing this parasite for 5, 10, 30 or 50 years is far more dangerous than careful treatment. Treatment side effects are low if the treatment is started at **20% of the suggested dose.**

I would appeal to you that one cannot be considered an expert in treating this potentially fatal infection by merely reading a few articles or guidelines. Nor is expertise acquired by diagnosing and treating the highly obvious, immensely ill, sickest 1% of patients as the "norm" in Babesia diagnosis. Expertise should require *at least* a review of 1500 articles over five years. The fact that parasite textbooks usually offer merely 1-2 pages about this infection shows that it is not mastered or understood even by those interested in parasites.

The cure of Babesia does not fit a set formula, but no one should be hopeless about reaching a full recovery. I have currently started a new, research-based, creative thinking textbook on **optimal Babesia treatments** for publication in 2012. It will discuss familiar treatments and offer ideas to maximize these options, but I will also add discussions on newer options for patients and clinicians who are not satisfied with the current options.

In summary, how can any certain medical or scientific Babesia position exist, when new species, sub-species or variants that infect humans are routinely emerging, and for which there is not even a direct test—regardless of sensitivity?

THE BABESIA CHECKLIST
James Schaller, M.D., M.A.R.
(Please Check Any Symptoms That Apply)

PSYCHIATRIC AND NEUROLOGICAL

☐ Family, friends or others report you look tired or foggy

☐ Slowed thinking

☐ Psychiatric label(s) given to a child or relative for all their troubles when clear medical problems exist as shown by abnormal laboratory results (I am not talking about basic organ failure labs, but the use of *wide testing which includes inflammation and anti-inflammation chemicals, hormones, nutrient levels, and other immune system chemicals*)

☐ Enlarged lymph nodes (but also in Lyme, Bartonella, other infections, high inflammation, tumors and other diseases)

☐ Brain troubles such as trouble keeping up with past routine life demands, lateness due to trouble with motivation and organization, and trouble with concentration [Any of these would be a positive]

☐ Memory troubles [this is not specific to one infection or one disease process.   For example, exposure to indoor mold's biological chemicals can decrease memory within an hour depending on the species mix.]

☐ Profound psychiatric illnesses [this is not limited to a single infection.]

HEART & CIRCULATORY SYSTEM

☐ A sudden loss of blood pressure

☐ Transfusions using blood that is not your own

☐ Anemia even if a non-infectious cause has been proposed

☐ Anemia without a clear explanation

☐ Severe chest wall pains

☐ A "heart attack" before the age of 55 (when you have three risk factors)

☐ A "heart attack" or infarct of the heart before the age of 60 years old, with only one risk factor. [Being male is **considered** a risk factor for many. Men **experience** heart damage sooner than women. Other risk factors include tobacco use or exposure, such as second hand smoke at home, diabetes, high blood pressure, high level of sticky cholesterol such as Lipoprotein (a) or high triglyceride levels, family history of heart attacks, limited physical activity, Obesity (might be defined as wearing pants over 39 inches if you are a man and over 34 inches if you a woman or a body fat or body mass index of 30 or higher), excess anger or routine poor handling of stress, and abuse of stimulant drugs such as cocaine or amphetamines. I would add a homocysteine laboratory level over 10, major depression, no vitamin K2 supplementation, a free dihydrotestosterone in the 10th percentile or lower, fragmented or poor sleep [which increases inflammation], a high C4a RIA, a MMPI in excess of 300 and a low VIP blood level.

MAJOR ORGANS

☐ A yellow hue on eyes, hands and skin (jaundice) with no other clear cause

☐ An enlarged liver (which sits under your right rib cage)

☐ An enlarged spleen (under your left rib cage).   **This is falsely believed to be a common human sign; actually it is very rare.**

☐ A ruptured spleen [rare but it gets fast medical attention and therefore is over-represented in medical articles]

☐ Dark urine [this is rarer than some articles intimate]

☐ An inability to urinate

☐ Shortness of breath [no clear asthma, pneumonia, COPD or other common cause]

☐ Pulmonary edema which is a high amount of fluid in the air sacs of the lungs, which leads to shortness of breath

☐ A stroke of any size or in any organ (the word stroke means tissue is unable to get oxygen). The stroke or infarct can be in the brain, retina, kidney, heart and many other tissues.

☐ An MRI, CT or other imaging study that shows dead tissue in any organ with no known cause

GENERAL MEDICAL

☐ Headaches with no clear cause

☐ Headaches which are hard to control and/or severe

☐ Headaches lasting over three years and which increase in pain despite treatments

☐ Weight gain in clear excess of diet and exercise

☐ Weight loss with reasonable eating and average exercise

☐ Excess fat in lower belly area that is in excess of lifestyle and activity

☐ Anorexia or a decrease in appetite

☐ Any decrease in appetite

☐ A poor appetite

☐ Fatigue in excess of that experienced by most people in the same age range

☐ Fatigue that produces need for sleep in excess of 8 ½ hours daily

☐ Fatigue with ongoing insomnia [consider the possibility of both Bartonella and Babesia in this case]

☐ Daytime sleep urgency despite nighttime sleep

☐ Night sweats

☐ Excessive perspiration during normal daily activity

☐ Hot flashes in a normal temperature room

☐ Intermittent fever

☐ Chills

☐ Any fever in excess of three days

☐ Spike of a fever over 100.5 after a possible tick bite

☐ Listlessness

☐ Swelling in limbs and other parts of body

☐ Waves of generalized itching [this sign of infection and inflammation is not limited just to Babesia.]

☐ Lumps or other types of tissue collection with no clear cause [Other tick and flea-borne infections can also cause these growths.]

☐ Wasting muscles

☐ The general wasting away of body tissue that is visible

☐ Profound bone loss in marked excess of that **expected at given age**

☐ Excess breast tissue in a man or boy

☐ Random stabbing pains

☐ Nausea or vomiting

☐ Any enhanced sense: sensitivity to light, touch, smells, taste or sound

☐ A sense of imbalance

☐ One or more medical problems with unclear cause(s), with changing or contradictory diagnoses, or which are eventually called "idiopathic"

☐ Two tick or flea infections with two positive tick or flea-borne viruses, bacteria or protozoa.   The presence of other infections such as tick-borne viruses or bacteria raises suspicion of a Babesia infection.

☐ The presence of one or more mystery illnesses after an evaluation by three quality physicians

LAB RESULTS

☐ Eosinophil Cationic Protein (ECP) level is in top 15% of normal. This is altered in perhaps 15-20% of Babesia patients.

☐ The ECP level is above normal.   (Other things can increase this lab, but it is an error that a Babesia infection is not on these lists).

□ The ECP level increases 30% or more in response to a protozoa killing medication in serial testing. (This test is about 40-60% sensitive and many patients have no change in this lab even with effective treatment).

□ The ECP level is below detectable levels.

□ Absolute Eosinophils in the low or high range [this is not definitive in any manner, but is a useful tool.]

□ A percentage of Eosinophils in low range or high normal range

□ Very high Eosinophils [rare with Babesia, but other findings suggest other possible causes]

□ A normal or low VEGF lab result in the presence of Bartonella

□ A TNF-alpha in excess of 1.0 in the presence of Bartonella

□ A CD57 or CD57/8 level that drops right after the start of a Babesia treatment, or which falls steadily with ongoing Babesia treatment

□ Hemolytic anemia with lab test showing positive blood products in your urine [this is not a routine finding.]

□ Your clinician understands the use of indirect testing and feels your lab pattern is suggestive of the presence of Babesia. This involves more than an ECP spike.

□ Since direct testing for Babesia by any lab misses many human species and is of variable reliability, and the common presence of Bartonella suppresses some antibody tests, a positive or "indeterminate" is likely a positive. Have you had an "indeterminate" or "borderline" Babesia result?

□ Bilirubin abnormality [elevated in perhaps 5 % of patients]

☐ Iron abnormalities in excess of normal [high or low levels. The finding of genetic disease that increases iron pathology does not necessarily rule out this finding.   The iron pathology can be genetic or acquired illness plus Babesia [See my HES cancer cure paper in Medscape in which the cancer-like eosinophils were primed by Babesia].

☐ After Babesia treatment with clear protozoa killing agents used also to kill malaria, IL-6 moves from very low to an increased level.

☐ After Babesia treatment with clear protozoa killing agents used also to kill malaria, IL-1B moves from very low to an increased level.

☐ Babesia creates and provokes changes in the human body chemistry.   Tests are being designed to identify chemicals only made by Babesia.   A sample is Babesia microti secreted antigen 1 (BmSA1).

☐ Any positive Epstein-Barr virus over the normal low level. You may have an infection, infections, or inflammation. It is not merely found in Babesia. [This is not a routine cause of fatigue].

☐ Autoimmunity testing is positive.   This is a stronger positive if there are two autoimmune results.   For example, a patient has a positive ANA and has antibodies against their thyroid system.

☐ Positive lab or skin testing placing patient's food sensitivity in top 5% of population

☐ Elevated monocytes

☐ Elevated neutrophils with no clear infection source

☐ Elevated C-reactive protein

☐ Elevated D-dimer

☐ An abnormally high ALT which is a liver enzyme increased by liver trauma, toxins or infections such as Babesia [a rare finding].

☐ Lymphocytopenia—low lymphocytes which are a type of infection-fighting white blood cell

☐ Thrombocytopenia—platelet number under 50,000

☐ A high lactate dehydrogenase or LDH. This enzyme measures tissue damage particularly found in the heart, liver, kidney, skeletal muscle, brain, blood cells and lungs.

REACTION OR CHANGES IN BODY

☐ React to any derivative of Artemisia (Sweet Wormwood). *Note: the reaction does not need to last more than a day and any immediate stomachaches or loose stools do not apply.

☐ React to a malaria drug. For example, ativoquone (Mepron), proguanil alone or with ativoquone (Malarone), artesunate, day 1-3 of artemesinin, a new high dose of artemesinin Day 1-2, artemeter, Alinia, clindamycin, quinine or azithromycin at 2,000 mg/day orally or at any dose IV for five straight days. (It requires profound wisdom for a clinician to distinguish between a side effect and a reaction caused by an effective Babesia treatment. For example, insomnia caused by the synthetic drug Larium is meaningless, since Larium has this as a side effect in uninfected patients. But fatigue, insomnia or severe headache resulting from a teaspoon of ativoquone (Mepron) on day one are very suspicious symptoms for a known protozoan like Babesia or Malaria or other similar infections that are newly identified genetically).

☐ Mood changes with any herb or drug that kills protozoa like Babesia, with the exception of Larium

☐ Muscle aches or joint aches/pain, especially worse after use of a protozoa killing medicine such as proquanil, Alinia, ativoquone, clindamycin, or one of many new emerging progressive natural medicine or synthetic malaria drug treatments

☐ Insomnia after taking a malaria killing herb or drug

☐ Anxiety and/or depression after taking a malaria killing herb or drug

☐ Rage or temporary personality regression right after use of a malaria killing herb or medication, e.g., ativoquone, Malarone, proguanil, artesunate, day 1-3 of artemesinin, artemeter, Alinia, clindamycin or azithromycin at 2,000 mg/day orally or at any dose IV for five straight days.

ENVIRONMENT

☐ Pets, farm animals or local relatives with ANY **clinical symptoms** of a tick-borne virus, bacteria or protozoa infection without a clear diagnosis

☐ The patient's **mother** is suspected of having or has been diagnosed with Babesia, STARI (Masterson's Disease), Neoehrlichia, Anaplasma, Lyme disease, Mycoplasmas, Q Fever, Rocky Mountain spotted fever (Rickettsia), tick-borne relapsing fever, Tularemia (bacteria), Ehrlichia, Protozoa FL1953, or viruses such as CMV, HHV-6, Coxsackie B Types 1, 2, 3, 4, 5, 6, Parvo B-19 or Powassan.

☐ **A sibling, father, spouse or child** with any tick borne infection who shared a residence or vacation with proximity to brush (wooded area)

☐ Exposure to outdoor environments with brush, wild grasses, wild streams, golf courses or woods *in excess of ten minutes in any location lived in or visited*

- [ ] **Pet(s) or family animals** of any type, e.g., horses, have had outdoor exposures to areas with brush, wild grasses, wild streams or woods.   If the pets were animals such as dogs, which can be given anti-tick and flea treatments, were these animals always *on schedule* with these treatments?

- [ ] Clear exposure to ticks in your current or past homes

- [ ] Clear exposure to ticks during vacations or other travels

- [ ] Have you ever had any type of tick bite?

- [ ] Have you ever found a tick on your clothing?

- [ ] Have you ever found a tick on your body?

- [ ] Have you been with others at a location in which they had ticks on their clothing or skin?

- [ ] Sexual contact is a debated form of communication of some tick and flea borne infections. I have no position. Isolation in a body fluid does not mean that is a route to spread the infection. If you and your healer feel this is a possible route of infection, has the patient had intimate contact with the sharing of body fluids with an infected person?

- [ ] You live in a state that has reports of any tick-borne infection in over 40 people. [Currently, this would usually be Lyme disease only].

- [ ] You live next to a state that has reports of any tick-borne infection in over 60 people. [Currently, this would usually be Lyme disease only].

- [ ] Many small mammals live near your home, exercise location, vacation locations or work.

A WORD ON MANUAL BLOOD EXAMINATIONS

No blood smear will be positive for Babesia unless you have a profound number of infected red blood cells. This is very rare. Therefore, **no blood smear should be considered negative unless it has been examined for at least thirty minutes.** While a 2-3 minute exam of large white blood cells may be fully sufficient to identify cancers and other diseases, a search for over eighty Babesia red blood cell presentations under 1000x, as found in my book, *Hematology Forms of Babesia,* requires at least thirty minutes. Unfortunately, in patients positive for Babesia, routine manual red blood smear exams with a clear request to look for Babesia under a microscope at 1,000x magnification have missed the Babesia at least 98% of the time.   In papers reporting clearly visualized Babesia in blood smears the patients tend to have immense infection, i.e., over 3% of red blood cells are infected.

However, if one privately contracts with a microbiologist, pathologist or can get a lab director to allow their staff to spend the extra time, the positive results on the blood smear increase with clearly positively infected patients. I know most laboratories are very overworked, but the notion that a blood slide is going to show an obvious tetrad or a classic X pattern is an error. Using slides from respected national or state sources, I found only by very careful exam, over fifty presentations of Babesia that are usually missed. Indeed, in my textbook on Babesia images most of the shapes had never been published.   No one in history had ever taken the time to look carefully at 200 slides and record each unique shape.   It is fairly stunning to write this and confirms that many tick and flea infections are clearly emerging and not yet mastered.

Please appreciate that stains help define whether a substance is what it appears to be.   For example, some in the alternative medicine school feel that Candida is a bad presence in the intestines and feel it often gets into the blood through defects in the intestinal wall.   While Candida is not a good presence for the intestine, I have found that some blood samples with items that look significantly like parts of Candida do not stain for cellulose and other components of yeasts. My point is that in the last ten years, in discussions or study, excellent pathologists and microbiologists have shown me the clear reason humanity has developed highly sophisticated staining techniques—they can be diagnostic and very cost effective. And some medical scientists are adding new technology to Babesia identification (discussed in my *Babesia 2009 Update* and my *Hematology of Babesia* text).

Babesia is an emerging infection. Any certainty claims or criticism about Babesia positions without extensive research and over 200 hours of reading is premature. Again, new Babesia species are emerging every one to four months.   Indeed, even a new protozoan has been found that looks like Babesia under a high powered microscope, but when it is genetically sequenced it is not Babesia or immature malaria, which can look similar.   It is a new infection and is presently called FL1953 and was genetically sequenced by Dr. Ellis and Dr. Fry. It looks like Babesia, but is not Babesia genetically.

Therefore, since human Babesia is a new emerging illness, this scale is meant merely to increase awareness of Babesia, an infection that can kill patients of any age. Writings in the past fifteen years have either seen Babesia as a mere "co-infection" or a footnote of a spirochete infection [i.e., Lyme]. Anything that can hide for a couple of decades, and then possibly kill you with a clot in your heart, brain or lungs or by other means, is not a casual infection.

Babesia cure claims should be made with the use of indirect testing birthed from extracts of superior journals read a minimum of five years. Currently, these many well-established indirect lab test patterns are not used or understood by immensely busy and smart clinicians working full-time. While this is fully understandable, I hope it may change in the coming decade.

Dr. Schaller is the author of 30 books and 27 top journal articles. His publications address issues in at least twelve fields of medicine.

He has published the most recent four textbooks on Babesia.

He has published on Babesia as a cancer primer under the supervision of the former editor of the *Journal of the American Medical Association (JAMA)*, and his entries on multiple tick and flea-borne infections, including Babesia [along with Bartonella and Lyme disease], were published in a respected infection textbook endorsed by the NIH Director of Infectious Disease.

Dr. Schaller has produced seven texts on tick and flea-borne infections based on his markedly unique full-time reading and study practice, which is not limited to either finite traditional or integrative progressive medicine. With a physician's medical license, he has been able to sort through many truth claims by ordering lab testing. He does not casually follow the dozens of yearly truth claims, without indirect testing laboratory proof. He has read full-time on these emerging problems for many years. He is rated a TOP and BEST physician (in the top 5 percent of doctors) by both physician peers and patients.

Bibliography (Babesia)

Abbas HM, Brenes RA, Ajemian MS, Scholand SJ. Successful conservative treatment of spontaneous splenic rupture secondary to Babesiosis: a case report and literature review. Conn Med. 2011 Mar;75(3):143-6. PMID:21500704

AbouLaila M, Sivakumar T, Yokoyama N, Igarashi I. Inhibitory effect of terpene nerolidol on the growth of Babesia parasites. Parasitol Int. 2010 Jun;59(2):278-82. Epub 2010 Feb 21. PMID:20178862

Aderinboye O, Syed SS. Congenital babesiosis in a four-week-old female infant. Pediatr Infect Dis J. 2010 Feb;29(2):188. PMID:20118748

Alekseev AN. [The possibility of the detection of one more tick-borne infection--babesiosis--on the territory of Russia].[Article in Russian]. Zh Mikrobiol Epidemiol Immunobiol. 2003 May-Jun;(3):39-43. PMID:12886630

Alekseev AN, Rudakov NV, Dubinina EV. [Possible types of tick-borne diseases and the predictive role of history data in their diagnosis (parasitological aspects of the problem)].[Article in Russian]. Med Parazitol (Mosk). 2004 Oct-Dec;(4):31-6. PMID:15689134

Alkhalil A, Hill DA, Desai SA. Babesia and plasmodia increase host erythrocyte permeability through distinct mechanisms. Cell Microbiol. 2007 Apr;9(4):851-60. Epub 2006 Nov 3. PMID:17087736

Arai S, Tsuji M, Kaiho I, Murayama H, Zamoto A, Wei Q, Okabe N, Kamiyama T, Ishihara C. Retrospective seroepidemiological survey for human babesiosis in an area in Japan where a tick-borne disease is endemic. J Vet Med Sci. 2003 Mar;65(3):335-40. PMID:12679563

Armstrong PM, Brunet LR, Spielman A, Telford SR 3rd. Risk of Lyme disease: perceptions of residents of a Lone Star tick-infested community. Bull World Health Organ. 2001;79(10):916-25. PMID:11693973

Arnez M, Luznik-Bufon T, Avsic-Zupanc T, Ruzic-Sabljic E, Petrovec M, Lotric-Furlan S, Strle F. Causes of febrile illnesses after a tick bite in Slovenian children. Pediatr Infect Dis J. 2003 Dec;22(12):1078-83. PMID:14688569

Asad S, Sweeney J, Mermel LA. Transfusion-transmitted babesiosis in Rhode Island. Transfusion. 2009 Dec;49(12):2564-73. Epub 2009 Sep 16. PMID:19761547

Babu RV, Sharma G. A 57-year-old man with abdominal pain, jaundice, and a history of blood transfusion. Chest. 2007 Jul;132(1):347-50. PMID:17625097

Barratt JL, Harkness J, Marriott D, Ellis JT, Stark D. Importance of nonenteric protozoan infections in immunocompromised people. Clin Microbiol Rev. 2010 Oct;23(4):795-836. PMID:20930074

Baumann D, Pusterla N, Péter O, Grimm F, Fournier PE, Schär G, Bossart W, Lutz H, Weber R. [Fever after a tick bite: clinical manifestations and diagnosis of acute tick bite-associated infections in northeastern Switzerland]. [Article in German] Dtsch Med Wochenschr. 2003 May 9;128(19):1042-7. PMID:12736854

Baumeister S, Wiesner J, Reichenberg A, Hintz M, Bietz S, Harb OS, Roos DS, Kordes M, Friesen J, Matuschewski K, Lingelbach K, Jomaa H, Seeber F. Fosmidomycin uptake into Plasmodium and Babesia-infected erythrocytes is facilitated by parasite-induced new permeability pathways. PLoS One. 2011 May 4;6(5):e19334. PMID:21573242

Belongia EA, Reed KD, Mitchell PD, Mueller-Rizner N, Vandermause M, Finkel MF, Kazmierczak JJ. Tickborne infections as a cause of nonspecific febrile illness in Wisconsin. Clin Infect Dis. 2001 May 15;32(10):1434-9. Epub 2001 Apr 17. PMID:11317244

Birkenheuer AJ, Whittington J, Neel J, Large E, Barger A, Levy MG, Breitschwerdt

EB. Molecular characterization of a Babesia species identified in a North American raccoon. J Wildl Dis. 2006 Apr;42(2):375-80. PMID:16870860

Blue D, Graves V, McCarthy L, Cruz J, Gregurek S, Smith D. Fatal transfusion-transmitted Babesia microti in the Midwest. Transfusion. 2009 Jan;49(1):8. Epub 2008 Aug 6. PMID:18694463

Braga W, Venasco J, Willard L, Moro MH. Ultrastructure of Babesia WA1 (Apicomplexa: Piroplasma) during infection of erythrocytes in a hamster model. J Parasitol. 2006 Oct;92(5):1104-7. PMID:17152960

Breitschwerdt EB, Maggi RG. A confusing case of canine vector-borne disease: clinical signs and progression in a dog co-infected with Ehrlichia canis and Bartonella vinsonii ssp. berkhoffii. Parasit Vectors. 2009 Mar 26;2 Suppl 1:S3. PMID:19426442

Brigden ML. Detection, education and management of the asplenic or hyposplenic patient. Am Fam Physician. 2001 Feb 1;63(3):499-506, 508. PMID:11272299

Buelvas F, Alvis N, Buelvas I, Miranda J, Mattar S. [A high prevalence of antibodies against Bartonella and Babesia microti has been found in villages and urban populations in Cordoba, Colombia].[Article in Spanish]. Rev Salud Publica (Bogota). 2008 Jan-Feb;10(1):168-77. PMID:18368229

Cacciò S, Cammà C, Onuma M, Severini C. The beta-tubulin gene of Babesia and Theileria parasites is an informative marker for species discrimination. Int J Parasitol. 2000 Oct;30(11):1181-5. PMID:11027785

Cangelosi JJ, Sarvat B, Sarria JC, Herwaldt BL, Indrikovs AJ. Transmission of Babesia microti by blood transfusion in Texas. Vox Sang. 2008 Nov;95(4):331-4. PMID:19138264

Cardoso L, Tuna J, Vieira L, Yisaschar-Mekuzas Y, Baneth G. Molecular detection of Anaplasma platys and Ehrlichia canis in dogs from the North of Portugal. Vet J. 2010 Feb;183(2):232-3. Epub 2008 Dec 3. PMID:19056304

Carter WJ, Yan Z, Cassai ND, Sidhu GS. Detection of extracellular forms of babesia in the blood by electron microscopy: a diagnostic method for differentiation from Plasmodium falciparum. Ultrastruct Pathol. 2003 Jul-Aug;27(4):211-6. PMID:12907365

Centeno-Lima S, do Rosário V, Parreira R, Maia AJ, Freudenthal AM, Nijhof AM, Jongejan F. A fatal case of human babesiosis in Portugal: molecular and phylogenetic analysis. Trop Med Int Health. 2003 Aug;8(8):760-4. PMID:12869099

Chatel G, Gulletta M, Matteelli A, Marangoni A, Signorini L, Oladeji O, Caligaris S. Short report: Diagnosis of tick-borne relapsing fever by the quantitative buffy coat fluorescence method. Am J Trop Med Hyg. 1999 May;60(5):738-9. PMID:10344644

Cichocka A, Skotarczak B. [Babesosis--difficulty of diagnosis]. [Article in Polish]. Wiad Parazytol. 2001;47(3):527-33. PMID:16894770

Clark IA, Budd AC, Hsue G, Haymore BR, Joyce AJ, Thorner R, Krause PJ. Absence of erythrocyte sequestration in a case of babesiosis in a splenectomized human patient. Malar J. 2006 Aug 4;5:69. PMID:16887045

Conrad PA, Kjemtrup AM, Carreno RA, Thomford J, Wainwright K, Eberhard M, Quick R, Telford SR 3rd, Herwaldt BL. Description of Babesia duncani n.sp. (Apicomplexa: Babesiidae) from humans and its differentiation from other piroplasms. Int J Parasitol. 2006 Jun;36(7):779-89. Epub 2006 May 4. PMID:16725142

Corpelet C, Vacher P, Coudore F, Laurichesse H, Conort N, Souweine B. Role of quinine in life-threatening Babesia divergens infection successfully treated with clindamycin. Eur J Clin Microbiol Infect Dis. 2005 Jan;24(1):74-5. PMID:15616840

Cunha BA, Cohen YZ, McDermott B. Fever of unknown origin (FUO) due to babesiosis in a immunocompetent host. Heart Lung. 2008 Nov-Dec;37(6):481-4. Epub 2008 Sep 30. PMID:18992633

Cunha BA, Nausheen S, Szalda D. Pulmonary complications of babesiosis: case report and literature review. Eur J Clin Microbiol Infect Dis. 2007 Jul;26(7):505-8. PMID:17558489

Dantas-Torres F, Figueredo LA. Canine babesiosis: a Brazilian perspective. Vet Parasitol. 2006 Nov 5;141(3-4):197-203. Epub 2006 Sep 8. PMID:16962707

Dantrakool A, Somboon P, Hashimoto T, Saito-Ito A. Identification of a new type of Babesia species in wild rats (Bandicota indica) in Chiang Mai Province, Thailand. J Clin Microbiol. 2004 Feb;42(2):850-4. PMID:14766871

Delbecq S, Precigout E, Schetters T, Gorenflot A. Babesia divergens: cloning of a Ran binding protein 1 homologue. Vet Parasitol. 2003 Jul 29;115(3):205-11. PMID:12935735

Dobroszycki J, Herwaldt BL, Boctor F, Miller JR, Linden J, Eberhard ML, Yoon JJ, Ali NM, Tanowitz HB, Graham F, Weiss LM, Wittner M. A cluster of transfusion-associated babesiosis cases traced to a single asymptomatic donor. JAMA. 1999 Mar 10;281(10):927-30. PMID:10078490

Dodd JD, Aquino SL, Sharma A. Babesiosis: CT and hematologic findings. J Thorac Imaging. 2007 Aug;22(3):271-3. PMID:17721341

Dorman SE, Cannon ME, Telford SR 3rd, Frank KM, Churchill WH. Fulminant babesiosis treated with clindamycin, quinine, and whole-blood exchange transfusion. Transfusion. 2000 Mar;40(3):375-80. PMID:10738042

Duh D, Jelovsek M, Avsic-Zupanc T. Evaluation of an indirect fluorescence immunoassay for the detection of serum antibodies against Babesia divergens in humans. Parasitology. 2007 Feb;134(Pt 2):179-85. Epub 2006 Oct 11. PMID:17032478

Dvoraková HM, Dvoráčková M. [Babesiosis, a little known zoonosis].[Article in Czech]. Epidemiol Mikrobiol Imunol. 2007 Nov;56(4):176-80. PMID:18072299

El-Bahnasawy MM, Morsy TA. Egyptian human babesiosis and
general review. J Egypt Soc Parasitol. 2008 Apr;38(1):265-72.
PMID:19143136

Eskow ES, Krause PJ, Spielman A, Freeman K, Aslanzadeh
J. Southern extension of the range of human babesiosis in the
eastern United States. J Clin Microbiol. 1999 Jun;37(6):2051-2.
PMID:10325378

Florescu D, Sordillo PP, Glyptis A, Zlatanic E, Smith B, Polsky
B, Sordillo E. Splenic infarction in human babesiosis: two
cases and discussion. Clin Infect Dis. 2008 Jan 1;46(1):e8-11.
PMID:18171204

Foppa IM, Krause PJ, Spielman A, Goethert H, Gern L, Brand B,
Telford SR 3rd. Entomologic and serologic evidence of zoonotic
transmission of Babesia microti, eastern Switzerland. Emerg Infect
Dis. 2002 Jul;8(7):722-6. PMID:12095442

Fox LM, Wingerter S, Ahmed A, Arnold A, Chou J, Rhein L, Levy
O. Neonatal babesiosis: case report and review of the literature.
Pediatr Infect Dis J. 2006 Feb;25(2):169-73. PMID:16462298

Froberg MK, Dannen D, Bakken JS. Babesiosis and HIV. Lancet.
2004 Feb 28;363(9410):704. PMID:15001329

Froberg MK, Dannen D, Bernier N, Shieh WJ, Guarner J, Zaki S.
Case report: spontaneous splenic rupture during acute parasitemia
of Babesia microti. Ann Clin Lab Sci. 2008 Autumn;38(4):390-2.
PMID:18988934

Gallagher LG, Chau S, Owaisi AS, Konczyk M, Bishop HS,
Arguin PM, Trenholme GM. An 84-year-old woman with fever
and dark urine. Clin Infect Dis. 2009 Jul 15;49(2):278, 310-1.
PMID:19538064

Gary AT, Webb JA, Hegarty BC, Breitschwerdt EB. The low seroprevalence of tick-transmitted agents of disease in dogs from southern Ontario and Quebec. Can Vet J. 2006 Dec;47(12):1194-200. PMID:17217089

Gern L, Lienhard R, Péter O. [Diseases and pathogenic agents transmitted by ticks in Switzerland].[Article in French]. Rev Med Suisse. 2010 Oct 13;6(266):1906-9. PMID:21089555

Goethert HK, Telford SR 3rd. Enzootic transmission of Babesia divergens among cottontail rabbits on Nantucket Island, Massachusetts. Am J Trop Med Hyg. 2003 Nov;69(5):455-60. PMID:14695079

Goo YK, Terkawi MA, Jia H, Aboge GO, Ooka H, Nelson B, Kim S, Sunaga F, Namikawa K, Igarashi I, Nishikawa Y, Xuan X. Artesunate, a potential drug for treatment of Babesia infection. Parasitol Int. 2010 Sep;59(3):481-6. Epub 2010 Jun 9. PMID:20541037

Guan G, Chauvin A, Yin H, Luo J, Moreau E. Course of infection by Babesia sp. BQ1 (Lintan) and B. divergens in sheep depends on the production of IFNgamma and IL10. Parasite Immunol. 2010 Feb;32(2):143-52. PMID:20070828

Gubernot DM, Lucey CT, Lee KC, Conley GB, Holness LG, Wise RP. Babesia infection through blood transfusions: reports received by the US Food and Drug Administration, 1997-2007. Clin Infect Dis. 2009 Jan 1;48(1):25-30. PMID:19035776

Gutman JD, Kotton CN, Kratz A. Case records of the Massachusetts General Hospital. Weekly clinicopathological exercises. Case 29-2003. A 60-year-old man with fever, rigors, and sweats. N Engl J Med. 2003 Sep 18;349(12):1168-75. PMID:13679532

Hamer SA, Tsao JI, Walker ED, Mansfield LS, Foster ES, Hickling GJ. Use of tick surveys and serosurveys to evaluate pet dogs as a sentinel species for emerging Lyme disease. Am J Vet Res. 2009 Jan;70(1):49-56. PMID:19119948

Han JI, Lee SJ, Jang HJ, Na KJ. Asymptomatic Babesia microti-like parasite infection in wild raccoon dogs (Nyctereutes procyonoides) in South Korea. J Wildl Dis. 2010 Apr;46(2):632-5. PMID:20688664

Harvey WT, Martz D. Motor neuron disease recovery associated with IV ceftriaxone and anti-Babesia therapy. Acta Neurol Scand. 2007 Feb;115(2):129-31. PMID:17212618

Häselbarth K, Tenter AM, Brade V, Krieger G, Hunfeld KP. First case of human babesiosis in Germany - Clinical presentation and molecular characterisation of the pathogen. Int J Med Microbiol. 2007 Jun;297(3):197-204. Epub 2007 Mar 12. PMID:17350888

Hatcher JC, Greenberg PD, Antique J, Jimenez-Lucho VE. Severe babesiosis in Long Island: review of 34 cases and their complications. Clin Infect Dis. 2001 Apr 15;32(8):1117-25. Epub 2001 Mar 26. PMID:11283800

Hemmer RM, Wozniak EJ, Lowenstine LJ, Plopper CG, Wong V, Conrad PA. Endothelial cell changes are associated with pulmonary edema and respiratory distress in mice infected with the WA1 human Babesia parasite. J Parasitol. 1999 Jun;85(3):479-89. PMID:10386441

Herman JH, Ayache S, Olkowska D. Autoimmunity in transfusion babesiosis: a spectrum of clinical presentations. J Clin Apher. 2010;25(6):358-61. Epub 2010 Sep 7. PMID:20824620

Hermanowska-Szpakowicz T, Skotarczak B, Kondrusik M, Rymaszewska A, Sawczuk M, Maciejewska A, Adamska M, Pancewicz S, Zajkowska J. Detecting DNAs of Anaplasma phagocytophilum and Babesia in the blood of patients suspected of Lyme disease. Ann Agric Environ Med. 2004;11(2):351-4. PMID:15627349

Herwaldt BL, Cacciò S, Gherlinzoni F, Aspöck H, Slemenda SB, Piccaluga P, Martinelli G, Edelhofer R, Hollenstein U, Poletti G, Pampiglione S, Löschenberger , Tura S, Pieniazek NJ. Molecular characterization of a non-Babesia divergens organism causing zoonotic babesiosis in Europe. Emerg Infect Dis. 2003 Aug;9(8):942-8. PMID:12967491

Herwaldt BL, McGovern PC, Gerwel MP, Easton RM, MacGregor RR. Endemic babesiosis in another eastern state: New Jersey. Emerg Infect Dis. 2003 Feb;9(2):184-8. PMID:12603988

Herwaldt BL, Neitzel DF, Gorlin JB, Jensen KA, Perry EH, Peglow WR, Slemenda SB,

Won KY, Nace EK, Pieniazek NJ, Wilson M. Transmission of Babesia microti in Minnesota through four blood donations from the same donor over a 6-month period. Transfusion. 2002 Sep;42(9):1154-8. PMID:12430672

Heyman P, Cochez C, Hofhuis A, van der Giessen J, Sprong H, Porter SR, Losson B, Saegerman C, Donoso-Mantke O, Niedrig M, Papa A. A clear and present danger: tick-borne diseases in Europe. Expert Rev Anti Infect Ther. 2010 Jan;8(1):33-50. PMID:20014900

Hildebrandt A, Hunfeld KP, Baier M, Krumbholz A, Sachse S, Lorenzen T, Kiehntopf M, Fricke HJ, Straube E. First confirmed autochthonous case of human Babesia microti infection in Europe. Eur J Clin Microbiol Infect Dis. 2007 Aug;26(8):595-601. PMID:17587072

Hilton E, DeVoti J, Benach JL, Halluska ML, White DJ, Paxton H, Dumler JS. Seroprevalence and seroconversion for tick-borne diseases in a high-risk population in the northeast United States. Am J Med. 1999 Apr;106(4):404-9. PMID:10225242

Hohenschild S. [Babesiosis--a dangerous infection for splenectomized children and adults].[Article in German]. Klin Padiatr. 1999 May-Jun;211(3):137-40. PMID:10412122

Holman PJ, Spencer AM, Droleskey RE, Goethert HK, Telford SR 3rd. In vitro cultivation of a zoonotic Babesia sp. isolated from eastern cottontail rabbits (Sylvilagus floridanus) on Nantucket Island, Massachusetts. J Clin Microbiol. 2005 Aug;43(8):3995-4001. PMID:16081941

Holman PJ, Spencer AM, Telford SR 3rd, Goethert HK, Allen AJ, Knowles DP, Goff WL. Comparative infectivity of Babesia divergens and a zoonotic Babesia divergens-like parasite in cattle. Am J Trop Med Hyg. 2005 Nov;73(5):865-70. PMID:16282295

Homer MJ, Aguilar-Delfin I, Telford SR 3rd, Krause PJ, Persing DH. Babesiosis. Clin Microbiol Rev. 2000 Jul;13(3):451-69. PMID:10885987

Homer MJ, Lodes MJ, Reynolds LD, Zhang Y, Douglass JF, McNeill PD, Houghton RL, Persing DH. Identification and characterization of putative secreted antigens from Babesia microti. J Clin Microbiol. 2003 Feb;41(2):723-9. PMID:12574273

Houghton RL, Homer MJ, Reynolds LD, Sleath PR, Lodes MJ, Berardi V, Leiby DA, Persing DH. Identification of Babesia microti-specific immunodominant epitopes and development of a peptide EIA for detection of antibodies in serum. Transfusion. 2002 Nov;42(11):1488-96. PMID:12421223

Hunfeld KP, Allwinn R, Peters S, Kraiczy P, Brade V. Serologic evidence for tick-borne pathogens other than Borrelia burgdorferi (TOBB) in Lyme borreliosis patients from midwestern Germany. Wien Klin Wochenschr. 1998 Dec 23;110(24):901-8. PMID:10048174

Hunfeld KP, Brade V. Zoonotic Babesia: possibly emerging pathogens to be considered for tick-infested humans in Central Europe. Int J Med Microbiol. 2004 Apr;293 Suppl 37:93-103. PMID:15146990

Hunfeld KP, Hildebrandt A, Gray JS. Babesiosis: recent insights into an ancient disease. Int J Parasitol. 2008 Sep;38(11):1219-37. Epub 2008 Mar 20. PMID:18440005

Hunfeld KP, Lambert A, Kampen H, Albert S, Epe C, Brade V, Tenter AM. Seroprevalence of Babesia infections in humans exposed to ticks in Midwestern Germany. J Clin Microbiol. 2002 Jul;40(7):2431-6. PMID:12089258

Hutchings CL, Li A, Fernandez KM, Fletcher T, Jackson LA, Molloy JB, Jorgensen WK, Lim CT, Cooke BM. New insights into the altered adhesive and mechanical properties of red blood cells parasitized by Babesia bovis. Mol Microbiol. 2007 Aug;65(4):1092-105. Epub 2007 Jul 19. PMID:17640278

Jackson LA, Waldron SJ, Weier HM, Nicoll CL, Cooke BM. Babesia bovis: culture of laboratory-adapted parasite lines and clinical isolates in a chemically defined medium. Exp Parasitol. 2001 Nov;99(3):168-74. PMID:11846527

Jahangir A, Kolbert C, Edwards W, Mitchell P, Dumler JS, Persing DH. Fatal pancarditis associated with human granulocytic Ehrlichiosis in a 44-year-old man. Clin Infect Dis. 1998 Dec;27(6):1424-7. PMID:9868655

Jeneby MM, Ngeiywa M, Yole DS, Mwenda JM, Suleman MA, Carlson HE. Enzootic simian piroplasm (Entopolypoides macaci) in wild-caught Kenyan non-human primates. J Med Primatol. 2008 Dec;37(6):329-36. Epub 2008 May 27. PMID:18507704

Kain KC, Jassoum SB, Fong IW, Hannach B. Transfusion-transmitted babesiosis in Ontario: first reported case in Canada. CMAJ. 2001 Jun 12;164(12):1721-3. PMID:11450217

Kim JY, Cho SH, Joo HN, Tsuji M, Cho SR, Park IJ, Chung GT, Ju JW, Cheun HI, Lee

HW, Lee YH, Kim TS. First case of human babesiosis in Korea: detection and characterization of a novel type of Babesia sp. (KO1) similar to ovine babesia. J Clin Microbiol. 2007 Jun;45(6):2084-7. Epub 2007 Mar 28. PMID:17392446

Kjemtrup AM, Conrad PA. A review of the small canine piroplasms from California: Babesia conradae in the literature. Vet Parasitol. 2006 May 31;138(1-2):112-7. Epub 2006 Mar 7. PMID:16522352

Kjemtrup AM, Wainwright K, Miller M, Penzhorn BL, Carreno RA. Babesia conradae, sp. Nov., a small canine Babesia identified in California. Vet Parasitol. 2006 May 31;138(1-2):103-11. Epub 2006 Mar 9. PMID:16524663

Kolören Z, Avşar C, Şekeroğlu ZA. [Diagnosis of protozoa by loop-mediated isothermal amplification: (LAMP)].[Article in Turkish]. Turkiye Parazitol Derg. 2010;34(4):207-11. PMID:21391196

Köster LS, Van Schoor M, Goddard A, Thompson PN, Matjila PT, Kjelgaard-Hansen M. C-reactive protein in canine babesiosis caused by Babesia rossi and its association with outcome. J S Afr Vet Assoc. 2009 Jun;80(2):87-91. PMID:19831269

Krause PJ. Babesiosis. Med Clin North Am. 2002 Mar;86(2):361-73. PMID:11982307

Krause PJ. Babesiosis diagnosis and treatment. Vector Borne Zoonotic Dis. 2003 Spring;3(1):45-51. PMID:12804380

Kumar S, Kumar R, Sugimoto C. A perspective on Theileria equi infections in donkeys. Jpn J Vet Res. 2009 Feb;56(4):171-80. PMID:19358444

Kuwayama DP, Briones RJ. Spontaneous splenic rupture caused by Babesia microti infection. Clin Infect Dis. 2008 May 1;46(9):e92-5. PMID:18419430

Lantos PM, Krause PJ. Babesiosis: similar to malaria but different. Pediatr Ann. 2002 Mar;31(3):192-7. PMID:11905293

Lee BP. Apnea, bradycardia and thrombocytopenia in a premature infant. Pediatr Infect Dis J. 2001 Aug;20(8):816, 820-2. PMID:11734753

Lee S, Carson K, Rice-Ficht A, Good T. Small heat shock proteins differentially affect Abeta aggregation and toxicity. Biochem Biophys Res Commun. 2006 Aug 25;347(2):527-33. Epub 2006 Jun 30. PMID:16828710

Leiby DA, Chung AP, Cable RG, Trouern-Trend J, McCullough J, Homer MJ, Reynolds LD, Houghton RL, Lodes MJ, Persing DH. Relationship between tick bites and the seroprevalence of Babesia microti and Anaplasma phagocytophila (previously Ehrlichia sp.) in blood donors. Transfusion. 2002 Dec;42(12):1585-91. PMID:12473139

Leiby DA, Chung AP, Gill JE, Houghton RL, Persing DH, Badon S, Cable RG. Demonstrable parasitemia among Connecticut blood donors with antibodies to Babesia microti. Transfusion. 2005 Nov;45(11):1804-10. PMID:16271108

Leiby DA, Gill JE. Transfusion-transmitted tick-borne infections: a cornucopia of threats. Transfus Med Rev. 2004 Oct;18(4):293-306. PMID:15497129

Leisewitz AL, Jacobson LS, de Morais HS, Reyers F. The mixed acid-base disturbances of severe canine babesiosis. J Vet Intern Med. 2001 Sep-Oct;15(5):445-52. PMID:11596731

Littman MP. Canine borreliosis. Vet Clin North Am Small Anim Pract. 2003 Jul;33(4):827-62. PMID:12910746

Loa CC, Adelson ME, Mordechai E, Raphaelli I, Tilton RC. Serological diagnosis of human babesiosis by IgG enzyme-linked immunosorbent assay. Curr Microbiol. 2004 Dec;49(6):385-9. PMID:15696612

Lodes MJ, Dillon DC, Houghton RL, Skeiky YA. Expression cloning. Methods Mol Med. 2004;94:91-106. PMID:14959824

Lodes MJ, Houghton RL, Bruinsma ES, Mohamath R, Reynolds LD, Benson DR, Krause PJ, Reed SG, Persing DH. Serological expression cloning of novel immunoreactive antigens of Babesia microti. Infect Immun. 2000 May;68(5):2783-90. PMID:10768973

Luo Y, Jia H, Terkawi MA, Goo YK, Kawano S, Ooka H, Li Y, Yu L, Cao S, Yamagishi J, Fujisaki K, Nishikawa Y, Saito-Ito A, Igarashi I, Xuan X. Identification and characterization of a novel secreted antigen 1 of Babesia microti and evaluation of its potential use in enzyme-linked immunosorbent assay and immunochromatographic test. Parasitol Int. 2011 Jun;60(2):119-25. Epub 2010 Nov 8. PMID:21070864

Lux JZ, Weiss D, Linden JV, Kessler D, Herwaldt BL, Wong SJ, Keithly J, Della-Latta P, Scully BE. Transfusion-associated babesiosis after heart transplant. Emerg Infect Dis. 2003 Jan;9(1):116-9. PMID:12533293

Marathe A, Tripathi J, Handa V, Date V. Human babesiosis--a case report. Indian J Med Microbiol. 2005 Oct;23(4):267-9. PMID:16327127

Marco I, Velarde R, Castellà J, Ferrer D, Lavín S. Presumptive Babesia ovis infection in a spanish ibex (Capra pyrenaica). Vet Parasitol. 2000 Jan;87(2-3):217-21. PMID:10622613

Marcu CB, Caracciolo E, Libertin C, Donohue T. Fulminant babesiosis manifested soon after coronary bypass surgery. Conn Med. 2005 Feb;69(2):67-8. PMID:15779600

Martinot M, Zadeh MM, Hansmann Y, Grawey I, Christmann D, Aguillon S, Jouglin M, Chauvin A, De Briel D. Babesiosis in immunocompetent patients, Europe. Emerg Infect Dis. 2011 Jan;17(1):114-6. PMID:21192869

Matsui T, Inoue R, Kajimoto K, Tamekane A, Okamura A, Katayama Y, Shimoyama M, Chihara K, Saito-Ito A, Tsuji M. [First documentation of transfusion-associated babesiosis in Japan].[Article in Japanese]. Rinsho Ketsueki. 2000 Aug;41(8):628-34. PMID:11020989

Matthews J, Rattigan E, Yee H. Case 29-2003: a 60-year-old man with fever, rigors, and sweats. N Engl J Med. 2003 Dec 18;349(25):2467; author reply 2467. PMID:14681519

Mbati PA, Hlatshwayo M, Mtshali MS, Mogaswane KR, De Waal TD, Dipeolu OO. Ticks and tick-borne diseases of livestock belonging to resource-poor farmers in the eastern Free State of South Africa. Exp Appl Acarol. 2002;28(1-4):217-24. PMID:14570134

Meer-Scherrer L, Adelson M, Mordechai E, Lottaz B, Tilton R. Babesia microti infection in Europe. Curr Microbiol. 2004 Jun;48(6):435-7. PMID:15170239

Meister J. Human babesiosis: a case study. Clin Excell Nurse Pract. 1999 Jul;3(4):214-6. PMID:10711060

Mitrović S, Kranjcić-Zec I, Arsić-Arsenijević V, Dzamić A, Radonjić I. [Human babesiosis--recent discoveries]. [Article in Serbian]. Med Pregl. 2004 Jul-Aug;57(7-8):349-53. PMID:15626291

Montero E, Rodriguez M, Oksov Y, Lobo CA. Babesia divergens apical membrane antigen 1 and its interaction with the human red blood cell. Infect Immun. 2009 Nov;77(11):4783-93. Epub 2009 Aug 31. PMID:19720759

Moreno Giménez JC, Jiménez Puya R, Galán Gutiérrez M, Ortega Salas R, Dueñas Jurado JM. Erythema figuratum in septic babesiosis. J Eur Acad Dermatol Venereol. 2006 Jul;20(6):726-8. PMID:16836504

Mylonakis E. When to suspect and how to monitor babesiosis. Am Fam Physician. 2001 May 15;63(10):1969-74. PMID:11388711

Nagao E, Arie T, Dorward DW, Fairhurst RM, Dvorak JA. The avian malaria parasite Plasmodium gallinaceum causes marked structural changes on the surface of its host erythrocyte. J Struct Biol. 2008 Jun;162(3):460-7. Epub 2008 Mar 21. PMID:18442920

Narasimhan S, Montgomery RR, DePonte K, Tschudi C, Marcantonio N, Anderson JF, Sauer JR, Cappello M, Kantor FS, Fikrig E. Disruption of Ixodes scapularis anticoagulation by using RNA interference. Proc Natl Acad Sci U S A. 2004 Feb 3;101(5):1141-6. Epub 2004 Jan 26. PMID:14745044

Ngo V, Civen R. Babesiosis acquired through blood transfusion, California, USA. Emerg Infect Dis. 2009 May;15(5):785-7. PMID:19402969

Nicholson GT, Walsh CA, Madan RP. Transfusion-associated babesiosis in a 7-month-old infant after bidirectional Glenn procedure. Congenit Heart Dis. 2010 Nov-Dec;5(6):607-13. PMID:21106022

Nishisaka M, Yokoyama N, Xuan X, Inoue N, Nagasawa H, Fujisaki K, Mikami T, Igarashi I. Characterisation of the gene encoding a protective antigen from Babesia microti identified it as eta subunit of chaperonin containing T-complex protein 1. Int J Parasitol. 2001 Dec;31(14):1673-9. PMID:11730795

Nohýnková E, Kubek J, Měst'ánková O, Chalupa P, Hubálek Z. [A case of Babesia microti imported into the Czech Republic from the USA].[Article in Czech]. Cas Lek Cesk. 2003;142(6):377-81. PMID:12924039

Oleson CV, Sivalingam JJ, O'Neill BJ, Staas WE Jr. Transverse myelitis secondary to coexistent Lyme disease and babesiosis. J Spinal Cord Med. 2003 Summer;26(2):168-71. PMID:12828297

Oliveira TM, Furuta PI, de Carvalho D, Machado RZ. A study of cross-reactivity in serum samples from dogs positive for Leishmania sp., Babesia canis and Ehrlichia canis in enzyme-linked immunosorbent assay and indirect fluorescent antibody test. Rev Bras Parasitol Vet. 2008 Jan-Mar;17(1):7-11. PMID:18554433

Ooka H, Terkawi MA, Goo YK, Luo Y, Li Y, Yamagishi J, Nishikawa Y, Igarashi I, Xuan X. Babesia microti: molecular and antigenic characterizations of a novel 94-kDa protein (BmP94). Exp Parasitol. 2011 Jan;127(1):287-93. Epub 2010 Jun 25. PMID:20599995

Pancewicz S, Moniuszko A, Bieniarz E, Puciło K, Grygorczuk S, Zajkowska J, Czupryna P, Kondrusik M, Swierzbińska-Pijanowska R. Anti-Babesia microti antibodies in foresters highly exposed to tick bites in Poland. Scand J Infect Dis. 2011 Mar;43(3):197-201. Epub 2010 Dec 9. PMID:21142620

Pantanowitz L, Aufranc S 3rd, Monahan-Earley R, Dvorak A, Telford SR 3rd. Transfusion medicine illustrated. Morphologic hallmarks of Babesia. Transfusion. 2002 Nov;42(11):1389. PMID:12421208

Pendse S, Bilyk JR, Lee MS. The ticking time bomb. Surv Ophthalmol. 2006 May-Jun;51(3):274-9. PMID:16644367

Perdrizet GA, Olson NH, Krause PJ, Banever GT, Spielman A, Cable RG. Babesiosis in a renal transplant recipient acquired through blood transfusion. Transplantation. 2000 Jul 15;70(1):205-8. PMID:10919602

Permin A, Yelifari L, Bloch P, Steenhard N, Hansen NP, Nansen P. Parasites in cross-bred pigs in the Upper East region of Ghana. Vet Parasitol. 1999 Nov;87(1):63-71. PMID:10628701

Precigout E, Delbecq S, Vallet A, Carcy B, Camillieri S, Hadj-Kaddour K, Kleuskens J, Schetters T, Gorenflot A. Association between sequence polymorphism in an epitope of Babesia divergens Bd37 exoantigen and protection induced by passive transfer. Int J Parasitol. 2004 Apr;34(5):585-93. PMID:15064123

Prince HE, Lapé-Nixon M, Patel H, Yeh C. Comparison of the Babesia duncani (WA1) IgG detection rates among clinical sera submitted to a reference laboratory for WA1 IgG testing and blood donor specimens from diverse geographic areas of the United States. Clin Vaccine Immunol. 2010 Nov;17(11):1729-33. Epub 2010 Sep 22. PMID:20861326

Qi C, Zhou D, Liu J, Cheng Z, Zhang L, Wang L, Wang Z, Yang D, Wang S, Chai T. Detection of Babesia divergens using molecular methods in anemic patients in Shandong Province, China. Parasitol Res. 2011 Jul;109(1):241-5. Epub 2011 Apr 19. PMID:21503639

Quintão-Silva MG, Melo MN, Ribeiro MF. Comparison of duplex PCR and microscopic techniques for the identification of Babesia bigemina and Babesia bovis in engorged female ticks of Boophilus microplus. Zoonoses Public Health. 2007;54(3-4):147-51. PMID:17456146

Raju M, Salazar JC, Leopold H, Krause PJ. Atovaquone and azithromycin treatment for babesiosis in an infant. Pediatr Infect Dis J. 2007 Feb;26(2):181-3. PMID:17259886

Ramharter M, Walochnik J, Lagler H, Winkler S, Wernsdorfer WH, Stoiser B, Graninger W. Clinical and molecular characterization of a near fatal case of human babesiosis in Austria. J Travel Med. 2010 Nov-Dec;17(6):416-8. PMID:21050324

Rech A, Bittar CM, de Castro CG, Azevedo KR, dos Santos RP, Machado AR, Schwartsmann G, Goldani L, Brunetto AL. Asymptomatic babesiosis in a child with hepatoblastoma. J Pediatr Hematol Oncol. 2004 Mar;26(3):213. PMID:15125618

Reis C, Cote M, Paul RE, Bonnet S. Questing ticks in suburban forest are infected by at least six tick-borne pathogens. Vector Borne Zoonotic Dis. 2011 Jul;11(7):907-16. Epub 2010 Dec 15. PMID:21158500

Reis SP, Maddineni S, Rozenblit G, Allen D. Spontaneous splenic rupture secondary to Babesia microti infection: treatment with splenic artery embolization. J Vasc Interv Radiol. 2011 May;22(5):732-4. PMID:21514529

Ríos L, Alvarez G, Blair S. Serological and parasitological study and report of the first case of human babesiosis in Colombia. Rev Soc Bras Med Trop. 2003 Jul-Aug;36(4):493-8. Epub 2003 Aug 13. PMID:12937727

Rosenblatt JE. Laboratory diagnosis of infections due to blood and tissue parasites. Clin Infect Dis. 2009 Oct 1;49(7):1103-8. PMID:19691431

Ryan R, Krause PJ, Radolf J, Freeman K, Spielman A, Lenz R, Levin A. Diagnosis of babesiosis using an immunoblot serologic test. Clin Diagn Lab Immunol. 2001 Nov;8(6):1177-80. PMID:11687460

Saito-Ito A, Dantrakool A, Kawai A, Yano Y, Takada N. [Babesiosis].[Article in Japanese]. Nihon Rinsho. 2003 Feb;61 Suppl 2:623-8. PMID:12722292

Saito-Ito A, Tsuji M, Wei Q, He S, Matsui T, Kohsaki M, Arai S, Kamiyama T, Hioki K, Ishihara C. Transfusion-acquired, autochthonous human babesiosis in Japan: isolation of Babesia microti-like parasites with hu-RBC-SCID mice. J Clin Microbiol. 2000 Dec;38(12):4511-6. PMID:11101588

Sambri V, Marangoni A, Storni E, Cavrini F, Moroni A, Sparacino M, Cevenini R. [Tick borne zoonosis: selected clinical and diagnostic aspects].[Article in Italian]. Parassitologia. 2004 Jun;46(1-2):109-13. PMID:15305697

Schaller JL, Burkland GA, Langhoff PJ. Are various Babesia species a missed cause for hypereosinophilia? A follow-up on the first reported case of imatinib mesylate for idiopathic hypereosinophilia. MedGenMed. 2007 Feb 27;9(1):38. PMID:17435644

Schetters TP, Eling WM. Can Babesia infections be used as a model for cerebral malaria? Parasitol Today. 1999 Dec;15(12):492-7. PMID:10557150

Schoeler GB, Manweiler SA, Wikel SK. Ixodes scapularis: effects of repeated infestations with pathogen-free nymphs on macrophage and T lymphocyte cytokine responses of BALB/c and C3H/HeN mice. Exp Parasitol. 1999 Aug;92(4):239-48. PMID:10425152

Schoeman JP. Canine babesiosis. Onderstepoort J Vet Res. 2009 Mar;76(1):59-66. PMID:19967929

Schoeman JP, Herrtage ME. Adrenal response to the low dose ACTH stimulation test and the cortisol-to-adrenocorticotrophic hormone ratio in canine babesiosis. Vet Parasitol. 2008 Jul 4;154(3-4):205-13. Epub 2008 Apr 7. PMID:18468798

Semel ME, Tavakkolizadeh A, Gates JD. Babesiosis in the immediate postoperative period after splenectomy for trauma. Surg Infect (Larchmt). 2009 Dec;10(6):553-6. PMID:19622029

Sethi S, Alcid D, Kesarwala H, Tolan RW Jr. Probable congenital babesiosis in infant, new jersey, USA. Emerg Infect Dis. 2009 May;15(5):788-91. PMID:19402971

Setty S, Khalil Z, Schori P, Azar M, Ferrieri P. Babesiosis. Two atypical cases from Minnesota and a review. Am J Clin Pathol. 2003 Oct;120(4):554-9. PMID:14560566

Sherr VT. Human babesiosis--an unrecorded reality. Absence of formal registry undermines its detection, diagnosis and treatment, suggesting need for immediate mandatory reporting. Med Hypotheses. 2004;63(4):609-15. PMID:15325004

Shoemaker RC, Hudnell HK, House DE, Van Kempen A, Pakes GE; COL40155 Study Team. Atovaquone plus cholestyramine in patients coinfected with Babesia microti and Borrelia burgdorferi refractory to other treatment. Adv Ther. 2006 Jan-Feb;23(1):1-11. PMID:16644602

Skotarczak B. [Babesiosis of human and domestic dog; ethiology, pathogenesis, diagnostics].[Article in Polish]. Wiad Parazytol. 2007;53(4):271-80. PMID:18441872

Skotarczak B, Cichocka A. Isolation and amplification by polymerase chain reaction DNA of Babesia microti and Babesia divergens in ticks in Poland. Ann Agric Environ Med. 2001;8(2):187-9. PMID:11748876

Skotarczak B, Sawczuk M. [Occurrence of Babesia microti in ticks Ixodes ricinus on selected areas of western Pomerania].[Article in Polish]. Wiad Parazytol. 2003;49(3):273-80. PMID:16889031

Sréter T, Sréterné Lancz Z, Széll Z, Egyed L. [Rickettsia helvetica: an emerging tick-borne pathogen in Hungary and Europe]. [Article in Hungarian]. Orv Hetil. 2005 Dec 11;146(50):2547-52. PMID:16440500

Sréter T, Kálmán D, Sréterné Lancz Z, Széll Z, Egyed L. [Babesia microti and Anaplasma phagocytophilum: two emerging zoonotic pathogens in Europe and Hungary].[Article in Hungarian]. Orv Hetil. 2005 Mar 27;146(13):595-600. PMID:15856623

Stańczak J, Myjak P, Bajer A, Siński E, Wedrychowicz H, Majewska AC, Gołab E, Budak A. [Usefulness of the molecular techniques for detecting and/or identifing of parasites and fungi in humans and animals or pathogens transmitted by ticks. Part III].[Article in Polish]. Wiad Parazytol. 2001;47(3):465-75. PMID:16894762

Stricker RB. Counterpoint: long-term antibiotic therapy improves persistent symptoms associated with lyme disease. Clin Infect Dis. 2007 Jul 15;45(2):149-57. Epub 2007 Jun 5. PMID:17578772

Stricker RB, Lautin A, Burrascano JJ. Lyme disease: point/ counterpoint. Expert Rev Anti Infect Ther. 2005 Apr;3(2):155-65. PMID:15918774

Taiwo B, Lee C, Venkat D, Tambar S, Sutton SH. Can tumor necrosis factor alpha blockade predispose to severe babesiosis? Arthritis Rheum. 2007 Feb 15;57(1):179-81. PMID:17266091

Tajima T, Zhi N, Lin Q, Rikihisa Y, Horowitz HW, Ralfalli J, Wormser GP, Hechemy KE. Comparison of two recombinant major outer membrane proteins of the human granulocytic ehrlichiosis agent for use in an enzyme-linked immunosorbent assay. Clin Diagn Lab Immunol. 2000 Jul;7(4):652-7. PMID:10882667

Talour K, Karam A, Dreux N, Lemasson G, Gilbert D, Abasq C, Misery L. Incipiens linear IgA disease with IgA antibodies directed against 200-kDa epidermal antigens. Eur J Dermatol. 2011 May-Jun;21(3):411-2. PMID:21515442

Terkawi MA, Jia H, Zhou J, Lee EG, Igarashi I, Fujisaki K, Nishikawa Y, Xuan X. Babesia gibsoni ribosomal phosphoprotein P0 induces cross-protective immunity against B. microti infection in mice. Vaccine. 2007 Mar 1;25(11):2027-35. Epub 2006 Dec 8. PMID:17229504

Tonnetti L, Eder AF, Dy B, Kennedy J, Pisciotto P, Benjamin RJ, Leiby DA. Transfusion-transmitted Babesia microti identified through hemovigilance. Transfusion. 2009 Dec;49(12):2557-63. Epub 2009 Jul 16. PMID:19624607

Topolovec J, Puntarić D, Antolović-Pozgain A, Vuković D, Topolovec Z, Milas J, Drusko-Barisić V, Venus M. Serologically detected "new" tick-borne zoonoses in eastern Croatia. Croat Med J. 2003 Oct;44(5):626-9. PMID:14515426

Torina A, Caracappa S. Anaplasmosis in cattle in Italy. Vet Res Commun. 2007 Aug;31 Suppl 1:73-8. PMID:17682850

Torina A, Vicente J, Alongi A, Scimeca S, Turlá R, Nicosia S, Di Marco V, Caracappa S, de la Fuente J. Observed prevalence of tick-borne pathogens in domestic animals in Sicily, Italy during 2003-2005. Zoonoses Public Health. 2007;54(1):8-15. PMID:17359441

Torres-Vélez FJ, Nace EK, Won KY, Bartlett J, Eberhard M, Guarner J. Development of an immunohistochemical assay for the detection of babesiosis in formalin-fixed, paraffin-embedded tissue samples. Am J Clin Pathol. 2003 Dec;120(6):833-8. PMID:14671971

Tsuji N, Miyoshi T, Battsetseg B, Matsuo T, Xuan X, Fujisaki K. A cysteine protease is critical for Babesia spp. transmission in Haemaphysalis ticks. PLoS Pathog. 2008 May 16;4(5):e1000062. PMID:18483546

Tuo W, Estes DM, Brown WC. Comparative effects of interleukin-12 and interleukin-4 on cytokine responses by antigen-stimulated memory CD4+ T cells of cattle: IL-12 enhances IFN-gamma production, whereas IL-4 has marginal effects on cytokine expression. J Interferon Cytokine Res. 1999 Jul;19(7):741-9. PMID:10454344

van Duivenvoorde LM, Voorberg-van der Wel A, van der Werff NM, Braskamp G, Remarque EJ, Kondova I, Kocken CH, Thomas AW. Suppression of Plasmodium cynomolgi in rhesus macaques by coinfection with Babesia microti. Infect Immun. 2010 Mar;78(3):1032-9. Epub 2010 Jan 4. PMID:20048045

Van Solingen RM, Evans J. Lyme disease. Curr Opin Rheumatol. 2001 Jul;13(4):293-9. PMID:11555731

Vannier E, Gewurz BE, Krause PJ. Human babesiosis. Infect Dis Clin North Am. 2008 Sep;22(3):469-88, viii-ix. PMID:18755385

Vannier E, Krause PJ. Update on babesiosis. Interdiscip Perspect Infect Dis. 2009;2009:984568. Epub 2009 Aug 27. PMID:19727410

Vyas JM, Telford SR, Robbins GK. Treatment of refractory Babesia microti infection with atovaquone-proguanil in an HIV-infected patient: case report. Clin Infect Dis. 2007 Dec 15;45(12):1588-90. PMID:18190320

Wang TJ, Liang MH, Sangha O, Phillips CB, Lew RA, Wright EA, Berardi V, Fossel AH, Shadick NA. Coexposure to Borrelia burgdorferi and Babesia microti does not worsen the long-term outcome of lyme disease. Clin Infect Dis. 2000 Nov;31(5):1149-54. Epub 2000 Nov 6. PMID:11073744

Weinberg GA. Laboratory diagnosis of ehrlichiosis and babesiosis. Pediatr Infect Dis J. 2001 Apr;20(4):435-7. PMID:11332670

Weiss LM. Babesiosis in humans: a treatment review. Expert Opin Pharmacother. 2002 Aug;3(8):1109-15. PMID:12150690

Wójcik-Fatla A, Cisak E, Chmielewska-Badora J, Zwoliński J, Buczek A, Dutkiewicz

J. Prevalence of Babesia microti in Ixodes ricinus ticks from Lublin region (eastern Poland). Ann Agric Environ Med. 2006;13(2):319-22. PMID:17196008

Wong WS, Chung JY, Wong KF. Images in haematology. Human babesiosis. Br J Haematol. 2008 Feb;140(4):364. Epub 2007 Nov 27. PMID:18042268

Wormser GP, Lombardo G, Silverblatt F, El Khoury MY, Prasad A, Yelon JA, Sanda A, Karim S, Coku L, Savino JA. Babesiosis as a cause of fever in patients undergoing a splenectomy. Am Surg. 2011 Mar;77(3):345-7. PMID:21375849

Wormser GP, Prasad A, Neuhaus E, Joshi S, Nowakowski J, Nelson J, Mittleman A, Aguero-Rosenfeld M, Topal J, Krause PJ. Emergence of resistance to azithromycin-atovaquone in immunocompromised patients with Babesia microti infection. Clin Infect Dis. 2010 Feb 1;50(3):381-6. PMID:20047477

Yabsley MJ, Davidson WR, Stallknecht DE, Varela AS, Swift PK, Devos JC Jr, Dubay SA. Evidence of tick-borne organisms in mule deer (Odocoileus hemionus) from the western United States. Vector Borne Zoonotic Dis. 2005 Winter;5(4):351-62. PMID:16417431

Yabsley MJ, Romines J, Nettles VF. Detection of Babesia and Anaplasma species in rabbits from Texas and Georgia, USA. Vector Borne Zoonotic Dis. 2006 Spring;6(1):7-13. PMID:16584322

Yamasaki M, Tajima M, Yamato O, Hwang SJ, Ohta H, Maede Y. Heat shock response of Babesia gibsoni heat shock protein 70. J Parasitol. 2008 Feb;94(1):119-24. PMID:18372630

Yoshinari NH, Abrão MG, Bonoldi VL, Soares CO, Madruga CR, Scofield A, Massard CL, da Fonseca AH. Coexistence of antibodies to tick-borne agents of babesiosis and Lyme borreliosis in patients from Cotia county, State of São Paulo, Brazil. Mem Inst Oswaldo Cruz. 2003 Apr;98(3):311-8. Epub 2003 Jul 18. PMID:12886408

Yu DH, Li YH, Yoon JS, Lee JH, Lee MJ, Yu IJ, Chae JS, Park JH. Ehrlichia chaffeensis infection in dogs in South Korea. Vector Borne Zoonotic Dis. 2008 Jun;8(3):355-8. PMID:18399775

Zamoto A, Tsuji M, Kawabuchi T, Wei Q, Asakawa M, Ishihara C. U.S.-type Babesia microti isolated from small wild mammals in Eastern Hokkaido, Japan. J Vet Med Sci. 2004 Aug;66(8):919-26. PMID:15353841

Zamoto A, Tsuji M, Wei Q, Cho SH, Shin EH, Kim TS, Leonova GN, Hagiwara K, Asakawa M, Kariwa H, Takashima I, Ishihara C. Epizootiologic survey for Babesia microti among small wild mammals in northeastern Eurasia and a geographic diversity in the beta-tubulin gene sequences. J Vet Med Sci. 2004 Jul;66(7):785-92. PMID:15297749

Zhao Y, Love KR, Hall SW, Beardell FV. A fatal case of transfusion-transmitted babesiosis in the State of Delaware. Transfusion. 2009 Dec;49(12):2583-7. Epub 2009 Nov 9. PMID:19906041

Zivkovic Z, Torina A, Mitra R, Alongi A, Scimeca S, Kocan KM, Galindo RC, Almazán C, Blouin EF, Villar M, Nijhof AM, Mani R, La Barbera G, Caracappa S, Jongejan F, de la Fuente J. Subolesin expression in response to pathogen infection in ticks. BMC Immunol. 2010 Feb 19;11:7. PMID:20170494

Zobba R, Parpaglia ML, Spezzigu A, Pittau M, Alberti A. First molecular identification and phylogeny of a Babesia sp. from a symptomatic sow (Sus scrofa Linnaeus 1758). J Clin Microbiol. 2011 Jun;49(6):2321-4. Epub 2011 Apr 13. PMID:21490184

LYME DISEASE SYMPTOM CHECKLIST
James Schaller, M.D., M.A.R.

INTRODUCTION

The following checklist is not meant to be complete or authoritative. Information about Lyme disease is constantly emerging and changing. Therefore any checklist is intended for use as a starting point. In traditional medicine, a physician performs a complete history and physical. Labs and studies **assist** in clarifying the differential diagnosis. In Lyme disease, much debate exists about laboratory kits, the alteration of kits to have fewer possible bands, and which labs are optimally sensitive and specific. This checklist is not intended to address that issue or treatment.

Over 200 animals carry the Ixodes tick, which is the most commonly known insect spreading Lyme disease. With so many vectors, the underlying assumption behind this checklist is that Lyme is not rare in North America, Europe, South America, Russia, Africa or Asia.

We know Lyme disease is highly under-reported. One study showed only 1 in 40 family doctors reported it.

Immediately upon biting, the tick transmits a pain killer, antihistamine and an anti-coagulant. Based on animal studies, it is also possible the bulls-eye rash is less common than assumed, in part because injections of spirochete related material in laboratory animals only show a rash with the **second** injection. With this background, I would appeal, that if a young or middle aged adult experiences a bite, and has profound symptoms, is it possible this was a small number of infectious particles igniting a larger number from 2, 5 or 20 years earlier? I am not asking for an answer, just for the possibility to be considered.

This checklist is offered with the sincere wish that others will improve on it. It is this author's personal belief that tick and flea-borne infection medicine is as specialized as HIV and Hepatitis medical science and treatment.

Some of the checklist materials might be new to you, which underscores the need for another scale to add to the ones currently in existence. This list is based on a massive review of thousands of papers over a decade of full-time reading, 2012 science revelations, and/or massive chart reviews. Since modern Lyme disease seems to focus on tick-borne disease and other laboratory testing, we will start with lab testing considerations. If a lab test has a value or a percentage, the numbers chosen are intended to avoid missing those positive patients who otherwise would be overlooked. The concern is about physicians and other healthcare workers not treating an infected patient, who over time can experience disability or even death at a frequency that is impossible to determine.

THE LYME DISEASE CHECKLIST
James Schaller, M.D., M.A.R.
(Please Check Any Symptoms That Apply)

LABORATORY TESTING — INDIRECT AND DIRECT

☐ Vitamin D level is in the lowest 20%.   If you supplement, it should be in top 50%.

☐ CD57 or CD58 is in the lowest 20th percentile.

☐ Free testosterone is in 10th percentile or below.

☐ In 5% of patients the testosterone or free testosterone is over the normal range.

☐ DHEA is in lower 20%. Or rarely is it fully over the top level.

☐ Free dihydrotestosterone is in the lowest 20th percentile or well over the normal range.

☐ Epstein Barr Virus is abnormal in any measure. [This virus is believed to be positive over normal positive levels in the presence of infections or high inflammation.]

☐ On the Western Blot, IgG or IgM any *species specific* band at any blood level, e.g., 18, 21, 23, 30, 31, 34, 37, 39, 83, 93.

☐ A free T3 level under 2.8 [the normal bottom range in 1990 was 2.6; the influx of large numbers of elderly patients reset the healthy "normal" range].

☐ Positive for viruses such as CMV, HHV-6, Coxsackie B Types 1, 2, 3, 4, 5, 6, Parvo B-19 or Powassan virus

☐ Positive for Mycoplasma, e.g. mycoplasma pneumonia

☐ The patient is positive for infections other than **routine** Lyme, [that is **Borrelia burgdorferi sensu stricto,** Borrelia **afzelii** and Borrelia **garinii**]. Some of the other infections also carried by infectious ticks, fleas or other vectors include Babesia (duncani, microti or other), Anaplasma (HGA), Ehrlichia (various species/strains), Neoehrlichia, Rocky Mountain or other Spotted Fevers, Brucellosis, Q-fever, STARI (Master's Disease), Malaria, and Bartonella [e.g., B. henselae, B. quintana, B. elizabethae and B. melophagi].   Once tests are commercially available for testing all forms of protozoa affecting humans, including FL1953, all Bartonella species, and Borrelia miyamotoi and other Lyme species, reporting should increase.

☐ IL-B is in lowest 10th percentile.

☐ IL-6 is in lowest 10th percentile.

☐ TNF-alpha is under 2, or in lowest 20th percentile.

☐ A WBC count was, or is, under 4.5.

☐ Eosinophil level in the CBC manual exam is either at 0-1 or 6-7.

☐ Total manual Eosinophil level is 140 or less.

☐ X-ray or other study shows cartilage defects in excess of injury or age median.

☐ If a full auto-immunity panel is run with at least eight different tests, two are positive; for example, you have a positive anti-gliadin and a positive thyroid peroxidase.

☐ Positive or near positive (borderline) ELISA, PCR, or a positive tissue biopsy; or a tick from your body is positive for Lyme or other tick infection

☐ Lab tests show high inflammation, e.g., a high C4a, elevated cholesterol and C-peptide. These are never specific just for Lyme.

☐ Lab tests show a MSH level under 30 [the reference range of 0-40 is due to the increase of very sick patients tested, and 40-85 is a better reference range which was used before the flood of the sick reset the range of normal]. MSH is an anti-inflammatory hormone.

☐ VIP is under 20. This is an anti-inflammation chemical.

BODY EXAMINATION RESULTS

☐ Weight loss or gain in excess of 20 pounds in 12 weeks

☐ A round or oval rash with a dark center was or is present in a loose "bulls-eye pattern" or other size and shape rashes that have no other cause after exposure to ticks and vectors

☐ Healing is slow after scratches or surgery. For example, after a cat scratch, flea bite or tick bite the mark is still visible later.

☐ Skin on arms, hands or feet has a texture like rice paper.

☐ Clear reaction and effect is seen with antibiotic treatment. Specifically, a marked improvement or worsening of a serious medical problem or function is observed with a spirochete killing treatment, e.g., doxycycline, tetracycline, minocycline, any penicillin such as amoxicillin, azithromycin, clarithromycin or cefuroxime.

☐ Presence of skin tags, red papules of any size, excess blood vessels compared to peers, and stretch marks with color or in significant excess of peers.

☐ Moles and raised or hard plaques in excess of the few on normal skin

☐ Areas of skin with ulcerations such as those seen in syphilis, but at any location on the body

☐ Areas of clear hypo-pigmentation and hyper-pigmentation

☐ Positive ACA (Acrodermatitis chronica atrophicans) which is a sign of long term untreated Lyme disease. Some report ACA begins as a reddish-blue patch of discolored skin, often of the hands or feet. It may include the back in some patients. The lesion slowly atrophies over months to years, with many developing skin that is thin, dry, hairless, wrinkled and abnormally colored. The color of the extremities such as hands and feet can be red, dark red, brown, dark blue or purple.

Sample Neurological Exam

☐ Patient's short-term memory is poor. For example, if asked to recall these numbers—23, 5, 76, 43 and 68—the patient cannot recall them.

☐ Patient cannot reverse four numbers, so if given—18, 96, 23 and 79—the patient cannot do it.

☐ If asked to subtract 17 from 120, (college graduate), it cannot be done in a timely manner. If a high school graduate, subtract 7 from 100 and continue to subtract by 7 four times in 20 seconds.

☐ Light headedness upon standing quickly in excess of peers, and with no clear cause

☐ Dizziness unrelated to position

☐ Dizziness made worse by Lyme killing antibiotics

☐ Trouble doing a nine step **heel to toe straight line walk test** with fingers slightly in pockets [The patient should not sway or need their hands pulled out to prevent a fall].   In patients with past experience in skating, skiing, dance or ballet this should be *very easy* and is rarely a challenge to such people. If it is not easy, it is suspicious medically, but not only for Lyme disease.

☐ Trouble performing a one leg lift, in which one leg is lifted 15 inches off the ground in front of you, as you count, e.g., "one Mississippi, two Mississippi, etc."

☐ Positive nystagmus [your eye jerks when you look right or left]

PATIENT'S REPORTED PHYSICAL HISTORY

Psychiatric & Neurological

☐ Mild to severe neurological disorders or psychiatric disorders

☐ A very profound neurological disease which does not clearly fit the labs, studies and course of the illness

☐ A moderate or severe medical, psychiatric or neurological illness.   [Many severe disorders can be associated with spirochetes such as those causing syphilis, and some propose that Lyme is also related to a well-known serious brain disease.]

☐ Severe medical, psychiatric or neurology illness with uncommon features, such as Parkinson's disease, appearing at a young age

☐ Facial paralysis (Bell's palsy)

☐ Personality has changed negatively and significantly for no clear reason.

☐ Psychosis at any age, but especially after 40 years of age when *usually* it would have already manifested itself

☐ Severe anxiety

☐ Mania or profound rage

☐ Depression with minimal genetic risk

☐ Depression or anxiety that did not exist when you were less than 25 years of age

☐ Irritability

☐ Any one of the following: paranoia, dementia, schizophrenia, bipolar disorder, panic attacks, major depression, anorexia nervosa or obsessive-compulsive disorder

☐ Adult onset ADHD/ADD [Primary psychiatric biological ADD or ADHD is present at 7 years of age. Adult onset may be a sign of a medical condition.]

☐ Increased verbal or physical fighting with others

☐ Functioning at work or in parenting is at least 20% reduced

☐ Patience and relational skills are decreased by 20% or more

☐ A mild to profound decrease of insight, i.e., an infected patient does not see their decreased function, failed treatment or personality change

☐ A new eccentric rigidity to hearing new medical or other important information

☐ Difficulty thinking or concentrating

☐ Poor memory and reduced ability to concentrate

☐ Increasingly difficult to recall names of people or things

☐ Difficulty speaking or reading

☐ Difficulty finding the words to express what you want to say

☐ Inability to learn new information as well as in the past [receptive learning]

☐ Repeating stories or forgetting information told to close relations, such as a spouse, roommate, sibling, best friend or parent

☐ Confusion without a clear reason

☐ An addiction that results in relapse in spite of sincere, reasonable and serious efforts to stop

☐ Fatigue in excess of normal, or fatigue that is getting worse

☐ Trouble sleeping including mild to severe insomnia and disrupted sleep

☐ Sleep in excess of 9 hours a day or night, or sleeping in excess of 9 hours every day if allowed

☐ Trouble falling asleep

☐ Trouble staying asleep [Taking a 5 minute bathroom break does not count]

Major Organs

☐ Gastritis or stomach sensitivity not caused by H. Pylori

☐ Intestinal troubles that are unable to be fully managed and/or which have no clear diagnosis

☐ Nausea without a clear reason

☐ Ear problems such as pain or increased ear "pressure"

☐ *Any trouble* with the senses (vision, sound, touch, taste or smell). The use of corrective lenses or contacts does not count, unless the prescription is changed more than expected.

☐ Buzzing or ringing in ears

☐ Double vision, floaters, dry eyes, or other vision trouble

☐ Conjunctivitis (pinkeye) or occasional damage to deep tissue in the eyes

☐ Bladder dysfunction of any kind

☐ Treatment resistant interstitial cystitis

☐ Blood clots fast when you get a cut, or you have a diagnosed problem with clotting. This may also be seen in blood draws where blood draw needle clots when blood is being removed. If on a blood thinner, blood thinness level goes up and down too much.

☐ Cardiac impairment

☐ Chest pain with all labs and studies in normal range

☐ Occasional rapid heartbeats (palpitations)

☐ Heart block/heart murmur

☐ Heart valve prolapse

☐ Shortness of breath with no clear cause on pulmonary function tests, examination, lab testing, X-rays, MRI's, etc.

☐ Air hunger or feelings of shortness of breath

Skin

☐ Numbness, tingling, burning, or shock sensations in an area of skin

☐ One or more troublesome skin sensations that move over months or years and do not always stay in one location

☐ Rash or rashes without a simple and obvious cause

☐ Rashes that persist despite treatment

☐ Eccentric itching with no clear cause

☐ Hair loss with no clear cause

Musculoskeletal

☐ Muscle pain or cramps

☐ Muscle spasms

☐ Muscle wasting without a clear cause

☐ Trouble with your jaw muscle(s) or joint insomnia (TMJ)

☐ Joint defects in one joint with no clear cause if 20 or younger

☐ Joint defects in two joints or more if 35 or younger

☐ Joint defects in three or more locations if younger than 55 with no clear trauma

☐ Swelling or pain (inflammation) in the joints [Most patients *never* have joint disease.]

☐ Joint pain that shifts location

☐ Neck stiffness

☐ Chronic arthritis with or without episodes of swelling, redness, and fluid buildup

General Medical

☐ Gaining or losing weight in a manner clearly inconsistent with diet and exercise

☐ New or more food allergies than ten years ago

☐ Feel worse after eating breads, pasta or sweets

☐ No longer tolerate or enjoy alcohol

☐ Anti-histamines are bothersome, more so than in the past.

☐ Reaction to medications is excessive (you are very "sensitive" to medications)

☐ Your response to antibiotics is significantly positive and you feel more functional, *or you have the opposite reaction* and feel worse, feeling ill, fatigued or agitated.

☐ Chronic pain in excess of what seems reasonable

☐ Nerve pain without a clear cause

☐ Sensitivity to lights, sounds, touch, smell or unusual tastes

☐ Sensitivity to cleaning chemicals, fragrances and perfumes

☐ Headaches that do not respond fully to treatment, or which are getting worse

☐ New allergies or increased allergies over those of your peers

☐ Any autoimmunity--Lyme and other tick infections, over many years, increase inflammation and decrease anti-inflammation chemicals. We believe this leads to increased food sensitivities, increased autoimmunity and a heightened sensitivity to various chemicals and medications.

☐ Day time sweats

- ☐ Night time sweats

- ☐ Chills

- ☐ Flu-like symptoms

- ☐ Abnormal menstrual cycle

- ☐ Decreased or increased libido

- ☐ Increased motion sickness

- ☐ Fainting

- ☐ A spinning sensation or vertigo

- ☐ Illnesses that come and go and decrease functioning with no certain cause

- ☐ Serious illnesses that undermine function with no clear cause, and which affect more than one body organ

- ☐ An abnormal lab result, physical exam finding or illness that is given many diagnoses or has no clear cause

ENVIRONMENT

- ☐ Someone in your neighborhood within 400 yards in any direction of your dwelling has been diagnosed with a tick borne infection [This includes vacation locations].

- ☐ You have someone living with you with any type of tick-borne infection—this assumes they were not merely tested for one infection. [It is not proven that the small Lyme-carrying ticks only carry Lyme, and it is possible some carry other infections without carrying Lyme at all.

- ☐ You have removed any ticks *from your body* in your lifetime at any location.

☐ You have removed ticks *from your clothing* in your lifetime at any location.

☐ After a tick or bug bite, you had a fever for at least 48 hours.

☐ After a tick or bug bite, you were ill.

☐ Grew up or played in areas with many small wild mammals

☐ When you are in a room that has visible mold or smells like mold and you start to feel ill, you do not return to your baseline health in 24 hours.

☐ Any discomfort *within two minutes* of being in a musty or moldy location. This may be a sign of chronic untreated infection, because a mere 30 inhalations of mold debris causes systemic effects in your body

☐ *Pets or farm animals* positive with ANY tick borne virus, bacteria or protozoa, or clinical symptoms without a clear diagnosis or cause

☐ The patient's **mother** is suspected of having or has been diagnosed with Babesia, Ehrlichia, Rocky Mountain Spotted Fever, Anaplasma, Lyme, Bartonella or other tick borne disease based on newer direct and indirect testing, or clinical signs and symptoms.

☐ **A sibling, father, spouse or child** with any tick borne infection

☐ **Casual or work-related exposure to outdoor environments** with brush, wild grasses, wild streams or woods (Examples- golf courses, parks, gardens, river banks, swamps, etc.)

☐ Pets, e.g., horses, dogs or cats, have had **outdoor exposures** to areas such as brush, wild grasses, wild streams or woods.

☐ You played in grass in the past.

☐ You have been bitten by fleas.

☐ You have been scratched by a cat or dog.

FINAL WORDS

Some of the above listed signs and symptoms fit other infections that may be more common than Lyme disease. Unfortunately, the research and experience indicating diverse infections carried by the Ixodes and other ticks is ignored so a small number of symptoms and signs were added to this checklist. Further, "testing" usually involves one test for a mono-infection—Borrelia or Lyme. Ticks and other vectors should never be assumed to carry only Lyme disease.

Please note that when we are talking about the Ixodes tick we are *not* referring to this as a "deer tick" since it has over 200 vectors (Ostfeld). **Many of the tick reduction options presently suggested are not successful in accomplishing their goals.** Reducing deer populations, once thought to reduce tick populations and incidence of Lyme disease, may simply increase tick numbers in mammals and other carriers that live closer to humans.

All healers have their familiar way of thinking, testing and treating. Kuhn has shown we are all biased and struggle to be objective...and fail. Certainty is simply impossible in medical science. Further, tick and flea infections have almost infinite pathological effects because the human body and these clusters of infections are so complex. I have not suggested a grid or a set number of symptoms, because one would not fit this list. Simply, the goal of this checklist is to have you think broadly.

You cannot use this checklist to diagnose Lyme disease or to rule it out.

A Lyme checklist is very medically important, since it is still an emerging illness and can sometimes disable or increase mortality risk in patients of any age if not diagnosed and treated early in the infection.

Writings in the past fifteen years have either viewed Babesia and Bartonella as mere "co-infections," or a footnote of a spirochete infection [i.e., Lyme]. Either infection can hide for decades, and then possibly disable or kill a person by causing a clot, heart arrhythmia or by other means.

The detection of Lyme from stained tissue samples or blood is very difficult. Currently, the well-established indirect lab test patterns presented are not used or understood by all health care professionals.   While this is fully understandable, I hope it may change in the coming decade. Tick infections have *systemic impacts* on the body, and are not limited to effects reported in journal articles, a few books or any national or international guidelines.

Dr. Schaller has published the four most recent textbooks on Babesia and the only recent textbook in any language on Bartonella.   His most recent book on Lyme, Babesia and Bartonella includes a "researchers only" list of over 2,600 references considered to be **a start** for basic education in tick infection medicine.

He published articles on both Babesia as a cancer primer and Bartonella as a profound psychiatric disease under the supervision of the former editor of the *Journal of the American Medical Association (JAMA)*. He also published entries on multiple tick and flea-borne infections, including Babesia, Bartonella and Lyme disease, in a respected infection textbook endorsed by the NIH Director of Infectious Disease.

Dr. Schaller is the author of seven texts on tick and flea-borne infections. He is rated a BEST physician, an honor that is awarded to only 1 in 20 physicians by physician peers. He is also rated a TOP physician by patients, again ranking in the top 5 percent of physicians.

Copyright © 2011 JAMES SCHALLER, M.D., M.A.R. version 25.

This form may not be altered if it is printed or posted, in any manner, without written permission. It can be printed for free to assist in diagnostic reflections, as long as no line is redacted or altered, including the introduction or final paragraphs. Dr. Schaller does not claim that this is a flawless or final form, and defers all diagnostic decisions to your licensed health professional.

Bibliography (Lyme Disease)

Aalto A, Sjöwall J, Davidsson L, Forsberg P, Smedby O. Brain magnetic resonance imaging does not contribute to the diagnosis of chronic neuroborreliosis. Acta Radiol. 2007 Sep;48(7):755-62. PMID:17729007

Aberer E. [Neuroborreliosis or Borrelia hysteria. This case becomes a nightmare!].[Article in German]. MMW Fortschr Med. 2006 Nov 9;148(45):8. PMID:17615738

Aboul-Enein F, Kristoferitsch W. Normal pressure hydrocephalus or neuroborreliosis? Wien Med Wochenschr. 2009;159(1-2):58-61. PMID:19225737

Alaedini A, Latov N. Antibodies against OspA epitopes of Borrelia burgdorferi cross-react with neural tissue. J Neuroimmunol. 2005 Feb;159(1-2):192-5. Epub 2004 Nov 26. PMID:15652419

Angelakis E, Billeter SA, Breitschwerdt EB, Chomel BB, Raoult D. Potential for tick-borne bartonellosis. Emerg Infect Dis. 2010 Mar;16(3):385-91.

Auwaerter PG. Point: antibiotic therapy is not the answer for patients with persisting symptoms attributable to lyme disease. Clin Infect Dis. 2007 Jul 15;45(2):143-8. Epub 2007 Jun 5. PMID:17578771

Banarer M, Cost K, Rychwalski P, Bryant KA. Chronic lymphocytic meningitis in an adolescent. J Pediatr. 2005 Nov;147(5):686-90. PMID:16291364

Baneth G, Breitschwerdt EB, Hegarty BC, Pappalardo B, Ryan J. A survey of tick-borne bacteria and protozoa in naturally exposed dogs from Israel. Vet Parasitol. 1998 Jan 31;74(2-4):133-42.

Barbour AG. Laboratory aspects of Lyme borreliosis. Clin Microbiol Rev 1988 Oct;1(4):415-31.

Barie PS. Warning! Danger Will Robinson! Lyme disease clinical practice guidelines of the Infectious Diseases Society of America, activist patients, antitrust law, and prosecutorial zeal. Surg Infect (Larchmt). 2007 Apr;8(2):147-50. PMID:17437359

Batinac T, Petranovic D, Zamolo G, Petranovic D, Ruzic A. Lyme borreliosis and multiple sclerosis are associated with primary effusion lymphoma. Med Hypotheses. 2007;69(1):117-9. Epub 2007 Jan 2. PMID:17197115

Begon E. [Lyme arthritis, Lyme carditis and other presentations potentially associated to Lyme disease].[Article in French]. Med Mal Infect. 2007 Jul-Aug;37(7-8):422-34. Epub 2007 Aug 14. PMID:17698309

Benhnia MR, Wroblewski D, Akhtar MN, Patel RA, Lavezzi W, Gangloff SC, Goyert SM, Dvoráková J, Celer V. [Pharmacological aspects of Lyme borreliosis].[Article in Czech]. Ceska Slov Farm. 2004 Jul;53(4):159-64. PMID:15369225

Bhate C, Schwartz RA. Lyme disease: Part II. Management and prevention. J Am Acad Dermatol. 2011 Apr;64(4):639-53; quiz 654, 653. PMID:21414494

Biesiada G, Czapiel J, Sobczyk-Krupiarz I, Garlicki A, Mach T. Neuroborreliosis with extrapyramidal symptoms: a case report. Pol Arch Med Wewn. 2008 May;118(5):314-7. PMID:18619183

Billeter SA, Levy MG, Chomel BB, Breitschwerdt EB. Vector transmission of Bartonella species with emphasis on the potential for tick transmission. Med Vet Entomol. 2008 Mar;22(1):1-15.

Bitar I, Lally EV. Musculoskeletal manifestations of Lyme disease. Med Health R I. 2008 Jul;91(7):213-5. PMID:18705221

Blanc F. [Epidemiology of Lyme borreliosis and neuroborreliosis in France].[Article in French]. Rev Neurol (Paris). 2009 Aug-Sep;165(8-9):694-701. Epub 2009 May 17. PMID:19447458

Blanc F; GEBLY. [Neurologic and psychiatric manifestations of Lyme disease].[Article in French]. Med Mal Infect. 2007 Jul-Aug;37(7-8):435-45. Epub 2007 Mar 9. PMID:17350199

Bransfield RC, Wulfman JS, Harvey WT, Usman AI. The association between tick-borne infections, Lyme borreliosis and autism spectrum disorders. Med Hypotheses. 2008;70(5):967-74. Epub 2007 Nov 5. PMID:17980971

Brehm M, Rellecke P, Strauer BE. [Inflammatory cardiac diseases by primary extracardial diseases].[Article in German]. Internist (Berl). 2008 Jan;49(1):27-33. PMID:17992497

Breitschwerdt EB. Feline bartonellosis and cat scratch disease. Vet Immunol Immunopathol. 2008 May 15;123(1-2):167-71. Epub 2008 Jan 19. Review.

Breitschwerdt EB, Atkins CE, Brown TT, Kordick DL, Snyder PS. Bartonella vinsonii subsp. berkhoffii and related members of the alpha subdivision of the Proteobacteria in dogs with cardiac arrhythmias, endocarditis, or myocarditis. J Clin Microbiol. 1999 Nov;37(11):3618-26.

Breitschwerdt EB, Blann KR, Stebbins ME, Muñana KR, Davidson MG, Jackson HA, Willard MD. Clinicopathological abnormalities and treatment response in 24 dogs seroreactive to Bartonella vinsonii (berkhoffii) antigens. J Am Anim Hosp Assoc. 2004 Mar-Apr;40(2):92-101.

Breitschwerdt EB, Hegarty BC, Hancock SI. Sequential evaluation of dogs naturally infected with Ehrlichia canis, Ehrlichia chaffeensis, Ehrlichia equi, Ehrlichia ewingii, or Bartonella vinsonii. J Clin Microbiol. 1998 Sep;36(9):2645-51.

Breitschwerdt EB, Hegarty BC, Maggi R, Hawkins E, Dyer P. Bartonella species as a potential cause of epistaxis in dogs. J Clin Microbiol. 2005 May;43(5):2529-33.

Breitschwerdt EB, Kordick DL. Bartonellosis. J Am Vet Med Assoc. 1995 Jun 15;206(12):1928-31. Review.

Breitschwerdt EB, Kordick DL. Bartonella infection in animals: carriership, reservoir potential, pathogenicity, and zoonotic potential for human infection. Clin Microbiol Rev. 2000 Jul;13(3):428-38. Review.

Breitschwerdt EB, Kordick DL, Malarkey DE, Keene B, Hadfield TL, Wilson K. Endocarditis in a dog due to infection with a novel Bartonella subspecies. J Clin Microbiol. 1995 Jan;33(1):154-60.

Breitschwerdt EB, Maggi RG. A confusing case of canine vector-borne disease: clinical signs and progression in a dog co-infected with Ehrlichia canis and Bartonella vinsonii ssp. berkhoffii. Parasit Vectors. 2009 Mar 26;2 Suppl 1:S3.

Breitschwerdt EB, Maggi RG. Comparative medical features of canine and human bartonellosis. Clin Microbiol Infect. 2009 Dec;15 Suppl 2:106-7. Epub 2009 Apr 30.

Breitschwerdt EB, Maggi RG, Cadenas MB, de Paiva Diniz PP. A groundhog, a novel Bartonella sequence, and my father's death. Emerg Infect Dis. 2009 Dec;15(12):2080-6.

Breitschwerdt EB, Maggi RG, Chomel BB, Lappin MR. Bartonellosis: an emerging infectious disease of zoonotic importance to animals and human beings. J Vet Emerg Crit Care (San Antonio). 2010 Feb;20(1):8-30. Review.

Breitschwerdt EB, Maggi RG, Duncan AW, Nicholson WL, Hegarty BC, Woods CW. Bartonella species in blood of immunocompetent persons with animal and arthropod contact. Emerg Infect Dis. 2007 Jun;13(6):938-41.

Breitschwerdt EB, Maggi RG, Farmer P, Mascarelli PE. Molecular evidence of perinatal transmission of Bartonella vinsonii subsp. berkhoffii and Bartonella henselae to a child. J Clin Microbiol. 2010 Jun;48(6):2289-93. Epub 2010 Apr 14.

Breitschwerdt EB, Maggi RG, Lantos PM, Woods CW, Hegarty BC, Bradley JM. Bartonella vinsonii subsp. berkhoffii and Bartonella henselae bacteremia in a father and daughter with neurological disease. Parasit Vectors. 2010 Apr 8;3(1):29.

Breitschwerdt EB, Maggi RG, Nicholson WL, Cherry NA, Woods CW. Bartonella sp. bacteremia in patients with neurological and neurocognitive dysfunction. J Clin Microbiol. 2008 Sep;46(9):2856-61. Epub 2008 Jul 16.

Breitschwerdt EB, Maggi RG, Robert Mozayeni B, Hegarty BC, Bradley JM, Mascarelli PE. PCR amplification of Bartonella koehlerae from human blood and enrichment blood cultures. Parasit Vectors. 2010 Aug 24;3:76.

Breitschwerdt EB, Maggi RG, Sigmon B, Nicholson WL. Isolation of Bartonella quintana from a woman and a cat following putative bite transmission. J Clin Microbiol. 2007 Jan;45(1):270-2. Epub 2006 Nov 8.

Breitschwerdt EB, Maggi RG, Varanat M, Linder KE, Weinberg G. Isolation of Bartonella vinsonii subsp. berkhoffii genotype II from a boy with epithelioid hemangioendothelioma and a dog with hemangiopericytoma. J Clin Microbiol. 2009 Jun;47(6):1957-60. Epub 2009 Apr 15.

Breitschwerdt EB, Mascarelli PE, Schweickert LA, Maggi RG, Hegarty BC, Bradley JM, Woods CW. Hallucinations, sensory neuropathy, and peripheral visual deficits in a young woman infected with Bartonella koehlerae. J Clin Microbiol. 2011 Sep;49(9):3415-7. Epub 2011 Jul 6.

Breitschwerdt EB, Sontakke S, Cannedy A, Hancock SI, Bradley JM. Infection with Bartonella weissii and detection of Nanobacterium antigens in a North Carolina beef herd. J Clin Microbiol. 2001 Mar;39(3):879-82.

Breitschwerdt EB, Suksawat J, Chomel B, Hegarty BC. The immunologic response of dogs to Bartonella vinsonii subspecies berkhoffii antigens: as assessed by Western immunoblot analysis. J Vet Diagn Invest. 2003 Jul;15(4):349-54.

Brtkova J, Jirickova P, Kapla J, Dedic K,, Pliskova L. Borrelia arthritis and chronic myositis accompanied by typical chronic dermatitis. JBR-BTR. 2008 May-Jun;91(3):88-9. PMID:18661710

Burns RB, Hartman EE. A 58-year-old man with a diagnosis of chronic Lyme disease, 1 year later. JAMA. 2003 Dec 24;290(24):3247. PMID:14693878

Caimano MJ, Radolf JD, Sellati TJ. Signaling through CD14 attenuates the inflammatory response to Borrelia burgdorferi, the agent of Lyme disease. J Immunol. 2005 Feb 1;174(3):1539-48. PMID:15661914

Calza L, Manfredi R, Chiodo F. [Tick-borne infections]. [Article in Italian]. Recenti Prog Med. 2004 Sep;95(9):403-13. PMID:15473378

Cameron D. Obstacles to trials of chronic Lyme disease in actual practice. Minerva Med. 2009 Oct;100(5):435-6. PMID:19910896

Cameron DJ. Clinical trials validate the severity of persistent Lyme disease symptoms. Med Hypotheses. 2009 Feb;72(2):153-6. Epub 2008 Nov 13. PMID:19013025

Cameron DJ. Proof that chronic lyme disease exists. Interdiscip Perspect Infect Dis. 2010;2010:876450. Epub 2010 May 25. PMID:20508824

Cerar T, Ruzic-Sabljic E, Cimperman J, Strle F. Comparison of immunofluorescence assay (IFA) and LIAISON in patients with different clinical manifestations of Lyme borreliosis. Wien Klin Wochenschr. 2006 Nov;118(21-22):686-90. PMID:17160608

Chandra A, Wormser GP, Klempner MS, Trevino RP, Crow MK, Latov N, Alaedini A. Anti-neural antibody reactivity in patients with a history of Lyme borreliosis and persistent symptoms. Brain Behav Immun. 2010 Aug;24(6):1018-24. Epub 2010 Mar 18th PMID:20227484

Chernogor LI, Arbatskaia EV, Danchinova GA, Kozlova IV, Gorina MO, Suntsova OV, Chaporgina EA, Belikov SI, Borisov VA. [Clinical and laboratory characterization of Ixodes tick-borne borreliosis in the Baikal area].[Article in Russian]. Zh Mikrobiol Epidemiol Immunobiol. 2005 Nov-Dec;(6):60-2. PMID:16438378

Chomel BB, Boulouis HJ, Maruyama S, Breitschwerdt EB. Bartonella spp. in pets and effect on human health. Emerg Infect Dis. 2006 Mar;12(3):389-94. PMID 16704774

Clarissou J, Song A, Bernedo C, Guillemot D, Dinh A, Ader F, Perronne C, Salomon J. Efficacy of a long-term antibiotic treatment in patients with a chronic Tick Associated Poly-organic Syndrome (TAPOS). Med Mal Infect. 2009 Feb;39(2):108-15. Epub 2009 Jan 4. PMID:19124209

Comer JA, Diaz T, Vlahov D, Monterroso E, Childs JE. Evidence of rodent-associated Bartonella and Rickettsia infections among intravenous drug users from Central and East Harlem, New York City. Am J Trop Med Hyg. 2001 Dec;65(6):855-60. PMID:11791987

Comer JA, Flynn C, Regnery RL, Vlahov D, Childs JE. Antibodies to Bartonella species in inner-city intravenous drug users in Baltimore, Md. Arch Intern Med. 1996 Nov 25;156(21):2491-5. PMID:8944742

Coyle PK. Lyme disease. In: Feldmann E, ed. Current diagnosis in neurology. St Louis:Mosby,1994; pp 110-4.

Coyle PK ed. Lyme Disease. St. Louis:Mosby Year Book 1993; pp 187-91.

Clark JR, Carlson RD, Sasaki CT, Pachner AR, Steere AC. Facial paralysis in Lyme disease. Laryngoscope 1985 Nov;95(11):1341-5.

Créange A. [Clinical manifestations and epidemiological aspects leading to a diagnosis of Lyme borreliosis: neurological and psychiatric manifestations in the course of Lyme borreliosis]. [Article in French]. Med Mal Infect. 2007 Jul-Aug;37(7-8):532-9. Epub 2007 Mar 26. PMID:17368785 da Franca I, Santos L, Mesquita T, Collares-Pereira M, Baptista S, Vieira L, Viana I, Vale E, Prates C. Lyme borreliosis in Portugal caused by Borrelia lusitaniae? Clinical report on the first patient with a positive skin isolate. Wien Klin Wochenschr. 2005 Jun;117(11-12):429-32. PMID:16053200

Danz B, Kreft B, Radant K, Marsch WCh, Fiedler E. Skin-coloured facial oedema as an initial manifestation of acrodermatitis chronica atrophicans. J Eur Acad Dermatol Venereol. 2008 Jun;22(6):751-3. PMID:18482035

Dattwyler RJ, Halperin JJ, Volkman DJ, Luft BJ. Treatment of late Lyme borreliosis - randomized comparison of ceftriaxone and penicillin. Lancet 1988 May 28;1(8596):1191-4.

Dattwyler RJ, Luft BJ, Maladorno D, et al. Treatment of late Lyme disease - a comparison of 2 weeks vs 4 weeks of ceftriaxone. VII International Congress on Lyme Borreliosis. San Francisco, June, 1996.

Dattwyler RJ, Wormser GP, Rush TJ, Finkel MF, Schoen RT, Grunwaldt E, Franklin M, Hilton E, Bryant GL, Agger WA, Maladorno D. A comparison of two treatment regimens of ceftriaxone in late Lyme disease. Wien Klin Wochenschr. 2005 Jun;117(11-12):393-7. PMID:16053194

de Freitas MR. Infectious neuropathy. Curr Opin Neurol. 2007 Oct;20(5):548-52. PMID:17885443

De Heller-Milev M, Peter O, Panizzon RG, Laffitte E. [Borrelial erythema of the face].[Article in French]. Ann Dermatol Venereol. 2008 Dec;135(12):852-4. Epub 2008 Oct 26. PMID:19084697

DeLong A. Lyme disease. Med Health R I. 2008 Dec;91(12):390; author reply 390. PMID:19170319

DePietropaolo DL, Powers JH, Gill JM, Foy AJ. Diagnosis of Lyme disease. Del Med J. 2006 Jan;78(1):11-8. PMID:16548394

Dillon R, O'Connell S, Wright S. Lyme disease in the U.K.: clinical and laboratory features and response to treatment. Clin Med. 2010 Oct;10(5):454-7. PMID:21117376

Djukic M, Schmidt-Samoa C, Nau R, von Steinbüchel N, Eiffert H, Schmidt H. The diagnostic spectrum in patients with suspected chronic Lyme neuroborreliosis--the experience from one year of a university hospital's Lyme neuroborreliosis outpatients clinic. Eur J Neurol. 2011 Apr;18(4):547-55. Epub 2010 Oct 27. PMID:20977545

Drancourt M, Tran-Hung L, Courtin J, Lumley H, Raoult D. Bartonella quintana in a 4000-year-old human tooth. J Infect Dis. 2005 Feb 15;191(4):607-11.

Dressler F, Whalen JA, Reinhardt BN, Steere A. Western blotting in the serodiagnosis of Lyme disease. J Infect Dis 1993 Feb;167(2):392-400.

Egle UT. [Chronic borreliosis? No, psychosomatic illness! (interview by Dr. med. Brigitte Moreano)].[Article in German]. MMW Fortschr Med. 2005 May 26;147(21):15. PMID:15966166

Einecke U. [Winter pause was too short--ticks are already becoming mobile].[Article in German]. MMW Fortschr Med. 2008 Mar 13;150(11):12-4. PMID:18447267

Ekerfelt C, Andersson M, Olausson A, Bergström S, Hultman P. Mercury exposure as a model for deviation of cytokine responses in experimental Lyme arthritis: HgCl2 treatment decreases T helper cell type 1-like responses and arthritis severity but delays eradication of Borrelia burgdorferi in C3H/HeN mice. Clin Exp Immunol. 2007 Oct;150(1):189-97. Epub 2007 Aug 2. PMID:17672870

Emedicine Health. Lyme Disease Symptoms. http://www.emedicinehealth.com/lyme_disease/page3_em.htm#Lyme Disease Symptoms

Eskow E, Rao RV, Mordechai E. Concurrent infection of the central nervous system by Borrelia burgdorferi and Bartonella henselae: evidence for a novel tick-borne disease complex. Arch Neurol. 2001 Sep;58(9):1357-63.

Fallon BA, Levin ES, Schweitzer PJ, Hardesty D. Inflammation and central nervous system Lyme disease. Neurobiol Dis. March 2010, 37 (3) :534-41. Epub 2009 Nov 26. PMID:19944760

Fallon BA, Lipkin RB, Corbera KM, Yu S, Nobler MS, Keilp JG, Petkova E, Lisanby SH, Moeller JR, Slavov I, Van Heertum R, Mensh BD, Sackeim HA. Regional cerebral blood flow and metabolic rate in persistent Lyme encephalopathy. Arch Gen Psychiatry. 2009 May;66(5):554-63. PMID:19414715

Fallon BA, Nields JA. Lyme Disease: A Neuropsychiatric Illness. Am J Psychiatry 1994 Nov;151(11):1571-83. PMID:7943444

Feder HM Jr, Abeles M, Bernstein M, Whitaker-Worth D, Grant-Kels JM. Diagnosis, treatment, and prognosis of erythema migrans and Lyme arthritis. Clin Dermatol. 2006 Nov-Dec;24(6):509-20. PMID:17113969

Feder HM Jr , Gerber MA, Luger SW, Ryan SW. Persistence of serum antibodies to Borrelia burgdorferi in patients treated for Lyme disease. Clin Infect Dis 1992 Nov;15(5):788-93.

Feder HM Jr, Johnson BJ, O'Connell S, Shapiro ED, Steere AC, Wormser GP; Ad Hoc International Lyme Disease Group, Agger WA, Artsob H, Auwaerter P, Dumler JS, Bakken JS, Bockenstedt LK, Green J, Dattwyler RJ, Munoz J, Nadelman RB, Schwartz I, Draper T, McSweegan E, Halperin JJ, Klempner MS, Krause PJ, Mead P, Morshed M, Porwancher R, Radolf JD, Smith RP Jr, Sood S, Weinstein A, Wong SJ, Zemel L. A critical appraisal of "chronic Lyme disease". N Engl J Med. 2007 Oct 4;357(14):1422-30. PMID:17914043

Fingerle V, Huppertz HI. [Lyme borreliosis in children. Epidemiology, diagnosis, clinical treatment, and therapy].[Article in German]. Hautarzt. 2007 Jun;58(6):541-50, quiz 551-2. PMID:17729432

Fingerle V, Wilske B. [Stage-oriented treatment of Lyme borreliosis].[Article in German]. MMW Fortschr Med. 2006 Jun 22;148(25):39-41. PMID:16859159

Finkel MJ, Halperin JJ. Nervous system Lyme neuroborreliosis revisited. Arch Neurol 1992 Jan;49(1):102-7.

Fomenko NV, Romanova EV, Mel'nikova OV, Chernousova NIa, Epikhina TI. [Detection of Borrelia DNA in the Borrelia burgdorferi sensu lato complex in the blood of patients with Ixodes tick-borne borrelios].[Article in Russian]. Klin Lab Diagn. 2006 Aug;(8):35-7. PMID:17087247

Fürst B, Glatz M, Kerl H, Müllegger RR. The impact of immunosuppression on erythema migrans. A retrospective study of clinical presentation, response to treatment and production of Borrelia antibodies in 33 patients. Clin Exp Dermatol. 2006 Jul;31(4):509-14. Erratum in Clin Exp Dermatol. 2006 Sep;31(5):751. PMID:16716151

Gheorghiev C, De Montleau F, Defuentes G. [Alcohol and epilepsy: a case report between alcohol withdrawal seizures and neuroborreliosis].[Article in French]. Brain. 2011 Jun;37(3):231-7. Epub 2010 December 3. PMID:21703439

Ghosh S, Huber BT. Clonal diversification in OspA-specific antibodies from peripheral circulation of a chronic Lyme arthritis patient. J Immunol Methods. 2007 Apr 10;321(1-2):121-34. Epub 2007 Feb 6. PMID:17307198

Ghosh S, Seward R, Costello CE, Stollar BD, Huber BT. Autoantibodies from synovial lesions in chronic, antibiotic treatment-resistant Lyme arthritis bind cytokeratin-10. J Immunol. 2006 Aug 15;177(4):2486-94. PMID:16888010

Ghosh S, Steere AC, Stollar BD, Huber BT. In situ diversification of the antibody repertoire in chronic Lyme arthritis synovium. J Immunol. 2005 Mar 1;174(5):2860-9. PMID:15728496

Ginsberg L, Kidd D. Chronic and recurrent meningitis. Pract Neurol. 2008 Dec;8(6):348-61. PMID:19015295

Girschick HJ, Morbach H, Tappe D. Treatment of Lyme borreliosis. Arthritis Res Ther. 2009;11(6):258. Epub 2009 Dec 17. PMID:20067594

Gouveia EA, Alves MF, Mantovani E, Oyafuso LK, Bonoldi VL, Yoshinari NH. Profile of patients with Baggio-Yoshinari Syndrome admitted at "Instituto de Emilio Ribas Infectologia ". Rev Inst Med Trop Sao Paulo. 2010 Dec;52(6):297-303. PMID:21225212

Grabe HJ, Spitzer C, Luedemann J, Guertler L, Kramer A, John U, Freyberger HJ, Völzke H. No association of seropositivity for anti-Borrelia IgG antibody with mental and physical complaints. Nord J Psychiatry. 2008;62(5):386-91. PMID:18752103

Grygorczuk S, Hermanowska-Szpakowicz T, Kondrusik M, Pancewicz S, Zajkowska J. [Ehrlichiosis--a disease rarely recognized in Poland].[Article in Polish]. Wiad Lek. 2004;57(9-10):456-61. PMID:15765762

Grygorczuk S, Pancewicz S, Zajkowska J, Kondrusik M, Moniuszko A. [Articular symptoms in Lyme borreliosis]. [Article in Polish]. Pol Merkur Lekarski. 2008 June: 24 (144) :542-4. PMID:18702339

Grygorczuk S, Pancewicz S, Zajkowska J, Kondrusik M, Swierzbińska R, Moniuszko A, Pawlak-Zalewska W. [Reinfection in Lyme borreliosis].[Article in Polish]. Pol Merkur Lekarski. 2008 Sep;25(147):257-9. PMID:19112844

Grygorczuk S, Zajkowska J, Panasiuk A, Kondrusik M, Chmielewski T, Swierzbińska R, Pancewicz S, Flisiak R, Tylewska-Wierzbanowska S. [Activity of the caspase-3 in the culture of peripheral blood mononuclear cells stimulated with Borrelia burgdorferi antigens].[Article in Polish]. Przegl Epidemiol. 2008;62(1):85-91. PMID:18536229

Grygorczuk S, Zajkowska J, Swierzbińska R, Pancewicz S, Kondrusik M, Hermanowska-Szpakowicz T. [Concentrations of soluble factors participating in regulation of apoptosis of lymphocyte from patients with chronic lyme arthritis (preliminary report)].[Article in Polish]. Pol Merkur Lekarski. 2006 Jan;20(115):49-52. PMID:16617735

Hagberg L, Dotevall L. Neuroborreliosis with bad reputation. This is no mystical, difficult-to-treat infection!].[Article in Swedish]. Lakartidningen. 2007 Nov 28-Dec 4;104(48):3621-2. PMID:18193671

Halperin JJ. Prolonged Lyme disease treatment: enough is enough. Neurology. 2008 Mar 25;70(13):986-7. Epub 2007 Oct 10. PMID:17928578

Halperin JJ. Lyme Disease: An Evidence-Based Approach (Advances in Molecular and Cellular Biology Series). Wallingford, Oxfordshire, UK:CABI. 2011.

Halperin JJ, Krupp LB, Golightly MG, Volkman DJ. Lyme borreliosis-associated encephalopathy. Neurology 1990 Sep;40(9):1340-3.

Halperin JJ, Logigian EL, Finkel MF, Pearl RA. Practice parameters for the diagnosis of patients with nervous system Lyme borreliosis (Lyme disease). Neurology 1996 Mar;46(3):619-27. PMID:8618656

Halperin JJ, Shapiro ED, Logigian E, Belman AL, Dotevall
L, Wormser GP, Krupp L, Gronseth G, Bever CT Jr; Quality
Standards Subcommittee of the American Academy of Neurology.
Practice parameter: treatment of nervous system Lyme disease
(an evidence-based review): report of the Quality Standards
Subcommittee of the American Academy of Neurology. Neurology.
2007 Jul 3;69(1):91-102. Epub 2007 May 23. Erratum in
Neurology. 2008 Apr 1;70(14):1223. PMID:17522387

Hamblin T. Is chronic lymphocytic leukemia a response to
infectious agents? Leuk Res. 2006 Sep;30(9):1063-4. Epub 2006
Jan 6. PMID:16406017

Hamlen R. Lyme borreliosis: perspective of a scientist-patient.
Lancet Infect Dis. 2004 Oct;4(10):603-4. PMID:15451481

Hanses F, Audebert FX, Glück T, Salzberger B, Ehrenstein BP.
[Suspected borreliosis - what's behind it?].[Article in German].
Dtsch Med Wochenschr. Aug 2011;136(33):1652-5. Epub 2011
Aug 10th PMID:21833884

Harrer T, Geissdörfer W, Schoerner C, Lang E, Helm G.
Seronegative Lyme neuroborreliosis in a patient on treatment for
chronic lymphatic leukemia. Infection. 2007 Apr;35(2):110-3.
PMID:17401717

Hassler D, Schnauffer M, Ehrfeld H, Müller E. Disappearance of
specific immune response after successful therapy of chronic Lyme
borreliosis. Int J Med Microbiol. 2004 Apr;293 Suppl 37:161-4.
PMID:15147000

Hausotter W. [Appraisal of Lyme borreliosis].[Article in German]
Versicherungsmedizin. 2004 Mar 1;56(1):25-9. PMID:15049470

Hendrickx G, De Boeck H, Goossens A, Demanet C, Vandenplas Y. Persistent synovitis in children with Lyme arthritis: two unusual cases. An immunogenetic approach. Eur J Pediatr. 2004 Nov;163(11):646-50. Epub 2004 Jul 28. PMID:15503133

Hendrickx G, Demanet C, Vandenplas Y. Persistent synovitis in two children with Lyme arthritis linked with HLA-DRB1*1104. Eur J Pediatr. 2006 Jun;165(6):420-1. Epub 2006 Mar 4. PMID:16518608

Hodzic E, Feng S, Holden K, Freet KJ, Barthold SW. Persistence of Borrelia burgdorferi following antibiotic treatment in mice. Antimicrob Agents Chemother. 2008 May;52(5):1728-36. Epub 2008 Mar 3. PMID:18316520

Holmes KD. An appraisal of "chronic Lyme disease". N Engl J Med. 2008 Jan 24;358(4):429; author reply 430-1. PMID:18219749

Hoppa E, Bachur R. Lyme disease update. Curr Opin Pediatr. 2007 Jun;19(3):275-80. PMID:17505186

Horneff G. [Juvenile arthritides].[Article in German]. Z Rheumatol. 2010 Oct;69(8):719-35; quiz 736-7. PMID:20798949

Hospach T, Langendörfer M, Kalle TV, Tewald F, Wirth T, Dannecker GE. Mimicry of lyme arthritis by synovial hemangioma. Rheumatol Int. 2009 Dec 16. [Epub ahead of print] PMID:20013264

Hurley RA, Taber KH. Acute and chronic Lyme disease: controversies for neuropsychiatry. J Neuropsychiatry Clin Neurosci. 2008 Winter;20(1):iv-6. PMID:18305280

Hytönen J, Hartiala P, Oksi J, Viljanen MK. Borreliosis: recent research, diagnosis, and management. Scand J Rheumatol. 2008 May-Jun;37(3):161-72. PMID:18465449

The International Lyme and Associated Diseases Society (ILADS), Evidence-based guidelines for the management of Lyme disease. Expert Rev Anti-infect Ther, 2004. 2(Suppl): p. S1-S13.

Jacomo V, Kelly PJ, Raoult D (2002). Natural history of Bartonella infections (an exception to Koch's postulate). Clin Diagn Lab Immunol. 2002 Jan;9(1):8-18. PMID:11777823

Jakobs M, Morawietz L, Rothschenk H, Hopf T, Weiner S, Schausten H, Krukemeyer

MG, Krenn V. [Synovitis score: value of histopathological diagnostics in unclear arthritis.   Case reports from rheumatological pathological practice].[Article in German]. Z Rheumatol. 2007 Dec;66(8):706-12. PMID:18000669

Jarefors S, Janefjord CK, Forsberg P, Jenmalm MC, Ekerfelt C. Decreased up-regulation of the interleukin-12Rbeta2-chain and interferon-gamma secretion and increased number of forkhead box P3-expressing cells in patients with a history of chronic Lyme borreliosis compared with asymptomatic Borrelia-exposed individuals. Clin Exp Immunol. 2007 Jan;147(1):18-27. PMID:17177959

Johnson BJ, Robbins KE, Bailey RE, Cao BL, Sviat SL, Craven RB, Mayer LW, Dennis DT. Serodiagnosis of Lyme disease: Accuracy of a two-step approach using a flagella-based ELISA and immunoblotting. J Infect Dis 1996 Aug;174(2):346-53. PMID:8699065

Johnson L, Aylward A, Stricker RB. Healthcare access and burden of care for patients with Lyme disease: a large United States survey. Health Policy. 2011 Sep;102(1):64-71. Epub 2011 Jun 14. PMID:21676482

Johnson M, Feder HM Jr. Chronic Lyme disease: a survey of Connecticut primary care physicians. J Pediatr. 2010 Dec;157(6):1025-1029. e1-2. Epub 2010 Sep 1. PMID:20813379

Kaiser R. [Clinical courses of acute and chronic neuroborreliosis following treatment with ceftriaxone].[Article in German]. Nervenarzt. 2004 Jun;75(6):553-7. PMID:15257378

Kalac M, Suvic-Krizanic V, Ostojic S, Kardum-Skelin I, Barsic B, Jaksica B. Central nervous system involvement of previously undiagnosed chronic lymphocytic leukemia in a patient with neuroborreliosis. Int J Hematol. 2007 May;85(4):323-5. PMID:17483076

Kaminsky A. Erythema figuratum. [Article in English, Spanish]. Proceedings Dermosifiliogr. 2009 Dec;100 Suppl 2:88-109. PMID:20096167

Kaplan FR, Jones-Woodward L. Lyme encephalopathy: a neuropsychological perspective. Semin Neurol 1997 Mar;17(1):31-7.

Karlsson M, Hovind-Hougen K, Svenungsson B, Stiernstedt G. Cultivation and characterization of spirochetes from cerebrospinal fluid of patients with Lyme borreliosis. J Clin Microbiol 1990 Mar;28(3):473-9.

Katchanov J, Siebert E, Klingebiel R, Endres M. Infectious vasculopathy of intracranial large- and medium-sized vessels in neurological intensive care unit: a clinical-radiological study. Neurocrit Care. 2010 Jun;12(3):369-74. PMID:20146025

Keller TL, Halperin JJ, Whitman M. PCR detection of Borrelia burgdorferi DNA in cerebrospinal fluid of Lyme neuroborreliosis patients. Neurology 1992 Jan;42(1):32-42.

Kemperman MM, Bakken JS, Kravitz GR. Dispelling the chronic Lyme disease myth. Minn Med. 2008 Jul;91(7):37-41. PMID:18714930

Kestelyn PG. An eye on inflammatory eye disease. Acta Clin Belg. 2005 Sep-Oct;60(5):270-5. PMID:16398326

Kisand KE, Prükk T, Kisand KV, Lüüs SM, Kalbe I, Uibo R. Propensity to excessive proinflammatory response in chronic Lyme borreliosis. APMIS. 2007 Feb;115(2):134-41. PMID:17295680

Kiser, K. In the Lyme light. Minn Med. 2009 Nov;92(11):10-2. PMID:20069988

Klimkiewicz Wolańska-E, Szymanska J, Bachanek T. Orofacial symptoms related to boreliosis--case report. Agric Environ Med Ann. 2010 Dec;17(2):319-21. PMID:21186776

Kohler J, Kern U, Kasper J, Rhese-Kupper B, Thoden U. Chronic central nervous system involvement in Lyme borreliosis. Neurology 1988 Jun;38(6):863-7.

Kordick DL, Breitschwerdt EB. Intraerythrocytic presence of Bartonella henselae. J Clin Microbiol. 1995 Jun;33(6):1655-6.

Kordick DL, Breitschwerdt EB. Relapsing bacteremia after blood transmission of Bartonella henselae to cats. Am J Vet Res. 1997 May;58(5):492-7.

Kordick DL, Breitschwerdt EB. Persistent infection of pets within a household with three Bartonella species. Emerg Infect Dis. 1998 Apr-Jun;4(2):325-8.

Kordick SK, Breitschwerdt EB, Hegarty BC, Southwick KL, Colitz CM, Hancock SI, Bradley JM, Rumbough R, Mcpherson JT, MacCormack JN. Coinfection with multiple tick-borne pathogens in a Walker Hound kennel in North Carolina. J Clin Microbiol. 1999 Aug;37(8):2631-8.

Krause A, Fingerle V. [Lyme borreliosis].[Article in German]. Z Rheumatol. 2009 May;68(3):239-52, quiz 253-4. PMID:19387665

Krause A, Herzer P. [Early diagnosis of Lyme arthritis].[Article in German]. Z Rheumatol. 2005 Nov;64(8):531-7. PMID:16328757

Kremer S, Holl N, Schmitt E, De Sèze J, Moser T, Dieterich JL Mann. [Imaging of non-traumatic and non-tumoral cord lesions]. [Article in French]. J Radiol. 2010 Sep;91(9 Pt 2):969-87. PMID:20814389

Kruger H, Kohlhepp W, Konig S. Follow-up of antibiotically treated and untreated neuroborreliosis. Acta Neurol Scand 1990 Jul;82(1):59-67.

Krupp LB. Lyme disease. In: Samuels MA, Feske S, eds. Office practice of neurology. London:Churchill-Livingstone, 1996; pp 383-7.

Kuenzle S, von Büdingen HC, Meier M, Harrer MD, Urich E, Becher B, Goebels N. Pathogen specificity and autoimmunity are distinct features of antigen-driven immune responses in neuroborreliosis. Infect Immun. 2007 Aug;75(8):3842-7. Epub 2007 May 21. PMID:17517881

Kuhn TS. The structures of scientific revolutions. Chicago: University Of Chicago Press; 3rd edition;1996. Summarized: http://des.emory.edu/mfp/Kuhn.html

LaFleur RL, Dant JC, Wasmoen TL, Callister SM, Jobe DA, Lovrich SD, Warner TF, Abdelmagid OR, Schell RF. Bacterin that induces anti-OspA and anti-OspC borreliacidal antibodies provides a high level of protection against canine Lyme disease. Clin Vaccine Immunol. 2009 Feb;16(2):253-9. Epub 2008 Dec 3. PMID:19052162

Lantos PM. Chronic Lyme disease: the controversies and the science. Expert Rev Anti Infect Ther. 2011 Jul;9(7):787-97. PMID:21810051

Lappin MR, Breitschwerdt E, Brewer M, Hawley J, Hegarty B, Radecki S. Prevalence of Bartonella species antibodies and Bartonella species DNA in the blood of cats with and without fever. J Feline Med Surg. 2009 Feb;11(2):141-8. Epub 2008 Aug 29.

Lee G, Xiang Z, Brannagan TH 3rd, Chin RL, Latov N. Differential gene expression in chronic inflammatory demyelinating polyneuropathy (CIDP) skin biopsies. J Neurol Sci. 2010 Mar 15;290(1-2):115-22. Epub 2009 Nov 17. PMID:19922956

Lesnicar G, Zerdoner D. Temporomandibular joint involvement caused by Borrelia Burgdorferi. J Craniomaxillofac Surg. 2007 Dec;35(8):397-400. Epub 2007 Oct 17. PMID:17942315

Leverkus M., Finner AM, Pokrywka A, Franke I, Gollnick H. Metastatic squamous cell carcinoma of the ankle in long-standing untreated acrodermatitis chronica atrophicans. Dermatology. 2008;217(3):215-8. Epub 2008 Jul 8. PMID:18607109

Liang FT, Brown EL, Wang T, Iozzo RV, Fikrig E. Protective niche for Borrelia burgdorferi to evade humoral immunity. Am J Pathol. 2004 Sep;165(3):977-85. PMID:15331421

Lins H, Wallesch CW, Wunderlich MT. Sequential analyses of neurobiochemical markers of cerebral damage in cerebrospinal fluid and serum in CNS infections. Acta Neurol Scand. 2005 Nov;112(5):303-8. PMID:16218912

Listernick R. A 17-year-old boy previously diagnosed with chronic Lyme disease. Patient complained of low-grade fevers, headaches, pharyngitis, and suspected his mother was trying to poison him. Pediatr Ann. 2004 Aug;33(8):494-8. PMID:15354601

Ljøstad U, Mygland A. [Lyme borreliosis in adults].[Article in Norwegian]. Tidsskr Nor Laegeforen. 2008 May 15;128(10):1175-8. PMID:18480867

Ljøstad U, Mygland A. Remaining complaints 1 year after treatment for acute Lyme neuroborreliosis; frequency, pattern and risk factors. Eur J Neurol. 2010 Jan;17(1):118-23. Epub 2009 Jul 23. PMID:19645771

Logigian EL. Neurologic manifestations of Lyme disease. In: Rahn QW, Evans J, eds. Lyme disease. Philadelphia:ACP, 1998; pp 89-106.

Logigian EL, Kaplan RF, Steere AC. Chronic neurologic manifestations of Lyme disease. N Engl J Med 1990 Nov;323(21):1438-44.

Lu B, PereiraPerrin M. A novel immunoprecipitation strategy identifies a unique functional mimic of the glial cell line-derived neurotrophic factor family ligands in the pathogen Trypanosoma cruzi. Infect Immun. 2008 Aug, 76 (8) :3530-8. Epub 2008 Jun 9. PMID:18541656

Lukashova LV, Karpova MR, Pirogova NP, Kiiutsina TA, Lepekhin AV, Perevozchikova TV, Faĭt EA. [Functional status of peripheral blood monocyte in patients with Ixodes tick-borne borreliosis accompanied by opisthorchiasis].[Article in Russian]. Zh Mikrobiol Epidemiol Immunobiol. 2006 Mar-Apr;(2):81-3. PMID:16758907

Maco V, Maguiña C, Tirado A, Maco V, Vidal JE. Carrion's disease (Bartonellosis bacilliformis) confirmed by histopathology in the High Forest of Peru. Rev Inst Med Trop Sao Paulo. 2004 May-Jun;46(3):171-4. PMID:15286824

Maggi RG, Breitschwerdt EB. Isolation of bacteriophages from Bartonella vinsonii subsp. berkhoffii and the characterization of Pap31 gene sequences from bacterial and phage DNA. J Mol Microbiol Biotechnol. 2005;9(1):44-51.

Maggi RG, Breitschwerdt EB. Potential limitations of the 16S-23S rRNA intergenic region for molecular detection of Bartonella species. J Clin Microbiol. 2005 Mar;43(3):1171-6.

Maloney E. Chronic lyme disease counterpoint. Minn Med. 2008 Aug;91(8):6-7. PMID:18773702

Maloney EL. An appraisal of "chronic Lyme disease". N Engl J Med. 2008 Jan 24;358(4):428-9; author reply 430-1. PMID:18219748

Maloney EL. Article shed no light. Minn Med. 2010 Jan;93(1):6-7. PMID:20191722

Markeljević J, Sarac H, Rados M. Tremor, seizures and psychosis as presenting symptoms in a patient with chronic Lyme neuroborreliosis (LNB). Coll Antropol. 2011 Jan;35 Suppl 1:313-8. PMID:21648354

Marques A. Chronic Lyme disease: a review. Infect Dis Clin North Am. 2008 Jun;22(2):341-60, vii-viii. PMID:18452806

Martí-Martínez S, Martín-Estefanía C, Turpín-Fenoll L, Pampliega-Pérez A, Reus-Bañuls S, García-Barragán N, Villarubia-Lor B. [Bilateral papilloedema as the initial symptom of POEMS syndrome].[Article in Spanish]. Rev Neurol. 2006 Nov 1-15;43(9):531-4. PMID:17072808

Mayer L, Merz S. An appraisal of "chronic Lyme disease". Engl J Med. 2008 Jan 24;358(4):428; author reply 430-1. PMID:18216368

Mayo Clinic Staff. Lyme Disease Symptoms. http://www.mayoclinic.com/health/lyme-disease/DS00116/DSECTION=symptoms

McGill S, Hjelm E, Rajs J, Lindquist O, Friman G. Bartonella spp. antibodies in forensic samples from Swedish heroin addicts. Ann N Y Acad Sci. 2003 Jun;990:409-13. PMID:12860665

Mervin P. Don't deny treatment. Minn Med. 2009 Dec;92(12):6. PMID:20092159

Michau TM, Breitschwerdt EB, Gilger BC, Davidson MG. Bartonella vinsonii subspecies berkhoffi as a possible cause of anterior uveitis and choroiditis in a dog. Vet Ophthalmol. 2003 Dec;6(4):299-304.

Michel JM, Sellal F. ["Reversible" dementia in 2011].[Article in French]. Old Geriatr Psychol neuropsychiatrist. 2011 Jun;9(2):211-25. PMID:21690030

Miklossy J. Chronic inflammation and amyloidogenesis in Alzheimer's disease -- role of Spirochetes. J Alzheimers Dis. 2008 May;13(4):381-91. PMID:18487847

Miklossy J, Kasas S, Zurn AD, McCall S, Yu S, McGeer PL. Persisting atypical and cystic forms of Borrelia burgdorferi and local inflammation in Lyme neuroborreliosis. J Neuroinflammation. 2008 Sep 25;5:40. PMID:18817547

Miklossy J, Khalili K, Gern L, Ericson RL, Darekar P, Bolle L, Hurlimann J, Paster BJ. Borrelia burgdorferi persists in the brain in chronic lyme neuroborreliosis and may be associated with Alzheimer disease. J Alzheimers Dis. 2004 Dec;6(6):639-49; discussion 673-81. PMID:15665404

Miller JC, von Lackum K, Woodman ME, Stevenson B. Detection of Borrelia burgdorferi gene expression during mammalian infection using transcriptional fusions that produce green fluorescent protein. Microb Pathog. 2006 Jul;41(1):43-7. Epub 2006 May 24. PMID:16723206

Mitty J, Margolius D. Updates and controversies in the treatment of Lyme disease. Med Health R I. 2008 Jul;91(7):219, 222-3. PMID:18705223

Moniuszko A, Czupryna P, Zajkowska J, Pancewicz SA, Grygorczuk S, Kondrusik M. [Post Lyme syndrome as a clinical problem]. [Article in Polish]. Pol Merkur Lekarski. 2009 Mar;26(153):227-30. PMID:19388538

Morales SC, Breitschwerdt EB, Washabau RJ, Matise I, Maggi RG, Duncan AW. Detection of Bartonella henselae DNA in two dogs with pyogranulomatous lymphadenitis. J Am Vet Med Assoc. 2007 Mar 1;230(5):681-5.

Mosbacher M, Elliott SP, Shehab Z, Pinnas JL, Klotz JH, Klotz SA. Cat scratch disease and arthropod vectors: more to it than a scratch? J Am Board Fam Med. 2010 Sep-Oct;23(5):685-6. PMID:20823366

Mulleger RR, Millner MM, Stanek, Spork KD. Penicillin G and ceftriaxone in the treatment of neuroborreliosis in children - a prospective study. Infection 1991 Jul-Aug;19(4):279-83.

Mygland A, Skarpaas T, Ljøstad U. Chronic polyneuropathy and Lyme disease. Eur J Neurol. 2006 Nov;13(11):1213-5. PMID:17038034

Nadelman RB, Arlen Z, Wormser GP. Life threatening complications of empiric ceftriaxone for 'seronegative' Lyme disease. South Med J 1991 Oct;84(10):1263-5.

Nafeev AA Klimova LV. [Clinical manifestations of neuroborreliosis in the Volga region].[Article in Russian]. Ter Arkh. 2010;82(11):68-70. PMID:21381354

Narayan K, Dail D, Li L, Cadavid D, Amrute S, Fitzgerald-Bocarsly P, Pachner AR. The nervous system as ectopic germinal center: CXCL13 and IgG in lyme neuroborreliosis. Ann Neurol. 2005 Jun;57(6):813-23. PMID:15929033

Nau R, Christian HJ, Eiffert H. Lyme disease--current state of knowledge. Dtsch Arztebl Int. 2009 Jan;106(5):72-81, 82 quiz, I. Epub 2009 Jan 30. PMID:19562015

Nigrovic LE, Thompson KM. The Lyme vaccine: a cautionary tale. Epidemiol Infect. 2007 Jan;135(1):1-8. Epub 2006 Aug 8. PMID:16893489

[No authors listed] [Differential aspects of multiple sclerosis and chronic borrelial encephalomyelitis].[Article in Russian]. Nevrol Zh Im SS Korsakova Psikhiatr. 2011;111(7):8-12. PMID:21947065

Nocton JJ, Bloom BJ, Rutledge BJ, Logigian EL, Schmid CH, Steere AC. Detection of Borrelia burgdorferi DNA by polymerase chain reaction in cerebrospinal fluid in Lyme neuroborreliosis. J Infect Dis 1996 Sep;174(3):623-7.

Nygård K, Brantsaeter AB, Mehl R. Disseminated and chronic Lyme borreliosis in Norway, 1995 - 2004. Euro Surveill. 2005 Oct;10(10):235-8. PMID:16282646

Ogrinc K, Logar M, Lotric-Furlan S, Cerar D, Ruzić-Sabljić E, Strle F. Doxycycline versus ceftriaxone for the treatment of patients with chronic Lyme borreliosis. Wien Klin Wochenschr. 2006 Nov;118(21-22):696-701. PMID:17160610

Oksi J, Nikoskelainen J, Hiekkanen H, Lauhio A, Peltomaa M, Pitkäranta A, Nyman D, Granlund H, Carlsson SA, Seppälä I, Valtonen V, Viljanen M. Duration of antibiotic treatment in disseminated Lyme borreliosis: a double-blind, randomized, placebo-controlled, multicenter clinical study. Eur J Clin Microbiol Infect Dis. 2007 Aug;26(8):571-81. PMID:17587070

Ostendorf GM. [No work disability in supposed post-borreliosis syndrome. On the decision of the OLG Saarbrücken of 19 May 2010].[Article in German].Versicherungsmedizin. 2011 Jun 1;63(2):106-7. PMID:21698949

Ostfeld RS. Lyme Disease: The Ecology of a Complex System. New York: Oxford University Press. 2011

Pachner AR. Lyme neuroborreliosis. In: Johnson RT, Griffin JW, eds. Current therapy in neurologic disease. St Louis: Mosby, 1997; pp 140-6.

Pachner AR, Delaney E. The polymerase chain reaction in the diagnosis of Lyme neuroborreliosis. Ann Neurol 1993 Oct;34(4):544-50.

Pachner AR, Duray P, Steere AC. Central nervous system manifestations of Lyme disease. Arch Neurol. 1989 Jul;46(7):790-5.

Pachner AR, Steere AC. The triad of neurologic manifestations of Lyme disease: meningitis, cranial neuritis, and radiculoneuritis. Neurology. 1985 Jan;35(1):47-53.

Pancewicz S, Popko J, Rutkowski R, Knaś M, Grygorczuk S, Guszczyn T, Bruczko M, Szajda S, Zajkowska J, Kondrusik M, Sierakowski S, Zwierz K. Activity of lysosomal exoglycosidases in serum and synovial fluid in patients with chronic Lyme and rheumatoid arthritis. Scand J Infect Dis. 2009;41(8):584-9. PMID:19513935

Papo T. [Could aspecific symptoms be related to Borrelia infection?].[Article in French]. Med Mal Infect. 2007 Jul-Aug;37(7-8):507-10. Epub 2007 Mar 13. PMID:17360137

Parish JM. Sleep-related problems in common medical conditions. Chest. 2009 Feb;135(2):563-72. PMID:19201722

Parker M, Turhan V, Aslan M, Musellim B, Hot Topic Y, Ertugrul B. [First report of three culture confirmed human Lyme cases in Turkey].[Article in Turkish]. Find Antimicrob. 2010 Jan;44(1):133-9. PMID:20455410

Persecă T, Feder A, Molnar GB. [Results of etiologic diagnosis in clinical syndrome consistent with acute and chronic borreliosis]. [Article in Romanian]. Rev Med Chir Soc Med Nat Iasi. 2008 Apr-Jun;112(2):496-501. PMID:19295026

Pfister HW. [Clinical aspects of neuroborreliosis].[Article in German]. MMW Fortschr Med. 2010 Jul 1;152(25-27):31-4; quiz 35. PMID:20672660

Pfister HW, Rupprecht TA. Clinical aspects of neuroborreliosis and post-Lyme disease syndrome in adult patients. Int J Med Microbiol. 2006 May;296 Suppl 40:11-6. Epub 2006 Mar 9. PMID:16524775

Phillips SE, Burrascano JJ, Harris NS, Johnson L, Smith PV, Stricker RB. Chronic infection in 'post-Lyme borreliosis syndrome'. Int J Epidemiol. 2005 Dec;34(6):1439-40; author reply 1440-3. Epub 2005 Nov 30. PMID:16319107

Pourel J. [Clinical diagnosis of Lyme borreliosis in case of joint and muscular presentations].[Article in French]. Med Mal Infect. 2007 Jul-Aug;37(7-8):523-31. Epub 2007 Mar 26. PMID:17368783

Przytuła L, Gińdzieńska-Sieśkiewicz E, Sierakowski S. [Diagnosis and treatment of Lyme arthritis].[Article in Polish]. Przegl Epidemiol. 2006;60 Suppl 1:125-30. PMID:16909789

Puéchal X. [Non antibiotic treatments of Lyme borreliosis].[Article in French]. Med Mal Infect. 2007 Jul-Aug;37(7-8):473-8. Epub 2007 Mar 21. PMID:17376627

Puius YA, Kalish RA. Lyme arthritis: pathogenesis, clinical presentation, and management. Infect Dis Clin North Am. 2008 Jun;22(2):289-300, vi-vii. PMID:18452802

Reik L Jr. Lyme Disease and the Nervous System. New York:Thieme Medical Publishers. 1991, pp 57-61.

Reik L Jr. Neurologic aspects of North American Lyme disease. In Lyme Disease, ed. Patricia K. Coyle, M.D. St. Louis:Mosby-Year Book Inc. 1993, pp.101-112.

Renaud I, Cachin C, Gerster JC. Good outcomes of Lyme arthritis in 24 patients in an endemic area of Switzerland. Joint Bone Spine. 2004 Jan;71(1):39-43. PMID:14769519

Reshetova GG, Zaripova TN, Titskaia EV, Moskvin VS, Udintsev SN. [Physical factors in rehabilitation treatment of patients with Ixodes tick-borne borreliosis with primary lesions of the joints]. [Article in Russian]. Vopr Kurortol Fizioter Lech Fiz Kult. 2004 Nov-Dec;(6):10-3. PMID:15717529

Roche Lanquetot MO, Ader F, Durand MC, Carlier R, Defferriere H, Dinh A, Herrmann JL, Guillemot D, Perrone C, Salomon J. [Results of a prospective standardized study of 30 patients with chronic neurological and cognitive disorders after tick bites]. [Article in French]. Med Mal Infect. 2008 Oct;38(10):543-8. PMID:18722064

Rolain JM, Brouqui P, Koehler JE, Maguina C, Dolan MJ, Raoult D. Recommendations for treatment of human infections caused by Bartonella species. Antimicrob Agents Chemother. 2004 Jun;48(6):1921-33. PMID:15155180

Rorat M, Kuchar E, Szenborn L, Małyszczak K. [Growing boreliosis anxiety and its reasons].[Article in Polish]. Psychiatr Pol 2010 Nov-Dec;44(6):895-904. PMID:21449171

Rossi M. [Late manifestations of Lyme borreliosis].[Article in German]. Ther Umsch. 2005 Nov;62(11):745-9. PMID:16350537

Roth J, Scheer I, Kraft S, Keitzer R, Riebel T. Uncommon synovial cysts in children. Eur J Pediatr. 2006 Mar;165(3):178-81. Epub 2005 Dec 13. PMID:16344992

Rudenko N, Golovchenko M, Růzek D, Piskunova N, Mallátová N, Grubhoffer L. Molecular detection of Borrelia bissettii DNA in serum samples from patients in the Czech Republic with suspected borreliosis. FEMS Microbiol Lett. March 2009, 292 (2) :274-81. Epub 2009 Jan 28. PMID:19187198

Samuels DS, Radolf JD, eds. Borrelia: Molecular Biology, Host Interaction and Pathogenesis. Norfolk, UK: Caister Academic Press. 2010.

Savely VR. Update on lyme disease: the hidden epidemic. Brews J Nurs. 2008 Jul-Aug;31(4):236-40. PMID:18641487

Savely V. Lyme disease: a diagnostic dilemma. Nurse Pract. 2010 Jul;35(7):44-50. PMID:20555245

Schaller J. The Diagnosis, Treatment and Prevention of Bartonella: Atypical Bartonella Treatment Failures and 40 Hypothetical Physical Exam Findings – Full Color Edition. Volume I-II. Tampa, FL:Hope Academic Press. 2008.

Schaller J. Babesia. in Encyclopedia of Plagues, Pestilence and Pandemics. Ed. J. Bryre. Westport, CT: Greenwood Press; 2008.

Schaller J. Bartonella. in Encyclopedia of Plagues, Pestilence and Pandemics. Ed. J. Bryre, Westport, CT: Greenwood Press; 2008

Schaller J. Lyme Disease. in Encyclopedia of Plagues, Pestilence and Pandemics. Ed. J. Bryre. Westport, CT: Greenwood Press; 2008

Schaller J. Babesia 2009 Supplement and Update. Tampa, FL:Hope Academic Press. 2009.

Schaller JL. Artemisin, Artesunate, Artemisinic Acid and Other Derivatives of Artemisia Used for Malaria, Babesia and Cancer. Tampa, FL: Hope Academic Press. 2006.

Schaller JL. The Health Care Professional's Guide to the Treatment and Diagnosis of Human Babesiosis, An Extensive Review of New Human Species and Advanced Treatments. Tampa, FL: Hope Academic Press. 2006.

Schaller JL, Burkland GA. Case report: rapid and complete control of idiopathic hypereosinophilia with imatinib mesylate. MedGenMed. 2001;3(5):9.

Schaller JL, Burkland GA, Langhoff PJ. Are various Babesia species a missed cause for hypereosinophilia? A follow-up on the first reported case of imatinib mesylate for idiopathic hypereosinophilia. MedGenMed. 2007 Feb 27;9(1):38.

Schaller JL, Burkland GA, Langhoff PJ. Do bartonella infections cause agitation, panic disorder, and treatment-resistant depression? MedGenMed. 2007 Sep 13;9(3):54.

Scheffer RE, Linden S. Concurrent medical conditions with pediatric bipolar disorder. Curr Opin Psychiatry. 2007 Jul;20(4):398-401. PMID:17551356

Schnarr S, Franz JK, Krause A, Zeidler H. Infection and musculoskeletal conditions: Lyme borreliosis. Best Pract Res Clin Rheumatol. 2006 Dec;20(6):1099-118. PMID:17127199

Schutzer SE, Angel TE, Liu T, Schepmoes AA, TR Clauss, JN Adkins, DG Camp, Holland BK, Bergquist J, Coyle PK, Smith RD, Fallon BA, Natelson BH. Distinct cerebrospinal fluid proteomes differentiate post-treatment lyme disease from chronic fatigue syndrome. PLoS One. 2011 Feb 23;6(2):e17287. PMID:21383843

Schweighofer CD, Fätkenheuer G, Staib P, Hallek M, Reiser M. Lyme disease in a patient with chronic lymphocytic leukemia mimics leukemic meningeosis. Onkologie. 2007 Nov;30(11):564-6. Epub 2007 Oct 16. PMID:17992027

Science Daily (Jan 6, 2009). New Bartonella Species That Infects Humans Discovered. Available at http://www.sciencedaily.com/releases/2009/01/090106145006.htm

Shapiro ED. Tick-borne diseases. Adv Pediatr Infect Dis. 1997;13:187-218. Review.

Shapiro ED. Long-term outcomes of persons with Lyme disease. Vector Borne Zoonotic Dis. 2002 Winter;2(4):279-81.

Shapiro ED, Gerber MA. Lyme disease and facial nerve palsy. Arch Pediatr Adolesc Med. 1997 Dec;151(12):1183-4.

Sherr VT. Human babesiosis--an unrecorded reality. Absence of formal registry undermines its detection, diagnosis and treatment, suggesting need for immediate mandatory reporting. Med Hypotheses. 2004;63(4):609-15. PMID:15325004

Sherr VT. Munchausen's syndrome by proxy and Lyme disease: medical misogyny or diagnostic mystery? Med Hypotheses. 2005;65(3):440-7. PMID:15925450

Siegel DM. Chronic arthritis in adolescence. Adolesc Med State Art Rev. 2007 May;18(1):47-61, viii. PMID:18605390

Sigal LH. Summary of the first 100 patients seen at a Lyme disease referral center. Am J Med 1990 Jun;88(6):577-83. PMID:2346158

Sigal LH. Current recommendations for the treatment of Lyme disease. Drugs 1992 May;43(5):683-99. PMID:1379147

Sigal LH. Long-term consequences of Lyme disease. In: Rahn QW, Evans J, eds. Lyme disease. Philadelphia:ACP, 1998; pp 137-53.

Sigal LH, Hassett AL. Commentary: 'What's in a name? That which we call a rose by any other name would smell as sweet.' Shakespeare W. Romeo and Juliet, II, ii(47-48). Int J Epidemiol. 2005 Dec;34(6):1345-7. Epub 2005 Sep 2. PMID:16143662

Simakova AI, Popov AF, Dadalova OB. [Ixodes tick-borne borreliosis with erythema nodosum].[Article in Russian]. Med Parazitol (Mosk). 2005 Oct-Dec;(4):31-2. PMID:16445235

Sjöwall J, Carlsson A, Vaarala O, Bergström S, Ernerudh J, Forsberg P, Ekerfelt C. Innate immune responses in Lyme borreliosis: enhanced tumour necrosis factor-alpha and interleukin-12 in asymptomatic individuals in response to live spirochetes. Clin Exp Immunol. 2005 Jul;141(1):89-98. PMID:15958074

Skotarczak B. Canine ehrlichiosis. Ann Agric Environ Med. 2003;10(2):137-41. PMID:14677903

Smith HM, Reporter R, Rood MP, Linscott AJ, Mascola LM, Hogrefe W, Purcell RH. Prevalence study of antibody to ratborne pathogens and other agents among patients using a free clinic in downtown Los Angeles. J Infect Dis. 2002 Dec 1;186(11):1673-6. PMID:12447746

Smith IS, Rechlin DP. Delayed diagnosis of neuroborreliosis presenting as bell palsy and meningitis. J Am Osteopath Assoc. 2010 Aug;110(8):441-4. PMID: 20805550

Sobek V, Birkner N, Falk I, Würch A, Kirschning CJ, Wagner H, Wallich R, Lamers

MC, Simon MM. Direct Toll-like receptor 2 mediated co-stimulation of T cells in the mouse system as a basis for chronic inflammatory joint disease. Arthritis Res Ther. 2004;6(5):R433-46. Epub 2004 Jul 19. PMID:15380043

Sood SK ed. Lyme Borreliosis in Europe and North America: Epidemiology and Clinical Practice. Hoboken New Jersey: Wiley and Sons, Inc., 2011.

Speelman P, de Jongh BM, Wolfs TF, Wittenberg J; Kwaliteitsinstituut voor de

Gezondheidszorg (CBO). [Guideline 'Lyme borreliosis'].[Article in Dutch]. Ned Tijdschr Geneeskd. 2004 Apr 3;148(14):659-63. PMID:15106316

Sréter T, Sréterné Lancz Z, Széll Z, Egyed L. [Rickettsia helvetica: an emerging tick-borne pathogen in Hungary and Europe]. [Article in Hungarian]. Orv Hetil. 2005 Dec 11;146(50):2547-52. PMID:16440500

Steere AC. Musculoskeletal manifestations of Lyme disease. Am J Med. 1995 Apr 24;98(4A):44S-48S; discussion 48S-51S. Review.

Steere AC, Bartenhagen NH, Craft JE, Hutchinson GJ, Newman JH, Rahn DW, Sigal LH, Spieler PN, Stenn KS, Malawista SE. The early clinical manifestations of Lyme disease. Ann Intern Med. 1983 Jul;99(1):76-82.

Steere AC, Berardi VP, Weeks KE, Logigian EL, Ackermann R. Evaluation of the intrathecal antibody response to Borrelia burgdorferi as a diagnostic test for Lyme neuroborreliosis. J Infect Dis. 1990 Jun;161(6):1203-9.

Steere AC, Gibofsky A, Patarroyo ME, Winchester RJ, Hardin JA, Malawista SE. Chronic Lyme arthritis. Clinical and immunogenetic differentiation from rheumatoid arthritis. Ann Intern Med. 1979 Jun;90(6):896-901.

Steere AC, Malawista SE, Bartenhagen NH, Spieler PN, Newman JH, Rahn DW, Hutchinson GJ, Green J, Snydman DR, Taylor E. The clinical spectrum and treatment of Lyme disease. Yale J Biol Med. 1984 Jul-Aug;57(4):453-61.

Steere AC, Sikand VK. The presenting manifestations of Lyme disease and the outcomes of treatment. N Engl J Med. 2003 Jun 12;348(24):2472-4.

Sterman AB, Nelson S, Barclay P. Demyelinating neuropathy accompanying Lyme disease. Neurology 1982 Nov;32(11):1302-5.

Storch A, Vladimirtsev VA, Tumani H, Wellinghausen N, Haas A, Krivoshapkin VG, Ludolph AC. Viliuisk encephalomyelitis in Northeastern Siberia is not caused by Borrelia burgdorferi infection. Neurol Sci. 2008 Feb;29(1):11-4. Epub 2008 Apr 1. PMID:18379734

Stricker RB. Counterpoint: long-term antibiotic therapy improves persistent symptoms associated with lyme disease. Clin Infect Dis. 2007 Jul 15;45(2):149-57. Epub 2007 Jun 5. PMID:17578772

Stricker RB, Johnson L. Lyme disease: a turning point. Expert Rev Anti Infect Ther. 2007 Oct;5(5):759-62. PMID:17914908

Stricker RB, Johnson L. Chronic Lyme disease and the 'Axis of Evil'. Future Microbiol. 2008 Dec;3(6):621-4. PMID:19072179

Stricker RB, Johnson L. Gender bias in chronic lyme disease. J Womens Health (Larchmt). 2009 Oct;18(10):1717-8; author reply 1719-20. PMID:19857097

Stricker RB, Johnson L. Lyme disease diagnosis and treatment: lessons from the AIDS epidemic. Minerva Med. 2010 Dec;101(6):419-25. PMID: 21196901

Stricker RB, Johnson L. Lyme disease: the next decade. Infect Drug Resist. 2011;4:1-9. Epub 2011 Jan 7. PMID:21694904

Stricker RB, Lautin A, Burrascano JJ. Lyme disease: point/ counterpoint. Expert Rev Anti Infect Ther. 2005 Apr;3(2):155-65. PMID:15918774

Stricker RB, Savely VR, Motanya NC, Giclas PC. Complement split products c3a and c4a in chronic lyme disease. Scand J Immunol. 2009 Jan;69(1):64-9. PMID:19140878

Summers BA, Straubinger AF, Jacobson RH, Chang YF, Appel MJ, Straubinger RK. Histopathological studies of experimental lyme disease in the dog. J Comp Pathol. 2005 Jul;133(1):1-13. PMID:15904927

Tauber SC, Ribes S, Ebert S, Heinz T, Fingerle V, Bunkowski S, Kugelstadt D, Spreer A, Jahn O, Eiffert H, Nau R. Long-term intrathecal infusion of outer surface protein C from Borrelia burgdorferi causes axonal damage. J Neuropathol Exp Neurol. 2011 Sep;70(9):748-57. PMID:21865883

Taylor RS, Simpson IN. Review of treatment options for lyme borreliosis. J Chemother. 2005 Sep;17 Suppl 2:3-16. PMID:16315580

Telford SR III, Wormser GP. Bartonella spp. transmission by ticks not established. Emerg Infect Dis. 2010 Mar;16(3):379-84.

Tory HO, Zurakowski D, Sundel RP. Outcomes of children treated for Lyme arthritis: results of a large pediatric cohort. J Rheumatol. 2010 May;37(5):1049-55. Epub 2010 Apr 1. PMID:20360182

Treib J, Woessner R, Dobler G, Fernandez A, Hozler G, Schimrigk K. Clinical value of specific intrathecal production of antibodies. Acta virol 1997 Feb;41(1):27-30.

Tuuminen T, Hedman K, Söderlund-Venermo M, Seppälä I. Acute parvovirus B19 infection causes nonspecificity frequently in Borrelia and less often in Salmonella and Campylobacter serology, posing a problem in diagnosis of infectious arthropathy. Clin Vaccine Immunol. 2011 Jan;18(1):167-72. Epub 2010 Nov 24. PMID:21106777

Vel'gin SO, Protas II, Ponomarev VV, Drakina SA, Shcherba VV. [Clinical polymorphism of neuroborreliosis at a late stage of the disease].[Article in Russian]. Zh Nevrol Psikhiatr Im S S Korsakova. 2006;106(3):48-51. PMID:16608111

Vojdani A. Antibodies as predictors of complex autoimmune diseases and cancer. Int J Immunopathol Pharmacol. 2008 Jul-Sep;21(3):553-66. Erratum in Int J Immunopathol Pharmacol. 2008 Oct-Dec;21(4):following 1051. PMID:18831922

Volkman DJ. An appraisal of "chronic Lyme disease". N Engl J Med. 2008 Jan 24;358(4):429; author reply 430-1. PMID:18219750

Wagner V, Zima E, Geller L, Merkely B. [Acute atrioventricular block in chronic Lyme disease].[Article in Hungarian]. Orv Hetil. 2010 Sep 26;151(39):1585-90. PMID:20840915

Wahlberg P, Nyman D. [Chronic Lyme borreliosis--fact or fiction?]. [Article in Finnish]. Duodecim. 2009;125(12):1269-76. PMID:19711595

WebMD. Lyme Disease Symptoms. http://arthritis.webmd.com/tc/lyme-disease-symptoms

Weintraub P. Cure Unknown: Inside the Lyme Epidemic. New York:Saint Martin's Griffin, 2009.

Weissenbacher S, Ring J, Hofmann H. Gabapentin for the symptomatic treatment of chronic neuropathic pain in patients with late-stage lyme borreliosis: a pilot study. Dermatology. 2005;211(2):123-7. PMID:16088158

Weissmann G. "Chronic Lyme" and other medically unexplained syndromes. FASEB J. 2007 Feb;21(2):299-301. PMID:17267382

Widhe M, Jarefors S, Ekerfelt C, Vrethem M, Bergstrom S, Forsberg P, Ernerudh J. Borrelia-specific interferon-gamma and interleukin-4 secretion in cerebrospinal fluid and blood during Lyme borreliosis in humans: association with clinical outcome. J Infect Dis. 2004 May 15;189(10):1881-91. Epub 2004 Apr 26. PMID:15122525

Wielgat P, Pancewicz S, Hermanowska-Szpakowicz T, Kondrusik M, Zajkowska J, Grygorczuk S, Popko J, Zwierz K. [Activity of lysosomal exoglycosidases in serum of patients with chronic borrelia arthritis].[Article in Polish]. Przegl Epidemiol. 2004;58(3):451-8. PMID:15730009

Wormser GP. Treatment and prevention of Lyme disease, with emphasis on antimicrobial therapy for neuroborreliosis and vaccination. Semin Neurol. 1997 Mar;17(1):45-52. Review.

Wormser GP, Schwartz I. Antibiotic treatment of animals infected with Borrelia burgdorferi. Clin Microbiol Rev. 2009 Jul;22(3):387-95. PMID:19597005

Wormser GP, Shapiro ED. Implications of gender in chronic Lyme disease. J Womens Health (Larchmt). 2009 Jun;18(6):831-4. PMID:19514824

Zajkowska J, Czupryna P, Pancewicz SA, Kondrusik M, Moniuszko A. Acrodermatitis chronica atrophicans. Lancet Infect Dis. 2011 Oct;11(10):800. PMID:21958583

Zajkowska JM, Kondrusik M, Pancewicz SA, Grygorczuk S, Jamiołkowski J, Stalewska J. [Comparison of test with antigen VlsE (C6) with tests with recombinant antigens in patients with Lyme borreliosis].[Article in Polish]. Pol Merkur Lekarski. 2007 Aug;23(134):95-9. PMID:18044336

Zajkowska JM, Swierzbińska R, Pancewicz SA, Kondrusik M, Hermanowska-Szpakowicz T. [Concentration of soluble CD4, CD8, CD25 receptors as well IFN-gamma and IL-4 released by lymphocyte of chronic Lyme patients cultured with 3 genotypes of Borrelia burgdorferi].[Article in Polish]. Pol Merkur Lekarski. 2004 May;16(95):447-50. PMID:15518424

Zalaudek I, Leinweber B, Kerl H, Müllegger RR. Acrodermatitis chronica atrophicans in a 15-year-old girl misdiagnosed as venous insufficiency for 6 years. 173. J Am Acad Dermatol. 2005 Jun;52(6):1091-4. PMID:15928636

Zeaiter Z, Liang Z, Raoult D. Genetic classification and differentiation of Bartonella species based on comparison of partial ftsZ gene sequences. J Clin Microbiol. 2002 Oct;40(10):3641-7. PMID:12354859

Zu-Rhein GM, Lo SC, Hulette CM, Powers JM. A novel cerebral microangiopathy with endothelial cell atypia and multifocal white matter lesions: a direct mycoplasmal infection? J Neuropathol Exp Neurol. 2007 Dec;66(12):1100-17. PMID:18090919

A Bibliography of Selected References for Researchers and Academicians Dedicated to Tick and Flea-borne Infection Science

Abbas HM, Brenes RA, Ajemian MS, Scholand SJ. Successful conservative treatment of spontaneous splenic rupture secondary to Babesiosis: a case report and literature review. Conn Med. 2011 Mar;75(3):143-6. Review.

Abdad MY, Stenos J, Graves S. Rickettsia felis, an emerging flea-transmitted human pathogen. Emerg Health Threats J. 2011; 4: 10. Published online 2011 July 1.

Abdollahi-Roodsaz S, Joosten LA, Roelofs MF, Radstake TR, Matera G, Popa C, van der Meer JW, Netea MG, van den Berg WB. Inhibition of Toll-like receptor 4 breaks the inflammatory loop in autoimmune destructive arthritis. Arthritis Rheum. 2007 Sep;56(9):2957-67.

Aberer E, Fingerle V, Wutte N, Fink-Puches R, Cerroni L. Within European margins. Lancet. 2011 Jan 8;377(9760):178.

Aberer E, Klade H Cutaneous manifestations of Lyme borreliosis. Infection. 1991 Jul-Aug;19(4):284-6.

Aberer E, Kersten A, Klade H, Poitschek C, Jurecka W. Heterogeneity of Borrelia burgdorferi in the skin. 1996. American Journal of Dermatopathology, 18(6):571-9.

Aboudharam G, Fournier PE, Drancourt M, Raoult D, Foucault C, Brouqui P. Molecular detection of Bartonella quintana DNA in the dental pulp of a homeless patient. Eur J Clin Microbiol Infect Dis. 2004 Dec;23(12):920-2.

Aboudharam G, Vu DL, Davoust B, Drancourt M, Raoult D. Molecular detection of Bartonella spp. in the dental pulp of stray cats buried for a year. Microb Pathog. 2005 Jan;38(1):47-51. Epub 2004 Dec 8.

AbouLaila M, Sivakumar T, Yokoyama N, Igarashi I. Inhibitory effect of terpene nerolidol on the growth of Babesia parasites. Parasitol Int. 2010 Jun;59(2):278-82. Epub 2010 Feb 21.

Abrams Y. Complications of coinfection with Babesia and Lyme disease after splenectomy. J Am Board Fam Med. 2008 Jan-Feb;21(1):75-7.

Accorinti M. Ocular bartonellosis. Int J Med Sci. 2009;6(3):131-2. Epub 2009 Mar 19.

Ackermann R, Rehse-Kupper B, Gollmer E, Schmidt R. Chronic neurologic manifestations of erythema migrans borreliosis. Annals of the New York Academy of Sciences, 539:16-23. 1988.

Ackermann R, Kabatzki J, Boisten HP, Steere AC, Grodzicki RL, Hartung S, Runne U. [Spirochete etiology of erythema chronicum migrans disease]. [Article in German]. Dtsch Med Wochenschr. 1984 Jan 20;109(3):92-7.

Ackermann R, Kabatzki J, Boisten HP, Steere AC, Grodzicki RL, Hartung S, Runne U. Ixodes ricinus spirochete and European erythema chronicum migrans disease. Yale J Biol Med. 1984 Jul-Aug;57(4):573-80.

Adamska M. [Bartonella spp. as a zoonotic pathogens transmitting by blood-feeding arthropods].[Article in Polish]. Wiad Parazytol. 2010;56(1):1-9. Review.

Adelson ME, Rao RV, Tilton RC, Cabets K, Eskow E, Fein L, Occi JL, Mordechai E. Prevalence of Borrelia burgdorferi, Bartonella spp., Babesia microti, and Anaplasma phagocytophila in Ixodes scapularis ticks collected in Northern New Jersey. J Clin Microbiol. 2004 Jun;42(6):2799-801.

Aderinboye O, Syed SS. Congenital babesiosis in a four-week-old female infant. Pediatr Infect Dis J. 2010 Feb;29(2):188.

Adham FK, El-Samie-Abd EM, Gabre RM, El Hussein H. Detection of tick blood parasites in Egypt using PCR assay II- Borrelia burgdorferi sensu lato. J Egypt Soc Parasitol. 2010 Dec;40(3):553-64.

Adjei G. Clinical neurotoxicity of artemisinin drugs in malaria treatment. In: Program and abstracts of the 4th Multilateral Initiative on Malaria conference. 2005.

Agger W. Case KL, Bryant GL, Callister SM. Lyme disease: clinical features, classification, and epidemiology in the upper midwest. 1991. Medicine (Baltimore) Mar;70(2):83-90.

Aguero-Rosenfeld ME, Donnarumma L, Zentmaier L, Jacob J, Frey M, Noto R, Carbonaro CA, Wormser GP. Seroprevalence of antibodies that react with Anaplasma phagocytophila, the agent of human granulocytic ehrlichiosis, in different populations in Westchester County, New York. J Clin Microbiol. 2002 Jul;40(7):2612-5.

Aguero-Rosenfeld ME, Nowakowski J, Bittker S, Cooper D, Nadelman RB, Wormser GP. Evolution of the serologic response to Borrelia burgdorferi in treated patients with culture-confirmed erythema migrans. J Clin Microbiol. 1996 Jan;34(1):1-9.

Aguero-Rosenfeld ME, Nowakowski J, McKenna DF, Carbonaro CA, Wormser GP. Serodiagnosis in early Lyme disease. J Clin Microbiol. 1993 Dec;31(12):3090-5. Erratum in: J Clin Microbiol 1994 Mar;32(3):860.

Aguero-Rosenfeld ME, Roberge J, Carbonaro CA, Nowakowski J, Nadelman RB, Wormser GP. Effects of OspA vaccination on Lyme disease serologic testing. J Clin Microbiol. 1999 Nov;37(11):3718-21.

Aguero-Rosenfeld ME, Wang G, Schwartz I, Wormser GP. Diagnosis of lyme borreliosis. Clin Microbiol Rev. 2005 Jul;18(3):484-509. Review.

Aguirre AA. Wild canids as sentinels of ecological health: a conservation medicine perspective. Parasit Vectors. 2009; 2(Suppl 1): S7. Published online 2009 March 26.

Ahmed JS. The role of cytokines in immunity and immuno-pathogenesis of pirolasmoses. Parasitol Res. 2002;88(13 Suppl 1): S48-50

Akiyama M. Risk management and measuring productivity with POAS--Point of Act System--a medical information system as ERP (Enterprise Resource Planning) for hospital management. Methods Inf Med. 2007;46(6):686-93.

Akin E, Aversa J, Steere AC. Expression of adhesion molecules in synovia of patients with treatment-resistant lyme arthritis. Infect Immun. 2001 Mar;69(3):1774-80.

Akin E, McHugh GL, Flavell RA, Fikrig E, Steere AC. The immunoglobulin (IgG) antibody response to OspA and OspB correlates with severe and prolonged Lyme arthritis and the IgG response to P35 correlates with mild and brief arthritis. Infect Immun. 1999 Jan;67(1):173-81.

Alberti A, Zobba R, Chessa B, Addis MF, Sparagano O, Pinna Parpaglia ML, Cubeddu T, Pintori G, Marco Pittau M. Equine and Canine Anaplasma phagocytophilum Strains Isolated on the Island of Sardinia (Italy) Are Phylogenetically Related to Pathogenic Strains from the United States. Appl Environ Microbiol. 2005 October; 71(10): 6418–6422.

Alcantara V, Rolain JM, Eduardo AG, Raul MJ, Raoult D. Molecular detection of Bartonella quintana in human body lice from Mexico City. Clin Microbiol Infect. 2009 Dec;15 Suppl 2:93-4. Epub 2009 Sep 28.

Al-Kappany YM, Lappin MR, Kwok OC, Abu-Elwafa SA, Hilali M, Dubey JP. Seroprevalence of Toxoplasma gondii and concurrent Bartonella spp., feline immunodeficiency virus, feline leukemia virus, and Dirofilaria immitis infections in Egyptian cats. J Parasitol. 2011 Apr;97(2):256-8. Epub 2010 Oct 14.

Alonso-Coello P, García JM, Solà I. [Limitations and subterfuges of criticism of evidence based medicine].[Article in Spanish]. Med Clin (Barc). 2005 Feb 19;124(6):237; author reply 237-8.

Al-Qudah AA, Mostratos A, Quesnel LB. A proposed life cycle for the Reiter treponeme. 1983. Journal of Applied Bacteriology, 55:417-428.

Alban PS, Johnson PW, Nelson DR. Serum-starvation-induced changes in protein synthesis and morphology of Borrelia burgdorferi. 2000. Microbiology, Jan;146 (Pt 1):119-27.

Alban PS, Nelson DR. Serum starvation-induced cyst formation in Borrelia burgdorferi under defined conditions. Presented at the 1999 International Conference on Lyme disease in Munich, Germany.

Alinia. Package Insert. Accessed 2006 September 10. Available from: http://www.romark.com.

Alkhalil A, Hill DA, Desai SA. Babesia and plasmodia increase host erythrocyte permeability through distinct mechanisms. Cell Microbiol. 2007 Apr;9(4):851-60. Epub 2006 Nov 3.

Alpert B, Esin J, Sivak SL, Wormser GP. Incidence and prevalence of Lyme disease in a suburban Westchester County community. N Y State J Med. 1992 Jan;92(1):5-8.

Alpert JE, Papakostas G, Mischoulon D, et al. S-adenosyl-L-methionine (SAMe) as an adjunct for resistant major depressive disorder: an open trial following partial or nonresponse to selective serotonin reuptake inhibitors or venlafaxine. J Clin Psychopharmacol. 2004;24(6):661-664.

Alter HJ, Stramer SL, Dodd RY. Emerging infectious diseases that threaten the blood supply. Semin Hematol. 2007 Jan;44(1):32-41. Review.

American Medical Association, Code of Medical Ethics.

Ames JR, Ryan MD, Klayman DL. Charge transfer and oxy radicals in antimalarial action. J. Free Rad Biol. Med. 1985;1:353-61.

Amsbaugh S, Huiras E, Wang NS, Wever A, Warren S. Bacillary angiomatosis associated with pseudoepitheliomatous hyperplasia. Am J Dermatopathol. 2006 Feb;28(1):32-5.

Anand KP, Anand A, Kashyap AS. Dr Victor Babes, discoverer of Babesia. Stamps issued on babesiosis, 7th International Congress of Protozoology, stamp--Kenya 1985. J Assoc Physicians India. 2008 Oct;56:808.

Ananjeva LP, Skripnikova IA, Barskova VG, Steere AC. Clinical and serologic features of Lyme borreliosis in Russia. J Rheumatol. 1995 Apr;22(4):689-94.

Ananjeva LP, Skripnikova IA, Barskova VG, Steere AC. [The clinical and serological manifestations of Lyme disease in Russia]. [Article in Russian]. Ter Arkh. 1995;67(11):38-42.

Anbu AT, Foulerton M, McMaster P, Bakalinova D. Basal ganglia involvement in a child with cat-scratch disease. Pediatr Infect Dis J. 2003 Oct;22(10):931-2.

Anderson JF, Mintz ED, Gadbaw JL, Magnerelli LA. Babesia microti, human babesiosis, and Borrelia burgdorferi in Connecticut. J Clin Microbiol. 1991;29:2779-83.

Anfosso L, Efferth T, Albini A, Pfeffer U. Microarray expression profiles of angiogenesis-related genes predict tumor cell response to artemisinins. Pharmacogenomics J. 2006;6:269-78. Epub 2006 Jan 24.

Angel TE, Luft BJ, Yang X, Nicora CD, Camp DG 2nd, Jacobs JM, Smith RD. Proteome analysis of Borrelia burgdorferi response to environmental change. PLoS One. 2010 Nov 2;5(11):e13800.

Angel-Moreno A, Hernández-Cabrera M, Pérez-Arellano JL. Kikuchi's disease or Kikuchi's syndrome? Clin Infect Dis. 2006 Feb 15;42(4):578-9; author reply 579-80.

Angelakis E, Billeter SA, Breitschwerdt EB, Chomel BB, Raoult D. Potential for tick-borne bartonelloses. Emerg Infect Dis. 2010 Mar;16(3):385-91. Review.

Angelakis E, Biswas S, Taylor C, Raoult D, Rolain JM. Heterogeneity of susceptibility to fluoroquinolones in Bartonella isolates from Australia reveals a natural mutation in gyrA. J Antimicrob Chemother. 2008 Jun;61(6):1252-5. Epub 2008 Mar 10.

Angelakis E, Edouard S, La Scola B, Raoult D. Bartonella henselae in skin biopsy specimens of patients with cat-scratch disease. Emerg Infect Dis. 2010 Dec;16(12):1963-5.

Angelakis E, Khamphoukeo K, Grice D, Newton PN, Roux V, Aplin K, Raoult D, Rolain JM. Molecular detection of Bartonella species in rodents from the Lao PDR. Clin Microbiol Infect. 2009 Dec;15 Suppl 2:95-7. Epub 2009 Apr 3.

Angelakis E, Lepidi H, Canel A, Rispal P, Perraudeau F, Barre I, Rolain JM, Raoult D. Human case of Bartonella alsatica lymphadenitis. Emerg Infect Dis. 2008 Dec;14(12):1951-3.

Angelakis E, Pulcini C, Waton J, Imbert P, Socolovschi C, Edouard S, Dellamonica P, Raoult D. Scalp eschar and neck lymphadenopathy caused by Bartonella henselae after Tick Bite. Clin Infect Dis. 2010 Feb 15;50(4):549-51.

Angelakis E, Raoult D, Rolain JM. Molecular characterization of resistance to fluoroquinolones in Bartonella henselae and Bartonella quintana. J Antimicrob Chemother. 2009 Jun;63(6):1288-9. Epub 2009 Apr 15.

Angelakis E, Rolain JM, Raoult D, Brouqui P. Bartonella quintana in head louse nits. FEMS Immunol Med Microbiol. 2011 Jul;62(2):244-6. Epub 2011 May 5.

Angelakis E, Roux V, Raoult D, Rolain JM.Real-time PCR strategy and detection of bacterial agents of lymphadenitis. Eur J Clin Microbiol Infect Dis. 2009 Nov;28(11):1363-8. Epub 2009 Aug 14.

Anghel G, De Rosa L, Ruscio C, et al. Efficacy of imatinib mesylate in a patient with idiopathic hypereosinophilic syndrome and severe heart involvement. Tumori. 2005;91(1):67-70.

Angibaud G, Balague JP, Lafontan JF. Bartonella hensalae encephalopathy. Presse Med. 2005;34(4):297-298.

Anigstein L, Anigstein DM. Effects of selected tissue antisera-- spleen-bone marrow, brain, thyroid, pancreas, pituitary, thymus, etc.--in vivo or in vitro: a review covering 30 years researches at the University of Texas Medical Branch. Tex Rep Biol Med. 1974 Summer;32(2):369-90. Review.

Antonara S, Chafel RM, LaFrance M, Coburn J. Borrelia burgdorferi Adhesins Identified Using In Vivo Phage Display. Mol Microbiol. 2007 October; 66(1): 262–276. Published online 2007 September 3.

Antonara S, Ristow L, Coburn J. Adhesion mechanisms of Borrelia burgdorferi. Adv Exp Med Biol. 2011;715:35-49. Review.

Arav-Boger R, Crawford T, Steere AC, Halsey NA. Cerebellar ataxia as the presenting manifestation of Lyme disease. Pediatr Infect Dis J. 2002 Apr;21(4):353-6.

Arimitsu Y, Seki M, Nakao M, Miyamoto K. Comparison of antibody titers against borrelial strains isolated in Japan by the microcapsule agglutination test for serological studies of early Lyme disease. Microbiol Immunol. 1994;38(4):269-72.

Armengol CE, Hendley JO. Cat-scratch disease encephalopathy: a cause of status epilepticus in school-aged children. J Pediatr. 1999 May;134(5):635-8.

Armstrong PM, Katavolos P, Caporale DA, Smith RP, Spielman A, Telford SR III. Diversity of Babesia infecting deer ticks (Ixodes dammini). Am J Trop Med Hyg. 1998;58:739-42.

Arvand M, Feil EJ, Giladi M, Boulouis HJ, Viezens J. Multi-locus sequence typing of Bartonella henselae isolates from three continents reveals hypervirulent and feline-associated clones. PLoS One. 2007 Dec 19;2(12):e1346.

Arvand M, Raoult D, Feil EJ. Multi-locus sequence typing of a geographically and temporally diverse sample of the highly clonal human pathogen Bartonella quintana. PLoS One. 2010 Mar 19;5(3):e9765.

Arvand M, Schäd SG. Isolation of Bartonella henselae DNA from the peripheral blood of a patient with cat scratch disease up to 4 months after the cat scratch injury. J Clin Microbiol. 2006 Jun;44(6):2288-90.

Arvand M, Schubert H, Viezens J. Emergence of distinct genetic variants in the population of primary Bartonella henselae isolates. Microbes Infect. 2006 Apr;8(5):1315-20. Epub 2006 Mar 15.

Arvand M, Viezens J. Evaluation of pulsed-field gel electrophoresis and multi-locus sequence typing for the analysis of clonal relatedness among Bartonella henselae isolates. Int J Med Microbiol. 2007 Jul;297(4):255-62. Epub 2007 Mar 30.

Asad S, Sweeney J, Mermel LA. Transfusion-transmitted babesiosis in Rhode Island. Transfusion. 2009 Dec;49(12):2564-73. Epub 2009 Sep 16.

Asano T, Ichiki K, Koizumi S, Kaizu K, Hatori T, Fujino O. High prevalence of antibodies against Bartonella henselae with cervical lymphadenopathy in children. Pediatr Int. 2010 Aug;52(4):533-5.

Asch ES, Bujak DI, Weiss M, Peterson MG, Weinstein A. Lyme disease: an infectious and postinfectious syndrome. J Rheumatol. 1994 Mar;21(3):454-61.

Asensio Sanchez VM, Corral Azor A, Bartolome Aragon A, De Paz Garcia M. [Diplopia as the first manifestation of Lyme disease]. [Article in Spanish]. Arch Soc Esp Oftalmol. 2003 Jan;78(1):51-4.

Asensio-Sánchez VM, Rodríguez-Delgado B, García-Herrero E, Cabo-Vaquera V, García-Loygorri C. [Serous macular detachment as an atypical sign in cat scratch disease].[Article in Spanish]. Arch Soc Esp Oftalmol. 2006 Dec;81(12):717-9. Review.

Atamanyuk I, Raja SG, Kostolny M. Bartonella henselae endocarditis of percutaneously implanted pulmonary valve: a case report. J Heart Valve Dis. 2011 Jan;20(1):94-7.

Atlas E, Novak SN, Duray PH, Steere AC. Lyme myositis: muscle invasion by Borrelia burgdorferi. Ann Intern Med. 1988 Aug 1;109(3):245-6.

Atovaquone. Drug Facts and Comparisons 2006. Wolters Kluwer Health. St. Louis, Missouri; p.1915.

Augustijns P, D'Hulst A, Van Daele J, Kinget R. Transport of artemisinin and sodium artesunate in Caco-2 intestinal epithelial cells. J Pharm Sci. 1996 Jun;85(6):577-9.

Ault P, Cortes J, Koller C, Kaled ES, Kantarjian H. Response of idiopathic hypereosinophilic syndrome to treatment with imatinib mesylate. Leuk Res. 2002;26(9):881-884.

Aupy B, Conessa C, Clement P, Roguet E, Poncet JL. [Cat scratch disease: a diagnosis to be aware of!]. [Article in French]. Rev Laryngol Otol Rhinol (Bord). 2008;129(1):53-6.

Auwaerter PG, Bakken JS, Dattwyler RJ, Dumler JS, Halperin JJ, McSweegan E, Nadelman RB, O'Connell S, Shapiro ED, Sood SK, Steere AC, Weinstein A, Wormser GP. Antiscience and ethical concerns associated with advocacy of Lyme disease. Lancet Infect Dis. 2011 Sep;11(9):713-9.

Auwaerter PG, Bakken JS, Dattwyler RJ, Dumler JS, Halperin JJ, McSweegan E, Nadelman RB, O'Connell S, Sood SK, Weinstein A, Wormser GP. Scientific evidence and best patient care practices should guide the ethics of Lyme disease activism. J Med Ethics. 2011 Feb;37(2):68-73. Epub 2010 Nov 21.

Awad A. Case 1-1998: a boy with a seizure. N Engl J Med. 1998;338(21):1549-1550.

Axford JS, Rees DH, Mageed RA, Wordsworth P, Alavi A, Steere AC. Increased IgA rheumatoid factor and V(H)1 associated cross reactive idiotype expression in patients with Lyme arthritis and neuroborreliosis. Ann Rheum Dis. 1999 Dec;58(12):757-61.

Axford JS, Watts RA, Long AA, Isenberg DA, Steere AC. Expression of public idiotypes in patients with Lyme arthritis. Ann Rheum Dis. 1993 Mar;52(3):199-205.

"Babesiosis". Family Practice Notebook.com. Available from: http://fnotebook.com/ID219.htm. Accessed June 30, 2006.

Babu RV, Sharma G. A 57-year-old man with abdominal pain, jaundice, and a history of blood transfusion. Chest. 2007 Jul;132(1):347-50.

Bachmann M, Horn K, Rudloff I, Goren I, Holdener M, Christen U, Darsow N, Hunfeld KP, Koehl U, Kind P, Pfeilschifter J, Kraiczy P, Mühl H. Early Production of IL-22 but Not IL-17 by Peripheral Blood Mononuclear Cells Exposed to live Borrelia burgdorferi: The Role of Monocytes and Interleukin-1. PLoS Pathog. 2010 October; 6(10): e1001144. Published online 2010 October 14.

Backert S, Meyer TF. Type IV secretion systems and their effectors in bacterial pathogenesis. Curr Opin Microbiol. 2006 Apr;9(2):207-17. Epub 2006 Mar 9. Review.

Bacon RM, Biggerstaff BJ, Schriefer ME, Gilmore RD Jr, Philipp MT, Steere AC, Wormser GP, Marques AR, Johnson BJ. Serodiagnosis of Lyme disease by kinetic enzyme-linked immunosorbent assay using recombinant VlsE1 or peptide antigens of Borrelia burgdorferi compared with 2-tiered testing using whole-cell lysates. J Infect Dis. 2003 Apr 15;187(8):1187-99. Epub 2003 Apr 2.

Badiaga S, Brouqui P, Raoult D. Autochthonous epidemic typhus associated with Bartonella quintana bacteremia in a homeless person. Am J Trop Med Hyg. 2005 May;72(5):638-9.

Badiaga S, Raoult D, Brouqui P. Preventing and controlling emerging and reemerging transmissible diseases in the homeless. Emerg Infect Dis. 2008 Sep;14(9):1353-9.

Bai HM, Yang FL, Yang H, Zhang Q. [Study on Bartonella species in rodents in western Yunnan, China].[Article in Chinese]. Zhonghua Liu Xing Bing Xue Za Zhi. 2005 Nov;26(11):868-70.

Bai Y, Kosoy MY, Boonmar S, Sawatwong P, Sangmaneedet S, Peruski LF. Enrichment culture and molecular identification of diverse Bartonella species in stray dogs. Vet Microbiol. 2010 Dec 15;146(3-4):314-9. Epub 2010 May 12.

Bai Y, Kosoy MY, Lerdthusnee K, Peruski LF, Richardson JH. Prevalence and genetic heterogeneity of Bartonella strains cultured from rodents from 17 provinces in Thailand. Am J Trop Med Hyg. 2009 Nov;81(5):811-6.

Bai Y, Kosoy M, Martin A, Ray C, Sheff K, Chalcraft L, Collinge SK. Characterization of Bartonella strains isolated from black-tailed prairie dogs (Cynomys ludovicianus). Vector Borne Zoonotic Dis. 2008 Spring;8(1):1-5.

Bai Y, Kosoy M, Recuenco S, Alvarez D, Moran D, Turmelle A, Ellison J, Garcia DL, Estevez A, Lindblade K, Rupprecht C. Bartonella spp. in Bats, Guatemala. Emerg Infect Dis. 2011 Jul;17(7):1269-72.

Bai Y, Montgomery SP, Sheff KW, Chowdhury MA, Breiman RF, Kabeya H, Kosoy MY. Bartonella strains in small mammals from Dhaka, Bangladesh, related to Bartonella in America and Europe. Am J Trop Med Hyg. 2007 Sep;77(3):567-70.

Bajard A, Chabaud S, Pérol D, Boissel JP, Nony P. Revisiting the level of evidence in randomized controlled clinical trials: A simulation approach. Contemp Clin Trials. 2009. Sep;30(5):400-10. Epub 2009 Jul 1.

Baker J, Ruiz-Rodriguez R, Whitfeld M, Heon V, Berger TG. Bacillary angiomatosis: a treatable cause of acute psychiatric symptoms in human immunodeficiency virus infection. J Clin Psychiatry. 1995;56(4):161-166.

Bakken LL, Case KL, Callister SM, et al. Performance of 45 laboratories participating in a proficiency testing program for Lyme Disease serology. JAMA. 1992;268:891-895.

Balakrishnan N, Menon T, Fournier PE, Raoult D. Bartonella quintana and Coxiella burnetii as causes of endocarditis, India. Emerg Infect Dis. 2008 Jul;14(7):1168-9.

Balfour A. The infective granule in certain protozoal infections, as illustrated by the spirochaetosis of Sudanese fowl. 1911. British Medical Journal, 1:752.

Baltimore RS, Shapiro ED. Lyme disease. Pediatr Rev. 1994 May;15(5):167-73; quiz 174. Review.

Baneth G, Breitschwerdt EB, Hegarty BC, Pappalardo B, Ryan J. A survey of tick-borne bacteria and protozoa in naturally exposed dogs from Israel. Vet Parasitol. 1998 Jan 31;74(2-4):133-42.

Baneth G, Kordick DL, Hegarty BC, Breitschwerdt EB. Comparative seroreactivity to Bartonella henselae and Bartonella quintana among cats from Israel and North Carolina. Vet Microbiol. 1996 May;50(1-2):95-103.

Bangchang K, Le TD, Thrinh KA, Karbwang J. Phamacokinetics of a single oral dose of dihydroartemisinin in Vietnamese healthy volunteers. Southeast Asian J Trop Med Public Health. 1999;30:11-6.

Banik S, Terekhova D, Iyer R, Pappas CJ, Caimano MJ, Radolf JD, Schwartz I. BB0844, an RpoS-regulated protein, is dispensable for Borrelia burgdorferi infectivity and maintenance in the mouse-tick infectious cycle. Infect Immun. 2011 Mar;79(3):1208-17. Epub 2010 Dec 20.

Bapiro TE, Sayi J, Hasler JA, Jande M, Rimoy G, Masselle A, Masimirembwa CM. Artemisinin and thiabendazole are potent inhibitors of cytochrome P450 1A2 (CYP1A2) activity in humans. Eur J Clin Pharmacol. 2005;61:755-61. [Epub 2005 Oct 29].

Bar KJ, Jochum T, Hager F, Meissner W, Sauer H. Painful hallucinations and somatic delusions in a patient with the possible diagnosis of neuroborreliosis. Clin J Pain, 21(4):362-3. 2005.

Barber RM, Li Q, Diniz PP, Porter BF, Breitschwerdt EB, Claiborne MK, Birkenheuer AJ, Levine JM, Levine GJ, Chandler K, Kenny P, Nghiem P, Wei S, Greene CE, Kent M, Platt SR, Greer K, Schatzberg SJ. Evaluation of brain tissue or cerebrospinal fluid with broadly reactive polymerase chain reaction for Ehrlichia, Anaplasma, spotted fever group Rickettsia, Bartonella, and Borrelia species in canine neurological diseases (109 cases). J Vet Intern Med. 2010 Mar-Apr;24(2):372-8.

Barbet AF. Persistence mechanisms in tick-borne diseases. Onderstepoort J Vet Res. 2009 Mar;76(1):53-8.

Barbier F, Fournier PE, Dauge MC, Gallien S, Raoult D, Andremont A, Ruimy R. Bartonella quintana coinfection in Staphylococcus aureus endocarditis: usefulness of screening in high-risk patients? Clin Infect Dis. 2009 May 1;48(9):1332-3.

Barbour AG, Bunikis J, Travinsky B, Hoen AG, Diuk-Wasser MA, Fish D, Tsao JI. Niche partitioning of Borrelia burgdorferi and Borrelia miyamotoi in the same tick vector and mammalian reservoir species. Am J Trop Med Hyg. 2009 Dec;81(6):1120-31.

Barbour AG, Burgdorfer W, Grunwaldt E, Steere AC. Antibodies of patients with Lyme disease to components of the Ixodes dammini spirochete. J Clin Invest. 1983 Aug;72(2):504-15.

Barbour AG, Jasinskas A, Kayala MA, Davies DH, Steere AC, Baldi P, Felgner PL. A genome-wide proteome array reveals a limited set of immunogens in natural infections of humans and white-footed mice with Borrelia burgdorferi. Infect Immun. 2008 Aug;76(8):3374-89. Epub 2008 May 12.

Barbour AG, Hayes SF. Biology of Borrelia species. 1986. Microbiol Rev, 50:381-400.

Barbour AG, Putteet-Driver AD, Bunikis J. Horizontally acquired genes for purine salvage in Borrelia spp. causing relapsing fever. Infect Immun. 2005 Sep;73(9):6165-8.

Barbour AG, Todd WJ, Stoenner HG. Action of penicillin on Borrelia hermsii. 1982. Antimicrobial Agents & Chemotherapy, 21:823-9.

Barnett W, Sigmund D, Roelcke U, Mundt C. Endogenous paranoid-hallucinatory syndrome caused by Borrelia encephalitis. Nervenarzt, 62(7):445-7. 1991.

Barratt JL, Harkness J, Marriott D, Ellis JT, Stark D. Importance of nonenteric protozoan infections in immunocompromised people. Clin Microbiol Rev. 2010 Oct;23(4):795-836. Review.

Barthold SW, de Souza MS, Janotka JL, Smith AL, Persing DH. Chronic Lyme borreliosis in the laboratory mouse. Am J Path. 1993;143(3):959-71.

Barthold SW, Hodzic E, Imai D, Feng S, Yang X, Luft BJ. Ineffectiveness of Tigecycline against persistent Borrelia Burgdorferi. 2010. Antimicro Agents Chemother, 54(2):643-51.

Barthold SW, Moody KD, Terwilliger GA, Duray PH, Jacoby RO, Steere AC. Experimental Lyme arthritis in rats infected with Borrelia burgdorferi. J Infect Dis. 1988 Apr;157(4):842-6.

Barthold SW, Moody KD, Terwilliger GA, Jacoby RO, Steere AC. An animal model for Lyme arthritis. Ann N Y Acad Sci. 1988;539:264-73.

Bartosik K, Lachowska-Kotowska P, Szymańska J, Pabis A, Buczek A. Lyme borreliosis in south-eastern Poland: relationships with environmental factors and medical attention standards. Ann Agric Environ Med. 2011 Jun;18(1):131-7.

Baspinar O, Bayraktaroglu Z, Karsligil T, Bayram A, Coskun Y. A rare cause of anemia and thrombocytopenia in a newborn: congenital malaria. Turk J Pediatr. Department of Pediatrics, Gaziantep University Faculty of Medicine, Gaziantep, Turkey. 2006 Jan-Mar;48(1):63-5.

Bass JW, Vincent JM, Person DA. The expanding spectrum of Bartonella infections: II. Cat-scratch disease. Pediatr Infect Dis J. 1997;16(2):163-179.

Battafarano DF, Combs JA, Enzenauer RJ, Fitzpatrick JE. Chronic septic arthritis caused by Borrelia burgdorferi. 1993. Clinical Orthop, 297:238-41.

Battisti JM, Minnick MF. Laboratory maintenance of Bartonella quintana. Curr Protoc Microbiol. 2008 Aug;Chapter 3:Unit 3C.1.1-3C.1.13.

Battisti JM, Sappington KN, Smitherman LS, Parrow NL, Minnick MF. Environmental signals generate a differential and coordinated expression of the heme receptor gene family of Bartonella quintana. Infect Immun. 2006 Jun;74(6):3251-61.

Battisti JM, Smitherman LS, Sappington KN, Parrow NL, Raghavan R, Minnick MF. Transcriptional regulation of the heme binding protein gene family of Bartonella quintana is accomplished by a novel promoter element and iron response regulator. Infect Immun. 2007 Sep;75(9):4373-85. Epub 2007 Jun 18.

Batty KT, Davis TM, Thu LT, Binh TQ, Anh TK, Ilett KF. Selective high-performance liquid chromatographic determination of artesunate and alpha- and beta-dihydroartemisinin in patients with falciparum malaria. J Chromatogr B Biomed Appl. 1996 Mar 3;677:345-350.

Batty KT, Thu LT, Davis TM, Ilett KF, Mai TX, Hung NC, Tien NP, Powell SM, Thien HV, Binh TQ, Kim NV. A pharmacokinetic and pharmacodynamic study of intravenous vs oral artesunate in uncomplicated falciparum malaria. Br J Clin Pharmacol. 1998 Feb;45:123-9.

Batty KT, Iletr KE, Powell SM, Martin J, Davis TM. Relative bioavailability of artesunate and dihydroartemisinin: investigations in the isolated perfused rat liver and in healthy Caucasian volunteers. Am J Trop Med Hyg. 2002;66:130-6.

Baty G, Lanotte P, Hocqueloux L, Prazuck T, Bret L, Romano M, Mereghetti L. [PCR rDNA 16S used for the etiological diagnosis of blood culture negative endocarditis].[Article in French]. Med Mal Infect. 2010 Jun;40(6):358-62. Epub 2009 Sep 30. Review.

Bauer J, Leitz G, Palmedo G, Hugel H. Anetoderma: Another facet of Lyme disease? J Am Acad Dermatol. 2003 May;48(5 Suppl):S86-8.

Baumeister S, Wiesner J, Reichenberg A, Hintz M, Bietz S, Harb OS, Roos DS, Kordes M, Friesen J, Matuschewski K, Lingelbach K, Jomaa H, Seeber F. Fosmidomycin uptake into Plasmodium and Babesia-infected erythrocytes is facilitated by parasite-induced new permeability pathways. PLoS One. 2011 May 4;6(5):e19334.

Bayard-Mc Neeley M, Bansal A, Chowdhury I, Girao G, Small CB, Seiter K, Nelson J, Liveris D, Schwartz I, Mc Neeley DF, Wormser GP, Aguero-Rosenfeld ME. In vivo and in vitro studies on Anaplasma phagocytophilum infection of the myeloid cells of a patient with chronic myelogenous leukaemia and human granulocytic ehrlichiosis. J Clin Pathol. 2004 May; 57(5): 499–503.

Bayer ME, Zhang L, Bayer MH. Borrelia burgdorferi DNA in the urine of treated patients with chronic Lyme disease symptoms. A PCR study of 97 cases. Infection. 1996 Sep-Oct;24(5):347-53.

Baylor P, Garoufi A, Karpathios T, Lutz J, Mogelof J, Moseley D. Transverse myelitis in 2 patients with Bartonella henselae infection (cat scratch disease). Clin Infect Dis. 2007 Aug 15;45(4):e42-5. Epub 2007 Jul 5.

Bazovska S, Durovska J, Derdakova M, Taragelova V, Pancak J, Zaborska M, Traubner P. The genospecies B. burgdorferi s.l., isolated from ticks and from neurological patients with suspected Lyme borreliosis. Neuro Endocrinol Lett. 2011;32(4):491-5.

Bazovská S, Durovská J, Pancák J, Záborská M, Derdáková M. [Lyme borreliosis and demyelinating disease of the central nervous system].[Article in Czech]. Epidemiol Mikrobiol Imunol. 2011 Feb;60(1):45-7.

Beard AW, Maggi RG, Kennedy-Stoskopf S, Cherry NA, Sandfoss MR, DePerno CS, Breitschwerdt EB. Bartonella spp. in feral pigs, southeastern United States. Emerg Infect Dis. 2011 May;17(5):893-5.

Beare PA, Sandoz KM, Omsland A, Rockey DD, Heinzen RA. Advances in Genetic Manipulation of Obligate Intracellular Bacterial Pathogens. Front Microbiol. 2011; 2: 97. Prepublished online 2011 March 14. Published online 2011 May 2.

Beck R, Vojta L, Curkovi S, Mrljak V, Margaleti J, Habrun B. Molecular survey of Babesia microti in wild rodents in central Croatia. Vector Borne Zoonotic Dis. 2011 Jan;11(1):81-3.

Becker CA, Malandrin L, Depoix D, Larcher T, David PH, Chauvin A, Bischoff E, Bonnet S. Identification of three CCp genes in Babesia divergens: novel markers for sexual stages parasites. Mol Biochem Parasitol. 2010 Nov;174(1):36-43. Epub 2010 Jul 21.

Becker JL. Vector-borne illnesses and the safety of the blood supply. Curr Hematol Rep. 2003 Nov;2(6):511-7. Review.

Beermann C, Wunderli-Allenspach H, Groscurth P, Filgueira L. Lipoproteins from Borrelia burgdorferi applied in liposomes and presented by dendritic cells induce CD8(+) T lymphocytes in vitro. 2000. Cell Immunology, May 1;201(2):124-131.

Begley DW, Edwards TE, Raymond AC, Smith ER, Hartley RC, Abendroth J, Sankaran B, Lorimer DD, Myler PJ, Staker BL, Stewart LJ. Inhibitor-bound complexes of dihydrofolate reductase-thymidylate synthase from Babesia bovis. Acta Crystallogr Sect F Struct Biol Cryst Commun. 2011 Sep 1;67(Pt 9):1070-7. Epub 2011 Aug 16.

Behera AK, Hildebrand E, Szafranski J, Hung HH, Grodzinsky AJ, Lafyatis R, Koch AE, Kalish R, Perides G, Steere AC, Hu LT. Role of aggrecanase 1 in Lyme arthritis. Arthritis Rheum. 2006 Oct;54(10):3319-29.

Behera AK, Hildebrand E, Scagliotti J, Steere AC, Hu LT. Induction of host matrix metalloproteinases by Borrelia burgdorferi differs in human and murine lyme arthritis. Infect Immun. 2005 Jan;73(1):126-34.

Bellissimo-Rodrigues F, da Fonseca BA, Martinez R. Bacillary angiomatosis in a pregnant woman. Int J Gynaecol Obstet. 2010 Oct;111(1):85-6. Epub 2010 Jul 21.

Belloni B, Andres C, Ring J, Hofmann H. [5-yr-old with borrelial lymphocytoma].[Article in German]. MMW Fortschr Med. 2011 Mar 10;153(10):40.

Belongia EA. Epidemiology and impact of coinfections acquired from Ixodes ticks. Vector Borne Zoonotic Dis. 2002 Winter;2(4):265-73.

Ben Slama L, Hasni W, Royer B. [Cat-scratch disease localisation in the parotid gland]. [Article in French]. Rev Stomatol Chir Maxillofac. 2008 Jun;109(3):183-6. Epub 2008 Jun 3.

Benach JL, Bosler EM, Hanrahan JP, Coleman JL, Habicht GS, Bast TF, Cameron DJ, Ziegler JL, Barbour AG, Burgdorfer W, Edelman R, Kaslow RA. Spirochetes isolated from the blood of two patients with Lyme disease. N Engl J Med. 1983 Mar 31;308(13):740-2.

Benach JL, Coleman JL, Habicht GS, MacDonald A, Grunwaldt E, Giron JA. Serological evidence for simultaneous occurrences of Lyme disease and babesiosis. J Infect Dis. 1985 Sept;152(3):473-7.

Benach JL, Coleman JL. Overview of spirochetal infections. In "Lyme Disease," ed. P. Coyle, M.D. St. Louis; Mosby-Year Book, Inc. 1993.

Benakis A, Binh TQ, Keundjian A, Scheiwe MW. Pharmacokinetics/Pharmacodynamics findings after repeated administration of ARTESUNATE thermostable suppositories (RECTOCAPS) in Vietnamese patients with uncomplicated malaria. Eur J Drug Metab Pharmacokinet. 2006 Jan-Mar;31(1):41-5.

Ben-Ami R, Ephros M, Avidor B, Katchman E, Varon M, Leibowitz C, Comaneshter D, Giladi M. Cat-scratch disease in elderly patients. Clin Infect Dis. 2005 Oct 1;41(7):969-974.

Benoit VM, Fischer JR, Lin YP, Parveen N, Leong JM. Allelic variation of the Lyme disease spirochete adhesin DbpA influences spirochetal binding to decorin, dermatan sulfate, and mammalian cells. Infect Immun. 2011 Sep;79(9):3501-9. Epub 2011 Jun 27.

Benslimani A, Fenollar F, Lepidi H, Raoult D. Bacterial zoonoses and infective endocarditis, Algeria. Emerg Infect Dis. 2005 Feb;11(2):216-24.

Bentzel DE, Espinosa BJ, Canal E, Blazes DL, Hall ER. Susceptibility of owl monkeys (Aotus nancymaae) to experimental infection with Bartonella bacilliformis. Comp Med. 2008 Feb;58(1):76-80.

Berardi VP, Weeks KE, Steere AC. Serodiagnosis of early Lyme disease: analysis of IgM and IgG antibody responses by using an antibody-capture enzyme immunoassay. J Infect Dis. 1988 Oct;158(4):754-60.

Berger BW. Treating erythema chronicum migrans of Lyme disease. 1986. Journal of Am Acad Dermatology, Sep;15(3):459-63.

Berger BW. Treatment of erythema chronicum migrans of Lyme disease. 1988. Annals of the New York Academy of Sciences, 539:346-51.

Berger BW, Kaplan MH, Rotherberg IR, Barbour AG. Isolation and characterization of the Lyme disease spirochete from the skin of patients with erythema chronicum migrans. J Am Acad Dermatol, 13:444-449. 1985.

Berger TG, Dieckmann D, Efferth T, Schultz ES, Funk JO, Baur A, Schuler G. Artesunate in the treatment of metastatic uveal melanoma–first experiences. Oncol. Rep. 2005;14:1599-603.

Berghoff J, Viezens J, Guptill L, Fabbi M, Arvand M. Bartonella henselae exists as a mosaic of different genetic variants in the infected host. Microbiology. 2007 Jul;153(Pt 7):2045-51.

Berglund EC, Ehrenborg C, Vinnere Pettersson O, Granberg F, Näslund K, Holmberg M, Andersson SG. Genome dynamics of Bartonella grahamii in micro-populations of woodland rodents. BMC Genomics. 2010 Mar 4;11:152.

Berglund EC, Ellegaard K, Granberg F, Xie Z, Maruyama S, Kosoy MY, Birtles RJ, Andersson SG. Rapid diversification by recombination in Bartonella grahamii from wild rodents in Asia contrasts with low levels of genomic divergence in Northern Europe and America. Mol Ecol. 2010 Jun;19(11):2241-55. Epub 2010 May 6.

Berglund EC, Frank AC, Calteau A, Vinnere Pettersson O, Granberg F, Eriksson AS, Näslund K, Holmberg M, Lindroos H, Andersson SG. Run-off replication of host-adaptability genes is associated with gene transfer agents in the genome of mouse-infecting Bartonella grahamii. PLoS Genet. 2009 Jul;5(7):e1000546. Epub 2009 Jul 3.

Berguiga M, Abouzeid H, Bart PA, Guex-Crosier Y. Severe occlusive vasculitis as a complication of cat scratch disease. Klin Monbl Augenheilkd. 2008 May;225(5):486-7.

Bernit E, Veit V, La Scola B, Tissot-Dupont H, Gachon J, Raoult D, Harlé JR. Bartonella quintana and Mycobacterium tuberculosis coinfection in an HIV-infected patient with lymphadenitis. J Infect. 2003 May;46(4):244-6.

Berrich M, Kieda C, Grillon C, Monteil M, Lamerant N, Gavard J, Boulouis HJ, Haddad N. Differential effects of Bartonella henselae on human and feline macro- and micro-vascular endothelial cells. PLoS One. 2011;6(5):e20204. Epub 2011 May 27.

Bertrand E, Szpak GM, Pilkowska E, Habib N, Lipczynska-Lojkowska W, et al. Central nervous system infection caused by Borrelia burgdorferi. Clinico-pathological correlation of three post-mortem cases. Folia Neuropathol; 37(1):43-51. 1999.

Bhambhani N, Disla E, Cuppari G. Lyme disease presenting with sequential episodes of ruptured baker cysts. J Clin Rheumatol, 12(3). 2006.

Bhate C, Schwartz RA. Lyme disease: Part I. Advances and perspectives. J Am Acad Dermatol. 2011 Apr;64(4):619-36; quiz 637-8. Review.

Bhattacharya D, Bensaci M, Luker KE, Luker G, Wisdom S, Telford SR, Hu LT. Development of a baited oral vaccine for use in reservoir-targeted strategies against Lyme disease. Vaccine. 2011 Oct 13;29(44):7818-25. Epub 2011 Aug 2

Bhatti Z, Berenson CS. Adult systemic cat scratch disease associated with therapy for hepatitis C. BMC Infect Dis. 2007 Feb 23;7:8.

Bhengsri S, Baggett HC, Peruski LF Jr, Morway C, Bai Y, Fisk TL, Sitdhirasdr A, Maloney SA, Dowell SF, Kosoy M. Bartonella spp. infections, Thailand. Emerg Infect Dis. 2010 Apr;16(4):743-5.

Bhengsri S, Baggett HC, Peruski LF, Morway C, Bai Y, Fisk TL, Sitdhirasdr A, Maloney SA, Dowell SF, Kosoy M. Bartonella seroprevalence in rural Thailand. Southeast Asian J Trop Med Public Health. 2011 May;42(3):687-92.

Bhide MR, Mucha R, Mikula I Jr, Kisova L, Skrabana R, Novak M, Mikula I Sr. Novel mutations in TLR genes cause hyporesponsiveness to Mycobacterium avium subsp. paratuberculosis infection. BMC Genet. 2009; 10: 21. Published online 2009 May 26.

Bialasiewicz AA, Huk W, Druschky KF, Naumann GO. Borrelia burgdorferi infection with bilateral optic neuritis and intracerebral demyelinization lesions. Klin Monbl Augenheilkd. 1989 Aug;195(2):91-4.

Bianda JC, Dedes W. [Positive polymerase chain reaction for Bartonella henselae in conjunctival granuloma].[Article in German]. Klin Monbl Augenheilkd. 2009 Apr;226(4):347. Epub 2009 Apr 21.

Biddinger PD, Isselbacher EM, Fan D, Shepard JA. Case records of the Massachusetts General Hospital. Weekly clinicopathological exercises. Case 5-2005. A 53-year-old man with depression and sudden shortness of breath. N Engl J Med. 2005 Feb 17;352(7):709-16.

Bihl F, Castelli D, Marincola F, Dodd RY, Brander C. Transfusion-transmitted infections. J Transl Med. 2007; 5: 25. Published online 2007 June 6.

Billeter SA, Blanton HL, Little SE, Levy MG, Breitschwerdt EB. Detection of Rickettsia amblyommii in association with a tick bite rash. Vector Borne Zoonotic Dis. 2007 Winter;7(4):607-10.

Billeter SA, Diniz PP, Battisti JM, Munderloh UG, Breitschwerdt EB, Levy MG. Infection and replication of Bartonella species within a tick cell line. Exp Appl Acarol. 2009 Nov;49(3):193-208. Epub 2009 Feb 26.

Billeter SA, Levy MG, Chomel BB, Breitschwerdt EB. Vector transmission of Bartonella species with emphasis on the potential for tick transmission. Med Vet Entomol. 2008 Mar;22(1):1-15. Review.

Billeter SA, Miller MK, Breitschwerdt EB, Levy MG. Detection of two Bartonella tamiae-like sequences in Amblyomma americanum (Acari: Ixodidae) using 16S-23S intergenic spacer region-specific primers. J Med Entomol. 2008 Jan;45(1):176-9.

Birtles RJ. Bartonellae as elegant hemotropic parasites. Ann N Y Acad Sci. 2005 Dec;1063:270-9. Review.

Birtles RJ, Canales J, Ventosilla P, Alvarez E, Guerra H, Llanos-Cuentas A, Raoult D, Doshi N, Harrison TG. Survey of Bartonella species infecting intradomicillary animals in the Huayllacallán Valley, Ancash, Peru, a region endemic for human bartonellosis. Am J Trop Med Hyg. 1999 May;60(5):799-805.

Birtles RJ, Fry NK, Ventosilla P, Cáceres AG, Sánchez E, Vizcarra H, Raoult D. Identification of Bartonella bacilliformis genotypes and their relevance to epidemiological investigations of human bartonellosis. J Clin Microbiol. 2002 Oct;40(10):3606-12.

Birtles RJ, Hazel SM, Bennett M, Bown K, Raoult D, Begon M. Longitudinal monitoring of the dynamics of infections due to Bartonella species in UK woodland rodents. Epidemiol Infect. 2001 Apr;126(2):323-9.

Birtles RJ, Hazel S, Bown K, Raoult D, Begon M, Bennett M. Subtyping of uncultured bartonellae using sequence comparison of 16 S/23 S rRNA intergenic spacer regions amplified directly from infected blood. Mol Cell Probes. 2000 Apr;14(2):79-87.

Birtles RJ, Raoult D. Comparison of partial citrate synthase gene (gltA) sequences for phylogenetic analysis of Bartonella species. Int J Syst Bacteriol. 1996 Oct;46(4):891-7.

Biswas S, Maggi RG, Papich MG, Breitschwerdt EB. Molecular mechanisms of Bartonella henselae resistance to azithromycin, pradofloxacin and enrofloxacin. J Antimicrob Chemother. 2010 Mar;65(3):581-2. Epub 2009 Dec 18.

Biswas S, Maggi RG, Papich MG, Keil D, Breitschwerdt EB. Comparative activity of pradofloxacin, enrofloxacin, and azithromycin against Bartonella henselae isolates collected from cats and a human. J Clin Microbiol. 2010 Feb;48(2):617-8. Epub 2009 Dec 9.

Biswas S, Raoult D, Rolain JM. Molecular characterization of resistance to macrolides in Bartonella henselae. Antimicrob Agents Chemother. 2006 Sep;50(9):3192-3.

Biswas S, Raoult D, Rolain JM. Molecular mechanisms of resistance to antibiotics in Bartonella bacilliformis. J Antimicrob Chemother. 2007 Jun;59(6):1065-70. Epub 2007 Apr 21.

Biswas S, Raoult D, Rolain JM. A bioinformatic approach to understanding antibiotic resistance in intracellular bacteria through whole genome analysis. Int J Antimicrob Agents. 2008 Sep;32(3):207-20. Epub 2008 Jul 10. Review.

Biswas S, Raoult D, Rolain JM. Molecular mechanism of gentamicin resistance in Bartonella henselae. Clin Microbiol Infect. 2009 Dec;15 Suppl 2:98-9.

Biswas S, Raoult D, Rolain JM. Molecular characterisation of resistance to rifampin in Bartonella quintana. Clin Microbiol Infect. 2009 Dec;15 Suppl 2:100-1. Epub 2009 Dec 24.

Biswas S, Rolain JM. Bartonella infection: treatment and drug resistance. Future Microbiol. 2010 Nov;5(11):1719-31. Review.

Bitam I, Dittmar K, Parola P, Whiting MF, Raoult D. Fleas and flea-borne diseases. Int J Infect Dis. 2010 Aug;14(8):e667-76. Epub 2010 Mar 1. Review.

Bitam I, Rolain JM, Kernif T, Baziz B, Parola P, Raoult D. Bartonella species detected in rodents and hedgehogs from Algeria. Clin Microbiol Infect. 2009 Dec;15 Suppl 2:102-3. Epub 2009 Dec 24.

Black JR, Herrington DA, Hadfield TL, Wear DJ, Margileth AM, Shigekawa B. Life-threatening cat-scratch disease in an immunocompromised host. Arch Intern Med. 1986 Feb;146(2):394-6.

Bladen HA, Hampp EG. Ultrastructure of Treponema microdentium and Borrelia vincentii. 1964. Journal of Bacteriology, 87:1180-1191.

Blaho VA, Zhang Y, Hughes-Hanks JM, Brown CR. 5-Lipoxygenase-deficient mice infected with Borrelia burgdorferi develop persistent arthritis. J Immunol. 2011 Mar 1;186(5):3076-84. Epub 2011 Jan 26.

Blakeley J, Jankovic J. Secondary paroxysmal dyskinesias. Mov Disord. 2002 Jul;17(4):726-34.

Blanco JR, Jado I, Marín M, Sanfeliu I, Portillo A, Anda P, Pons I, Oteo JA. [Microbiological diagnosis of emerging bacterial pathogens: Anaplasma, Bartonella, Rickettsia, and Tropheryma whipplei].[Article in Spanish]. Enferm Infecc Microbiol Clin. 2008 Nov;26(9):573-80. Review.

Blanco JR, Pérez-Martínez L, Vallejo M, Santibáñez S, Portillo A, Oteo JA. Prevalence of rickettsia felis-like and Bartonella Spp. in Ctenocephalides felis and Ctenocephalides canis from La Rioja (Northern Spain). Ann N Y Acad Sci. 2006 Oct;1078:270-4.

Blanco JR, Raoult D. [Diseases produced by Bartonella].[Article in Spanish]. Enferm Infecc Microbiol Clin. 2005 May;23(5):313-9; quiz 320. Review.

Blaschitz M, Narodoslavsky-Gföller M, Kanzler M, Stanek G, Walochnik J. Babesia species occurring in Austrian Ixodes ricinus ticks. Appl Environ Microbiol. 2008 Aug;74(15):4841-6. Epub 2008 Jun 6.

Blue D, Graves V, McCarthy L, Cruz J, Gregurek S, Smith D. Fatal transfusion-transmitted Babesia microti in the Midwest. Transfusion. 2009 Jan;49(1):8. Epub 2008 Aug 6.

Bloom BJ, Wyckoff PM, Meissner HC, Steere AC. Neurocognitive abnormalities in children after classic manifestations of Lyme disease. Pediatr Infect Dis J. 1998 Mar;17(3):189-96.

Bodner RA, Lynch T, Lewis L, Kahn D. Serotonin syndrome. Neurology. 1995 Feb;45(2):219-223.

Boggs SR, Fisher RG. Bone pain and fever in an adolescent and his sibling. Cat scratch disease (CSD). Pediatr Infect Dis J. 2011 Jan;30(1):89, 93-4.

Boillat N, Greub G. [Cat scratch disease and other human infections caused by Bartonella species].[Article in French]. Rev Med Suisse. 2008 Apr 9;4(152):901-7. Review.

Bolton JG, Galeckas KJ, Satter EK. Inoculation bartonellosis in an adult: a case report. Cutis. 2010 Jan;85(1):37-42.

Bolz DD, Sundsbak RS, Ma Y, Akira S, Weis JH, Schwan TG, Weis JJ. Dual Role of MyD88 in Rapid Clearance of Relapsing Fever Borrelia spp. Infect Immun. 2006 December; 74(12): 6750–6760. Published online 2006 October 9.

Bonatti H, Mendez J, Guerrero I, Krishna M, Ananda-Michel J, Yao J, Steers JL, Hellinger W, Dickson RC, Alvarez S. Disseminated Bartonella infection following liver transplantation. Transpl Int. 2006 Aug;19(8):683-7.

Bonhomme CJ, Nappez C, Raoult D. Microarray for serotyping of Bartonella species. BMC Microbiol. 2007 Jun 25;7:59.

Bonilla DL, Kabeya H, Henn J, Kramer VL, Kosoy MY. Bartonella quintana in body lice and head lice from homeless persons, San Francisco, California, USA. Emerg Infect Dis. 2009 Jun;15(6):912-5.

Bonnet S, Brisseau N, Hermouet A, Jouglin M, Chauvin A. Experimental in vitro transmission of Babesia sp. (EU1) by Ixodes ricinus. Vet Res. 2009 May-Jun;40(3):21. Epub 2009 Feb 13.

Bonnet S, Jouglin M, Malandrin L, Becker C, Agoulon A, L'hostis M, Chauvin A. Transstadial and transovarial persistence of Babesia divergens DNA in Ixodes ricinus ticks fed on infected blood in a new skin-feeding technique. Parasitology. 2007 Feb;134(Pt 2):197-207. Epub 2006 Nov 1.

Boonjakuakul JK, Gerns HL, Chen YT, Hicks LD, Minnick MF, Dixon SE, Hall SC, Koehler JE. Proteomic and immunoblot analyses of Bartonella quintana total membrane proteins identify antigens recognized by sera from infected patients. Infect Immun. 2007 May;75(5):2548-61. Epub 2007 Feb 16.

Boralevi F, Léauté-Labrèze C, Lepreux S, Barbarot S, Mazereeuw-Hautier J, Eschard C, Taïeb A; Groupe de Recherche Clinique en Dermatologie Pédiatrique. Idiopathic facial aseptic granuloma: a multicentre prospective study of 30 cases. Br J Dermatol. 2007 Apr;156(4):705-8.

Borboli S, Afshari NA, Watkins L, Foster CS. Presumed oculoglandular syndrome from Bartonella quintana. Ocul Immunol Inflamm. 2007 Jan-Feb;15(1):41-3.

Borgoiakov VIu, Fomenko NV, Panov VV, Chikova ED. [Study on the infection of taiga ticks with Borrelia in the territory of Novosibirsk Scientific Center SB PAS].[Article in Russian]. Parazitologiia. 2010 Nov-Dec;44(6):543-56.

Bos MP, Tefsen B, Geurtsen J, Tommassen J. Identification of an outer membrane protein required for the transport of lipopolysaccharide to the bacterial cell surface. Proc Natl Acad Sci U S A. 2004 June 22; 101(25): 9417–9422. Published online 2004 June 10.

Bouchouicha R, Durand B, Monteil M, Chomel BB, Berrich M, Arvand M, Birtles RJ, Breitschwerdt EB, Koehler JE, Maggi R, Maruyama S, Kasten R, Petit E, Boulouis HJ, Haddad N. Molecular epidemiology of feline and human Bartonella henselae isolates. Emerg Infect Dis. 2009 May;15(5):813-6.

Boudová L, Kazakov DV, Hes O, Sůvová B,, Neprasova P, Treska V, Fakan F, Michal M. [Pseudolymphoma of the breast nipple. The problem overview.].[Article in Czech]. Rozhl Chir. 2005 Feb;84(2):66-9.

Boulouis HJ, Barrat F, Bermond D, Bernex F, Thibault D, Heller R, Fontaine JJ, Piémont Y, Chomel BB. Kinetics of Bartonella birtlesii infection in experimentally infected mice and pathogenic effect on reproductive functions. Infect Immun. 2001 Sep;69(9):5313-7.

Boulouis HJ, Chang CC, Henn JB, Kasten RW, Chomel BB. Factors associated with the rapid emergence of zoonotic Bartonella infections. Vet Res. 2005;36(3):383-410.

Boulouis HJ, Haddad N, Vayssier-Taussat M, Maillard R, Chomel B. [Persistent Bartonella infection: epidemiological and clinical implications]. [Article in French]. Bull Acad Natl Med. 2007 Jun;191(6):1037-44; discussion 1047-9.

Bourré-Tessier J, Milord F, Pineau C, Vinet E. Indigenous Lyme disease in Quebec. J Rheumatol. 2011 Jan;38(1):183.

Bradbury CA, Lappin MR. Evaluation of topical application of 10% imidacloprid-1% moxidectin to prevent Bartonella henselae transmission from cat fleas. J Am Vet Med Assoc. 2010 Apr 15;236(8):869-73.

Bradley JF, Johnson RC, Goodman JL. The persistence of spirochetal nucleic acids in active Lyme arthritis. 1994. Annals of Internal Medicine, 120(6):487-9.

Braga W, Venasco J, Willard L, Moro MH. Ultrastructure of Babesia WA1 (Apicomplexa: Piroplasma) during infection of erythrocytes in a hamster model. J Parasitol. 2006 Oct;92(5):1104-7.

Branda JA, Aguero-Rosenfeld ME, Ferraro MJ, Johnson BJ, Wormser GP, Steere AC. 2-tiered antibody testing for early and late Lyme disease using only an immunoglobulin G blot with the addition of a VlsE band as the second-tier test. Clin Infect Dis. 2010 Jan 1;50(1):20-6.

Branda JA, Linskey K, Kim YA, Steere AC, Ferraro MJ. Two-tiered antibody testing for Lyme disease with use of 2 enzyme immunoassays, a whole-cell sonicate enzyme immunoassay followed by a VlsE C6 peptide enzyme immunoassay. Clin Infect Dis. 2011 Sep;53(6):541-7.

Branigan P, Rao J, Rao J, Gerard H, Hudson A, Williams W, Arayssi T, Pando J, Bayer M, Rothfuss S, Clayburne G, Sieck M, Schumacher HR. PCR evidence for Borrelia burgdorferi DNA in synovium in absence of positive serology. Arthritis Rheum. 1997 Sep;40(9 Suppl):S270.

Braschler T, Demierre N, Nascimento E, Silva T, Oliva AG, Renaud P. Continuous separation of cells by balanced dielectrophoretic forces at multiple frequencies. Lab Chip. 2008 Feb;8(2):280-6. Epub 2007 Nov 15.

Breathnach AS, Hoare JM, Eykyn SJ. Culture-negative endocarditis: contribution of bartonella infections. Heart. 1997 May;77(5):474-6.

Brecht A, Stiegler T, Lange J, de Groot K. [Generalized lymphadenitis associated with Hashimoto's thyroiditis].[Article in German]. Dtsch Med Wochenschr. 2007 Apr 20;132(16):874-7.

Breier F, Khanakah G, Stanek G, Kunz G, Aberer E, et al. Isolation and polymerase chain reaction typing of Borrelia afzelii from a skin lesion in a seronegative patient wtih generalized ulcerating bullous lichen sclerosus et atrophicus. Br J Dermatol. 2001 Feb;144(2):387-92.

Breitschwerdt EB. Feline bartonellosis and cat scratch disease. Vet Immunol Immunopathol. 2008 May 15;123(1-2):167-71. Epub 2008 Jan 19. Review.

Breitschwerdt EB, Maggi RG. A confusing case of canine vector-borne disease: clinical signs and progression in a dog co-infected with Ehrlichia canis and Bartonella vinsonii ssp. berkhoffii. Parasit Vectors. 2009 Mar 26;2 Suppl 1:S3.

Breitschwerdt EB, Maggi RG. Comparative medical features of canine and human bartonellosis. Clin Microbiol Infect. 2009 Dec;15 Suppl 2:106-7. Epub 2009 Apr 30.

Breitschwerdt EB, Maggi RG, Cadenas MB, de Paiva Diniz PP. A groundhog, a novel Bartonella sequence, and my father's death. Emerg Infect Dis. 2009 Dec;15(12):2080-6.

Breitschwerdt EB, Maggi RG, Chomel BB, Lappin MR. Bartonellosis: an emerging infectious disease of zoonotic importance to animals and human beings. J Vet Emerg Crit Care (San Antonio). 2010 Feb;20(1):8-30. Review.

Breitschwerdt EB, Maggi RG, Duncan AW, Nicholson WL, Hegarty BC, Woods CW. Bartonella species in blood of immunocompetent persons with animal and arthropod contact. Emerg Infect Dis. 2007 Jun;13(6):938-41.

Breitschwerdt EB, Maggi RG, Farmer P, Mascarelli PE. Molecular evidence of perinatal transmission of Bartonella vinsonii subsp. berkhoffii and Bartonella henselae to a child. J Clin Microbiol. 2010 Jun;48(6):2289-93. Epub 2010 Apr 14.

Breitschwerdt EB, Maggi RG, Lantos PM, Woods CW, Hegarty BC, Bradley JM. Bartonella vinsonii subsp. berkhoffii and Bartonella henselae bacteremia in a father and daughter with neurological disease. Parasit Vectors. 2010 Apr 8;3(1):29.

Breitschwerdt EB, Maggi RG, Nicholson WL, Cherry NA, Woods CW. Bartonella sp. bacteremia in patients with neurological and neurocognitive dysfunction. J Clin Microbiol. 2008 Sep;46(9):2856-61. Epub 2008 Jul 16.

Breitschwerdt EB, Maggi RG, Robert Mozayeni B, Hegarty BC, Bradley JM, Mascarelli PE. PCR amplification of Bartonella koehlerae from human blood and enrichment blood cultures. Parasit Vectors. 2010 Aug 24;3:76.

Breitschwerdt EB, Maggi RG, Sigmon B, Nicholson WL. Isolation of Bartonella quintana from a woman and a cat following putative bite transmission. J Clin Microbiol. 2007 Jan;45(1):270-2. Epub 2006 Nov 8.

Breitschwerdt EB, Maggi RG, Varanat M, Linder KE, Weinberg G. Isolation of Bartonella vinsonii subsp. berkhoffii genotype II from a boy with epithelioid hemangioendothelioma and a dog with hemangiopericytoma. J Clin Microbiol. 2009 Jun;47(6):1957-60. Epub 2009 Apr 15.

Brenneis C, Scherfler C, Engelhardt K, Helbok R, Brössner G, Beer R, Lackner P, Walder G, Pfausler B, Schmutzhard E. Encephalitis lethargica following Bartonella henselae infection. J Neurol. 2007 Apr;254(4):546-7. Epub 2007 Mar 12.

Brenner SA, Rooney JA, Manzewitsch P, Regnery RL. Isolation of Bartonella (Rochalimaea) henselae: effects of methods of blood collection and handling. J Clin Microbiol. 1997 Mar;35(3):544-7.

Brewer TG, Grate SJ, Peggins JO, Weina PJ, Petras JM, Levine BS, Heiffer MH, Schuster BG. Fatal neurotoxicity of arteether and artemether. Am J Trop Med Hyg. 1994 Sept;51(3):251-9.

Bridwell KH, Berven S, Edwards C 2nd, Glassman S, Hamill C, Schwab F. The problems and limitations of applying evidence-based medicine to primary surgical treatment of adult spinal deformity. Spine (Phila Pa 1976). 2007 Sep 1;32(19 Suppl):S135-9. Review.

Brinar VV, Habek M. Rare infections mimicking MS. Clin Neurol Neurosurg. 2010 Sep;112(7):625-8. Epub 2010 May 2.

Brinck T, Hansen K, Olesen J. Headache resembling tension-type headache as the single manifestation of Lyme neuroborreliosis. Cephalalgia. 1993 Jun;13(3):207-9.

Brinkane A, Crickx L, Leroy Terquem E, Mauger C, Akpan T, Bergheul S, Peschard S, Raheriarisoa H, Gaudin B, Levy R. [Encephalopathy during cat scratch disease in an adult].[Article in French]. Rev Med Interne. 2001 Jun;22(6):589-90.

Brinkerhoff RJ, Folsom-O'Keefe CM, Streby HM, Bent SJ, Tsao K, Diuk-Wasser MA. Regional variation in immature Ixodes scapularis parasitism on North American songbirds: implications for transmission of the Lyme pathogen, Borrelia burgdorferi. J Med Entomol. 2011 Mar;48(2):422-8.

Brisson D, Baxamusa N, Schwartz I, Wormser GP. Biodiversity of Borrelia burgdorferi strains in tissues of Lyme disease patients. PLoS One. 2011;6(8):e22926. Epub 2011 Aug 4.

Brogan GX, Homan CS, Viccellio P. The enlarging clinical spectrum of Lyme disease: Lyme cerebral vasculitis, a new disease entity. Ann Emerg Med. 1990 May;19(5):572-6.

Brook I. The bacteriology of salivary gland infections. Oral Maxillofac Surg Clin North Am. 2009 Aug;21(3):269-74. Review.

Brorson O, Brorson SH. Susceptibility of motile and cystic forms of Borrelia burgdorferi to ranitidine bismuth citrate. Int Microbiol. 2001 Dec;4(4):209-15.

Brorson O, Brorson SH, Henriksen TH, Skogen PR, Schoyen R. Association between multiple sclerosis and cystic structures in cerebrospinal fluid. Infection. 2001 Dec;29(6):315-9.

Brorson O, Brorson S. An in vitro study of the susceptibility of mobile and cystic forms of Borrelia burgdorferi to metronidazole. APMIS. 1999 Jun;107(6):566-576.

Brorson O, Brorson S. A rapid method for generating cystic forms of Borrelia burgdorferi, and their reversal to mobile spirochetes. APMIS. 1998 Dec;106(12):1131-1141.

Brorson O, Brorson S. In vitro conversion of Borrelia burgdorferi to cystic forms in spinal fluid, and transformation to mobile spirochetes by incubation in BSK-H medium. Infection. 1998 May-Jun;26(3):144-50.

Brorson O, Brorson SH. Transformation of cystic forms of Borrelia burgdorferi to normal mobile spirochetes. Infection. 1997 Jul-Aug;25:240-6.

Brouqui P. Arthropod-borne diseases associated with political and social disorder. Annu Rev Entomol. 2011 Jan;56:357-74. Review.

Brouqui P, Bacellar F, Baranton G, Birtles RJ, Bjoërsdorff A, Blanco JR, Caruso G, Cinco M, Fournier PE, Francavilla E, Jensenius M, Kazar J, Laferl H, Lakos A, Lotric Furlan S, Maurin M, Oteo JA, Parola P, Perez-Eid C, Peter O, Postic D, Raoult D, Tellez A, Tselentis Y, Wilske B; ESCMID Study Group on Coxiella, Anaplasma, Rickettsia and Bartonella; European Network for Surveillance of Tick-Borne Diseases. Guidelines for the diagnosis of tick-borne bacterial diseases in Europe. Clin Microbiol Infect. 2004 Dec;10(12):1108-32.

Brouqui P, Houpikian P, Dupont HT, Toubiana P, Obadia Y, Lafay V, Raoult D. Survey of the seroprevalence of Bartonella quintana in homeless people. Clin Infect Dis. 1996 Oct;23(4):756-9.

Brouqui P, Lascola B, Roux V, Raoult D. Chronic Bartonella quintana bacteremia in homeless patients. N Engl J Med. 1999 Jan 21;340(3):184-9.

Brouqui P, Raoult D. Bartonella quintana invades and multiplies within endothelial cells in vitro and in vivo and forms intracellular blebs. Res Microbiol. 1996 Nov-Dec;147(9):719-31.

Brouqui P, Raoult D. Endocarditis due to rare and fastidious bacteria. Clin Microbiol Rev. 2001 Jan;14(1):177-207. Review.

Brouqui P, Raoult D. New insight into the diagnosis of fastidious bacterial endocarditis. FEMS Immunol Med Microbiol. 2006 Jun;47(1):1-13. Review.

Brouqui P, Raoult D. Arthropod-borne diseases in homeless. Ann N Y Acad Sci. 2006 Oct;1078:223-35. Review.

Brouqui P, Stein A, Dupont HT, Gallian P, Badiaga S, Rolain JM, Mege JL, La Scola B, Berbis P, Raoult D. Ectoparasitism and vector-borne diseases in 930 homeless people from Marseilles. Medicine (Baltimore). 2005 Jan;84(1):61-8.

Brown JS Jr. Geographic correlation of schizophrenia to ticks and tick-borne encephalitis. Schizophr Bull. 1994;20(4):755-75

Bruckner DA, Garcia LS, Shimizu RY, Goldstein EJ, Murray PM, Lazar GS. Babesiosis: problems in diagnosis using autoanalyzers. Am J Clin Pathol. 1985 Apr;83(4):520-1.

Brueckner Randomized Dose-Ranging Study of the Safety and Efficacy of WR 238605 (Tafenoquine) in the Prevention of Relapse of Plasmodium vivax Malaria in Thailand. J Infect Dis. 1999 Oct;180(4):1282-7.

Bruneval P, Choucair J, Paraf F, Casalta JP, Raoult D, Scherchen F, Mainardi JL. Detection of fastidious bacteria in cardiac valves in cases of blood culture negative endocarditis. J Clin Pathol. 2001 Mar;54(3):238-40.

Brunner JL, Cheney L, Keesing F, Killilea M, Logiudice K, Previtali A, Ostfeld RS. Molting success of Ixodes scapularis varies among individual blood meal hosts and species. J Med Entomol. 2011 Jul;48(4):860-6.

Bryksin AV, Godfrey HP, Carbonaro CA, Wormser GP, Aguero-Rosenfeld ME, Cabello FC. Borrelia burgdorferi BmpA, BmpB, and BmpD proteins are expressed in human infection and contribute to P39 immunoblot reactivity in patients with Lyme disease. Clin Diagn Lab Immunol. 2005 Aug;12(8):935-40.

Buchmann AU, Kempf VA, Kershaw O, Gruber AD. Peliosis hepatis in cats is not associated with Bartonella henselae infections. Vet Pathol. 2010 Jan;47(1):163-6.

Buchmann AU, Kershaw O, Kempf VA, Gruber AD. Does a feline leukemia virus infection pave the way for Bartonella henselae infection in cats? J Clin Microbiol. 2010 Sep;48(9):3295-300. Epub 2010 Jul 7.

Buchholz BM, Bauer AJ. Membrane TLR Signaling Mechanisms in the Gastrointestinal Tract during Sepsis. Neurogastroenterol Motil. 2010 March;22(3):232–245.

Buelvas F, Alvis N, Buelvas I, Miranda J, Mattar S. [A high prevalence of antibodies against Bartonella and Babesia microti has been found in villages and urban populations in Cordoba, Colombia].[Article in Spanish]. Rev Salud Publica (Bogota). 2008 Jan-Feb;10(1):168-77.

Bunikis J, Tsao J, Garpmo U, Berglund J, Fish D, Barbour AG. Typing of Borrelia relapsing fever group strains. Emerg Infect Dis. 2004 Sep;10(9):1661-4.

Bunnell JE, Price SD, Das A, Shields TM, Glass GE. Geographic information systems and spatial analysis of adult Ixodes scapularis (Acari: Ixodidae) in the MiddleAtlantic region of the USA. J Med Entomol. 2003;40(4):570-6.

Burbelo PD, Bren KE, Ching KH, Coleman A, Yang X, Kariu T, Iadarola MJ, Pal U. Antibody Profiling of Borrelia burgdorferi Infection in Horses. Clin Vaccine Immunol. 2011 Sep;18(9):1562-7. Epub 2011 Jul 20.

Burgdorfer W. (Discoverer of Borrelia burgdorferi) Keynote Address - The Complexity of Vector-borne Spirochetes. 12th International Conference on Lyme Disease and Other Spirochetal and Tick-Borne Disorders. New York City, April 9-10, 1999. Full text available online at: www.medscape.com/medscape/cno/1999/lyme/Story.cfm? story_id=534.

Burgess EC, Gendron-Fitzpatrick A, Wright WO. Arthritis and systemic disease caused by Borrelia burgdorferi infection in a cow. J Am Vet Med Assoc. 1987 Dec 1;191(11):1468-70.

Burkhard C, Gleichmann M, Wilhelm H. Optic nerve lesion following neuroborreliosis: a case report. Eur J Ophthalmol. 2001 Apr-Jun;11(2):203-6.

Burk O, Arnold KA, Nussler AK, Schaeffeler E, Efimova E, Avery BA, Avery MA, Fromm MF, Eichelbaum M. Antimalarial artemisinin drugs induce cytochrome P450 and MDR1 expression by activation of xenosensors pregnane X receptor and constitutive androstane receptor. Mol Pharmacol. 2005;67:1954-65. [Epub 2005 Mar 10].

Burri C, Dupasquier C, Bastic V, Gern L. Pathogens of emerging tick-borne diseases, Anaplasma phagocytophilum, Rickettsia spp., and Babesia spp., in ixodes ticks collected from rodents at four sites in Switzerland (Canton of Bern). Vector Borne Zoonotic Dis. 2011 Jul;11(7):939-44. Epub 2011 Mar 21.

Butler AR, Gilbert BC, Hulme P, Irvine LR, Rendon L, Whitwood AC. EPR evidence for the involvement of free radicals in the iron-catalysed decomposition of quinghaosu (artemisinin) and some derivatives; antimalarial action of some polycyclic endoperoxides. Free Radic Res. 1998 May;28(5):471-6.

Butterfield JH. Interferon treatment for hypereosinophilic syndromes and systemic mastocytosis. Acta Haematol. 2005;114(1):26-40.

Byrd RP Jr, Roy TM. Babesiosis in Missouri. Ann Intern Med. 1997 Jan 15;126(2):172.

Byrnes V, Chopra S, Koziel MJ. Resolution of chronic hepatitis C following parasitosis. World J Gastroenterol. 2007 Aug 21;13(31):4268-9.

Cabezos J, Bada JL. The diagnosis of malaria by the thick film and the QBC: a comparative study of both technics. Med Clin (Barc). 1993 Jun 12;101(3):91-4.

Cadavid D, O'Neill T, Schaefer H, Pachner AR. Localization of Borrelia burgdorferi in the nervous system and other organs in a nonhuman primate model of Lyme disease. Lab Invest. 2000 Jul;80(7):1043-54.

Cadenas MB, Bradley J, Maggi RG, Takara M, Hegarty BC, Breitschwerdt EB. Molecular characterization of Bartonella vinsonii subsp. berkhoffii genotype III. J Clin Microbiol. 2008 May;46(5):1858-60. Epub 2008 Mar 26.

Cadenas MB, Maggi RG, Diniz PP, Breitschwerdt KT, Sontakke S, Breithschwerdt EB. Identification of bacteria from clinical samples using Bartonella alpha-Proteobacteria growth medium. J Microbiol Methods. 2007 Nov;71(2):147-55. Epub 2007 Aug 24.

Caimano MJ, Kenedy MR, Kairu T, Desrosiers DC, Harman M, Dunham-Ems S, Akins DR, Pal U, Radolf JD. The hybrid histidine kinase Hk1 is part of a two-component system that is essential for survival of Borrelia burgdorferi in feeding Ixodes scapularis ticks. Infect Immun. 2011 Aug;79(8):3117-30. Epub 2011 May 23.

Calderaro A, Montecchini S, Gorrini C, Piccolo G, Chezzi C, Dettori G. Presence of anti-Borrelia burgdorferi antibodies and Borrelia burgdorferi sensu lato DNA in samples of subjects in an area of the Northern Italy in the period 2002-2008. Diagn Microbiol Infect Dis. 2011 Aug;70(4):455-60. Epub 2011 Mar 11.

Calvo de Mora A, Garcia Castellano JM, Herrera C and Jimenez-Alonso J. [Human babesiosis: report of a case with fatal outcome]. [Article in Spanish]. Med Clin (Barc). 1985 Oct 19;85(12):515-6.

Calza L, Manfredi R, Chiodo F. Infective endocarditis: a review of the best treatment options. Expert Opin Pharmacother. 2004 Sep;5(9):1899-916. Review.

Cameron D, Gaito A, Harris N, Bach G, Bellovin S, Bock K, Bock S, Burrascano J, Dickey C, Horowitz R, Phillips S, Meer-Scherrer L, Raxlen B, Sherr V, Smith H, Smith P, Stricker R; ILADS Working Group. Evidence-based guidelines for the management of Lyme disease. Expert Rev Anti Infect Ther. 2004;2(1 Suppl):S1-13.

Campbell GL, Fritz CL, Fish D, Nowakowski J, Nadelman RB, Wormser GP. Estimation of the incidence of Lyme disease. Am J Epidemiol. 1998 Nov 15;148(10):1018-26.

Campbell RE, Rosahn PD. The morphology and staining characteristics of Treponema pallidum. Review of the literature and description of a new technique for staining the organisms in tissues.Yale J Biol Med. 1950 Jul;22(6):527-43.

Camponovo F, Meier C. Neuropathy of vasculitic origin in a case of Garin-Boujadoux-Bannwarth syndrome with positive borrelia antibody response. J Neurol. 1986 Apr;233(2):69-72.

Campos Franco J, Mallo González N, López Rodríquez R, Pérez Pampín E. [Cat-scratch disease].[Article in Spanish]. Med Clin (Barc). 2007 Sep 8;129(8):320.

Cangelosi JJ, Sarvat B, Sarria JC, Herwaldt BL, Indrikovs AJ. Transmission of Babesia microti by blood transfusion in Texas. Vox Sang. 2008 Nov;95(4):331-4.

Capo C, Amirayan-Chevillard N, Brouqui P, Raoult D, Mege JL. Bartonella quintana bacteremia and overproduction of interleukin-10: model of bacterial persistence in homeless people. J Infect Dis. 2003 Mar 1;187(5):837-44. Epub 2003 Feb 24.

Caponetti G, Pantanowitz L. Cat-scratch disease lymphadenitis. Ear Nose Throat J. 2007 Aug;86(8):449-50.

Caponetti GC, Pantanowitz L, Marconi S, Havens JM, Lamps LW, Otis CN. Evaluation of immunohistochemistry in identifying Bartonella henselae in cat-scratch disease. Am J Clin Pathol. 2009 Feb;131(2):250-6.

Cardoso L, Tuna J, Vieira L, Yisaschar-Mekuzas Y, Baneth G. Molecular detection of Anaplasma platys and Ehrlichia canis in dogs from the North of Portugal. Vet J. 2010 Feb;183(2):232-3. Epub 2008 Dec 3.

Carithers HA. Cat-scratch disease. An overview based on a study of 1,200 patients. Am J Dis Child. 1985 Nov;139(11):1124-33.

Carithers HA, Margileth AM. Cat-scratch disease. Acute encephalo-pathy and other neurologic manifestations. Am J Dis Child. 1991 Jan;145(1):98-101.

Carlberg H, Naito S. Lyme borreliosis--a review and present situation in Japan. J Dermatol. 1991 Mar;18(3):125-42. Review.

Carlson D, Hernandez J, Bloom BJ, Coburn J, Aversa JM, Steere AC. Lack of Borrelia burgdorferi DNA in synovial samples from patients with antibiotic treatment-resistant Lyme arthritis. Arthritis Rheum. 1999 Dec;42(12):2705-9.

Cartwright, M.J., S.E. Martin, and S.T. Donta. A novel neurotoxin (Bbtox1) of Borrelia burgdorferi. Meeting of the American Society for Microbiology. May 1999. Chicago.

Carucci LR, Halvorsen RA. Hepatic peliosis (bacillary angiomatosis) in AIDS: CT findings. Abdom Imaging. 2006 Mar-Apr;31(2):253; author reply 254.

Carvalho TL, Ribolla PE, Curi RA, Mota LS. Characterization and transcriptional analysis of the promoter region of the Duffy blood group, chemokine receptor (DARC) gene in cattle. Vet Immunol Immunopathol. 2009 Dec 15;132(2-4):153-9. Epub 2009 Jun 6.

Cary NR, Fox B, Wright DJ, Cutler SJ, Shapiro LM, Grace AA. Fatal Lyme carditis and endodermal heterotopia of the atrioventricular node. Postgrad Med J. 1990 Feb;66(772):134-6.

Casalta JP, Gouriet F, Richet H, Thuny F, Habib G, Raoult D. Prevalence of Coxiella burnetii and Bartonella species as cases of infective endocarditis in Marseilles (1994-2007). Clin Microbiol Infect. 2009 Dec;15 Suppl 2:152-3. Epub 2009 Sep 28.

Case JB, Chomel B, Nicholson W, Foley JE. Serological survey of vector-borne zoonotic pathogens in pet cats and cats from animal shelters and feral colonies. J Feline Med Surg. 2006 Apr;8(2):111-7. Epub 2006 Jan 23.

Case records of the Massachusetts General Hospital. Weekly clinicopathological exercises. Case 22-1992. A 6 1/2-year-old girl with status epilepticus, cervical lymphadenopathy, pleural effusions, and respiratory distress. N Engl J Med. 1992 May 28;326(22):1480-9.

Case records of the Massachusetts General Hospital. Weekly clinicopathological exercises. Case 1-1998. An 11-year-old boy with a seizure. N Engl J Med. 1998;338(2):112-9. Erratum in: N Engl J Med 1998 Feb 12;338(7):483.

Casjens SR, Fraser-Liggett CM, Mongodin EF, Qiu WG, Dunn JJ, Luft BJ, Schutzer SE. Whole genome sequence of an unusual Borrelia burgdorferi sensu lato isolate. J Bacteriol. 2011 Mar;193(6):1489-90. Epub 2011 Jan 7.

Casolari C, Pecorari M, Balli F, Fabio G, Gennari W, Sabbatini AM, Nanni N, Migaldi M, Guaraldi N, Tagliazucchi S, Alù M, Bertoli G, Fabio R, Portolani M. Unusual concurrent detection by polymerase chain reaction of Bartonella henselae and parvovirus b19 in an immunocompetent child with erythema nodosum and hepatic granulomatous disease. Diagn Microbiol Infect Dis. 2007 Sep;59(1):81-4. Epub 2007 May 29.

Cassarino DS, Quezado MM, Ghatak NR, Duray PH. Lyme-associated parkinsonism: a neuropathologic case study and review of the literature. Arch Pathol Lab Med, 127(9):1204-6. 2003.

Celebi B. [Bartonella henselae and its infections]. [Article in Turkish]. Mikrobiyol Bul. 2008 Jan;42(1):163-75. Review.

Centers for Disease Control and Prevention (CDC). Encephalitis associated with cat scratch disease--Broward and Palm Beach Counties, Florida, 1994. MMWR Morb Mortal Wkly Rep. 1994;43(49):909, 915-6.

Cerar D, Cerar T, Ruzić-Sabljić E, Wormser GP, Strle F. Subjective symptoms after treatment of early Lyme disease. Am J Med. 2010 Jan;123(1):79-86.

Cerimele F, Brown LF, Bravo F, Ihler GM, Kouadio P, Arbiser JL. Infectious Angiogenesis: Bartonella bacilliformis Infection Results in Endothelial Production of Angiopoetin-2 and Epidermal Production of Vascular Endothelial Growth Factor. Am J Pathol. 2003 Oct;163(4):1321-7.

Cerroni L, Zochling N, Putz B, Kerl H. Infection by Borrelia burgdorferi and cutaneous B-cell lymphoma. J Cutan Pathol. 1997 Sep;24(8):457-61.

Cervantes JL, Dunham-Ems SM, La Vake CJ, Petzke MM, Sahay B, Sellati TJ, Radolf JD, Salazar JC. Phagosomal signaling by Borrelia burgdorferi in human monocytes involves Toll-like receptor (TLR) 2 and TLR8 cooperativity and TLR8-mediated induction of IFN-ß Proc Natl Acad Sci U S A. 2011 March 1;108(9):3683-8. Published online 2011 February 14.

Chae JS, Yu do H, Shringi S, Klein TA, Kim HC, Chong ST, Lee IY, Foley J. Microbial pathogens in ticks, rodents and a shrew in northern Gyeonggi-do near the DMZ, Korea. J Vet Sci. 2008 Sep;9(3):285-93.

Chai CL, Lu QY, Sun JM, Jiang LP, Ling F, Zhang LJ, Zheng SG, Zhang H, Ge JH. [Sero-epidemiologic investigation on tick-borne diseases of humans and domestic animals in Zhejiang province]. [Article in Chinese]. Zhonghua Liu Xing Bing Xue Za Zhi. 2010 Oct;31(10):1144-1147.

Chaloner GL, Harrison TG, Coyne KP, Aanensen DM, Birtles RJ. Multilocus sequence typing of Bartonella henselae in the United Kingdom indicates that only a few, uncommon sequence types are associated with zoonotic disease. J Clin Microbiol. 2011 Jun;49(6):2132-7. Epub 2011 Apr 6.

Chaloner GL, Palmira Ventosilla, Birtles RJ. Multi-locus sequence analysis reveals profound genetic diversity among isolates of the human pathogen Bartonella bacilliformis. PLoS Negl Trop Dis. 2011 Jul;5(7):e1248. Epub 2011 Jul 19.

Chamorro A, Alonso P, Arrizabalaga J, Carné X, Camps V. [Limitations of evidence-based medicine: the case of stroke]. [Article in Spanish]. Med Clin (Barc). 2001 Mar 10;116(9):343-9.

Chan L, Reilly KM, Snyder HS. An unusual presentation of cat scratch encephalitis. J Emerg Med. 1995;13(6):769-772.

Chancellor MB, Dato VM, Yang JY. Lyme disease presenting as urinary retention. J Urol. 1990 Jun;143(6):1223-4.

Chancellor MB, McGinnis DE, Shenot PJ, Kiilholma P, Hirsch IH. Urinary dysfunction in Lyme disease. J Urol. 1993 Jan;149(1):26-30.

Chanchamroen S, Kewcharoenwong C, Susaengrat W, Ato M, Lertmemongkolchai G. Human Polymorphonuclear Neutrophil Responses to Burkholderia pseudomallei in Healthy and Diabetic Subjects. Infect Immun. 2009 Jan;77(1): 456–463. Published online 2008 October 27.

Chandra A, Latov N, Wormser GP, Marques AR, Alaedini A. Epitope mapping of antibodies to VlsE protein of Borrelia burgdorferi in post-Lyme disease syndrome. Clin Immunol. 2011 Oct;141(1):103-10. Epub 2011 Jul 2.

Chandra A, Wormser GP, Klempner MS, Trevino RP, Crow MK, Latov N, Alaedini A. Anti-neural antibody reactivity in patients with a history of Lyme borreliosis and persistent symptoms. Brain Behav Immun. 2010 Aug;24(6):1018-24. Epub 2010 Mar 18.

Chandra A, Wormser GP, Marques AR, Latov N, Alaedini A. Anti-Borrelia burgdorferi antibody profile in post-Lyme disease syndrome. Clin Vaccine Immunol. 2011 May;18(5):767-71. Epub 2011 Mar 16.

Chandrashekar R, Mainville CA, Beall MJ, O'Connor T, Eberts MD, Alleman AR, Gaunt SD, Breitschwerdt EB. Performance of a commercially available in-clinic ELISA for the detection of antibodies against Anaplasma phagocytophilum, Ehrlichia canis, and Borrelia burgdorferi and Dirofilaria immitis antigen in dogs. Am J Vet Res. 2010 Dec;71(12):1443-50.

Chang CC, Chen YJ, Tseng CS, Lai WL, Hsu KY, Chang CL, Lu CC, Hsu YM. A comparative study of the interaction of Bartonella henselae strains with human endothelial cells. Vet Microbiol. 2011 Apr 21;149(1-2):147-56. Epub 2010 Oct 7.

Chang CC, Lee CC, Maruyama S, Lin JW, Pan MJ. Cat-scratch disease in veterinary-associated populations and in its cat reservoir in Taiwan. Vet Res. 2006 Jul-Aug;37(4):565-77. Epub 2006 Apr 28.

Chang YF, Ku Y, Chang CF, Chang CD, McDonough SP, Divers T, Pough M, Torres A. Antibiotic treatment of experimentally Borrelia burgdorferi-infected ponies. Vet Microbiol. 2005 May 20;107(3-4):285-94.

Chapes SK, Ganta RR. Defining the Immune Response to Ehrlichia species Using Murine Models. Vet Parasitol. 2008 Dec 20;158(4):344–359. Published online 2008 October 17.

Chauhan VS, Sterka DG Jr, Gray DL, Bost KL, Marriott I. Neurogenic Exacerbation of Microglial and Astrocyte Responses to Neisseria meningitidis and Borrelia burgdorferi. J Immunol. 2008 Jun 15;180(12):8241-9.

Chausov EV, Ternovoĭ VA, Protopopova EV, Konovalova SN, Kononova IuV, Pershikova NL, Moskovitina NS, Romanenko VN, Ivanova NV, Bol'shakova NP, Moskvitin SS, Korobitsyn IG, Gashkov SI, Tiuten'kov OIu, Kuranova VN, Kravchenko LB, Suchkova NG, Agulova LP, Loktev VB. [Genetic diversity of ixodid tick-borne pathogens in Tomsk City and suburbs].[Article in Russian]. Parazitologiia. 2009 Sep-Oct;43(5):374-88.

Chehrenama M, Zagardo MT, Koski CL. Subarachnoid hemorrhage in a patient with Lyme disease. Neurology. 1997 Feb;48(2):520-3.

Chen HH, Zhou HJ, Fang X. Inhibition of human cancer cell line growth and human umbilical vein endothelial cell angiogenesis by artemisinin derivatives in vitro. Pharmacol Res. 2003 Sep;48:231-6.

Chen HH, Zhou HJ, Wang WQ, Wu GD. Antimalarial dihydroartemisinin also inhibits angiogenesis. Cancer Chemother Pharmacol. 2004 May;53(5):423-32.

Chen HH, Zhou HJ, Wu GD, Lou XE. Inhibitory effects of artesunate on angiogenesis and on expressions of vascular endothelial growth factor and VEGF receptor KDR/flk-1. Pharmacology. 2004 May;71(1):1-9.

Chen J, Field JA, Glickstein L, Molloy PJ, Huber BT, Steere AC. Association of antibiotic treatment-resistant Lyme arthritis with T cell responses to dominant epitopes of outer surface protein A of Borrelia burgdorferi. Arthritis Rheum. 1999 Sep;42(9):1813-22.

Chen S, Zückert WR. Probing the Borrelia burgdorferi Surface Lipoprotein Secretion Pathway Using a Conditionally Folding Protein Domain. J Bacteriol. 2011 Sep 30. [Epub ahead of print]

Chen TC, Lin WR, Lu PL, Lin CY, Chen YH. Cat scratch disease from a domestic dog. J Formos Med Assoc. 2007 Feb;106(2 Suppl):S65-68. Review.

Chen YD, Lin BY, Zhang JX. [Study on inducing an artemisinin-resistant line of Plasmodium berghei.]. [Article in Chinese]. Zhongguo Ji Sheng Chong Xue Yu Ji Sheng Chong Bing Za Zhi. 2002;20(1):37-8.

Cherinet Y, Tomlinson R. Cat scratch disease presenting as acute encephalopathy. Emerg Med J. 2008 Oct;25(10):703-4.

Cherry NA, Diniz PP, Maggi RG, Hummel JB, Hardie EM, Behrend EN, Rozanski E, Defrancesco TC, Cadenas MB, Breitschwerdt EB. Isolation or molecular detection of Bartonella henselae and Bartonella vinsonii subsp. berkhoffii from dogs with idiopathic cavitary effusions. J Vet Intern Med. 2009 Jan-Feb;23(1):186-9.

Cherry NA, Liebisch G, Liebisch A, Breitschwerdt EB, Jones SL, Ulrich R, Allmers E, Wolf P, Hewicker-Trautwein M. Identification of Bartonella henselae in a horse from Germany. Vet Microbiol. 2011 Jun 2;150(3-4):414-5. Epub 2011 Feb 18.

Cherry NA, Maggi RG, Cannedy AL, Breitschwerdt EB. PCR detection of Bartonella bovis and Bartonella henselae in the blood of beef cattle. Vet Microbiol. 2009 Mar 30;135(3-4):308-12. Epub 2008 Sep 21.

Cherry NA, Maggi RG, Rossmeisl JH, Hegarty BC, Breitschwerdt EB. Ecological Diversity of Bartonella Species Infection Among Dogs and Their Owner in Virginia. Vector Borne Zoonotic Dis. 2011 Jul 7. [Epub ahead of print]

Cheuk W, Chan AK, Wong MC, Chan JK. Confirmation of diagnosis of cat scratch disease by immunohistochemistry. Am J Surg Pathol. 2006 Feb;30(2):274-5.

Cheung VW, Moxham JP. Cat scratch disease presenting as acute mastoiditis. Laryngoscope. 2010;120 Suppl 4:S222. Review.

China Cooperative Research Group on Qinghaosu and its Derivatives as Antimalarials. J Tradit Chin Med. 1982 Mar;2(1):9-16.

Chiao JW, Villalon P, Schwartz I, Wormser GP. Modulation of lymphocyte proliferative responses by a canine Lyme disease vaccine of recombinant outer surface protein A (OspA). FEMS Immunol Med Microbiol. 2000 Jul;28(3):193-6.

Chiaraviglio L, Duong S, Brown DA, Birtles RJ, Kirby JE. An immunocompromised murine model of chronic Bartonella infection. Am J Pathol. 2010 Jun;176(6):2753-63. Epub 2010 Apr 15.

Chinnadurai SK, Birkenheuer AJ, Blanton HL, Maggi RG, Belfiore N, Marr HS, Breitschwerdt EB, Stoskopf MK. Prevalence of selected vector-borne organisms and identification of Bartonella species DNA in North American river otters (Lontra canadensis). J Wildl Dis. 2010 Jul;46(3):947-50.

Chmielewski T, Podsiadly E, Tylewska-Wierzbanowska S. Presence of Bartonella spp. in various human populations. Pol J Microbiol. 2007;56(1):33-38.

Choi P, Qin X, Chen EY, Inglis AF Jr, Ou HC, Perkins JA, Sie KC, Patterson K, Berry S, Manning SC. Polymerase chain reaction for pathogen identification in persistent pediatric cervical lymphadenitis. Arch Otolaryngol Head Neck Surg. 2009 Mar;135(3):243-8.

Chomel B. Tick-borne infections in dogs-an emerging infectious threat. Vet Parasitol. 2011 Jul 15;179(4):294-301.

Chomel BB, Boulouis HJ, Breitschwerdt EB. Cat scratch disease and other zoonotic Bartonella infections. J Am Vet Med Assoc. 2004 Apr 15;224(8):1270-9. Review.

Chomel BB, Boulouis HJ, Breitschwerdt EB, Kasten RW, Vayssier-Taussat M, Birtles RJ, Koehler JE, Dehio C. Ecological fitness and strategies of adaptation of Bartonella species to their hosts and vectors. Vet Res. 2009 Mar-Apr;40(2):29. Epub 2009 Mar 14. Review.

Chomel BB, Boulouis HJ, Maruyama S, Breitschwerdt EB. Bartonella spp. in pets and effect on human health. Emerg Infect Dis. 2006 Mar;12(3):389-94. Review.

Chomel BB, Henn JB, Kasten RW, Nieto NC, Foley J, Papageorgiou S, Allen C, Koehler JE. Dogs are more permissive than cats or guinea pigs to experimental infection with a human isolate of Bartonella rochalimae. Vet Res. 2009 Jul-Aug;40(4):27.

Chomel BB, Kasten RW. Bartonellosis, an increasingly recognized zoonosis. J Appl Microbiol. 2010 Sep;109(3):743-50. Review.

Chomel BB, Kasten RW, Henn JB, Molia S. Bartonella infection in domestic cats and wild felids. Ann N Y Acad Sci. 2006 Oct;1078:410-5.

Chomel BB, Kasten RW, Sykes JE, Boulouis HJ, Breitschwerdt EB. Clinical impact of persistent Bartonella bacteremia in humans and animals. Ann N Y Acad Sci. 2003 Jun;990:267-78. Review.

Chomel BB, Kasten RW, Williams C, Wey AC, Henn JB, Maggi R, Carrasco S, Mazet J, Boulouis HJ, Maillard R, Breitschwerdt EB. Bartonella endocarditis: a pathology shared by animal reservoirs and patients. Ann N Y Acad Sci. 2009 May;1166:120-6.

Chong CR, Sullivan DJ Jr. Inhibition of heme crystal growth by antimalarials and other compounds: implications for drug discovery. Biochem Pharmacol. 2003 Dec 1;66(11):2201-12.

Chopra I, Roberts M. Tetracycline antibiotics: mode of action, applications, molecular biology, and epidemiology of bacterial resistance. Microbiol Mol Biol Rev. 2001 Jun;65(2): 232–260.

Chu BC, Tam VT. A serologically proven case of cat-scratch disease presenting with neuroretinitis. Hong Kong Med J. 2009 Oct;15(5):391-3.

Ciceroni L, Pinto A, Ciarrocchi S, Ciervo A. Bartonella infections in Italy. Clin Microbiol Infect. 2009 Dec;15 Suppl 2:108-9. Epub 2009 Apr 30.

Cichocka A, Skotarczak B. [Babesosis--difficulty of diagnosis]. [Article in Polish]. Wiad Parazytol. 2001;47(3):527-33. Review.

Cieniuch S, Staczak J, Ruczaj A. The first detection of Babesia EU1 and Babesia canis canis in Ixodes ricinus ticks (Acari, Ixodidae) collected in urban and rural areas in northern Poland. Pol J Microbiol. 2009;58(3):231-6.

Cimmino MA, Moggiana GL, Parisi M, S. Accardo S. Treatment of Lyme arthritis. Infection. 1996 Jan-Feb;24:1:91-93.

Cimperman J, Maraspin V, Lotric-Furlan S, Ruzic-Sabljic E, Strle F. Lyme meningitis: a one-year follow up controlled study. Wien Klin Wochenschr. 1999 Dec 10;111(22-23):961-3.

Cimperman J, Maraspin V, Lotric-Furlan S, Ruzic-Sabljic E, Avsic-Zupanc T, Strle F. Diffuse reversible alopecia in patients with Lyme meningitis and tick-borne encephalitis. Wien Klin Wochenschr. 1999 Dec 10;111(22-23):976-7.

Clark IA. Does endotoxin cause both the disease and parasite death in acute malaria and babasiosis? Lancet. 1978 Jul 8;2(8080):75-7.

Clark IA, Alleva LM, Mills AC, Cowden WB. Pathogenesis of Malaria and Clinically Similar Conditions. Clin Microbiol Rev. 2004 July;17(3):509-39.

Clark IA, Budd AC, Hsue G, Haymore BR, Joyce AJ, Thorner R, Krause PJ. Absence of erythrocyte sequestration in a case of babesiosis in a splenectomized human patient. Malar J. 2006 Aug 4;5:69.

Clark JR, Carlson RD, Sasaki CT, Pachner AR, Steere AC. Facial paralysis in Lyme disease. Laryngoscope. 1985 Nov;95(11):1341-5.

Clark RL, White TE, A Clode S, Gaunt I, Winstanley P, Ward SA. Developmental toxicity of artesunate and an artesunate combination in the rat and rabbit. Birth Defects Res B Dev Reprod Toxicol. 2004 Dec; 71(6):380-94.

Clindamycin: Medline Plus. [Monograph on the Internet]. Available from: http://www.nlm.nih.gov/medlineplus/druginfo/medmaster/a682399.html.

Cockwill KR, Taylor SM, Philibert HM, Breitschwerdt EB, Maggi RG. Bartonella vinsonii subsp. berkhoffii endocarditis in a dog from Saskatchewan. Can Vet J. 2007 Aug; 48(8):839-44.

Codolo G, Amedei A, Steere AC, Papinutto E, Cappon A, Polenghi A, Benagiano M, Paccani SR, Sambri V, Del Prete G, Baldari CT, Zanotti G, Montecucco C, D'Elios MM, de Bernard M. Borrelia burgdorferi NapA-driven Th17 cell inflammation in lyme arthritis. Arthritis Rheum. 2008 Nov;58(11):3609-17.

Cohnstaedt LW, Beati L, Caceres AG, Ferro C, Munstermann LE. Phylogenetics of the phlebotomine sand fly group Verrucarum (Diptera: Psychodidae: Lutzomyia). Am J Trop Med Hyg. 2011 Jun;84(6):913-22.

Coipan EC, Vladimirescu AF. Ixodes ricinus ticks (Acari: Ixodidae): vectors for Lyme disease spirochetes in Romania. Exp Appl Acarol. 2011 Jul;54(3):293-300. Epub 2011 Mar 24.

Colborn JM, Kosoy MY, Motin VL, Telepnev MV, Valbuena G, Myint KS, Fofanov Y, Putonti C, Feng C, Peruski L. Improved detection of Bartonella DNA in mammalian hosts and arthropod vectors by real-time PCR using the NADH dehydrogenase gamma subunit (nuoG). J Clin Microbiol. 2010 Dec;48(12):4630-3. Epub 2010 Oct 6.

Coleman AS, Rossmann E, Yang X, Song H, Lamichhane CM, Iyer R, Schwartz I, Pal U. BBK07 immunodominant peptides as serodiagnostic markers of Lyme disease. Clin Vaccine Immunol. 2011 Mar;18(3):406-13. Epub 2010 Dec 22.

Collart P, Borel L, Durel P. Significance of spiral organisms found after treatment in late human and experimental syphilis. Br J Vener Dis. 1964 Jun;40:81-9.

Collier JA, Longmore JM. The reliability of the microscopic diagnosis of malaria in the field and in the laboratory. Ann Trop Med Parasitol. 1983 Apr;77(2):113-7.

Collins C, Shi C, Russell JQ, Fortner KA, Budd RC. Activation of T Cells by Borrelia burgdorferi is Indirect via a TLR- and Caspase-Dependent Pathway. J Immunol. 2008 Aug 15;181(4):2392-8.

Colović N, Bumbasirević L, Palibrk V, Vidović A, Colović M. [Neuroborreliosis in patient with aplastic anaemia secondary to therapy with ticlopidine].[Article in Serbian]. Srp Arh Celok Lek. 2010 Sep-Oct;138(9-10):632-4.

Colton L, Zeidner N, Lynch T, Kosoy MY. Human isolates of Bartonella tamiae induce pathology in experimentally inoculated immunocompetent mice. BMC Infect Dis. 2010 Jul 30;10:229.

Comer JA, Flynn C, Regnery RL, Vlahov D, Childs JE. Antibodies to Bartonella species in inner-city intravenous drug users in Baltimore, Md. Arch Intern Med. 1996;156(21):2491-5.

Commander NJ, Spencer SA, Wren BW, MacMillan AP. The identification of two protective DNA vaccines from a panel of five plasmid constructs encoding Brucella melitensis 16M genes. Vaccine. 2007 Jan 2;25(1):43-54. Epub 2006 Aug 4.

Commins MA, Goodger BV, Waltisbuhl DJ, Wright IG. Babesia bovis: studies of parameters influencing microvascular stasis of infected erythrocytes. Res Vet Sci. 1988 Mar;44(2):226-8.

Conrad DA. Treatment of cat-scratch disease. Curr Opin Pediatr. 2001 Feb;13(1):56-9.

Conrad PA, Kjemtrup AM, Carreno RA, Thomford J, Wainwright K, Eberhard M, Quick R, Telford SR 3rd, Herwaldt BL. Description of Babesia duncani n.sp. (Apicomplexa: Babesiidae) from humans and its differentiation from other piroplasms. Int J Parasitol. 2006 Jun;36(7):779-89

Cooke WD, Dattwyler RJ. Complications of Lyme borreliosis. Ann Rev Med. 1992;43:93-103.

Cools J, DeAngelo DJ, Gotlib J, et al. A tyrosine kinase created by fusion of the PDGFRA and FIP1L1 genes as a therapeutic target of imatinib in idiopathic hypereosinophilic syndrome. N Engl J Med. 2003 Mar 27;348(13):1201-14.

Cortes J, Ault P, Koller C, Thomas D, Ferrajoli A, Wierda W, Rios MB, Letvak L, Kaled ES, Kantarjian H. Efficacy of imatinib mesylate in the treatment of idiopathic hypereosinophilic syndrome. Blood. 2003 Jun 15;101(12):4714-6.

Costa V, Sommese L, Casamassimi A, Colicchio R, Angelini C, Marchesano V, Milone L, Farzati B, Giovane A, Fiorito C, Rienzo M, Picardi M, Avallone B, Marco Corsi M, Sarubbi B, Calabrò R, Salvatore P, Ciccodicola A, Napoli C. Impairment of circulating endothelial progenitors in Down syndrome. BMC Med Genomics. 2010 Sep 13;3:40.

Costello CM, Steere AC, Pinkerton RE, Feder HM Jr. A prospective study of tick bites in an endemic area for Lyme disease. Conn Med. 1989 Jun;53(6):338-40.

Costello CM, Steere AC, Pinkerton RE, Feder HM Jr. A prospective study of tick bites in an endemic area for Lyme disease. J Infect Dis. 1989 Jan;159(1):136-9.

Cotté V, Bonnet S, Le Rhun D, Le Naour E, Chauvin A, Boulouis HJ, Lecuelle B, Lilin T, Vayssier-Taussat M. Transmission of Bartonella henselae by Ixodes ricinus. Emerg Infect Dis. 2008 Jul;14(7):1074-80.

Coumou J, Hovius JW. [Lyme disease].[Article in Dutch]. Ned Tijdschr Tandheelkd. 2011 Jun;118(6):310-6. Review.

Coumou J, van der Poll T, Speelman P, Hovius JW. Tired of Lyme borreliosis. Lyme borreliosis in the Netherlands. Neth J Med. 2011 Mar;69(3):101-11. Review.

Courtney JW, Dryden RL, Montgomery J, Schneider BS, Smith G, Massung RF. Molecular characterization of Anaplasma phagocytophilum and Borrelia burgdorferi in Ixodes scapularis ticks from Pennsylvania. J Clin Microbiol 2003 Apr;41(4):1569-73.

Coutts WE, Coutts WR. Treponema pallidum buds, granules and cysts as found in human syphilitic chancres and seen in fixed unstained smears under darkground illumination. Am J Syph Gonorrhea Vener Dis. 1953 Jan;37(1):29-36.

Coyle PK. Neurologic complications of late and chronic Lyme disease. 9th Annual International Scientific Conference on Lyme Disease & Other Tick-Borne Disorders, Westin Copley Plaza Hotel, Boston, MA, April 19-20, 1996.

Coyle PK. Lyme disease. Curr Neurol Neurosci Rep. 2002 Nov; 2(6):479-87.

Coyle PK, Schutzer SE. Neurologic presentations in Lyme disease. Hosp Pract (Off Ed). 1991 Nov 15;26(11):55-66; discussion 66, 69-70.

Craft JE, Grodzicki RL, Steere AC. Antibody response in Lyme disease: evaluation of diagnostic tests. J Infect Dis. 1984 May;149(5):789-95.

Craft JE, Grodzicki RL, Shrestha M, Fischer DK, García-Blanco M, Steere AC. The antibody response in Lyme disease. Yale J Biol Med. 1984 Jul-Aug;57(4):561-5.

Craft JE, Fischer DK, Shimamoto GT, Steere AC. Antigens of Borrelia burgdorferi recognized during Lyme disease. Appearance of a new immunoglobulin M response and expansion of the immunoglobulin G response late in the illness. J Clin Invest. 1986 Oct;78(4):934-9.

Craven RB, Quan TJ, Bailey RE, Dattwyler R, Ryan RW, Sigal LH, Steere AC, Sullivan B, Johnson BJ, Dennis DT, Gubler DJ. Improved serodiagnostic testing for Lyme disease: results of a multicenter serologic evaluation. Emerg Infect Dis. 1996 Apr-Jun;2(2):136-40.

Creamer M, Foran J, Bell R. The Beck Anxiety Inventory in a non-clinical sample. Behav Res Ther. 1995;33(4):477-485.

Cross JR, Rossmeisl JH, Maggi RG, Breitschwerdt EB, Duncan RB. Bartonella-associated meningoradiculoneuritis and dermatitis or panniculitis in 3 dogs. J Vet Intern Med. 2008 May-Jun;22(3):674-8. Epub 2008 May 2.

Cruz M, Hansen K, Ernerudh J, Steere AC, Link H. Lyme arthritis: oligoclonal anti-Borrelia burgdorferi IgG antibodies occur in joint fluid and serum. Scand J Immunol. 1991 Jan;33(1):61-71.

Cunha BA, Barnett B, Sharma S, Talavera F, Sharma OP, Mylonakis E, Zevitz ME. Babesiosis. EMedicine. Accessed 2006 Jun 23.

Cunha BA, Cohen YZ, McDermott B. Fever of unknown origin (FUO) due to babesiosis in a immunocompetent host. Heart Lung. 2008 Nov-Dec;37(6):481-4. Epub 2008 Sep 30.

Cunha BA, Nausheen S, Szalda D. Pulmonary complications of babesiosis: case report and literature review. Eur J Clin Microbiol Infect Dis. 2007 Jul;26(7):505-8. Review.

Cuong BT, Binh VQ, Dai B, Duy DN, Lovell CM, Rieckmann KH, Edstein MD. Does gender, food or grapefruit juice alter the pharmacokinetics of primaquine in healthy subjects? Br J Clin Pharmacol. 2006 Jun;61(6):682-9.

Curi AL, Machado D, Heringer G, Campos WR, Lamas C, Rozental T, Gutierres A, Orefice F, Lemos E. Cat-scratch disease: ocular manifestations and visual outcome. Int Ophthalmol. 2010 Oct;30(5):553-8. Epub 2010 Jul 30.

Curi AL, Machado DO, Heringer G, Campos WR, Orefice F. Ocular manifestation of cat-scratch disease in HIV-positive patients. Am J Ophthalmol. 2006 Feb;141(2):400-1.

Curless RG, Schatz NJ, Bowen BC, Rodriguez Z, Ruiz A. Lyme neuroborreliosis masquerading as a brainstem tumor in a 15-year-old. Pediatr Neurol. 1996 Oct;15(3):258-60.

Curno O, Behnke JM, McElligott AG, Reader T, Barnard CJ. Mothers produce less aggressive sons with altered immunity when there is a threat of disease during pregnancy. Proc Biol Sci. 2009 Mar 22;276(1659):1047-54.

Czekalowki JW, Eaves G. Formation of granular structures by Leptospirae as revealed by the electron microscope. J Bacteriol. 1954 Jun;67:619-627.

Czell D, Rodic B, Imoberdorf R. [Neuroborreliosis--a disease with many faces].[Article in German]. Praxis (Bern 1994). 2011 May 11;100(10):607-12.

da Costa PS, Brigatte ME, Greco DB. Antibodies to Rickettsia rickettsii, Rickettsia typhi, Coxiella burnetii, Bartonella henselae, Bartonella quintana, and Ehrlichia chaffeensis among healthy population in Minas Gerais, Brazil. Mem Inst Oswaldo Cruz. 2005 Dec;100(8):853-9. Epub 2006 Jan 20.

Da Silva K, Chussid S. Cat scratch disease: clinical considerations for the pediatric dentist. Pediatr Dent. 2009 Jan-Feb;31(1):58-62.

Dabo SM, Confer AW, Anderson BE, Gupta S. Bartonella henselae Pap31, an extracellular matrix adhesin, binds the fibronectin repeat III13 module. Infect Immun. 2006 May;74(5):2513-21.

Dabo SM, Confer AW, Saliki JT, Anderson BE. Binding of Bartonella henselae to extracellular molecules: identification of potential adhesins. Microb Pathog. 2006 Jul;41(1):10-20. Epub 2006 May 24.

Dabrowska-Bień J, Pietniczka-Załeska M, Rowicki T. [Cat scratch disease--a diagnostic problem, case report].[Article in Polish]. Otolaryngol Pol. 2009 Mar-Apr;63(2):154-7.

Dadamessi I, Brazier F, Smail A, Delcenserie R, Dupas JL, Capron JP. Hepatic injuries related to Lyme disease. Study of 2 cases and a review of the literature. Gastroenterol Clin Biol, 25(2):193-196. 2001.

Dai J, Narasimhan S, Zhang L, Liu L, Wang P, Fikrig E. Tick histamine release factor is critical for Ixodes scapularis engorgement and transmission of the lyme disease agent. PLoS Pathog. 2010 Nov 24;6(11):e1001205.

Daffner KR, Saver JL, Biber MP. Lyme polyradiculoneuropathy presenting as increasing abdominal girth. Neurology. 1990 Feb;40:373-5.

Dandache P, Nadelman RB. Erythema migrans. Infect Dis Clin North Am. 2008 Jun;22(2):235-60, vi. Review.

Dantas-Torres F. The brown dog tick, Rhipicephalus sanguineus (Latreille, 1806) (Acari: Ixodidae): from taxonomy to control. Vet Parasitol. 2008 Apr 15;152(3-4):173-85. Epub 2008 Jan 3. Review.

Dantas-Torres F. Canine vector-borne diseases in Brazil. Parasit Vectors. 2008;1:25. Published online 2008 August 8.

Dantas-Torres F, Figueredo LA. Canine babesiosis: a Brazilian perspective. Vet Parasitol. 2006 Nov 5;141(3-4):197-203. Epub 2006 Sep 8. Review. Erratum in: Vet Parasitol. 2007 Sep 1;148(2):185. Dosage error in article text.

Dardenne S, Coche E, Weynand B, Poncelet A, Zech F, De Meyer M. High suspicion of bacillary angiomatosis in a kidney transplant recipient: a difficult way to diagnose--case report. Transplant Proc. 2007 Jan-Feb;39(1):311-3.

Das BB, Wasser E, Bryant KA, Woods CR, Yang SG, Zahn M. Culture negative endocarditis caused by Bartonella henselae in a child with congenital heart disease. Pediatr Infect Dis J. 2009 Oct;28(10):922-5.

Datta SC, Opp MR. Lipopolysaccharide-induced increases in cytokines in discrete mouse brain regions are detectable using Luminex xMAP® technology. J Neurosci Methods. 2008 Oct 30;175(1): 119–124. Published online 2008 August 14.

Dattwyler RJ, Halperin JJ. Failure of tetracycline therapy in early Lyme disease. Arthritis Rheum. 1987 Apr;30(4):448-50.

Dattwyler RJ, Halperin JJ, Volkman DJ, Luft BJ. Treatment of late Lyme borreliosis-randomized comparison of ceftriaxone and penicillin. Lancet. 1988 May 28;1(8596):1191-4.

Dattwyler RJ, Luft BJ, Kunkel MJ, Finkel MF, Wormser GP, Rush TJ, Grunwaldt E, Agger WA, Franklin M, Oswald D, Cockey L, Maladorno D. Ceftriaxone compared with doxycycline for the treatment of acute disseminated Lyme disease. N Engl J Med. 1997 Jul 31;337(5):289-94.

Dattwyler RJ, Volkman DJ, Luft BJ, Halperin JJ, Thomas J, Golightly MG. Seronegative Lyme disease. Dissociation of specific T-and B-lymphocyte responses to Borrelia burgdorferi. N Engl J Med. 1988 Dec 1;319(22):1441-6.

Dattwyler RJ, Volkman DJ, Luft BJ. Immunologic aspects of Lyme borreliosis. Rev Infect Dis. 1989 Sep-Oct;11 Suppl 6:S1494-8.

Dattwyler RJ, Wormser GP, Rush TJ, Finkel MF, Schoen RT, Grunwaldt E, Franklin M, Hilton E, Bryant GL, Agger WA, Maladorno D. A comparison of two treatment regimens of ceftriaxone in late Lyme disease. Wien Klin Wochenschr. 2005 Jun;117(11-12):393-7.

Dayan AD. Neurotoxicity and artemisinin compounds do the observations in animals justify limitation of clinical use? Med Trop (Mars). 1998;58(3 Suppl):32-7.

Dayan NE, Rubin LG, Di John D, Sood SK. Hypoglycorrhachia in Lyme meningitis. Pediatr Infect Dis J. 2004 Apr;23(4):370-1.

de Caprariis D, Dantas-Torres F, Capelli G, Mencke N, Stanneck D, Breitschwerdt EB, Otranto D. Evolution of clinical, haematological and biochemical findings in young dogs naturally infected by vector-borne pathogens. Vet Microbiol. 2011 Apr 21;149(1-2):206-12. Epub 2010 Oct 16.

De Clerck KF, Van Offel JF, Vlieghe E, Van Marck E, Stevens WJ. Bartonella endocarditis mimicking adult Still's disease. Acta Clin Belg. 2008 May-Jun;63(3):190-2.

De Koning J, Duray PH. Histopathology of human Lyme borreliosis. In Aspects of Lyme Borreliosis, ed. Klaus Weber, M.D., Willy Burgdorfer, Ph.D., M.D. Berlin Heidelberg:Springer-Verlag:pp 70-104. 1993.

de Kort JG, Robben SG, Schrander JJ, van Rhijn LW. Multifocal osteomyelitis in a child: a rare manifestation of cat scratch disease: a case report and systematic review of the literature. J Pediatr Orthop B. 2006 Jul;15(4):285-8. Review.

de La Blanchardière A, Fournier PE, Haustraete E, du Cheyron D, Lepage O, Verdon R. [Infective endocarditis due to Bartonella henselae following a rupture of a cerebral aneurysm].[Article in French]. Med Mal Infect. 2009 Jun;39(6):394-6. Epub 2008 Dec 18.

de Paiva Diniz PP, Schwartz DS, de Morais HS, Breitschwerdt EB. Surveillance for zoonotic vector-borne infections using sick dogs from southeastern Brazil. Vector Borne Zoonotic Dis. 2007 Winter;7(4):689-97.

de Saussure P, Bertolini D. [Functional bowel disorders: impact and limitations of evidence-based medicine].[Article in French]. Rev Med Suisse. 2006 Sep 6;2(77):1987-91. Review.

De Sousa R, Edouard-Fournier P, Santos-Silva M, Amaro F, Bacellar F, Raoult D. Molecular detection of Rickettsia felis, Rickettsia typhi and two genotypes closely related to Bartonella elizabethae. Am J Trop Med Hyg. 2006 Oct;75(4):727-31.

de Vries PJ, Dien TK. Clinical pharmacology and therapeutic potential of artemisinin and its derivatives in the treatment of malaria. Drugs. 1996 Dec;52(6):818-36.

Debarry JD, Kissinger JC. Jumbled genomes: missing apicomplexan synteny. Mol Biol Evol. 2011 Oct;28(10):2855-71. Epub 2011 Apr 19.

Defer G, Levy R, Brugieres P, Postic D, Degos JD. Lyme disease presenting as a stroke in the vertebrobasilar territory: MRI. Neuroradiology. 1993;35(7):529-31.

Dehio C. Infection-associated type IV secretion systems of Bartonella and their diverse roles in host cell interaction. Cell Microbiol. 2008 Aug;10(8):1591-8. Epub 2008 Jul 30. Review.

Dekkers MJ, Dees A, Weidema WF, Bartelsman M, Veeken H, Hart W. [Clinical thinking and decision making in practice. A man with abdominal pain, weight loss and fever].[Article in Dutch]. Ned Tijdschr Geneeskd. 2009 Jan 31;153(5):174-80.

Dekonenko EJ, Steere AC, Berardi VP, Kravchuk LN. Lyme borreliosis in the Soviet Union: a cooperative US-USSR report. J Infect Dis. 1988 Oct;158(4):748-53.

del Rio B, Seegers JF, Gomes-Solecki M. Immune Response to Lactobacillus plantarum Expressing Borrelia burgdorferi OspA Is Modulated by the Lipid Modification of the Antigen. PLoS One. 2010; 5(6): e11199. Published online 2010 June 18.

del Valle LJ, Flores L, Vargas M, García-de-la-Guarda R, Quispe RL, Ibañez ZB, Alvarado D, Ramírez P, Ruiz J. Bartonella bacilliformis, endemic pathogen of the Andean region, is intrinsically resistant to quinolones. Int J Infect Dis. 2010 Jun;14(6):e506-10. Epub 2009 Dec 6.

Delamater ED, Haanes M, Wiggall RH, Pillsbury DM. Studies on the life cycle of spirochetes. VIII. Summary and comparison of observations on various organisms. J Invest Dermatol. 1951 Apr;16(4):231-256.

Delamater ED, Newcomer VD, Haanes M, Wiggall RH. Studies on the life cycles of spirochaetes: I. The use of phase contrast microscopy. Am J Syph Gonorrhea Vener Dis. 1950 Mar;34(2):122-5.

Dell'Eva R, Pfeffer U, Vene R, Anfosso L, Forlani A, Albini A, Efferth T. Inhibition of angiogenesis in vivo and growth of Kaposi's sarcoma xenograft tumors by the anti-malarial artesunate. Biochem Pharmacol. 2004 Dec 15;68(12):2359-66.

Deloizy M, Devos P, Stekelorom T, Testard D, Belhadia A. Left sided sudden hemiparesis linked to a central form of Lyme disease. Rev Neurol (Paris). 2000 Dec;156(12):1154-6.

delos Santos JR, Boughan K, Bremer WG, Rizzo B, Schaefer JJ, Rikihisa Y, Needham GR, Capitini LA, Anderson DE, Oglesbee M, Ewing SA, Stich RW. Experimental infection of dairy calves with Ehrlichia chaffeensis. J Med Microbiol. 2007 Dec; 56(Pt 12):1660-8.

deLuise VP, Lesser RL, Scrimenti RJ. Lyme borreliosis. [Chapter 63] In Eye and Skin Disease, ed M.J. Mannis et al. Lippencot-Raven Publishers, Philadelphia. 1996.

Demaerel P, Crevits I, Casteels-Van Daele M, Baert AL. Meningo-radiculitis due to borreliosis presenting as low back pain only. Neuroradiology. 1998 Feb;40(2):126-7.

Dennis VA, Jefferson A, Singh SR, Ganapamo F, Philipp MT. Interleukin-10 Anti-Inflammatory Response to Borrelia burgdorferi, the Agent of Lyme Disease: a Possible Role for Suppressors of Cytokine Signaling 1 and 3. Infect Immun. 2006 Oct;74(10): 5780-9.

Depeyre C, Mancel E, Besson-Leaud L, Goursaud R. [Abrupt visual loss in children. Three case studies of ocular bartonellosis]. [Article in French]. J Fr Ophtalmol. 2005 Nov;28(9):968-75.

Derbyshire ET, Franssen FJ, de Vries E, Morin C, Woodrow CJ, Krishna S, Staines HM. Identification, expression and characterisation of a Babesia bovis hexose transporter. Mol Biochem Parasitol. 2008 Oct;161(2):124-9. Epub 2008 Jun 27.

Deretic V, Levine B. Autophagy, Immunity, and Microbial Adaptations. Cell Host Microbe. 2009 June 18; 5(6): 527–549.

Desenclos JC, Laporte A, Brouqui P. [Louse-borne infections in humans].[Article in French]. Med Mal Infect. 2011 Jun;41(6):295-300. Epub 2011 Mar 30. Review.

Di Rocco A, Rogers JD, Brown R, Werner P, Bottiglieri T. S-Adenosyl-Methionine improves depression in patients with Parkinson's disease in an open-label clinical trial. Mov Disord. 2000 Nov;15(6):1225-9.

DiCarlo EF, Kahn LB. Inflammatory diseases of the bones and joints. Semin Diagn Pathol. 2011 Feb;28(1):53-64. Review.

Dickinson GS, Piccone H, Sun G, Lien E, Gatto L, Alugupalli KR.Toll-Like Receptor 2 Deficiency Results in Impaired Antibody Responses and Septic Shock during Borrelia hermsii Infection. Infect Immun. 2010 Nov;78(11):4579-88. Published online 2010 August 9.

Diederen BM, Vermeulen MJ, Verbakel H, van der Zee A, Bergmans A, Peeters MF. Evaluation of an internally controlled real-time polymerase chain reaction assay targeting the groEL gene for the detection of Bartonella spp. DNA in patients with suspected cat-scratch disease. Eur J Clin Microbiol Infect Dis. 2007 Sep;26(9):629-33.

Dieterle L, Kubina FG, Staudacher T, Budingen HJ. Neuro-borreliosis or intervertebral disk prolapse? Dtsch Med Wochenschr. 1989 Oct 20;114(42);1602-6.

Dietrich F, Schmidgen T, Maggi RG, Richter D, Matuschka FR, Vonthein R, Breitschwerdt EB, Kempf VA. Prevalence of Bartonella henselae and Borrelia burgdorferi sensu lato DNA in ixodes ricinus ticks in Europe. Appl Environ Microbiol. 2010 Mar;76(5):1395-8. Epub 2010 Jan 8.

Dillon B, Iredell J, Breitschwerdt EB, Maggi RG. Potential limitations of the 16S-23S rRNA intergenic region for molecular detection of Bartonella species. J Clin Microbiol. 2005 Sep;43(9):4921-2.

Dinerman H, Steere AC. Lyme disease associated with fibromyalgia. Ann Intern Med. 1992 Aug 15;117(4):281-5.

Diniz PP, Beall MJ, Omark K, Chandrashekar R, Daniluk DA, Cyr KE, Koterski JF, Robbins RG, Lalo PG, Hegarty BC, Breitschwerdt EB. High prevalence of tick-borne pathogens in dogs from an Indian reservation in northeastern Arizona. Vector Borne Zoonotic Dis. 2010 Mar;10(2):117-23.

Diniz PP, Billeter SA, Otranto D, De Caprariis D, Petanides T, Mylonakis ME, Koutinas AF, Breitschwerdt EB. Molecular documentation of Bartonella infection in dogs in Greece and Italy. J Clin Microbiol. 2009 May;47(5):1565-7. Epub 2009 Mar 4.

Diniz PP, de Morais HS, Breitschwerdt EB, Schwartz DS. Serum cardiac troponin I concentration in dogs with ehrlichiosis. J Vet Intern Med. 2008 Sep-Oct;22(5):1136-43. Epub 2008 Jul 11.

Diniz PP, Maggi RG, Schwartz DS, Cadenas MB, Bradley JM, Hegarty B, Breitschwerdt EB. Canine bartonellosis: serological and molecular prevalence in Brazil and evidence of co-infection with Bartonella henselae and Bartonella vinsonii subsp. berkhoffii. Vet Res. 2007 Sep-Oct;38(5):697-710. Epub 2007 Jun 23.

Diniz PP, Wood M, Maggi RG, Sontakke S, Stepnik M, Breitschwerdt EB. Co-isolation of Bartonella henselae and Bartonella vinsonii subsp. berkhoffii from blood, joint and subcutaneous seroma fluids from two naturally infected dogs. Vet Microbiol. 2009 Sep 18;138(3-4):368-72. Epub 2009 Feb 4.

Diringer MN, Halperin JJ, Dattwyler RJ. Lyme meningoencephalitis--report of a severe, penicillin resistant case. Arthritis Rheum. 1987 Jun;30(6):705-8.

Disbrow GL, Baege AC, Kierpiec KA, Yuan H, Centeno JA, Thibodeaux CA, Hartmann D, Schlegel R. Dihydroartemisinin is cytotoxic to papillomavirus-expressing epithelial cells in vitro and in vivo. Cancer Res. 2005 Dec 1;65:10854-61.

Djukic M, Schmidt-Samoa C, Lange P, Spreer A, Neubieser K, Eiffert H, Nau R, Schmidt H. Cerebrospinal fluid findings in adults with acute Lyme neuroborreliosis. J Neurol. 2011 Sep 6. [Epub ahead of print]

Dobler G, Pfeffer M. Fleas as parasites of the family Canidae. Parasit Vectors. 2011 Jul 18;4:139.

Dodd JD, Aquino SL, Sharma A. Babesiosis: CT and hematologic findings. J Thorac Imaging. 2007 Aug;22(3):271-3.

Dodd RY. Emerging pathogens in transfusion medicine. Clin Lab Med. 2010 Jun;30(2):499-509. Epub 2010 May 6.

Dondorp AM, Omodeo-Sale F, Chotivanich K, Taramelli D, White NJ. Oxidative stress and rheology in severe malaria. Redox Rep. 2003;8:292-4.

Dong J, Olano JP, McBride JW, Walker DH. Emerging pathogens: challenges and successes of molecular diagnostics. J Mol Diagn. 2008 May;10(3):185-97. Epub 2008 Apr 10. Review.

Donnio A, Jean-Charles A, Merle H. Macular hole following Bartonella henselae neuroretinitis. Eur J Ophthalmol. 2008 May-Jun;18(3):456-8.

Donta ST. Tetracycline therapy for chronic Lyme disease. Clin Infect Dis Jul;25 Suppl 1:S52-6.

Donta ST. Treatment of chronic Lyme disease with macrolide antibiotics. In: Program and abstracts of the VIIIth International Conference on Lyme Borreliosis. 1999 June 20-24; Munich, Germany. [Abstract P193].

Donta ST. Macrolide therapy of chronic Lyme disease. Med Sci Monit. 2003 Nov;9(11):PI136-42.

Dorado Moles MJ, López-Ibor B, Figueredo MA, González Laguillo A. [Atypical cat scratch disease in an immunocompetent school-aged child].[Article in Spanish]. An Pediatr (Barc). 2007 Apr;66(4):418-9.

Dörbecker C, Sander A, Oberle K, Schülin-Casonato T. In vitro susceptibility of Bartonella species to 17 antimicrobial compounds: comparison of Etest and agar dilution. J Antimicrob Chemother. 2006 Oct;58(4):784-8. Epub 2006 Aug 17.

dos Santos AP, dos Santos RP, Biondo AW, Dora JM, Goldani LZ, de Oliveira ST, de Sá Guimarães AM, Timenetsky J, de Morais HA, González FH, Messick JB. Hemoplasma infection in HIV-positive patient, Brazil. Emerg Infect Dis. 2008 Dec;14(12):1922-4.

dos Santos RP, Cartell A, Goldani LZ. An HIV-positive patient with cervical lymphadenopathy and skin lesions. Clin Infect Dis. 2007 Mar 15;44(6):849, 884-5.

Dotevall L, Eliasson T, Hagberg L, Mannheimer C. Pain as presenting symptom in Lyme neuroborreliosis. Eur J Pain. 2003;7(3):235-9.

Drancourt M, Berger P, Terrada C, Bodaghi B, Conrath J, Raoult D, LeHoang P. High prevalence of fastidious bacteria in 1520 cases of uveitis of unknown etiology. Medicine (Baltimore). 2008 May;87(3):167-76.

Drancourt M, Bodaghi B, Lepidi H, Le Hoang P, Raoult D. Intraocular detection of Bartonella henselae in a patient with HLA-B27 uveitis. J Clin Microbiol. 2004 Apr;42(4):1822-5.

Drancourt M, Carrieri P, Gévaudan MJ, Raoult D. Blood agar and Mycobacterium tuberculosis: the end of a dogma. J Clin Microbiol. 2003 Apr;41(4):1710-1.

Drancourt M, Tran-Hung L, Courtin J, Lumley H, Raoult D. Bartonella quintana in a 4000-year-old human tooth. J Infect Dis. 2005 Feb 15;191(4):607-11. Epub 2005 Jan 10.

Drebber U, Kasper HU, Ratering J, Wedemeyer I, Schirmacher P, Dienes HP, Odenthal M. Hepatic granulomas: histological and molecular pathological approach to differential diagnosis--a study of 442 cases. Liver Int. 2008 Jul;28(6):828-34.

Dreier J, Vollmer T, Freytag CC, Bäumer D, Körfer R, Kleesiek K. Culture-negative infectious endocarditis caused by Bartonella spp.: 2 case reports and a review of the literature. Diagn Microbiol Infect Dis. 2008 Aug;61(4):476-83. Epub 2008 May 1. Review.

Dressler F, Ackermann R, Steere AC. Antibody responses to the three genomic groups of Borrelia burgdorferi in European Lyme borreliosis. J Infect Dis. 1994 Feb;169(2):313-8.

Dressler F, Yoshinari NH, Steere AC. The T-cell proliferative assay in the diagnosis of Lyme disease. Ann Intern Med. 1991 Oct 1;115(7):533-9.

Dressler F, Whalen JA, Reinhardt BN, Steere AC. Western blotting in the serodiagnosis of Lyme disease. J Infect Dis. 1993 Feb;167(2):392-400.

Drevets DA, Leenen PJ, Greenfield RA. Invasion of the Central Nervous System by Intracellular Bacteria. Clin Microbiol Rev. 2004 Apr;17(2):323-47.

Drouin EE, Glickstein L, Kwok WW, Nepom GT, Steere AC. Searching for borrelial T cell epitopes associated with antibiotic-refractory Lyme arthritis. Mol Immunol. 2008 Apr;45(8):2323-32. Epub 2008 Jan 11. Erratum in: Mol Immunol. 2008 Jul;45(12):3508.

Drouin EE, Glickstein L, Kwok WW, Nepom GT, Steere AC. Human homologues of a Borrelia T cell epitope associated with antibiotic-refractory Lyme arthritis. Mol Immunol. 2008 Jan;45(1):180-9. Epub 2007 Jun 6.

Drouin EE, Glickstein LJ, Steere AC. Molecular characterization of the OspA(161-175) T cell epitope associated with treatment-resistant Lyme arthritis: differences among the three pathogenic species of Borrelia burgdorferi sensu lato. J Autoimmun. 2004 Nov;23(3):281-92.

Drummond MR, Gilioli R, Velho PE. Bartonellosis diagnosis requires careful evaluation. Braz J Infect Dis. 2010 May-Jun;14(3):217.

Dubey JP, Lappin MR, Kwok OC, Mofya S, Chikweto A, Baffa A, Doherty D, Shakeri J, Macpherson CN, Sharma RN. Seroprevalence of Toxoplasma gondii and concurrent Bartonella spp., feline immunodeficiency virus, and feline leukemia virus infections in cats from Grenada, West Indies. J Parasitol. 2009 Oct;95(5):1129-33. Epub 2009 Apr 22.

Duchemin JB, Fournier PE, Parola P. [Fleas and diseases transmissible to man].[Article in French]. Med Trop (Mars). 2006 Feb;66(1):21-9.

Duh D, Jelovsek M, Avsic-Zupanc T. Evaluation of an indirect fluorescence immunoassay for the detection of serum antibodies against Babesia divergens in humans. Parasitology. 2007 Feb;134(Pt 2):179-85. Epub 2006 Oct 11.

Duijvestijn AM, Horst E, Pals ST, Rouse BN, Steere AC, Picker LJ, Meijer CJ, Butcher EC. High endothelial differentiation in human lymphoid and inflammatory tissues defined by monoclonal antibody HECA-452. Am J Pathol. 1988 Jan;130(1):147-55.

Dulebohn DP, Bestor A, Rego RO, Stewart PE, Rosa PA. Borrelia burgdorferi linear plasmid 38 is dispensable for completion of the mouse-tick infectious cycle. Infect Immun. 2011 Sep;79(9):3510-7. Epub 2011 Jun 27.

Dumler JS. Fitness and freezing: vector biology and human health. J Clin Invest. 2010 Sep 1;120(9):3087-90. Published online 2010 August 25.

Dummond R. Ticks and what you can do about them. Wilderness Press;Berkeley, CA: 2004. p.59-69.

Duncan AW, Maggi RG, Breitschwerdt EB. A combined approach for the enhanced detection and isolation of Bartonella species in dog blood samples: pre-enrichment liquid culture followed by PCR and subculture onto agar plates. J Microbiol Methods. 2007 May;69(2):273-81. Epub 2007 Feb 2.

Duncan AW, Maggi RG, Breitschwerdt EB. Bartonella DNA in dog saliva. Emerg Infect Dis. 2007 Dec;13(12):1948-50.

Duncan AW, Marr HS, Birkenheuer AJ, Maggi RG, Williams LE, Correa MT, Breitschwerdt EB. Bartonella DNA in the blood and lymph nodes of Golden Retrievers with lymphoma and in healthy controls. J Vet Intern Med. 2008 Jan-Feb;22(1):89-95.

Dunning Hotopp JC, Lin M, Madupu R, Crabtree J, Angiuoli SV, Eisen J, Seshadri R, Ren Q, Wu M, Utterback TR, Smith S, Lewis M, Khouri H, Zhang C, Niu H, Lin Q, Ohashi N, Zhi N, Nelson W, Brinkac LM, Dodson RJ, Rosovitz MJ, Sundaram J, Daugherty SC, Davidsen T, Durkin AS, Gwinn M, Haft DH, Selengut JD, Sullivan SA, Zafar N, Zhou L, Benahmed F, Forberger H, Halpin R, Mulligan S, Robinson J, White O, Rikihisa Y, Tettelin H. Comparative Genomics of Emerging Human Ehrlichiosis Agents. PLoS Genet. 2006 Feb; 2(2):e21. Published online 2006 February 17. Correction in: PLoS Genet. 2006 Dec; 2(12):e213.

Dupeyron A, Lecocq J, Jaulhac B, Isner-Horobeti ME, Vautravers P, Vautravers P, Cohen-Solal J, Sordet C, Kuntz JL. Sciatica, disk herniation, and neuroborreliosis: A report of four cases. Joint Bone Spine. 2004 Sep;71(5):433-7.

Dupouy-Camet J. [New drugs for the treatment of human parasitic protozoa]. [Article in French]. Parassitologia. 2004 Jun;46(1-2):81-4.

Durá Travé T, Yoldi Petri ME, Lavilla Oiz A, Molins Castiella T. [Neuroretinitis in cat-scratch disease].[Article in Spanish]. An Pediatr (Barc). 2010 Apr;72(4):290-1. Epub 2010 Mar 2.

Duray PH, Steere AC. The spectrum of organ and systems pathology in human Lyme disease. Zentralbl Bakteriol Mikrobiol Hyg A. 1986 Dec;263(1-2):169-78.

Duray PH, Steere AC. Clinical pathologic correlations of Lyme disease by stage. Ann N Y Acad Sci. 1988;539:65-79.

Duray PH. Clinical pathologic correlations of Lyme disease. Rev Infect Dis. 1989 Sep-Oct;11, Suppl. 6: S1487-93.

Duray PH, Johnson RC. The histopathology of experimentally infected hamsters with the Lyme disease spirochete, Borrelia burgdorferi. Proc Soc Exp Biol Med. 1986 Feb;181(2):263-9.

Duray PH. Visceral histopathology in Lyme borreliosis: new observations. Zentralbl Bacteriol 1989. (Suppl), 18:116-125.

Durupt F, Seve P, Roure C, Biron F, Raoult D, Broussolle C. Liver and spleen abscesses without endocarditis due to Bartonella quintana in an immunocompetent host. Eur J Clin Microbiol Infect Dis. 2004 Oct;23(10):790-1.

Dutta A, Schwarzwald HL, Edwards MS. Disseminated bartonellosis presenting as neuroretinitis in a young adult with human immunodeficiency virus infection. Pediatr Infect Dis J. 2010 Jul;29(7):675-7.

Dutton JS, Todd JL. A note on the morphology of Spirochaeta Duttoni. Lancet. 1907;2:1523.

Dvorakováá HM, Dvoráčková M. [Babesiosis, a little known zoonosis].[Article in Czech]. Epidemiol Mikrobiol Imunol. 2007 Nov;56(4):176-80. Review.

Dykhuizen DE, Brisson D, Sandigursky S, Wormser GP, Nowakowski J, Nadelman RB, Schwartz I. The propensity of different Borrelia burgdorferi sensu stricto genotypes to cause disseminated infections in humans. Am J Trop Med Hyg. 2008 May;78(5):806-10.

Dzelalija B, Medić A, Rode OD, Mazzi A. [Rash and purulent lymphadenitis in cat scratch disease].[Article in Croatian]. Acta Med Croatica. 2006 Dec;60(5):483-6.

Earl TJ. Cardiac manifestations of Lyme disease. Med Health R I. 2010 Nov;93(11):339-41.

Earnhart CG, Rhodes DV, Marconi RT. Disulfide-mediated oligomer formation in Borrelia burgdorferi outer surface protein C, a critical virulence factor and potential Lyme disease vaccine candidate. Clin Vaccine Immunol. 2011 Jun;18(6):901-6. Epub 2011 Apr 27.

Easterbrook JD, Kaplan JB, Vanasco NB, Reeves WK, Purcell RH, Kosoy MY, Glass GE, Watson J, Klein SL. A survey of zoonotic pathogens carried by Norway rats in Baltimore, Maryland, USA. Epidemiol Infect. 2007 Oct;135(7):1192-9. Epub 2007 Jan 15.

Eberhardt C, Engelmann S, Kusch H, Albrecht D, Hecker M, Autenrieth IB, Kempf VA. Proteomic analysis of the bacterial pathogen Bartonella henselae and identification of immunogenic proteins for serodiagnosis. Proteomics. 2009 Apr;9(7):1967-81.

Ecklund K, Vargas S, Zurakowki D, Sundel RP. MRI features of Lyme arthritis in children. Am J Roentgenol. 2005 Jun;184(6):1904-9.

Eckman MH, Steere AC, Kalish RA, Pauker SG. Cost effectiveness of oral as compared with intravenous antibiotic therapy for patients with early Lyme disease or Lyme arthritis. N Engl J Med. 1997 Jul 31;337(5):357-63.

Edouard S, Gonin K, Turc Y, Angelakis E, Socolovschi C, Raoult D. Eschar and neck lymphadenopathy caused by Francisella tularensis after a tick bite: a case report. J Med Case Reports. 2011 Mar 19;5:108.

Edouard S, Raoult D. [Bartonella henselae, an ubiquitous agent of proteiform zoonotic disease].[Article in French]. Med Mal Infect. 2010 Jun;40(6):319-30. Epub 2009 Dec 29. Review.

Edstein MD, Kocisko DA, Brewer TG, Walsh DS, Eamsila C, Charles BG. Population pharmacokinetics of the new antimalarial agent tafenoquine in Thai soldiers. Br J Clin Pharmacol. 2001 Dec;52(6):663-70.

Edstein MD, Kocisko DA, Walsh DS, Eamsila C, Charles BG, Rieckmann KH. Plasma concentrations of tafenoquine, a new long-acting antimalarial agent, in Thai soldiers receiving monthly prophylaxis. Clin Infect Dis. 2003 Dec 15;37(12):1654-8. Epub 2003 Nov 20.

Edstein MD, Nasveld PE, Kocisko DA, Kitchener SJ, Gatton ML, Rieckmann KH. Gender differences in gastrointestinal disturbances and plasma concentrations of tafenoquine in healthy volunteers after tafenoquine administration for post-exposure vivax malaria prophylaxis. Trans R Soc Trop Med Hyg. 2007 Mar;101(3):226-30. Epub 2006 Jun 30.

Edwards KS, Kanengiser S, Li KI, Glassman M. Lyme disease presenting as hepatitis and jaundice in a child. Pediatr Infect Dis J. 1990 Aug;9(8):592-3.

Efferth T, Dunstan H, Sauerbrey A, Miyachi H, Chitambar CR. The anti-malarial artesunate is also active against cancer. Int J Oncol. 2001 Apr;18(4):767-73.

Efferth T, Olbrich A, Bauer R. mRNA expression profiles for the response of human tumor cell lines to the antimalarial drugs artesunate, arteether, and artemether. Biochem Pharmacol. 2002 Aug 15;64(4):617-23.

Efferth T, Benakis A, Romero MR, Tomicic M, Rauh R, Steinbach D, Hafer R, Stamminger T, Oesch F, Kaina B, Marschall M. Enhancement of cytotoxicity of artemisinins toward cancer cells by ferrous iron. Free Radic Biol Med. 2004 Oct 1;37(7):998-1009.

Efferth T. Molecular pharmacology and pharmacogenomics of artemisinin and its derivatives in cancer cells. Curr Drug Targets. 2006 Apr;7(4):407-21.

Egan TJ. Chloroquine and primaquine: combining old drugs as a new weapon against falciparum malaria? Trends Parasitol. 2006 Jun;22(6):235-7. Epub 2006 Apr 3.

Eglantin F, Hamdad F, El Samad Y, Monge AS, Sevestre H, Eb F, Schmit JL. [The diagnosis of cat-scratch-disease-associated adenitis: diagnostic value of serology and polymerase chain reaction].[Article in French]. Pathol Biol (Paris). 2008 Nov-Dec;56(7-8):461-6. Epub 2008 Oct 7.

Ehrenborg C, Byström R, Hjelm E, Friman G, Holmberg M. High Bartonella spp. seroprevalence in a Swedish homeless population but no evidence of trench fever. Scand J Infect Dis. 2008;40(3):208-15. Epub 2007 Sep 6.

Ehrenborg C, Hagberg S, Alden J, Makitalo S, Myrdal G, Larsson E, Hjelm E, Friman G. First known case of Bartonella quintana endocarditis in Sweden. Scand J Infect Dis. 2009;41(1):73-5.

Eichhorn-Sens J, Bund T, Vogt PM. [Painful soft-tissue swelling of the upper arm].[Article in German]. Chirurg. 2008 Mar;79(3):249-51.

Eidlitz-Markus T, Zeharia A. Images in clinical medicine. Cat scratch disease lymphadenopathy. N Engl J Med. 2006 Apr 27;354(17):e17.

Eisen RJ, Gage KL. Transmission of Flea-Borne Zoonotic Agents. Annu Rev Entomol. 2010 Dec 15. [Epub ahead of print]

El-Bahnasawy MM, Morsy TA. Egyptian human babesiosis and general review. J Egypt Soc Parasitol. 2008 Apr;38(1):265-72.

Ellis TN, Kuehn MJ. Virulence and Immunomodulatory Roles of Bacterial Outer Membrane Vesicles. Microbiol Mol Biol Rev. 2010 March ;74(1): 81-94. Published online 2009 December 14.

Elsheikha HM, Khan NA. Protozoa traversal of the blood-brain barrier to invade the central nervous system. FEMS Microbiol Rev. 2010 Jul;34(4):532-53. Epub 2010 Feb 6. Review.

Embers ME, Wormser GP, Schwartz I, Martin DS, Philipp MT. Borrelia burgdorferi spirochetes that harbor only a portion of the lp28-1 plasmid elicit antibody responses detectable with the C6 test for Lyme disease. Clin Vaccine Immunol. 2007 Jan;14(1):90-3. Epub 2006 Nov 15.

Engel P, Dehio C. Genomics of host-restricted pathogens of the genus bartonella. Genome Dyn. 2009;6:158-69. Epub 2009 Aug 19.

Engel P, Salzburger W, Liesch M, Chang CC, Maruyama S, Lanz C, Calteau A, Lajus A, Médigue C, Schuster SC, Dehio C. Parallel evolution of a type IV secretion system in radiating lineages of the host-restricted bacterial pathogen Bartonella. PLoS Genet. 2011 Feb 10;7(2):e1001296.

Engelmann S, Silvie O, Matuschewski K. Disruption of Plasmodium sporozoite transmission by depletion of sporozoite invasion-associated protein 1. Eukaryot Cell. 2009 Apr;8(4):640-8. Epub 2009 Jan 30.

Eremeeva ME, Gerns HL, Lydy SL, Goo JS, Ryan ET, Mathew SS, Ferraro MJ, Holden JM, Nicholson WL, Dasch GA, Koehler JE. Bacteremia, fever, and splenomegaly caused by a newly recognized bartonella species. N Engl J Med. 2007 Jun 7;356(23):2381-7.

Eroğlu C, Candir N, Dervişoğlu A, Kefeli M. [A case of cat scratch disease].[Article in Turkish]. Mikrobiyol Bul. 2007 Oct;41(4):603-6.

Eskow ES, Krause PJ, Spielman A, Freeman K, Aslanzadeh J. Southern extension of the range of human babesiosis in the eastern United States. J Clin Microbiol. 1999 Jun;37(6):2051-2.

Eskow E, Rao RV, Mordechai E. Concurrent infection of the central nervous system by Borrelia burgdorferi and Bartonella henselae: evidence for a novel tick-borne disease complex. Arch Neurol. 2001 Sep;58(9):1357-63.

Espana A, Torrelo A, Guerrero A, Suarez J, Rocamora A, Ledo A. Periarticular fibrous nodules in Lyme borreliosis. Br J Dermatol. 1991 Jul;125(1):68-70.

Espinoza-León F, Arocha F, Hassanhi M, Arévalo J. [Using the polymerase chain reaction to Borrelia burgdorferi infection in localized scleroderma injure (morphea), in Venezuelan patients]. [Article in Spanish]. Invest Clin. 2010 Sep;51(3):381-90.

Espy MJ, Uhl JR, Sloan LM, Buckwalter SP, Jones MF, Vetter EA, Yao JD, Wengenack NL, Rosenblatt JE, Cockerill FR 3rd, Smith TF. Real-Time PCR in Clinical Microbiology: Applications for Routine Laboratory Testing. Clin Microbiol Rev. 2006 Jan;19(1):165–256. Correction in: Clin Microbiol Rev. 2006 July;19(3):595.

Estrada-Peña A, Acevedo P, Ruiz-Fons F, Gortázar C, de la Fuente J. Evidence of the Importance of Host Habitat Use in Predicting the Dilution Effect of Wild Boar for Deer Exposure to Anaplasma spp. PLoS ONE. 2008 Aug 20;3(8):e2999. Published online 2008 August 20.

European Academy of Paediatrics, Barcelona, Spain, October 7-10, 2006. Eur J Pediatr. 2006 Nov;165 Suppl 1:1–389. Published online 2006 December 20.

Ewing J. Note on involution forms of Spirochaete pallida in gummata. Proceedings of the New York Path. Soc., n.s. 7:166-171. 1907-8.

Eymin G, Zapata A, Andrade M, Aizman A, Rojas L, Rabagliati R. [Cat-scratch disease. Review of eight adult patients hospitalized for fever or adenopathy].[Article in Spanish]. Rev Med Chil. 2006 Oct;134(10):1243-8. Epub 2006 Dec 13.

Ezzelarab M, Yeh P, Wagner R, Cooper DK. Babesia as a complication of immunosuppression following pig-to-baboon heart transplantation. Xenotransplantation. 2007 Mar;14(2):162-5. Erratum in: Xenotransplantation. 2007 Jul;14(4):374.

Falagas ME, Klempner MS. Babesiosis in patients with AIDS: a chronic infection presenting as fever of unknown origin. Clin Infect Dis. 1996 May;22(5):809-812.

Falco RC, McKenna DF, Daniels TJ, Nadelman RB, Nowakowski J, Fish D, Wormser GP. Temporal relation between Ixodes scapularis abundance and risk for Lyme disease associated with erythema migrans. Am J Epidemiol. 1999 Apr 15;149(8):771-6.

Faller J, Thompson F, Hamilton W. Foot and ankle disorders resulting from Lyme disease. Foot & Ankle, (11)4:236-238 1991.

Fallon, BA. Testimony at public hearings in re Lyme disease for the State of Connecticut Department of Public Health. 2004: p. 134-153.

Fallon BA, Das S, Plutchok JJ, Tager F, Liegner K, Van Heertum R. Functional brain imaging and neuropsychological testing in Lyme disease. Clin Infect Dis. 1997 Jul;25 Suppl 1:S57-63. Review.

Fallon BA, Keilp JG, Corbera KM, Petkova E, Britton CB, Dwyer E, Slavov I, Cheng J, Dobkin J, Nelson DR, Sackeim HA. A randomized, placebo-controlled trial of repeated IV antibiotic therapy for Lyme encephalopathy. Neurology. 2008 Mar 25;70(13):992-1003. Epub 2007 Oct 10.

Fallon BA, Keilp J, Prohovnik I, Heertum RV, Mann JJ. Regional cerebral blood flow and cognitive deficits in chronic lyme disease. J Neuropsychiatry Clin Neurosci. 2003 Summer;15(3):326-32.

Fallon BA, Kochevar JM, Gaito A, Nields JA. The underdiagnosis of neuropsychiatric Lyme disease in children and adults. Psychiatr Clin North Am. 1998 Sep;21(3):693-703, viii. Review.

Fallon BA, Levin ES, Schweitzer PJ, Hardesty D. Inflammation and central nervous system Lyme disease. Neurobiol Dis. 2010 Mar;37(3):534-41. Epub 2009 Nov 26. Review.

Fallon BA, Lipkin RB, Corbera KM, Yu S, Nobler MS, Keilp JG, Petkova E, Lisanby SH, Moeller JR, Slavov I, Van Heertum R, Mensh BD, Sackeim HA. Regional cerebral blood flow and metabolic rate in persistent Lyme encephalopathy. Arch Gen Psychiatry. 2009 May;66(5):554-63.

Fallon BA, Nields JA. Lyme disease: a neuropsychiatric illness. Am J Psychiatry. 1994 Nov;151(11):1571-83. Review.

Fallon BA, Nields JA. Acute disseminated encephalomyelitis. J Neuropsychiatry Clin Neurosci. 1998 Summer;10(3):366-7.

Fallon BA, Nields JA, Burrascano JJ, Liegner K, DelBene D, Liebowitz MR. The neuropsychiatric manifestations of Lyme borreliosis. Psychiatr Q. 1992 Spring;63(1):95-117. Review.

Fallon BA, Nields JA, Parsons B, Liebowitz MR, Klein DF. Psychiatric manifestations of Lyme borreliosis. J Clin Psychiatry. 1993 Jul;54(7):263-8.

Fallon BA, Schwartzberg M, Bransfield R, Zimmerman B, Scotti A, Weber CA, Liebowitz MR. Late-stage neuropsychiatric Lyme borreliosis. Differential diagnosis and treatment. Psychosomatics. 1995 May-Jun;36(3):295-300.

Fallon BA, Tager F, Keilp J, Weiss N, Liebowitz MR, Fein L, Liegner K. Repeated antibiotic treatment in chronic Lyme disease. J Spirochetal Tick Dis. 1999;6:94-101.

Fallon J, Bujak DI, Guardino S, Weinstein A. The Fibromyalgia Impact Questionnaire: a useful tool in evaluating patients with post-Lyme disease syndrome. Arthritis Care Res. 1999 Feb;12(1):42-7.

Family-Pigné D, Mouchet B, Lousteau V, Borie MF, Deforges L, Lesprit P, Godeau B. [Hepatosplenic localization of cat scratch disease: two cases in immunocompetent adult patients].[Article in French]. Rev Med Interne. 2006 Oct;27(10):772-5. Epub 2006 Jul 7.

Fantham HB, Cantab MA. Spirochaetes and their granule phase. Br Med J. 1916 Mar 18;1(2881):409-11

Fardet L, Revuz J. [Synthetic antimalarials]. [Article in French]. Ann Dermatol Venereol. 2005 Aug-Sep;132(8-9 Pt 1):665-74.

Faul JL, Ruoss S, Doyle RL, Kao PN. Diaphragmatic paralysis due to Lyme disease. Eur Respir J, 13(3):700-2. 1999.

Faulde M, Hoffmann G. Vorkommen und Verhutung vertorassoziierter Erkrankungen des Menschen in Deutschland unter Berucksichtigung zoonotischer Aspekte. Bundesgesundheitsbl. – Gesundheitsforsch. – Gesundheitsschutz. 2001;44:116-136.

Feder HM Jr, Gerber MA, Krause PJ, Ryan R, Shapiro ED. Early Lyme disease: a flu-like illness without erythema migrans. Pediatrics. 1993 Feb;91(2):456-9. Review.

Feder HM Jr, Gerber MA, Luger SW, Ryan RW. Persistence of serum antibodies to Borrelia burgdorferi in patients treated for Lyme disease. Clin Infect Dis. 1992 Nov;15(5):788-93.

Feder HM Jr, Johnson BJ, O'Connell S, Shapiro ED, Steere AC, Wormser GP; Ad Hoc International Lyme Disease Group, Agger WA, Artsob H, Auwaerter P, Dumler JS, Bakken JS, Bockenstedt LK, Green J, Dattwyler RJ, Munoz J, Nadelman RB, Schwartz I, Draper T, McSweegan E, Halperin JJ, Klempner MS, Krause PJ, Mead P, Morshed M, Porwancher R, Radolf JD, Smith RP Jr, Sood S, Weinstein A, Wong SJ, Zemel L. A critical appraisal of "chronic Lyme disease". N Engl J Med. 2007 Oct 4;357(14):1422-30. Review

Feder HM Jr, Zalneraitis EL, Reik L Jr. Lyme disease: Acute focal meningoencephalitis in a child. Pediatrics. 1988. Dec;82(6):931-4.

Feng HM, Walker DH. Mechanisms of Immunity to Ehrlichia muris: a Model of Monocytotropic Ehrlichiosis. Infect Immun. 2004 Feb;72(2): 966-71.

Feng S, Kasten RW, Werner JA, Hodzic E, Barthold SW, Chomel BB. Immunogenicity of Bartonella henselae P26 in cats. Vet Immunol Immunopathol. 2009 Dec 15;132(2-4):251-6. Epub 2009 May 18.

Fenimore A, Varanat M, Maggi R, Schultheiss P, Breitschwerdt E, Lappin MR. Bartonella spp. DNA in cardiac tissues from dogs in Colorado and Wyoming. J Vet Intern Med. 2011 May-Jun;25(3):613-6.

Fenollar F, Lepidi H, Raoult D. Whipple's endocarditis: review of the literature and comparisons with Q fever, Bartonella infection, and blood culture-positive endocarditis. Clin Infect Dis. 2001 Oct 15;33(8):1309-16. Epub 2001 Sep 14. Review.

Fenollar F, Raoult D. Diagnosis of rickettsial diseases using samples dried on blotting paper. Clin Diagn Lab Immunol. 1999 Jul;6(4):483-8.

Fenollar F, Raoult D. Molecular genetic methods for the diagnosis of fastidious microorganisms. APMIS. 2004 Nov-Dec;112(11-12):785-807. Review.

Fenollar F, Sire S, Raoult D. Bartonella vinsonii subsp. arupensis as an agent of blood culture-negative endocarditis in a human. J Clin Microbiol. 2005 Feb;43(2):945-7. Erratum in: J Clin Microbiol. 2005 Sep;43(9):4923. Wilhelm, Nathalie [removed].

Fernández-González E, de Paz HD, Alperi A, Agúndez L, Faustmann M, Sangari FJ, Dehio C, Llosa M. Transfer of R388 derivatives by a pathogenesis-associated type IV secretion system into both bacteria and human cells. J Bacteriol. 2011 Sep 9. [Epub ahead of print]

Fernández-López R, Garcillán-Barcia MP, Revilla C, Lázaro M, Vielva L, de la Cruz F. Dynamics of the IncW genetic backbone imply general trends in conjugative plasmid evolution. FEMS Microbiol Rev. 2006 Nov;30(6):942-66. Epub 2006 Oct 6. Review.

Ferraro V, Mantoux F, Denis K, Lay-Macagno MA, Ortonne JP, Lacour JP. [Hallucinations during treatment with hydrochloroquine]. Ann Dermatol Venereol. 2004 May;131(5):471-3. [Article in French].

Ferreira JFS, Janick J. Distribution of artemisinin in Artemisia annua. In: Progress in new crops. Ed. J. Janick. Arlington, VA: ASHS Press. 1996; pp.579-584.

Ferrés G M, Abarca V K, Prado D P, Montecinos P L, Navarrete C M, Vial C PA. [Prevalence of Bartonella henselae antibodies in Chilean children, adolescents and veterinary workers].[Article in Spanish]. Rev Med Chil. 2006 Jul;134(7):863-7. Epub 2006 Aug 29.

Ferrés M, Abarca K, Godoy P, García P, Palavecino E, Méndez G, Valdés A, Ernst S, Thibaut J, Koberg J, Chanqueo L, Vial PA. [Presence of Bartonella henselae in cats: natural reservoir quantification and human exposition risk of this zoonoses in Chile].[Article in Spanish]. Rev Med Chil. 2005 Dec;133(12):1465-71. Epub 2006 Jan 27.

Ferris i TortajadaJ, Lopez-Andreu JA, Salcede-Vivo J, Sala-Lizarraga JA. Lyme borreliosis. [Letter]. 1995. Lancet. 1995 Jun 3;345(8962):1436-7.

Fikrig, E Narasimhan, S. Neelakanta, G, Pal U, Chen M, Flavell, R. Toll-Like Receptors 1 and 2 Heterodimers Alter Borrelia burgdorferi Gene Expression in Mice and Ticks. J Infect Dis. 2009 October 15; 200(8): 1331–1340.

Filgueira L, Beermann C, Groscurth P. Liposome-like vesicles from Borrelia burgdorferi modulate the function of human dendritic cells. J Invest Dermatol. 2000 ;114(1):23.

Final Diagnosis—Babesiosis. [cited 2006 Jul 3]. Available from: http://path.upmc.edu/cases/case332/dx. html.

Fisher W. Images in emergency medicine. Bartonella henselae lymphadenitis. Ann Emerg Med. 2007 Jul;50(1):90, 97.

Fishwick L, McLean WG, Edwards G, Ward SA. The toxicity of artemisinin and related compounds on neuronal and glial cells in culture. Chem. Biol. Interact. 1995 Jun 14;96(3):263-71.

Fishwick L, Edwards G, Ward SA, McLean WG. Binding of dihydroartemisinin to differentiating neuroblastoma cells and rat cortical homogenate. Neurotoxicology. 1998 Jun;19(3):405-12.

Fishwick L, Edwards G, Ward SA, McLean WG. Morphological and immunocytochemical effects of dihydroartemisinin on differentiating NB2a neuroblastoma cells. Neurotoxicology. 1998 Jun;19(3);393-403.

Fister RD, Weymouth LA, McLaughlin JC, et al. Comparative evaluation of three products for the detection of Borrelia burgdorferi antibody in human serum. J Clin Microbiol. 1989 Dec;27(12):2834-7.

Flach AJ, Lavoie PE. Episcleritis, conjunctivitis, and keratitis as ocular manifestations of Lyme disease. Ophthalmology. 1990 Aug;97(8):973-5.

Flodr P. [What is your diagnosis? 1. Lymphadenopathy in sarcoidosis. 2. Toxoplasmic lymphadenitis (Piringer-Kuchinkov). 3. Reactive (paraneoplastic) granulomatous lymphadenopathy. 4. Granulomatous cat-scratch lymphadenitis].[Article in Czech]. Cesk Patol. 2011 Jul;47(3):122-4.

Florescu D, Sordillo PP, Glyptis A, Zlatanic E, Smith B, Polsky B, Sordillo E. Splenic infarction in human babesiosis: two cases and discussion. Clin Infect Dis. 2008 Jan 1;46(1):e8-11.

Florin TA, Zaoutis TE, Zaoutis LB. Beyond cat scratch disease: widening spectrum of Bartonella henselae infection. Pediatrics. 2008 May;121(5):e1413-25. Epub 2008 Apr 28. Review.

Florin-Christensen M, Schnittger L. Piroplasmids and ticks: a long-lasting intimate relationship. Front Biosci. 2009 Jan 1;14:3064-73. Review.

Focus Technologies. Bartonella Antibody Panel, IFA (Serum). Code 4020. And Bartonella DNA, PCR. Code 47000. http://www.focusdx.com/focus/1-reference_laboratory/search_frame.asp?f=2. Accessed September 6, 2007.

Foley JE, Nieto NC. The ecology of tick-transmitted infections in the redwood chipmunk (Tamias ochrogenys). Ticks Tick Borne Dis. 2011 Jun;2(2):88-93.

Fomenko NV, Borgoiakov VIu, Panov VV. [Genetic features of Borrelia miyamotoi transmitted by Ixodes persulcatus].[Article in Russian]. Mol Gen Mikrobiol Virusol. 2011;(2):12-7.

Fomenko NV, Livanova NN, Borgoiakov VIu, Kozlova IV, Shulaikina IV, Pukhovskaia NM, Tokarevich KN, Livanov SG, Doroshchenko EK, Ivanov LI. [Detection of Borrelia miyamotoi in ticks Ixodes persulcatus from Russia]. [Article in Russian]. Parazitologiia. 2010 May-Jun;44(3):201-11.

Fonollosa A, Galdos M, Artaraz J, Perez-Irezabal J, Martinez-Alday N. Occlusive vasculitis and optic disk neovascularization associated with neuroretinitis. Ocul Immunol Inflamm. 2011 Feb;19(1):62-4. Epub 2010 Oct 31.

Font RL, Del Valle M, Mitchell BM, Boniuk M. Cat-scratch uveitis confirmed by histological, serological, and molecular diagnoses. Cornea. 2011 Apr;30(4):468-71.

Forbes SJ, Eschmann M, Mantis NJ. Inhibition of Salmonella enterica Serovar Typhimurium Motility and Entry into Epithelial Cells by a Protective Antilipopolysaccharide Monoclonal Immunoglobulin A Antibody. Infect Immun. 2008 Sep; 76(9):4137-44. Published online 2008 July 14.

Fouch B, Coventry S. A case of fatal disseminated Bartonella henselae infection (cat-scratch disease) with encephalitis. Arch Pathol Lab Med. 2007 Oct;131(10):1591-4.

Foucault C, Barrau K, Brouqui P, Raoult D. Bartonella quintana Bacteremia among Homeless People. Clin Infect Dis. 2002 Sep 15;35(6):684-9. Epub 2002 Aug 20.

Foucault C, Brouqui P, Raoult D. Bartonella quintana characteristics and clinical management. Emerg Infect Dis. 2006 Feb;12(2):217-23. Review.

Foucault C, La Scola B, Lindroos H, Andersson SG, Raoult D. Multispacer typing technique for sequence-based typing of Bartonella quintana. J Clin Microbiol. 2005 Jan;43(1):41-8.

Foucault C, Raoult D, Brouqui P. Randomized open trial of gentamicin and doxycycline for eradication of Bartonella quintana from blood in patients with chronic bacteremia. Antimicrob Agents Chemother. 2003 Jul;47(7):2204-7.

Foucault C, Rolain JM, Raoult D, Brouqui P. Detection of Bartonella quintana by direct immunofluorescence examination of blood smears of a patient with acute trench fever. J Clin Microbiol. 2004 Oct;42(10):4904-6.

Fouch B, Coventry S. A case of fatal disseminated Bartonella henselae infection (cat-scratch disease) with encephalitis. Arch Pathol Lab Med. 2007 Oct;131(10):1591-4.

Fournier PE, Couderc C, Buffet S, Flaudrops C, Raoult D. Rapid and cost-effective identification of Bartonella species using mass spectrometry. J Med Microbiol. 2009 Sep;58(Pt 9):1154-9. Epub 2009 Jun 15.

Fournier PE, Lelievre H, Eykyn SJ, Mainardi JL, Marrie TJ, Bruneel F, Roure C, Nash J, Clave D, James E, Benoit-Lemercier C, Deforges L, Tissot-Dupont H, Raoult D. Epidemiologic and clinical characteristics of Bartonella quintana and Bartonella henselae endocarditis: a study of 48 patients. Medicine (Baltimore). 2001 Jul;80(4):245-51.

Fournier PE, Mainardi JL, Raoult D. Value of microimmuno-fluorescence for diagnosis and follow-up of Bartonella endocarditis. Clin Diagn Lab Immunol. 2002 Jul;9(4):795-801.

Fournier PE, Minnick MF, Lepidi H, Salvo E, Raoult D. Experimental model of human body louse infection using green fluorescent protein-expressing Bartonella quintana. Infect Immun. 2001 Mar;69(3):1876-9.

Fournier PE, Ndihokubwayo JB, Guidran J, Kelly PJ, Raoult D. Human pathogens in body and head lice. Emerg Infect Dis. 2002 Dec;8(12):1515-8. Review.

Fournier PE, Robson J, Zeaiter Z, McDougall R, Byrne S, Raoult D. Improved culture from lymph nodes of patients with cat scratch disease and genotypic characterization of Bartonella henselae isolates in Australia. J Clin Microbiol. 2002 Oct;40(10):3620-4.

Fournier PE, Taylor C, Rolain JM, Barrassi L, Smith G, Raoult D. Bartonella australis sp. nov. from kangaroos, Australia. Emerg Infect Dis. 2007 Dec;13(12):1961-2.

Fournier PE, Thuny F, Richet H, Lepidi H, Casalta JP, Arzouni JP, Maurin M, Célard M, Mainardi JL, Caus T, Collart F, Habib G, Raoult D. Comprehensive diagnostic strategy for blood culture-negative endocarditis: a prospective study of 819 new cases. Clin Infect Dis. 2010 Jul 15;51(2):131-40.

Fox JW, Studley JK, Cohen DM. Recurrent expressive aphasia as a presentation of cat-scratch encephalopathy. Pediatrics. 2007 Mar;119(3):e760-3.

Fox LM, Wingerter S, Ahmed A, Arnold A, Chou J, Rhein L, Levy O. Neonatal babesiosis: case report and review of the literature. Pediatr Infect Dis J. 2006 Feb;25(2):169-73.

Fraenkel CJ, Garpmo U, Berglund J. Determination of novel Borrelia genospecies in Swedish Ixodes ricinus ticks. J Clin Microbiol. 2002 Sep;40(9):3308-12.

Franke J, Hildebrandt A, Meier F, Straube E, Dorn W. Prevalence of Lyme disease agents and several emerging pathogens in questing ticks from the German Baltic coast. J Med Entomol. 2011 Mar;48(2):441-4.

Franke J, Meier F, Moldenhauer A, Straube E, Dorn W, Hildebrandt A. Established and emerging pathogens in Ixodes ricinus ticks collected from birds on a conservation island in the Baltic Sea. Med Vet Entomol. 2010 Dec;24(4):425-32. Epub 2010 Sep 26.

Franz B, Kempf VA. Adhesion and host cell modulation: critical pathogenicity determinants of Bartonella henselae. Parasit Vectors. 2011 Apr 13;4:54. Published online 2011 April 13.

Freddi G, Romàn-Pumar JL. Evidence-based medicine: what it can and cannot do. Ann Ist Super Sanita. 2011;47(1):22-5. Review.

Fredrikson S, Link H. CNS-borreliosis selectively affecting central motor neurons. Acta Neurol Scand. 1988 Sep;78(3):181-4.

Frey M, Jaulhac B, Sibilia J, Monteil H, Kuntz JL, Vautravers P. [Detection of Borrelia burgdorferi DNA by gene amplification in the muscle of a patient with fibromyalgia].[Article in French]. Presse Med. 1995 Nov 11;24(34):1623.

Frey M, Jaulhac B, Piemont Y, Marcellin L, Boohs PM, Vautravers P, Jesel M, Kuntz JL, Monteil H, Sibilia J. Detection of Borrelia burgdorferi DNA in muscle of patients with chronic myalgia related to Lyme disease. Am J Med. 1998 Jun;104(6):591-4.

Froberg MK, Dannen D, Bernier N, Shieh WJ, Guarner J, Zaki S. Case report: spontaneous splenic rupture during acute parasitemia of Babesia microti. Ann Clin Lab Sci. 2008 Autumn;38(4):390-2.

Fried L, Arbiser JL. Application of Angiogenesis to Clinical Dermatology. Adv Dermatol. 2008; 24: 89–103.

Fryland L, Wilhelmsson P, Lindgren PE, Nyman D, Ekerfelt C, Forsberg P. Low risk of developing Borrelia burgdorferi infection in the south-east of Sweden after being bitten by a Borrelia burgdorferi-infected tick. Int J Infect Dis. 2011 Mar;15(3):e174-81. Epub 2010 Dec 17.

Fu J, Muttaiyah S, Pandey S, Thomas M. Two cases of endocarditis due to Bartonella henselae. N Z Med J. 2007 Jun 1;120(1255):U2558.

Füessl HS. [From tick bite to borreliosis: the dreaded small blood sucker].[Article in German]. MMW Fortschr Med. 2011 Jun 2;153(22):14-7.

Fujisawa K, Nakajima R, Jinnai M, Hirata H, Zamoto-Niikura A, Kawabuchi-Kurata T, Arai S, Ishihara C. Intron Sequences from the CCT7 Gene Exhibit Diverse Evolutionary Histories among the Four Lineages within the Babesia microti-Group, a Genetically Related Species Complex That Includes Human Pathogens. Jpn J Infect Dis. 2011 Sep;64(5):403-10.

Fukunaga M, Hamase A, Okada K, Inoue H, Tsuruta Y, Miyamoto K, Nakao M. Characterization of spirochetes isolated from ticks (Ixodes tanuki, Ixodes turdus, and Ixodes columnae) and comparison of the sequences with those of Borrelia burgdorferi sensu lato strains. Appl Environ Microbiol. 1996 Jul;62(7):2338-44.

Fukunaga M, Koreki Y. The flagellin gene of Borrelia miyamotoi sp. nov. and its phylogenetic relationship among Borrelia species. FEMS Microbiol Lett. 1995 Dec 15;134(2-3):255-8.

Fukunaga M, Okada K, Nakao M, Konishi T, Sato Y. Phylogenetic analysis of Borrelia species based on flagellin gene sequences and its application for molecular typing of Lyme disease borreliae. Int J Syst Bacteriol. 1996 Oct;46(4):898-905.

Fukunaga M, Sohnaka M, Nakao M, Miyamoto K. Evaluation of genetic divergence of borrelial isolates from Lyme disease patients in Hokkaido, Japan, by rRNA gene probes. J Clin Microbiol. 1993 Aug;31(8):2044-8.

Fukunaga M, Sohnaka M, Takahashi Y, Nakao M, Miyamoto K. Antigenic and genetic characterization of Borrelia species isolated from Ixodes persulcatus in Hokkaido, Japan. J Clin Microbiol. 1993 May;31(5):1388-91.

Fukunaga M, Takahashi Y, Tsuruta Y, Matsushita O, Ralph D, McClelland M, Nakao M. Genetic and phenotypic analysis of Borrelia miyamotoi sp. nov., isolated from the ixodid tick Ixodes persulcatus, the vector for Lyme disease in Japan. Int J Syst Bacteriol. 1995 Oct;45(4):804-10.

Fung BP, McHugh GL, Leong JM, Steere AC. Humoral immune response to outer surface protein C of Borrelia burgdorferi in Lyme disease: role of the immunoglobulin M response in the serodiagnosis of early infection. Infect Immun. 1994 Aug;62(8):3213-21.

Gabriel MW, Henn J, Foley JE, Brown RN, Kasten RW, Foley P, Chomel BB. Zoonotic Bartonella species in fleas collected on gray foxes (Urocyon cinereoargenteus). Vector Borne Zoonotic Dis. 2009 Dec;9(6):597-602.

Gajović O, Todorović Z, Nesić L, Lazić Z. [Lyme borreliosis-- diagnostic difficulties in interpreting serological results].[Article in Serbian]. Med Pregl. 2010 Nov-Dec;63(11-12):839-43. Review.

Galal AM, Ross SA, ElSohly MA, ElSohly HN, El-Feraly FS, Ahmed MS, McPhail AT. Deoxyartemisinin derivatives from photooxygenation of anhydrodeoxydihydroartemisinin and their cytotoxic evaluation. J Nat Prod. 2002 Feb;65(2):184-8.

Galiukov IA, Vasilenko FI, Lapidus MS, Anochin AS. [Early recurrence of neuroborreliosis with a fatal outcome].[Article in Russian]. Arkh Patol. 2010 Mar-Apr;72(2):36-7.

Gallagher LG, Chau S, Owaisi AS, Konczyk M, Bishop HS, Arguin PM, Trenholme GM. An 84-year-old woman with fever and dark urine. Clin Infect Dis. 2009 Jul 15;49(2):278, 310-1.

Gan JJ, Mandell AM, Otis JA, Holmuhamedova M, Perloff MD. Suspecting optic neuritis, diagnosing Bartonella cat scratch disease. Arch Neurol. 2011 Jan;68(1):122-6.

Gandhi G, Londoño D, Whetstine CR, Sethi N, Kim KS, Zückert WR, Cadavid D. Interaction of Variable Bacterial Outer Membrane Lipoproteins with Brain Endothelium. PLoS One. 2010 Oct 22;5(10):e13257. Published online 2010 October 22.

García FM. [About limitations (and subterfuges) of evidence based medicine].[Article in Spanish]. Med Clin (Barc). 2003 Feb 15;120(5):197; author reply 197-8.

García-Esteban C, Gil H, Rodríguez-Vargas M, Gerrikagoitia X, Barandika J, Escudero R, Jado I, García-Amil C, Barral M, García-Pérez AL, Bhide M, Anda P. Molecular method for Bartonella species identification in clinical and environmental samples. J Clin Microbiol. 2008 Feb;46(2):776-9. Epub 2007 Dec 19.

García-García JA, Baquerizo R, Vargas J, Mira JA, Merchante N, Macías J, Pineda JA. [Prevalence of serum antibodies against Bartonella ssp. in a health population from the south area of the Seville province].[Article in Spanish]. Rev Clin Esp. 2005 Nov;205(11):541-4.

Garcia-Monco JC, Gomez-Beldarrain M, Benach JL, Anda P, Alvarez J, Ojanguren J. Borrelia meningitis mimicking meningeal lymphoma. Neurology. 1994 Nov;44(11):2207.

García Moncó JC, Wheeler CM, Benach JL, Furie RA, Lukehart SA, Stanek G, Steere AC. Reactivity of neuroborreliosis patients (Lyme disease) to cardiolipin and gangliosides. J Neurol Sci. 1993 Jul;117(1-2):206-14.

García Puga JM, Ramos Ramos MV, Muwaqued Rodríguez F, Santos Pérez JL, Vega Pérez S. [Submandibular tumor].[Article in Spanish]. An Pediatr (Barc). 2006 May;64(5):503-4.

Gardner T. Lyme disease. In Infectious Diseases of the Fetus and Newborn Infant, Ed. JS Remington, JO Klein.Philadelphia:W.B. Saunders Company. 2001. pp. 519-641.

Garré L, Guaraglia W, Cuatz D, Kaufman S, Gil H, De Rosa AF. [Infective endocarditis due to Bartonella quintana].[Article in Spanish]. Medicina (B Aires). 2008;68(2):144-6. Erratum in: Medicina (B Aires). 2008;68(3):267.

Gary AT, Webb JA, Hegarty BC, Breitschwerdt EB. The low seroprevalence of tick-transmitted agents of disease in dogs from southern Ontario and Quebec. Can Vet J. 2006 Dec;47(12):1194-200.

Gaskin AA, Schantz P, Jackson J, Birkenheuer A, Tomlinson L, Gramiccia M, Levy M, Steurer F, Kollmar E, Hegarty BC, Ahn A, Breitschwerdt EB. Visceral leishmaniasis in a New York foxhound kennel. J Vet Intern Med. 2002 Jan-Feb;16(1):34-44.

Gasquet S, Maurin M, Brouqui P, Lepidi H, Raoult D. Bacillary angiomatosis in immunocompromised patients. AIDS. 1998 Oct 1;12(14):1793-803. Review.

Gasser R, Watzinger N, Eber B, Luha O, Reisinger E, Seinost G, Klein W. Coronary artery aneurysm in two patients with long-standing Lyme borreliosis. Lancet.1994 Nov 5;344(8932):1300-1.

Gasser R, Horn S, Reisinger E, Fischer L, Pokan R, Wendelin I, Klein W. First description of recurrent pericardial effusion associated with borrelia burgdorferi infection. Int J Cardiol. 1998 May 15;64(3):309-10.

Gassner F, van Vliet AJ, Burgers SL, Jacobs F, Verbaarschot P, Hovius EK, Mulder S, Verhulst NO, van Overbeek LS, Takken W. Geographic and temporal variations in population dynamics of Ixodes ricinus and associated Borrelia infections in The Netherlands. Vector Borne Zoonotic Dis. 2011 May;11(5):523-32. Epub 2010 Nov 17.

Gautam A, Dixit S, Philipp MT, Singh SR, Morici LA, Kaushal D, Dennis VA. Interleukin-10 Alters Effector Functions of Multiple Genes Induced by Borrelia burgdorferi in Macrophages to Regulate Lyme Disease Inflammation. Infect Immun. 2011 Sep 26. [Epub ahead of print]

Gebbers JO, Marder HP. Unusual in vitro formation of cyst-like structures associated with human intestinal spirochaetosis. Eur J Clin Microbiol Infect Dis. 1989 Apr;8(4):302-6.

Gellis SE, Stadecker MJ, Steere AC. Spirochetes in atrophic skin lesions accompanied by minimal host response in a child with Lyme disease. J Am Acad Dermatol. 1991 Aug;25(2 Pt 2):395-7.

Genchi C. Human babesiosis, an emerging zoonosis. Parassitologia. 2007 May;49 Suppl 1:29-31. Review.

Geng Z, Hou XX, Wan KL, Hao Q. [Isolation and identification of Borrelia burgdorferi sensu lato from ticks in six provinces in China].[Article in Chinese]. Zhonghua Liu Xing Bing Xue Za Zhi. 2010 Dec;31(12):1346-1348.

Genizi J, Kasis I, Schif A, Shahar E. Effect of high-dose methyl-prednisolone on brainstem encephalopathy and basal ganglia impairment complicating cat scratch disease. Brain Dev. 2007 Jul;29(6):377-9. Epub 2006 Dec 15.

George JG, Bradley JC, Kimbrough RC 3rd, Shami MJ. Bartonella quintana associated neuroretinitis. Scand J Infect Dis. 2006;38(2):127-8.

George TI, Manley G, Koehler JE, Hung VS, McDermott M, Bollen A. Detection of Bartonella henselae by polymerase chain reaction in brain tissue of an immunocompromised patient with multiple enhancing lesions. Case report and review of the literature. J Neurosurg. 1998 Oct;89(4):640-4. Review.

Georgilis K, Peacocke M, Klempner MS. Fibroblasts protect the Lyme disease spirochete, Borrelia burgdorferi, from ceftriaxone in vitro. J Infect Dis 1992. Aug;166(2):440-4.

Georgilis K, Steere AC, Klempner MS. Infectivity of Borrelia burgdorferi correlates with resistance to elimination by phagocytic cells. J Infect Dis. 1991 Jan;163(1):150-5.

Georgilis K, Noring R, Steere AC, Klempner MS. Neutrophil chemotactic factors in synovial fluids of patients with Lyme disease. Arthritis Rheum. 1991 Jun;34(6):770-5.

Gerber JE, Johnson JE, Scott MA, Madhusudhan KT. Fatal meningitis and encephalitis due to Bartonella henselae bacteria. J Forensic Sci. 2002 May;47(3):640-644.

Gerber MA, Shapiro ED. Diagnosis of Lyme disease in children. J Pediatr. 1992 Jul;121(1):157-62. Review.

Gerber MA, Shapiro ED, Bell GL, Sampieri A, Padula SJ. Recombinant outer surface protein C ELISA for the diagnosis of early Lyme disease. J Infect Dis. 1995 Mar;171(3):724-7.

Gerber MA, Shapiro ED, Burke GS, Parcells VJ, Bell GL. Lyme disease in children in southeastern Connecticut. Pediatric Lyme Disease Study Group. N Engl J Med. 1996 Oct 24;335(17):1270-4.

Gerber MA, Shapiro ED, Krause PJ, Cable RG, Badon SJ, Ryan RW. The risk of acquiring Lyme disease or babesiosis from a blood transfusion. J Infect Dis. 1994 Jul;170(1):231-4.

Gerber MA, Zemel LS, Shapiro ED. Lyme arthritis in children: clinical epidemiology and long-term outcomes. Pediatrics. 1998 Oct;102(4 Pt 1):905-8.

Gern L, Lienhard R, Péter O. [Diseases and pathogenic agents transmitted by ticks in Switzerland].[Article in French]. Rev Med Suisse. 2010 Oct 13;6(266):1906-9.

Gescher DM, Mallmann C, Kovacevic D, Schmiedel D, Borges AC, Schweickert B, Göbel UB, Moter A. A view on Bartonella quintana endocarditis--confirming the molecular diagnosis by specific fluorescence in situ hybridization. Diagn Microbiol Infect Dis. 2008 Jan;60(1):99-103. Epub 2007 Sep 21.

Ghosh S, Steere AC, Stollar BD, Huber BT. In situ diversification of the antibody repertoire in chronic Lyme arthritis synovium. J Immunol. 2005 Mar 1;174(5):2860-9.

Gigandet L, Stauffer E, Douet V, Rais O, Moret J, Gern L. Prevalence of three zoonotic Babesia species in Ixodes ricinus (Linné, 1758) nymphs in a suburban forest in Switzerland. Vector Borne Zoonotic Dis. 2011 Apr;11(4):363-6. Epub 2011 Mar 11.

Gil H, García-Esteban C, Barandika JF, Peig J, Toledo A, Escudero R, Jado I, Rodríguez-Vargas M, García-Amil C, Lobo B, Roales P, Rodríguez-Moreno I, Olmeda AS, García-Pérez AL, Anda P. Variability of Bartonella genotypes among small mammals in Spain. Appl Environ Microbiol. 2010 Dec;76(24):8062-70. Epub 2010 Oct 8.

Gillaspie D, Perkins I, Larsen K, McCord A, Pangonis S, Sweger D, Seleem MN, Sriranganathan N, Anderson BE. Plasmid-based system for high-level gene expression and antisense gene knockdown in Bartonella henselae. Appl Environ Microbiol. 2009 Aug;75(16):5434-6. Epub 2009 Jun 19.

Gillespie TN, Washabau RJ, Goldschmidt MH, Cullen JM, Rogala AR, Breitschwerdt EB. Detection of Bartonella henselae and Bartonella clarridgeiae DNA in hepatic specimens from two dogs with hepatic disease. J Am Vet Med Assoc. 2003 Jan 1;222(1):47-51, 35.

Ginsberg HS. Potential effects of mixed infections in ticks on transmission dynamics of pathogens: comparative analysis of published records. Exp Appl Acarol. 2008 Dec;46(1-4):29-41. Epub 2008 Jul 22.

Girard YA, Fedorova N, Lane RS. Genetic diversity of Borrelia burgdorferi and detection of B. bissettii-like DNA in serum of north-coastal California residents. J Clin Microbiol. 2011 Mar;49(3):945-54. Epub 2010 Dec 22.

Glauser TA, Brennan PJ, Galetta SL. Reversible Horner's syndrome and Lyme disease. J Clin Neuroophthalmol. 1989 Dec;9(4):225-8.

Gleich GJ, Leiferman KM, Pardanani A, Tefferi A, Butterfield JH. Treatment of hypereosinophilic syndrome with imatinib mesilate. Lancet. 2002 May 4;359(9317):1577-8.

Glickstein L, Moore B, Bledsoe T, Damle N, Sikand V, Steere AC. Inflammatory cytokine production predominates in early Lyme disease in patients with erythema migrans. Infect Immun. 2003 Oct;71(10):6051-3.

Goddard J, Varela-Stokes AS. Role of the lone star tick, Amblyomma americanum (L.), in human and animal diseases. Vet Parasitol. 2009 Mar 9;160(1-2):1-12. Epub 2008 Oct 28. Review.

Goellner MH, Agger WA, Burgess JH, Duray PH. Hepatitis due to recurrent Lyme disease. Ann Intern Med. 1988 May;108(5):707-8.

Góes TS, Góes VS, Ribeiro MF, Gontijo CM. Bovine babesiosis: anti-erythrocyte antibodies purification from the sera of naturally infected cattle. Vet Immunol Immunopathol. 2007 Apr 15;116(3-4):215-8. Epub 2007 Jan 16.

Gohil S, Kats LM, Sturm A, Cooke BM. Recent insights into alteration of red blood cells by Babesia bovis: moovin' forward. Trends Parasitol. 2010 Dec;26(12):591-9. Epub 2010 Jul 2. Review.

Goldberg NS, Forseter G, Nadelman RB, Schwartz I, Jorde U, McKenna D, Holmgren D, Bittker S, Montecalvo M, Wormser GP. Vesicular erythema migrans. Arch Dermatol. 1992 Nov;128(11):1495-8.

Gomes-Solecki MJ, Wormser GP, Dattwyler RJ. IFNgamma production in peripheral blood of early Lyme disease patients to hLFAalphaL (aa326-345). BMC Musculoskelet Disord. 2002 Oct 17;3:25.

Gomes-Solecki MJ, Wormser GP, Persing DH, Berger BW, Glass JD, Yang X, Dattwyler RJ. A first-tier rapid assay for the serodiagnosis of Borrelia burgdorferi infection. Arch Intern Med. 2001 Sep 10;161(16):2015-20.

Gomes-Solecki MJ, Wormser GP, Schriefer M, Neuman G, Hannafey L, Glass JD, Dattwyler RJ. Recombinant assay for serodiagnosis of Lyme disease regardless of OspA vaccination status. J Clin Microbiol. 2002 Jan;40(1):193-7.

Goo YK, Terkawi MA, Jia H, Aboge GO, Ooka H, Nelson B, Kim S, Sunaga F, Namikawa K, Igarashi I, Nishikawa Y, Xuan X. Artesunate, a potential drug for treatment of Babesia infection. Parasitol Int. 2010 Sep;59(3):481-6. Epub 2010 Jun 9.

Goodlad JR, Davidson MM, Hollowood K, Ling C, MacKenzie C, Christie I, Batstone PJ, Ho-Yen DO. Primary cutaneous B-cell lymphoma and Borrelia burgdorferi infection in patients from the Highlands of Scotland. Am J Surg Pathol. 2000 Sep;24(9):1279-85.

Goodman RA, Breitschwerdt EB. Clinicopathologic findings in dogs seroreactive to Bartonella henselae antigens. Am J Vet Res. 2005 Dec;66(12):2060-4.

Goossens HA, Maes JH, van den Bogaard AE. The prevalence of antibodies against B. burgdorferi, an indicator for Lyme borreliosis in dogs? A comparison of serological tests. Tijdschr Diergeneeskd. 2003 Nov 1;128(21):650-7.

Goossens HA, Nohlmans MK, van den Bogaard AE. Epstein-Barr virus and cytomegalovirus infections cause false-positive results in IgM two-test protocol for early Lyme borreliosis. Infection. 1999 May-Jun;27(3):231.

Goossens HA, van den Bogaard AE, Nohlmans MK. Evaluation of fifteen commercially available serological tests for diagnosis of Lyme borreliosis. Eur J Clin Microbiol Infect Dis. 1999 Aug;18(8):551-60.

Goossens HA, van den Bogaard AE, Nohlmans MK. Reduced specificity of combined IgM and IgG enzyme immunoassay testing for lyme borreliosis. Eur J Clin Microbiol Infect Dis. 2000 May;19(5):400-2.

Goossens HA, van den Bogaard AE, Nohlmans MK. Dogs as sentinels for human Lyme borreliosis in The Netherlands. J Clin Microbiol. 2001 Mar;39(3):844-8.

Goossens HA, van den Bogaard AE, Nohlmans MK. Serodiagnosis of Lyme borreliosis using detection of different immunoglobulin (sub)classes by enzyme-linked immunosorbent assay and Western blotting. Clin Lab. 2001;47(1-2):41-9.

Gordi T, Lepist EI. Toxicol Lett. 2004 Aug 1;151(3):489-90, author reply 491-2. Acta Trop. 2002 May;82(2)175-81.

Gordi T, Lepist EI. Artemisinin derivatives: toxic for laboratory animals, safe for humans? Toxicol Lett. 2004 Mar 1;147(2):99-107.

Gordi T, Xie R, Huong NV, Huong DX, Karlsson MO, Ashton M. A semiphysiological pharmacokinetic model for artemisinin in healthy subjects incorporating autoinduction of metabolism and saturable first-pass hepatic extraction. Br J Clin Pharmacol. 2005 Feb;59(2):189-98.

Goren JL, Stoll AL, Damico KE, Sarmiento IA, Cohen BM. Bioavailability and lack of toxicity of S-adenosyl-L-methionine (SAMe) in humans. Pharmacotherapy. 2004;24(11):1501-1507.

Gorenflot A, Moubri K, Precigout G, Carcy B, Schetters TP. Human babesiosis. Ann Trop Med Parisitol. Jun;92(4):489-501.

Gouriet F, Fenollar F, Patrice JY, Drancourt M, Raoult D. Use of shell-vial cell culture assay for isolation of bacteria from clinical specimens: 13 years of experience. J Clin Microbiol. 2005 Oct;43(10):4993-5002.

Gouriet F, Lepidi H, Habib G, Collart F, Raoult D. From cat scratch disease to endocarditis, the possible natural history of Bartonella henselae infection. BMC Infect Dis. 2007 Apr 18;7:30.

Gouriet F, Samson L, Delaage M, Mainardi JL, Meconi S, Drancourt M, Raoult D. Multiplexed whole bacterial antigen microarray, a new format for the automation of serodiagnosis: the culture-negative endocarditis paradigm. Clin Microbiol Infect. 2008 Dec;14(12):1112-8.

Gouveia EA, Alves MF, Mantovani E, Oyafuso LK, Bonoldi VL, Yoshinari NH. Profile of patients with Baggio-Yoshinari Syndrome admitted at "Instituto de Infectologia Emilio Ribas". Rev Inst Med Trop Sao Paulo. 2010 Dec;52(6):297-303.

Graves SF, Kobayashi SD, DeLeo FR. Community-associated methicillin-resistant Staphylococcus aureus immune evasion and virulence. J Mol Med (Berl). 2010 Feb;88(2):109-14. Published online 2010 January 5.

Gray GC, Johnson AA, Thornton SA, Smith WA, Knobloch J, Kelley PW, Obregon Escudero L, Arones Huayda M, Wignall FS. An epidemic of Oroya fever in the Peruvian Andes. Am J Trop Med Hyg. 1990 Mar;42(3):215-21.

Gray J, Zintl A, Hildebrandt A, Hunfeld KP, Weiss L. Zoonotic babesiosis: overview of the disease and novel aspects of pathogen identity. Ticks Tick Borne Dis. 2010 Mar;1(1):3-10. Epub 2009 Dec 24.

Greenberg HE, Ney G, Scharf SM, Ravdin L, Hilton E. Sleep quality in Lyme disease. Sleep. 1995 Dec;18(10):912-6.

Greenburg, S. G6PD Deficiency. [Monograph on the Internet] Available from: http://www.utoronto.ca/kids/ G6PD.htm.

Greengarten PJ, Tuininga AR, Morath SU, Falco RC, Norelus H, Daniels TJ. Occurrence of soil- and tick-borne fungi and related virulence tests for pathogenicity to Ixodes scapularis (Acari: Ixodidae). J Med Entomol. 2011 Mar;48(2):337-44.

Greer DM, Schaefer PW, Plotkin SR, Hasserjian RP, Steere AC. Case records of the Massachusetts General Hospital. Case 11-2007. A 59-year-old man with neck pain, weakness in the arms, and cranial-nerve palsies. N Engl J Med. 2007 Apr 12;356(15):1561-70.

Grellier P, Benach J, Labaied M, Charneau S, Gil H, Monsalve G, Alfonso R, Sawyer L, Lin L, Steiert M, Dupuis K. Photochemical inactivation with amotosalen and long-wavelength ultraviolet light of Plasmodium and Babesia in platelet and plasma components. Transfusion. 2008 Aug;48(8):1676-84. Epub 2008 May 22.

Greub G, Raoult D. Bartonella: new explanations for old diseases. J Med Microbiol. 2002 Nov;51(11):915-23. Review.

Grodzicki RL, Steere AC. Comparison of immunoblotting and indirect enzyme-linked immunosorbent assay using different antigen preparations for diagnosing early Lyme disease. J Infect Dis. 1988 Apr;157(4):790-7.

Gross D, Huber BT, Steere AC. Molecular mimicry and Lyme arthritis. Curr Dir Autoimmun. 2001;3:94-111. Review.

Gross DM, Forsthuber T, Tary-Lehmann M, Etling C, Ito K, Nagy ZA, Field JA, Steere AC, Huber BT. Identification of LFA-1 as a candidate autoantigen in treatment-resistant Lyme arthritis. Science. 1998 Jul 31;281(5377):703-6.

Gross DM, Steere AC, Huber BT. T helper 1 response is dominant and localized to the synovial fluid in patients with Lyme arthritis. J Immunol. 1998 Jan 15;160(2):1022-8.

Grumbkow PV, Zipp A, Seidenberg V, Fehren-Schmitz L, Kempf VA, Groß U, Hummel S. Brief communication: Evidence of Bartonella quintana infections in skeletons of a historical mass grave in Kassel, Germany. Am J Phys Anthropol. 2011 Jun 27. [Epub ahead of print]

Gruntar I, Malovrh T, Murgia R, Cinco M. Conversion of Borrelia garinii cystic forms to motile spirochetes in vivo. APMIS. 2001 May;109(5):383-8.

Gruppen LD, Rana GK, Arndt TS. A controlled comparison study of the efficacy of training medical students in evidence-based medicine literature searching skills. Acad Med. 2005. Oct;80(10):940-4.

Grzeszczuk A, Staczak J, Pogorzelska J, Prokopowicz D. [Diagnostics of human granulocytic anaplasmosis].[Article in Polish]. Wiad Parazytol. 2005;51(2):109-14. Review.

Grzeszczuk A, Ziarko S, Kovalchuk O, Staczak J. Etiology of tick-borne febrile illnesses in adult residents of North-Eastern Poland: report from a prospective clinical study. Int J Med Microbiol. 2006 May;296 Suppl 40:242-9. Epub 2006 Mar 10.

Guan G, Chauvin A, Yin H, Luo J, Moreau E. Course of infection by Babesia sp. BQ1 (Lintan) and B. divergens in sheep depends on the production of IFNgamma and IL10. Parasite Immunol. 2010 Feb;32(2):143-52.

Guay D. Update on clindamycin in the management of bacterial, fungal and protozoal infections. Expert Opin Pharmacother. 2007 Oct;8(14):2401-44. Review.

Gubernot DM, Lucey CT, Lee KC, Conley GB, Holness LG, Wise RP. Babesia infection through blood transfusions: reports received by the US Food and Drug Administration, 1997-2007. Clin Infect Dis. 2009 Jan 1;48(1):25-30.

Gubernot DM, Nakhasi HL, Mied PA, Asher DM, Epstein JS, Kumar S. Transfusion-transmitted babesiosis in the United States: summary of a workshop. Transfusion. 2009 Dec;49(12):2759-71. Epub 2009 Oct 10.

Guittet V, Ménager C, Missotte I, Duparc B, Verhaegen F, Duhamel JF. [Hepatic abscesses in childhood: retrospective study about 33 cases observed in New-Caledonia between 1985 and 2003].[Article in French]. Arch Pediatr. 2004 Sep;11(9):1046-53.

Gundi VA, Bourry O, Davous B, Raoult D, La Scola B. Bartonella clarridgeiae and B. henselae in dogs, Gabon. Emerg Infect Dis. 2004 Dec;10(12):2261-2.

Gundi VA, Davoust B, Khamis A, Boni M, Raoult D, La Scola B. Isolation of Bartonella rattimassiliensis sp. nov. and Bartonella phoceensis sp. nov. from European Rattus norvegicus. J Clin Microbiol. 2004 Aug;42(8):3816-8.

Gundi VA, Taylor C, Raoult D, La Scola B. Bartonella rattaustraliani sp. nov., Bartonella queenslandensis sp. nov. and Bartonella coopersplainsensis sp. nov., identified in Australian rats. Int J Syst Evol Microbiol. 2009 Dec;59(Pt 12):2956-61. Epub 2009 Jul 23.

Gunson TH, Oliver GF. Osler's nodes and Janeway lesions. Australas J Dermatol. 2007 Nov;48(4):251-5.

Guo BP, Teneberg S, Münch R, Terunuma D, Hatano K, Matsuoka K, Angström J, Borén T, Bergström S. Relapsing fever Borrelia binds to neolacto glycans and mediates rosetting of human erythrocytes. Proc Natl Acad Sci U S A. 2009 Nov 17;106(46):19280-5. Published online 2009 November 2.

Gupta D, Green J, Franco-Paredes C, Lerakis S. Challenges in the clinical management of blood-culture negative endocarditis: case of Bartonella henselae infection. Am J Med. 2011 Mar;124(3):e1-2.

Gupta PK, Patel R, Bhatti MT. Neuroretinitis secondary to concurrent infection with cat scratch disease and lyme disease. Eye (Lond). 2009 Jul;23(7):1607. Epub 2008 Sep 12.

Guptill L. Bartonellosis. Vet Microbiol. 2010 Jan 27;140(3-4):347-59. Epub 2009 Nov 18. Review.

Guptill L. Feline bartonellosis. Vet Clin North Am Small Anim Pract. 2010 Nov;40(6):1073-90. Review.

Guptill L, Wu CC, Glickman L, Turek J, Slater L, HogenEsch H. Extracellular Bartonella henselae and artifactual intraerythrocytic pseudoinclusions in experimentally infected cats. Vet Microbiol. 2000 Oct 1;76(3):283-290.

Gustaw K, Mirecka U. Dysarthria as the isolated clinical symptom of borreliosis--a case report. Ann Agric Environ Med. 2001;8(1):95-7.

Gutierrez MA, de Pablos C, Oterino A, Garcia Monco JC. Isolated posterior cord syndrome in Lyme disease: a clinico-neurophysiological study. Rev Neurol. Nov 16-30;33(10):954-7.

Gutierrez Y. Blood apicomplexa: plasmodium, Babesia and entopolypoides. In: Diagnostic Pathology of Parasitic Infections with Clinical Correlations. 9th ed. Philadelphia, PA: Lea Febiger; 1990, p. 146.

Guzel M, Celebi B, Yalcin E, Koenhemsi L, Mamak N, Pasa S, Atalay O. A Serological Investigation of Bartonella henselae Infection in Cats in Turkey. J Vet Med Sci. 2011 Jul 7. [Epub ahead of print]

H Fischer A, van der Loo B, M Shär G, Zbinden R, Duru F, Brunckhorst C, Rousson V, Delacrétaz Y E, Stuber T, Oechslin EN, Follath F, Jenni R. Serological evidence for the association of Bartonella henselae infection with arrhythmogenic right ventricular cardiomyopathy. Clin Cardiol. 2008 Oct;31(10):469-71.

Haapasalo K, Suomalainen P, Sukura A, Siikamaki H, Jokiranta TS. Fatal babesiosis in man, Finland, 2004. Emerg Infect Dis. 2010 Jul;16(7):1116-8.

Habyarimana F, Price CT, Santic M, Al-Khodor S, Kwaik YA. Molecular Characterization of the Dot/Icm-Translocated AnkH and AnkJ Eukaryotic-Like Effectors of Legionella pneumophila. Infect Immun. 2010 Mar;78(3):1123-34. Published online 2009 December 22.

Haddad FA, Nadelman RB. Lyme disease and the heart. Front Biosci. 2003 Sep 1;8:s769-82. Review.

Hagen K. [Risk of infections among orienteers].[Article in Norwegian]. Tidsskr Nor Laegeforen. 2009 Jun 25;129(13):1326-8. Review.

Hahn JS, Sum JM, Lee KP. Unusual MRI findings after status epilepticus due to cat-scratch disease. Pediatr Neurol. 1994 May;10(3):255-8.

Haider Z, Tsigrelis C, Baddour LM. 65-Year-Old Man With Persistent Fever. Mayo Clin Proc. 2009 Nov; 84(11):1017-20.

Hajjaji N, Hocqueloux L, Kerdraon R, Bret L. Bone infection in cat-scratch disease: a review of the literature. J Infect. 2007 May;54(5):417-21. Epub 2006 Nov 29. Review.

Halos L, Bord S, Cotté V, Gasqui P, Abrial D, Barnouin J, Boulouis HJ, Vayssier-Taussat M, Vourc'h G. Ecological Factors Characterizing the Prevalence of Bacterial Tick-Borne Pathogens in Ixodes ricinus Ticks in Pastures and Woodlands. Appl Environ Microbiol. 2010 Jul; 76(13):4413-20. Published online 2010 May 7.

Halperin JJ. Neuroborreliosis. Am J Med. 1995 Apr 24;98(4A):52S-56S; discussion 56S-59S. Review.

Halperin JJ. Nervous system Lyme disease. J R Coll Physicians Edinb. 2010 Sep;40(3):248-55. Review.

Halperin JJ. Nervous system lyme disease: is there a controversy? Semin Neurol. 2011 Jul;31(3):317-24. Epub 2011 Sep 30.

Halperin JJ. Neurologic manifestations of lyme disease. Curr Infect Dis Rep. 2011 Aug;13(4):360-6.

Halperin JJ, Golightly M. Lyme borreliosis in Bell's palsy. Long Island neuroborreliosis collaborative study group. Neurology. 1992 Jul;42(7):1268-70.

Halperin, JJ, Heyes MP. Neuroactive kynurenines in Lyme borreliosis. Neurology. 1992 Jan;42(1):43-50.

Halperin JJ, Kaplan GP, Brazinsky S, Tsai TF, Cheng T, Ironside A, Wu P, Delfiner J, Golightly M, et al. Immunologic reactivity against Borrelia burgdorferi in patients with motor neuron disease. Arch Neurol. 1990 May;47(5):586-94.

Halperin JJ, Little BW, Coyle PK, Dattwyler RJ. Lyme disease: cause of a treatable peripheral neuropathy. Neurology. 1987 Nov;37(11):1700-6.

Halperin J, Luft BJ, Volkman DJ, Dattwyler RJ. Lyme neuroborreliosis. Peripheral nervous system manifestations. Brain.1990 Aug;113 (Pt 4):1207-21.

Halperin JJ, Shapiro ED, Logigian E, Belman AL, Dotevall L, Wormser GP, Krupp L, Gronseth G, Bever CT Jr. Practice parameter: treatment of nervous system Lyme disease (an evidence-based review): report of the Quality Standards Subcommittee of the American Academy of Neurology. Neurology. 2007 Jul 3;69(1):91-102. Epub 2007 May 23. Erratum in: Neurology. 2008 Apr 1;70(14):1223.

Halperin JJ, Volkman DJ, Luft BJ, Dattwyler RJ. Carpal tunnel syndrome in Lyme borreliosis. Muscle Nerve. 1989 12(5):397-400. 1989.

Halperin JJ, Wormser GP. Of fleas and ticks on cats and mice... Arch Neurol. 2001 Sep;58(9):1345-7.

Hale BR, Owusu-Agyei S, Fryauff DJ, Koram KA, Adjuik M, Oduro AR, Prescott WR, Baird JK, Nkrumah F, Ritchie TL, Franke ED, Binka FN, Horton J, Hoffman SL. A randomized, double-blind, placebo-controlled, dose-ranging trial of tafenoquine for weekly prophylaxis against Plasmodium falciparum. Clin Infect Dis. 2003 Mar 1;36(5):541-9. [Epub. 2003 Feb 14].

Hamase A, Takahashi Y, Nohgi K, Fukunaga M. Homology of variable major protein genes between Borrelia hermsii and Borrelia miyamotoi. FEMS Microbiol Lett. 1996 Jul 1;140(2-3):131-7. Erratum in FEMS Microbiol Lett 1996 Oct 1;143(2-3):299.

Hamby CV, Llibre M, Utpat S, Wormser GP. Use of Peptide library screening to detect a previously unknown linear diagnostic epitope: proof of principle by use of lyme disease sera. Clin Diagn Lab Immunol. 2005 Jul;12(7):801-7.

Hamel MJ, Holtz T, Mkandala C, Kaimila N, Chizani N, Bloland P, Kublin J, Kazembe P, Steketee R. Efficacy of trimethoprim-sulfamethoxazole compared with sulfadoxine-pyrimethamine plus erythromycin for the treatment of uncomplicated malaria in children with integrated management of childhood illness dual classifications of malaria and pneumonia. Am J Trop Med Hyg. 2005 Sep;73(3):609-15.

Hamer SA, Hickling GJ, Sidge JL, Rosen ME, Walker ED, Tsao JI. Diverse Borrelia burgdorferi strains in a bird-tick cryptic cycle. Appl Environ Microbiol. 2011 Mar;77(6):1999-2007. Epub 2011 Jan 21.

Hamer SA, Roy PL, Hickling GJ, Walker ED, Foster ES, Barber CC, Tsao JI. Zoonotic pathogens in Ixodes scapularis, Michigan. Emerg Infect Dis. 2007 Jul;13(7):1131-3.

Hamer SA, Tsao JI, Walker ED, Hickling GJ. Invasion of the lyme disease vector Ixodes scapularis: implications for Borrelia burgdorferi endemicity. Ecohealth. 2010 Aug;7(1):47-63. Epub 2010 Mar 13.

Hamer SA, Tsao JI, Walker ED, Mansfield LS, Foster ES, Hickling GJ. Use of tick surveys and serosurveys to evaluate pet dogs as a sentinel species for emerging Lyme disease. Am J Vet Res. 2009 Jan;70(1):49-56.

Hammers-Berggren S, Gröndahl A, Karlsson M, von Arbin M, Carlsson A, Stiernstedt G. Screening for neuroborreliosis in patients with stroke. Stroke. 1993 Sep;24(9):1393-6.

Hampp EG, Scott D, Wyckoff RWG. Morphologic characteristics of certain cultured strains of oral spirochetes and Treponema pallidum as revealed by the electron microscope. J Bacteriol. 1948 Dec;56(6):755-69.

Han JI, Lee SJ, Jang HJ, Na KJ. Asymptomatic Babesia microti-like parasite infection in wild raccoon dogs (Nyctereutes procyonoides) in South Korea. J Wildl Dis. 2010 Apr;46(2):632-5.

Han S, Norimine J, Palmer GH, Mwangi W, Lahmers KK, Brown WC. Rapid deletion of antigen-specific CD4+ T cells following infection represents a strategy of immune evasion and persistence for Anaplasma marginale. J Immunol. 2008 Dec 1;181(11):7759.

Hanafusa Y, Cho KO, Kanemaru T, Wada R, Sugimoto C, Onuma M. Pathogenesis of Babesia caballi infection in experimental horses. J Vet Med Sci. 1998 Oct;60(10):1127-32.

Hanincová K, Liveris D, Sandigursky S, Wormser GP, Schwartz I. Borrelia burgdorferi sensu stricto is clonal in patients with early Lyme borreliosis. Appl Environ Microbiol. 2008 Aug;74(16):5008-14. Epub 2008 Jun 6.

Hannier S, Liversidge J, Sternberg JM, Bowman AS. Characterization of the B-cell inhibitory protein factor in Ixodes ricinus tick saliva: a potential role in enhanced Borrelia burgdoferi transmission. Immunology. 2004 Nov;113(3):401-8.

Hanscheid T, Melo-Cristino J, Grobusch MP, Pinto BG. Avoiding misdiagnosis of imported malaria: screening of emergency department samples with thrombocytopenia detects clinically unsuspected cases. J Travel Med. 2003 May-Jun;10(3):155-9.

Hansel Y, Ackerl M, Stanek G. ALS-like sequelae in chronic neuroborreliosis. Wien Med Wochenschr. 1995;145(7-8):186-8.

Hao GF, Li H, Sun Y, Ge RP, Qiao GQ, Li B, Tian WZ, Shi NX, Yang XY. [Detection of tick and tick-borne pathogen in some ports of Inner Mongolia].[Article in Chinese]. Zhonghua Liu Xing Bing Xue Za Zhi. 2009 Apr;30(4):365-7.

Hao Q, Hou X, Geng Z, Wan K. Distribution of Borrelia burgdorferi sensu lato in China. J Clin Microbiol. 2011 Feb;49(2):647-50. Epub 2010 Nov 24.

Hardin JA, Steere AC, Malawista SE. The pathogenesis of arthritis in Lyme disease: humoral immune responses and the role of intra-articular immune complexes. Yale J Biol Med. 1984 Jul-Aug;57(4):589-93.

Hardin JA, Steere AC, Malawista SE. Immune complexes and the evolution of Lyme arthritis. Dissemination and localization of abnormal C1q binding activity. N Engl J Med. 1979 Dec 20;301(25):1358-63.

Hardin JA, Walker LC, Steere AC, Trumble TC, Tung KS, Williams RC Jr, Ruddy S, Malawista SE. Circulating immune complexes in Lyme arthritis. Detection by the 125I-C1q binding, C1q solid phase, and Raji cell assays. J Clin Invest. 1979 Mar;63(3):468-77.

Harjacek M, Diaz-Cano S, Alman BA, Coburn J, Ruthazer R, Wolfe H, Steere AC. Prominent expression of mRNA for proinflammatory cytokines in synovium in patients with juvenile rheumatoid arthritis or chronic Lyme arthritis. J Rheumatol. 2000 Feb;27(2):497-503.

Harms CA, Maggi RG, Breitschwerdt EB, Clemons-Chevis CL, Solangi M, Rotstein DS, Fair PA, Hansen LJ, Hohn AA, Lovewell GN, McLellan WA, Pabst DA, Rowles TK, Schwacke LH, Townsend FI, Wells RS. Bartonella species detection in captive, stranded and free-ranging cetaceans. Vet Res. 2008 Nov-Dec;39(6):59. Epub 2008 Aug 23.

Harris PJ. Intracerebral bacillary angiomatosis in HIV. Ann Intern Med. 1992 Nov 1;117(9):795.

Harrison A, Montgomery WI, Bown KJ. Investigating the persistence of tick-borne pathogens via the R0 model. Parasitology. 2011 Apr 26:1-10. [Epub ahead of print]

Harrus S, Perlman-Avrahami A, Mumcuoglu KY, Morick D, Eyal O, Baneth G. Molecular detection of Ehrlichia canis, Anaplasma bovis, Anaplasma platys, Candidatus Midichloria mitochondrii and Babesia canis vogeli in ticks from Israel. Clin Microbiol Infect. 2011 Mar;17(3):459-63.

Hartel C, Schilling S, Neppert B, Tiemer B, Sperner J. Intracranial hypertension in neuroborreliosis. Dev Med Child Neurol. 2002;44(9):641-2.

Harvey RA, Misselbeck WJ, Uphold RE. Cat-scratch disease: an unusual cause of combative behavior. Am J Emerg Med. 1991;9(1):52-53.

Harvey WT, Martz D. Motor neuron disease recovery associated with IV ceftriaxone and anti-Babesia therapy. Acta Neurol Scand. 2007 Feb;115(2):129-31.

Häselbarth K, Tenter AM, Brade V, Krieger G, Hunfeld KP. First case of human babesiosis in Germany - Clinical presentation and molecular characterisation of the pathogen. Int J Med Microbiol. 2007 Jun;297(3):197-204. Epub 2007 Mar 12.

Hashimoto Y, Kawagishi N, Sakai H, Takahashi H, Matsuo S, Nakao M, Miyamoto K, Iizuka H. Lyme disease in Japan. Analysis of Borrelia species using rRNA gene restriction fragment length polymorphism. Dermatology. 1995;191(3):193-8.

Hashimoto Y, Takahashi H, Kishiyama K, Sato Y, Nakao M, Miyamoto K, Iizuka H. Lyme disease with facial nerve palsy: rapid diagnosis using a nested polymerase chain reaction-restriction fragment length polymorphism analysis. Br J Dermatol. 1998 Feb;138(2):304-9.

Hashimoto Y, Takahashi H, Matsuo S, Hirai K, Takemori N, Nakao M, Miyamoto K, Iizuka H. Polymerase chain reaction of Borrelia burgdorferi flagellin gene in Shulman syndrome. Dermatology. 1996;192(2):136-9.

Hasle G, Leinaas HP, Røed KH, Øines Ø. Transport of Babesia venatorum-infected Ixodes ricinus to Norway by northward migrating passerine birds. Acta Vet Scand. 2011 Jun 23;53:41.

Hassin GB, Diamond IB. Silver cells and spirochete-like formations in MS and other diseases of the central nervous system. Archives of Neurology & Psychiatry. 1939;41:471-483.

Hasslberger, S. Sweet Wormwood Heals Malaria. [monograph on the Internet]. Available from: http://www.newmediaexplorer.org/sepp/2004/07/17/sweet_wormwood_heals_malaria.htm. Accessed 2006 Aug 1.

Hassler D, Zöller L, Haude M, Hufnagel HD, Heinrich F, Sonntag HG. Cefotaxime versus penicillin in the late stage of Lyme disease-prospective, randomized therapeutic trial. Infection. 1990 Jan-Feb;18(1):16-20.

Hassler D, Riedel K, Zorn J, Preac-Mursic V. Pulsed High Dose Cefotaxime Therapy in Refractory Lyme Borreliosis (Letter). Lancet. 1991;338(8760):193.

Hatanaka K, Miyagishima T, Kamata T, Nakagawa M, Miura Y, Arai S, Kishimoto A, Kamishima Y, Shibata M, Choi GH, Kudo M, Okabe M, Tsukamoto T, Miyamoto K. [Occurrence of angioimmunoblastic T-cell lymphoma six months after onset of Lyme disease].[Article in Japanese]. Rinsho Ketsueki. 2000 Dec;41(12):1273-6.

Haupl T, Hahn G, Rittig M, Krause A, Schoerner C, Schonherr U, Kalden JR, Burmester GR. Persistence of Borrelia burgdorferi in ligamentous tissue from a patient with chronic Lyme borreliosis. Arthr Rheum. 1993;36(11):1621-6.

Hauser U, Krahl H, Peters H, Fingerle V, Wilske B. Impact of strain heterogeneity on Lyme disease serology in Europe: comparison of enzyme-linked immunosorbent assays using different species of Borrelia burgdorferi sensu lato. J Clin Microbiol. 1998 Feb;36(2):427-36.

Hauser U, Lehnert G, Wilske B. Diagnostic value of proteins of three Borrelia species (Borrelia burgdorferi sensu lato) and implications for development and use of recombinant antigens for serodiagnosis of Lyme borreliosis in Europe. Clin Diagn Lab Immunol. 1998 Jul;5(4):456-62.

Hauser U, Lehnert G, Wilske B. Validity of interpretation criteria for standardized Western blots (immunoblots) for serodiagnosis of Lyme borreliosis based on sera collected throughout Europe. J Clin Microbiol. 1999 Jul;37(7):2241-7.

Haven J, Vargas LC, Mongodin EF, Xue V, Hernandez Y, Pagan P, Fraser-Liggett CM, Schutzer SE, Luft BJ, Casjens SR, Qiu WG. Pervasive Recombination and Sympatric Genome Diversification Driven by Frequency-Dependent Selection in Borrelia burgdorferi, the Lyme disease Bacterium. Genetics. 2011 Sep 2. [Epub ahead of print]

Hawkins EC, Johnson LR, Guptill L, Marr HS, Breitschwerdt EB, Birkenheuer AJ. Failure to identify an association between serologic or molecular evidence of Bartonella infection and idiopathic rhinitis in dogs. J Am Vet Med Assoc. 2008 Aug 15;233(4):597-9.

Hawkins RC. The Evidence Based Medicine approach to diagnostic testing: practicalities and limitations. Clin Biochem Rev. 2005 May;26(2):7-18.

Hayes CN, Diez D, Joannin N, Honda W, Kanehisa M, Wahlgren M, Wheelock CE, Goto S. varDB: a pathogen-specific sequence database of protein families involved in antigenic variation. Bioinformatics. 2008 November 1; 24(21): 2564–2565. Published online 2008 September 6.

Hayes RK. From artemisinin to new artemisinin antimalarials: bio-synthesis, extraction, old and new derivatives, stereochemistry and medicinal chemistry requirements. Curr Top Med Chem. 2006;6(5):509-37.

Hayes SF, Burgdorfer W. Ultrastructure of Borrelia burgdorferi. In "Aspects of Lyme borreliosis," ed. K. Weber, W. Burgdorfer. Berlin; Springer-Verlag. 1993.

He M, Ouyang Z, Troxell B, Xu H, Moh A, Piesman J, Norgard MV, Gomelsky M, Yang XF. Cyclic di-GMP is essential for the survival of the lyme disease spirochete in ticks. PLoS Pathog. 2011 Jun;7(6):e1002133. Epub 2011 Jun 30.

Heinrich A, Khaw AV, Ahrens N, Kirsch M, Dressel A. Cerebral vasculitis as the only manifestation of Borrelia burgdorferi infection in a 17-year-old patient with basal ganglia infarction. Eur Neurol. 2003;50(2):109-112.

Heir GM, Fein LA. Lyme disease: considerations for dentistry. J Orofac Pain. 1996 Winter;10(1):74-86.

Heller R, Kubina M, Mariet P, et al. Bartonella alsatica sp. nov., a new Bartonella species isolated from the blood of wild rabbits. Int J Syst Bacteriol. 1999;49 Pt 1:283-288.

Hemsworth S, Pizer B. Pet ownership in immunocompromised children--a review of the literature and survey of existing guidelines. Eur J Oncol Nurs. 2006 Apr;10(2):117-27. Epub 2006 Apr 3. Review.

Henderson SO, Magana RN. Babesiosis. eMedicine from WebMD. http://www.emedicine.com/emerg/topic49.htm. Updated 2006 Mar 8. Accessed January 2, 2007.

Hendrickx G, De Boeck H, Goossens A, Demanet C, Vandenplas Y. Persistent synovitis in children with Lyme arthritis: two unusual cases. An immunogenetic approach. Eur J Pediatr. 2004 Nov;163(11):646-50. Epub 2004 Jul 28.

Henn JB, Chomel BB, Boulouis HJ, Kasten RW, Murray WJ, Bar-Gal GK, King R, Courreau JF, Baneth G. Bartonella rochalimae in raccoons, coyotes, and red foxes. Emerg Infect Dis. 2009 Dec;15(12):1984-7.

Henn JB, Gabriel MW, Kasten RW, Brown RN, Koehler JE, MacDonald KA, Kittleson MD, Thomas WP, Chomel BB. Infective endocarditis in a dog and the phylogenetic relationship of the associated "Bartonella rochalimae" strain with isolates from dogs, gray foxes, and a human. J Clin Microbiol. 2009 Mar;47(3):787-90. Epub 2008 Dec 24.

Henn JB, Vanhorn BA, Kasten RW, Kachani M, Chomel BB. Antibodies to Bartonella vinsonii subsp. Berkhoffii in Moroccan dogs. Am J Trop Med Hyg. 2006 Feb;74(2):222-3.

Henningsson AJ, Tjernberg I, Malmvall BE, Forsberg P, Ernerudh J. Indications of Th1 and Th17 responses in cerebrospinal fluid from patients with Lyme neuroborreliosis: a large retrospective study. J Neuroinflammation. 2011 Apr 20;8:36.

Hercík K, Hásová V, Janecek J, Branny P. Molecular evidence of Bartonella DNA in ixodid ticks in Czechia. Folia Microbiol (Praha). 2007;52(5):503-9.

Herman JH, Ayache S, Olkowska D. Autoimmunity in transfusion babesiosis: a spectrum of clinical presentations. J Clin Apher. 2010;25(6):358-61. Epub 2010 Sep 7.

Hernandez-Da-Mota S, Escalante-Razo F. Bartonellosis causing bilateral Leber neuroretinitis: a case report. Eur J Ophthalmol. 2009 Mar-Apr;19(2):307-9.

Herremans M, Bakker J, Vermeulen MJ, Schellekens JF, Koopmans MP. Evaluation of an in-house cat scratch disease IgM ELISA to detect Bartonella henselae in a routine laboratory setting. Eur J Clin Microbiol Infect Dis. 2009 Feb;28(2):147-52. Epub 2008 Aug 5.

Herremans M, Vermeulen MJ, Van de Kassteele J, Bakker J, Schellekens JF, Koopmans MP. The use of Bartonella henselae-specific age dependent IgG and IgM in diagnostic models to discriminate diseased from non-diseased in Cat Scratch Disease serology. J Microbiol Methods. 2007 Nov;71(2):107-13. Epub 2007 Sep 15.

Herwaldt B, Persing DH, Précigout EA, Goff WL, Mathiesen DA, Taylor PW, Eberhard ML, Gorenflot AF. A fatal case of babesiosis in Missouri: identification of another piroplasm that infects humans. Ann Intern Med. 1996 Apr 1;124(7):643-50.

Herwaldt BL, Caccio S, Gherlinzoni F, Aspock H, Slemenda SB, Piccaluga P, Martinelli G, Edelhofer R, Hollenstein U, Poletti G, Pampiglione S, Loschenberger K, Tura S, Pieniazek NJ. Molecular characterization of a non-Babesia divergens organism causing zoonotic babesiosis in Europe. Emerg Infect Dis. 2003;9:942-48.

Herwaldt BL, de Bruyn G, Pieniazek NJ, Homer M, Lofy KH, Slemenda SB, Fritsche TR, Persing DH, Limaye AP. Babesia divergens-like infection, Washington State. Emerg Infect Dis. 2004 Apr;10(4):622-9.

Herwaldt RM, Kjemtrup AM, Conrad PA, Barnes RC, Wilson M, McCarthy MG, Sayers MH, Eberhard ML. Transfusion-transmitted babesiosis in Washington State: first reported case caused by WA1-type parasite. J. Infect. Dis. 1997 May;175(5):1259-62.

Herzer P, Wilske B, Preac-Mursic V, Schierz G, Schattenkirchner M, Zollner N. Lyme arthritis: clinical features, serological, and radiographic findings of cases in Germany. Klin Wochenschr. 1986;64(5):206-15.

Herzer P. Joint manifestations. In Aspects of Lyme Borreliosis, ed. Klaus Weber, M.D., Willy Burgdorfer, Ph.D., M.D. Berlin Heidelberg:Springer-Verlag.1993. pp 168-184.

Hess A, Buchmann J, Zettl UK, Henschel S, Schlaefke D, Grau G, Benecke R. Borrelia burgdorferi central nervous system infection presenting as an organic schizophrenialike disorder. Biol Psychiatry. 1999 Mar 15;45(6):795.

Heyman P, Cochez C, Hofhuis A, van der Giessen J, Sprong H, Porter SR, Losson B, Saegerman C, Donoso-Mantke O, Niedrig M, Papa A. A clear and present danger: tick-borne diseases in Europe. Expert Rev Anti Infect Ther. 2010 Jan;8(1):33-50. Review.

Hien TT, Turner G, Mai NTH. Neuropathological assessment of artemether-treated severe malaria. Lancet. 2003;362:295-6.

Hildebrandt A, Hunfeld KP, Baier M, Krumbholz A, Sachse S, Lorenzen T, Kiehntopf M, Fricke HJ, Straube E. First confirmed autochthonous case of human Babesia microti infection in Europe. Eur J Clin Microbiol Infect Dis. 2007 Aug;26(8):595-601.

Hildebrandt A, Straube E, Neubauer H, Schmoock G. Coxiella burnetii and coinfections in Ixodes ricinus ticks in Central Germany. Vector Borne Zoonotic Dis. 2011 Aug;11(8):1205-7. Epub 2010 Dec 13.

Hilton E, Devoti J, Sood S. Recommendation to include OspA and OspB in the new immunoblotting criteria for serodiagnosis of Lyme disease. J Clin Microbiol. 1996 Jun;34(6):1353-4. Erratum in: J Clin Microbiol 1997 Oct;35(10):2713.

Hilton E, Smith C, Sood S. Ocular Lyme borreliosis diagnosed by polymerase chain reaction on vitreous fluid. Ann Intern Med. 1996 Sep 1;125(5):424-5.

Hilton E, Tramontano A, DeVoti J, Sood SK. Temporal study of immunoglobin M seroreactivity to Borrelia burgdorferi in patients treated for Lyme borreliosis. J Clin Microbiol. 1997 Mar;35(3):774-6.

Hindle E. On the life-cycle of spirochaeta gallinarum. Parasitology, Vol IV, pp. 463-477. 1912.

Hinrichsen VL, Whitworth UG, Breitschwerdt EB, Hegarty BC, Mather TN. Assessing the association between the geographic distribution of deer ticks and seropositivity rates to various tick-transmitted disease organisms in dogs. J Am Vet Med Assoc. 2001 Apr 1;218(7):1092-7.

Hinterseher I, Gäbel G, Corvinus F, Lück C, Saeger HD, Bergert H, Tromp G, Kuivaniemi H. Presence of Borrelia burgdorferi sensu lato antibodies in the serum of patients with abdominal aortic aneurysms. Eur J Clin Microbiol Infect Dis. 2011 Aug 13. [Epub ahead of print]

Hirai K, Takemori N, Yanagawa N, Namiki M, Iizuka H, Miyamoto K. Borrelia burgdorferi and Shulman syndrome. Lancet. 1992 Dec 12;340(8833):1472.

Hitt, J. The year in ideas: a to z.; evidence-based medicine. in New York Times (December 9, 2001, Sunday).

Hodzic, E, Feng S, Holden K, Freet K, Barthold SW. Persistence of Borrelia burgdorferi Following Antibiotic Treatment in Mice. 2008. Antimicro Agents Chemother, 52(5):1728-36.

Hoen AG, Rollend LG, Papero MA, Carroll JF, Daniels TJ, Mather TN, Schulze TL, Stafford KC 3rd, Fish D. Effects of tick control by acaricide self-treatment of white-tailed deer on host-seeking tick infection prevalence and entomologic risk for Ixodes scapularis-borne pathogens. Vector Borne Zoonotic Dis. 2009 Aug;9(4):431-8.

Hoey JG, Valois-Cruz F, Goldenberg H, Voskoboynik Y, Pfiffner J, Tilton RC, Mordechai E, Adelson ME. Development of an immunoglobulin M capture-based enzyme-linked immunosorbent assay for diagnosis of acute infections with Bartonella henselae. Clin Vaccine Immunol. 2009 Feb;16(2):282-4. Epub 2008 Dec 3.

Hofbauer GF, Kessler B, Kempf W, Nestle FO, Burg G, Dummer R. Multilesional primary cutaneous diffuse large b-cell lymphoma responsive to antibiotic treatment. Dermatology. 2001 ;203(2):168-70.

Hoffman RM, AboulHosn J, Child JS, Pegues DA. Bartonella endocarditis in complex congenital heart disease. Congenit Heart Dis. 2007 Jan-Feb;2(1):79-84.

Hofmann-Lehmann R, Meli ML, Dreher UM, Gönczi E, Deplazes P, Braun U, Engels M, Schüpbach J, Jörger K, Thoma R, Griot C, Stärk KD, Willi B, Schmidt J, Kocan KM, Lutz H. Concurrent Infections with Vector-Borne Pathogens Associated with Fatal Hemolytic Anemia in a Cattle Herd in Switzerland. J Clin Microbiol. 2004 August;42(8):3775-80.

Hofmeister E, Kolbert C, Abdulkarim A, Magera J et al. Cosegregatin of a novel Bartonella species with Borrelia burgdorferi and Babesia microti in Peromyscus leucopus. J Infect Dis. 1998;177:409-416.

Holman PJ. Phylogenetic and biologic evidence that Babesia divergens is not endemic in the United States. Ann N Y Acad Sci. 2006 Oct;1081:518-25.

Holmes NE, Opat S, Kelman A, Korman TM. Refractory Bartonella quintana bacillary angiomatosis following chemotherapy for chronic lymphocytic leukaemia. J Med Microbiol. 2011 Jan;60(Pt 1):142-6. Epub 2010 Oct 14.

Homer MJ, Aguiler-Delfin I, SR Telford III, PJ Krause and DH Persing. Babesiosis. Clin Microbiol Rev. 2000 Jul;13(3):451-69.

Horneff G, Huppertz HI, Müller K, Voit T, Karch H. Demonstration of Borrelia burgdorferi infection in a child with Guillain-Barré syndrome. Eur J Pediatr. 1993;152(10):810-2.

Horowitz HW, Aguero-Rosenfeld M, Dumler JS, McKenna DF, Hsieh TC, Wu J, Schwartz I, Wormser GP. Reinfection with the agent of human granulocytic ehrlichiosis. Ann Intern Med. 1998 Sep 15;129(6):461-3.

Horowitz HW, Dworkin B, Forseter G, Nadelman RB, Connolly C, Luciano BB, Nowakowski J, O'Brien TA, Calmann M, Wormser GP. Liver function in early Lyme disease. Hepatology. 1996 Jun;23(6):1412-7.

Horowitz HW, Pavia CS, Bittker S, Forseter G, Cooper D, Nadelman RB, Byrne D, Johnson RC, Wormser GP. Sustained cellular immune responses to Borrelia burgdorferi: lack of correlation with clinical presentation and serology. Clin Diagn Lab Immunol. 1994 Jul;1(4):373-8.

Horowitz HW, Sanghera K, Goldberg N, Pechman D, Kamer R, Duray P, Weinstein A. Dermatomyositis associated with Lyme disease: case report and review of Lyme myositis. Clin Infect Dis. 1994;18(2):166-71.

Horowitz HW, Wormser GP. Doxycycline revisited: an old medicine for emerging diseases. Arch Intern Med. 1998 Jan 26;158(2):192-3.

Hoshinari NH, Barros PJ, Yassuda P, Baggio D, Steere AC, Pagliarine RC, Cossermelli W. [Epidemiological study of Lyme disease in Brazil]. [Article in Portuguese]. Rev Hosp Clin Fac Med Sao Paulo. 1992 Mar-Apr;47(2):71-5. Review.

Houck JA, Hojgaard A, Piesman J, Kuchta RD. Low-density microarrays for the detection of Borrelia burgdorferi s.s. (the Lyme disease spirochete) in nymphal Ixodes scapularis. Ticks Tick Borne Dis. 2011 Mar;2(1):27-36. Epub 2010 Nov 27.

Houhamdi L, Parola P, Raoult D. [Lice and lice-borne diseases in humans].[Article in French]. Med Trop (Mars). 2005;65(1):13-23. Review.

Houhamdi L, Raoult D. Experimental infection of human body lice with Acinetobacter baumannii. Am J Trop Med Hyg. 2006 Apr;74(4):526-31.

Houtman PM, Tazelaar DJ. Joint and bone involvement in Dutch patients with Lyme borreliosis presenting with acrodermatitis chronica atrophicans. Neth J Med. 1999 Jan;54(1):5-9.

Houpikian P, Fournier PE, Raoult D. Phylogenetic position of Bartonella vinsonii subsp. arupensis based on 16S rDNA and gltA gene sequences. Int J Syst Evol Microbiol. 2001 Jan;51(Pt 1):179-82.

Houpikian P, Raoult D. Molecular phylogeny of the genus Bartonella: what is the current knowledge? FEMS Microbiol Lett. 2001 Jun 12;200(1):1-7. Review.

Houpikian P, Raoult D. 16S/23S rRNA intergenic spacer regions for phylogenetic analysis, identification, and subtyping of Bartonella species. J Clin Microbiol. 2001 Aug;39(8):2768-78.

Houpikian P, Raoult D. Diagnostic methods current best practices and guidelines for identification of difficult-to-culture pathogens in infective endocarditis. Infect Dis Clin North Am. 2002 Jun;16(2):377-92. Review.

Houpikian P, Raoult D. Western immunoblotting for Bartonella endocarditis. Clin Diagn Lab Immunol. 2003 Jan;10(1):95-102.

Houpikian P, Raoult D. Diagnostic methods. Current best practices and guidelines for identification of difficult-to-culture pathogens in infective endocarditis. Cardiol Clin. 2003 May;21(2):207-17. Review.

Houpikian P, Raoult D. Blood culture-negative endocarditis in a reference center: etiologic diagnosis of 348 cases. Medicine (Baltimore). 2005;84(3):162-173.

Hovind-Hougen K, Asbrink E, Stiernstedt G, Steere AC, Hovmark A. Ultrastructural differences among spirochetes isolated from patients with Lyme disease and related disorders, and from Ixodes ricinus. Zentralbl Bakteriol Mikrobiol Hyg A. 1986 Dec;263(1-2):103-11.

Hovius JW, Bijlsma MF, van der Windt GJ, Wiersinga WJ, Boukens BJ, Coumou J, Oei A, de Beer R, de Vos AF, van 't Veer C, van Dam AP, Wang P, Fikrig E, Levi MM, Roelofs JJ, van der Poll T. The Urokinase Receptor (uPAR) Facilitates Clearance of Borrelia burgdorferi. PLoS Pathog. 2009 May; 5(5): e1000447. Published online 2009 May 22.

Hovmark A, Asbrink E, Olsson I. Joint and bone involvement in Swedish patients with Ixodes ricinus-borne Borrelia infection. Zentralbl Bakteriol Mikrobiol Hyg A. 1986 Dec;263(1-2):275-84.

Howland RH. Limitations of evidence in the practice of evidence-based medicine. J Psychosoc Nurs Ment Health Serv. 2007 Nov;45(11):13-6. Review.

Hsieh JW, Tung KC, Chen WC, Lin JW, Chien LJ, Hsu YM, Wang HC, Chomel BB, Chang CC. Epidemiology of Bartonella infection in rodents and shrews in Taiwan. Zoonoses Public Health. 2010 Sep;57(6):439-46.

Hu LT, Eskildsen MA, Masgala C, Steere AC, Arner EC, Pratta MA, Grodzinsky AJ, Loening A, Perides G. Host metalloproteinases in Lyme arthritis. Arthritis Rheum. 2001 Jun;44(6):1401-10.

Huang H, Lin M, Wang X, Kikuchi T, Mottaz H, Norbeck A, Rikihisa Y. Proteomic Analysis of and Immune Responses to Ehrlichia chaffeensis Lipoproteins. Infect Immun. 2008 Aug;76(8):3405-14. Published online 2008 May 19.

Huang J, Dai L, Lei S, Liao DY, Wang XQ, Luo TY, Chen Y, Hang ZB, Li GD, Dong DD, Xu G, Gu ZC, Hao JL, Hua P, He L, Duan FL. [Application of Warthin-Starry stain, immunohistochemistry and transmission electron microscopy in diagnosis of cat scratch disease].[Article in Chinese]. Zhonghua Bing Li Xue Za Zhi. 2010 Apr;39(4):225-9.

Huang R, Liu Q, Li G, Li D, Song X, Birtles RJ, Zhao F. Bartonella quintana Infections in Captive Monkeys, China. Emerg Infect Dis. 2011 Sep;17(9):1707-9.

Huarcaya E, Best I, Rodriguez-Tafur J, Maguiña C, Solórzano N, Menacho J, Lopez De Guimaraes D, Chauca J, Ventosilla P. Cytokines and T-Lymphocute count in patients in the acute and chronic phases of Bartonella bacilliformis infection in an endemic area in peru: a pilot study. Rev Inst Med Trop Sao Paulo. 2011 Jun;53(3):149-54.

Huarcaya E, Maguina C, Best I, Solorzano N, Leeman L. Immunological response in cases of complicated and uncomplicated bartonellosis during pregnancy. Rev Inst Med Trop Sao Paulo. 2007 Sep-Oct;49(5):335-7.

Huarcaya E, Maguiña C, Torres R, Rupay J, Fuentes L. Bartonelosis (Carrion's Disease) in the pediatric population of Peru: an overview and update. Braz J Infect Dis. 2004 Oct;8(5):331-9. Epub 2005 Mar 17. Review.

Hudson BJ, Stewart M, Lennox VA, Fukunaga M, Yabuki M, et al. Culture-positive Lyme borreliosis. Med J Aust. 1998 May 18;168(10):500-2.

Huegli D, Moret J, Rais O, Moosmann Y, Erard P, Malinverni R, Gern L. Prospective study on the incidence of infection by Borrelia burgdorferi sensu lato after a tick bite in a highly endemic area of Switzerland. Ticks Tick Borne Dis. 2011 Sep;2(3):129-36. Epub 2011 Jul 28.

Hulinska D, Bartak P, Hercogova J, Hancil J, Basta J, Schramlova J. Electron microscopy of Langerhans cells and Borrelia burgdorferi in Lyme disease patients. Zbl Bakt. 1994;280:348-9.

Hulínská D, Votýpka J, Kríz B, Holínková N, Nováková J, Hulínský V. Phenotypic and genotypic analysis of Borrelia spp. isolated from Ixodes ricinus ticks by using electrophoretic chips and real-time polymerase chain reaction. Folia Microbiol (Praha). 2007;52(4):315-24.

Hunfeld KP, Brade V. Zoonotic Babesia: Possibly emerging pathogens to be considered for tick-infested humans in central Europe. Int. J. Med. Microbiol. 2004;S37:93-103.

Hunfeld KP, Hildebrandt A, Gray JS. Babesiosis: recent insights into an ancient disease. Int J Parasitol. 2008 Sep;38(11):1219-37. Epub 2008 Mar 20. Review.

Hunfeld KP, Lambert A, Kampen H, Albert S, Epe C, Brade V, Tenter AM. Seroprevalence of Babesia infections in humans exposed to ticks in midwestern Germany. J Clin Microbiol. 2002 Jul;40(7):2431-6.

Hunfeld KP, Ruzic-Sabljic E, Norris DE, Kraiczy P, Strle F. In Vitro Susceptibility Testing of Borrelia burgdorferi Sensu Lato Isolates Cultured from Patients with Erythema Migrans before and after Antimicrobial Chemotherapy. 2005. Antimicro Agents Chemother,49(4):1294-1301.

Hung le Q, de Vries PJ, Binh TQ, Giao PT, Nam NV, Holman R, Kager PA. Artesunate with mefloquine at various intervals for non-severe Plasmodium falciparum malaria. Am J Trop Med Hyg. 2004 Aug;71(2):160-6.

Hurwitz B, Clinical guidelines and the law. BMJ. 1995 Dec 9; 311(7019):1517-8.

Hussain S, Rathore MH. Cat scratch disease with epidural extension while on antimicrobial treatment. Pediatr Neurosurg. 2007;43(2):164-6.

Hutagalung R, Htoo H, Nwee P, Arunkamomkiri J, Zwang J, Carrara VI, Ashley E, Singhasivanon P, White NJ, Nosten F. A case-control auditory evaluation of patients treated with artemether-lumefantrine. Am J Trop Med Hyg. 2006 Feb;74(2):211-4.

Hutchings CL, Li A, Fernandez KM, Fletcher T, Jackson LA, Molloy JB, Jorgensen WK, Lim CT, Cooke BM. New insights into the altered adhesive and mechanical properties of red blood cells parasitized by Babesia bovis. Mol Microbiol. 2007 Aug;65(4):1092-105. Epub 2007 Jul 19.

Hyde JA, Weening EH, Chang M, Trzeciakowski JP, Höök M, Cirillo JD, Skare JT. Bioluminescent imaging of Borrelia burgdorferi in vivo demonstrates that the fibronectin-binding protein BBK32 is required for optimal infectivity. Mol Microbiol. 2011 Oct;82(1):99-113. Epub 2011 Aug 30.

Hyde JA, Weening EH, Skare JT. Genetic transformation of Borrelia burgdorferi. Curr Protoc Microbiol. 2011 Feb;Chapter 12:Unit 12C.4.

Igarashi I, Suzuki R, Waki S, et al. Roles of CD4(+) T cells and gamma interferon in protective immunity against Babesia microti infection in mice. Infect Immun. 1999;67(8):4143-8.

Il'ina TS, Bashkirov VN. [Interaction of bacteria of the genus Bartonella with the host: inhibition of apoptosis, induction of proliferation, and formation of tumors].[Article in Russian]. Mol Gen Mikrobiol Virusol. 2008;(3):3-11. Review.

Imai DM, Barr BC, Daft B, Bertone JJ, Feng S, Hodzic E, Johnston JM, Olsen KJ, Barthold SW. Lyme Neuroborreliosis in 2 Horses. Vet Pathol. 2011 Apr 1. [Epub ahead of print]

Imashuku S, Kakazu N, Ueda I, et al. Response to imatinib mesylate in a patient with idiopathic hypereosinophilic syndrome associated with cyclic eosinophil oscillations. Int J Hematol. 2005;81(4):310-4.

Incandela S, Raoult D, Vitale G, Micalizzi A, Mansueto P. Hepatosplenic cat-scratch fever with seropositivity for Bartonella quintana? Lancet Infect Dis. 2008 Nov;8(11):663.

Inoue K, Maruyama S, Kabeya H, Hagiya K, Izumi Y, Une Y, Yoshikawa Y. Exotic small mammals as potential reservoirs of zoonotic Bartonella spp. Emerg Infect Dis. 2009 Apr;15(4):526-32.

Inokuma H, Oyamada M, Kelly PJ, Jacobson LA, Fournier PE, Itamoto K, Okuda M, Brouqui P. Molecular Detection of a New Anaplasma Species Closely Related to Anaplasma phagocytophilum in Canine Blood from South Africa. J Clin Microbiol. 2005 June; 43(6): 2934-7.

Inoue K, Maruyama S, Kabeya H, Yamada N, Ohashi N, Sato Y, Yukawa M, Masuzawa T, Kawamori F, Kadosaka T, Takada N, Fujita H, Kawabata H. Prevalence and genetic diversity of Bartonella species isolated from wild rodents in Japan. Appl Environ Microbiol. 2008 Aug;74(16):5086-92. Epub 2008 Jul 7.

Inoue S, Gordon R, Berner G. Erythema chronicum migrans as the presenting manifestation of juvenile chronic myelocytic leukemia. Cutis. 1989;43(4):333-7.

The International Lyme and Associated Diseases Society (ILADS), Evidence-based guidelines for the management of Lyme disease. Expert Rev Anti-infect Ther, 2004. 2(Suppl): p. S1-S13.

Iori A, Gabrielli S, Calderini P, Moretti A, Pietrobelli M, Tampieri MP, Galuppi R, Cancrini G. Tick reservoirs for piroplasms in central and northern Italy. Vet Parasitol. 2010 Jun 24;170(3-4):291-6. Epub 2010 Feb 26.

Iralu J, Bai Y, Crook L, Tempest B, Simpson G, Mckenzie T, Koster F. Rodent-associated Bartonella febrile illness, Southwestern United States. Emerg Infect Dis. 2006 Jul;12(7):1081-6.

Irshad FA, Gordon RA. Bartonella henselae neuroretinitis in a 15-year-old girl with chronic myelogenous leukemia. J AAPOS. 2009 Dec;13(6):602-4.

Ishihara M, Ohno S, Ono H, Isogai E, Kimura K, Isogai H, Aoki K, et al. Seroprevalence of anti-Borrelia antibodies among patients with confirmed sarcoidosis in a region of Japan where Lyme borreliosis is endemic. Graefes Arch Clin Exp Ophthalmol. 1998;236(4):280-4.

Ishikawa T, Suzuki T, Shinoda M, Takashi H, Yamaguchi H, Suzuki T, Miyake N, Kamiya T. [A case of hepatosplenic cat scratch disease].[Article in Japanese]. Nihon Shokakibyo Gakkai Zasshi. 2006 Sep;103(9):1050-4.

Ismail N, Crossley EC, Stevenson HL, Walker DH. Relative Importance of T-Cell Subsets in Monocytotropic Ehrlichiosis: a Novel Effector Mechanism Involved in Ehrlichia-Induced Immunopathology in Murine Ehrlichiosis. Infect Immun. 2007 Sep;75(9):4608-20. Published online 2007 June 11.

Ismail N, Stevenson HL, Walker DH. Role of Tumor Necrosis Factor Alpha (TNF-α) and Interleukin-10 in the Pathogenesis of Severe Murine Monocytotropic Ehrlichiosis: Increased Resistance of TNF Receptor p55- and p75-Deficient Mice to Fatal Ehrlichial Infection. Infect Immun. 2006 Mar;74(3):1846-56.

Iyer R, Hardham JM, Wormser GP, Schwartz I, Norris SJ. Conservation and heterogeneity of vlsE among human and tick isolates of Borrelia burgdorferi. Infect Immun. 2000 Mar;68(3):1714-8.

Iyer R, Liveris D, Adams A, Nowakowski J, McKenna D, Bittker S, Cooper D, Wormser GP, Schwartz I. Characterization of Borrelia burgdorferi isolated from erythema migrans lesions: interrelationship of three molecular typing methods. J Clin Microbiol. 2001 Aug;39(8):2954-7.

Izri A, Depaquit J, Parola P. Phlebotomine sandflies and transmission of disease agents around the Mediterranean basin. Med Trop (Mars). 2006;66(5):429-435.

Jackson LA, Spach DH. Emergence of Bartonella quintana infection among homeless persons. Emerg Infect Dis. 1996;2(2):141-144.

Jacobi C, Schwark C, Kress B, Hug A, Storch-Hagenlocher B, Schwaninger M. Subarachnoid hemorrhage due to Borrelia burgdorferi-associated vasculitis. Eur J Neurol 2006;13(5):536-8.

Jacobs JC, Stevens M, Duray PH. Lyme disease simulating septic arthritis. JAMA, 256(9)-letters. 1986.

Jacobs, RA. Infectious Diseases: Spirochetal. Current Medical Diagnosis and Treatment, 39th edition. New York:Lange Medical Books/McGraw-Hill. 2000.

Jacomo V, Kelly PJ, Raoult D. Natural history of Bartonella infections (an exception to Koch's postulate). Clin Diagn Lab Immunol. 2002 Jan;9(1):8-18. Review.

Jacquemin L, Bazin C, Lamy C, Chubilleau C, Barale T, Daoudal P, Duhamel C. Babesiose (ou piroplasmose) humaine: a propos de trios observations recentes en France. Maghreb Informations Medicales. 1980;2:31-38.

Jaenson TG, Lindgren E. The range of Ixodes ricinus and the risk of contracting Lyme borreliosis will increase northwards when the vegetation period becomes longer. Ticks Tick Borne Dis. 2011 Mar;2(1):44-9. Epub 2010 Dec 13.

Jain VK, Hilton E, Maytal J, Dorante G, Ilowite NT, Sood SK. Immunoglobulin M immunoblot for diagnosis of Borrelia burgdorferi infection in patients with acute facial palsy. J Clin Microbiol. 1996 Aug;34(8):2033-5.

Jalkanen S, Steere AC, Fox RI, Butcher EC. A distinct endothelial cell recognition system that controls lymphocyte traffic into inflamed synovium. Science. 1986 Aug 1;233(4763):556-8.

James AM, Liveris D, Wormser GP, Schwartz I, Montecalvo MA, Johnson BJ. Borrelia lonestari infection after a bite by an Amblyomma americanum tick. J Infect Dis. 2001 Jun 15;183(12):1810-4. Epub 2001 May 17.

James FM, Engiles JB, Beech J. Meningitis, cranial neuritis, and radiculoneuritis associated with Borrelia burgdorferi infection in a horse. J Am Vet Med Assoc. 2010 Nov 15;237(10):1180-5.

Jardine C, Appleyard G, Kosoy MY, McColl D, Chirino-Trejo M, Wobeser G, Leighton FA. Rodent-associated Bartonella in Saskatchewan, Canada. Vector Borne Zoonotic Dis. 2005 Winter;5(4):402-9.

Jardine C, Waldner C, Wobeser G, Leighton FA. Effect of experimental ectoparasite control on bartonella infections in wild Richardson's ground squirrels. J Wildl Dis. 2006 Oct;42(4):750-8.

Jaruratanasirkul S, Hortiwakul R, Tantisarasart T, Phuenpathom N, Tussanasunthornwong S. Distribution of Azithromycin into brain tissue, cerebrospinal fluid, and aqueous humor of the eye. Antimicrob Agents Chemother. 1996 Mar;40(3):825-6.

Javed MZ, Srivastava M, Zhang S, Kandathil M. Concurrent babesiosis and ehrlichiosis in an elderly host. Mayo Clinic Proceeding 2001;76(5):563-5.

Jeanclaude D, Godmer P, Leveiller D, Pouedras P, Fournier PE, Raoult D, Rolain JM. Bartonella alsatica endocarditis in a French patient in close contact with rabbits. Clin Microbiol Infect. 2009 Dec;15 Suppl 2:110-1. Epub 2009 Apr 30.

Jeandel C, Perret C, Blain H, Jouanny P, Penin F, Laurain MC. Rhabdomyolysis with acute renal failure due to Borrelia burgdorferi. J Intern Med, 235(2):191-2. 1994.

Jeneby MM, Ngeiywa M, Yole DS, Mwenda JM, Suleman MA, Carlson HE. Enzootic simian piroplasm (Entopolypoides macaci) in wild-caught Kenyan non-human primates. J Med Primatol. 2008 Dec;37(6):329-36. Epub 2008 May 27.

Jenkins NE, Ferguson DJ, Alp NJ, Harrison TG, Bowler IC. Urban trench fever presenting as culture-negative endocarditis. QJM. 2009 Jan;102(1):63-5. Epub 2008 Oct 3.

Jensen WA, Fall MZ, Rooney J, Kordick DL, Breitschwerdt EB. Rapid identification and differentiation of Bartonella species using a single-step PCR assay. J Clin Microbiol. 2000 May;38(5):1717-22.

Jewett MW, Jain S, Linowski AK, Sarkar A, Rosa PA. Molecular characterization of the Borrelia burgdorferi in vivo-essential protein PncA. Microbiology. 2011 Oct;157(Pt 10):2831-40. Epub 2011 Jul 21.

Jiang G, Guo M, Wen Z. [Cat-scratch disease].[Article in Chinese]. Lin Chuang Er Bi Yan Hou Ke Za Zhi. 2005 Sep;19(18):820-2. Review.

Jiang S, Gilpin ME, Attia M, Ting YL, Berti PJ. Lyme disease enolpyruvyl-UDP-GlcNAc synthase: fosfomycin-resistant MurA from Borrelia burgdorferi, a fosfomycin-sensitive mutant, and the catalytic role of the active site Asp. Biochemistry. 2011 Mar 29;50(12):2205-12. Epub 2011 Feb 18.

Jiang Y, Hou XX, Geng Z, Hao Q, Wan KL. Interpretation criteria for standardized Western blot for the predominant species of Borrelia burgdorferi sensu lato in China. Biomed Environ Sci. 2010 Oct;23(5):341-9.

Johnson L, Aylward A, Stricker RB. Healthcare access and burden of care for patients with Lyme disease: a large United States survey. Health Policy. 2011 Sep;102(1):64-71. Epub 2011 Jun 14.

Johnson L, Stricker RB. Treatment of Lyme disease: a medicolegal assessment. Expert Rev Anti Infect Ther. 2004 Aug;2(4):533-57. Review.

Johnson L, Stricker RB. Attorney General forces Infectious Diseases Society of America to redo Lyme guidelines due to flawed development process. J Med Ethics. 2009 May;35(5):283-8.

Johnson L, Stricker RB. The Infectious Diseases Society of America Lyme guidelines: a cautionary tale about the development of clinical practice guidelines. Philos Ethics Humanit Med. 2010 Jun 9;5:9.

Johnson L, Stricker RB. Final report of the Lyme disease review panel of the Infectious Diseases Society of America: a pyrrhic victory? Clin Infect Dis. 2010 Nov 1;51(9):1108-9; author reply 1109-1.

Johnson R, Ramos-Vara J, Vemulapalli R. Identification of Bartonella henselae in an aborted equine fetus. Vet Pathol. 2009 Mar;46(2):277-81.

Johnson RC. Leptospira. In: Baron S, editor. Medical Microbiology. 4th edition. Galveston (TX): University of Texas Medical Branch at Galveston; 1996. Chapter 35.

Johnson RC, Kodner C, Jarnefeld J, Eck DK, Xu Y. Agents of Human Anaplasmosis and Lyme Disease at Camp Ripley, Minnesota. Vector Borne Zoonotic Dis. 2011 Aug 25. [Epub ahead of print]

Johnson ST, Cable RG, Leiby DA. Lookback investigations of Babesia microti-seropositive blood donors: seven-year experience in a Babesia-endemic area. Transfusion. 2011 Sep 12. [Epub ahead of print]

Johnson ST, Cable RG, Tonnetti L, Spencer B, Rios J, Leiby DA. Seroprevalence of Babesia microti in blood donors from Babesia-endemic areas of the northeastern United States: 2000 through 2007. Transfusion. 2009 Dec;49(12):2574-82. Epub 2009 Oct 10.

Johnston YE, Duray PH, Steere AC, Kashgarian M, Buza J, Malawista SE, Askenase PW. Lyme arthritis. Spirochetes found in synovial microangiopathic lesions. Am J Pathol. 1985 Jan;118(1):26-34.

Jones, JH. Bad Blood: The Tuskegee Syphilis Experiment, expanded edition (New York: Free Press, 1993).

Jones KL, Glickstein LJ, Damle N, Sikand VK, McHugh G, Steere AC. Borrelia burgdorferi genetic markers and disseminated disease in patients with early Lyme disease. J Clin Microbiol. 2006 Dec;44(12):4407-13. Epub 2006 Oct 11.

Jones KL, McHugh GA, Glickstein LJ, Steere AC. Analysis of Borrelia burgdorferi genotypes in patients with Lyme arthritis: High frequency of ribosomal RNA intergenic spacer type 1 strains in antibiotic-refractory arthritis. Arthritis Rheum. 2009 Jul;60(7):2174-82.

Jones KL, Muellegger RR, Means TK, Lee M, Glickstein LJ, Damle N, Sikand VK, Luster AD, Steere AC. Higher mRNA levels of chemokines and cytokines associated with macrophage activation in erythema migrans skin lesions in patients from the United States than in patients from Austria with Lyme borreliosis. Clin Infect Dis. 2008 Jan 1;46(1):85-92.

Jones KL, Seward RJ, Ben-Menachem G, Glickstein LJ, Costello CE, Steere AC. Strong IgG antibody responses to Borrelia burgdorferi glycolipids in patients with Lyme arthritis, a late manifestation of the infection. Clin Immunol. 2009 Jul;132(1):93-102. Epub 2009 Apr 2.

Jones SL, Maggi R, Shuler J, Alward A, Breitschwerdt EB. Detection of Bartonella henselae in the blood of 2 adult horses. J Vet Intern Med. 2008 Mar-Apr;22(2):495-8. Epub 2008 Mar 10.

Joseph JT, Roy SS, Shams N, Visintainer P, Nadelman RB, Hosur S, Nelson J, Wormser GP. Babesiosis in Lower Hudson Valley, New York, USA. Emerg Infect Dis. 2011 May;17(5):843-7.

Juchnowicz D, Rudnik I, Czernikiewicz A, Zajkowska J, Pancewicz SA. [Mental disorders in the course of Lyme borreliosis and tick-borne encephalitis].[Article in Polish]. Przegl Epidemiol. 2002;56 Suppl 1:37-50.

Just FT, Gilles J, Pradel I, Pfalzer S, Lengauer H, Hellmann K, Pfister K. Molecular evidence for Bartonella spp. in cat and dog fleas from Germany and France. Zoonoses Public Health. 2008 Oct;55(8-10):514-20. Epub 2008 May 16.

Kabacoff RI, Segal DL, Hersen M, Van Hasselt VB. Psychometric properties and diagnostic utility of the Beck Anxiety Inventory and the State-Trait Anxiety Inventory with older adult psychiatric outpatients. J Anxiety Disord. 1997;11(1):33-47.

Kabeya H, Colborn JM, Bai Y, Lerdthusnee K, Richardson JH, Maruyama S, Kosoy MY. Detection of Bartonella tamiae DNA in ectoparasites from rodents in Thailand and their sequence similarity with bacterial cultures from Thai patients. Vector Borne Zoonotic Dis. 2010 Jun;10(5):429-34.

Kabeya H, Tsunoda E, Maruyama S, Mikami T. Immune responses of immunocompetent and immunocompromised mice experimentally infected with Bartonella henselae. J Vet Med Sci. 2003 Apr;65(4):479-84.

Kaçar N, Taşli L, Demirkan N, Ergin C, Ergin S. HIV-negative case of bacillary angiomatosis with chronic hepatitis B. J Dermatol. 2010 Aug;37(8):722-5.

Kachur SP, Reller ME, Barber AM, Barat LM, Koumans EH, Parise ME, Roberts J, Ruebush TK 2nd, Zucker JR. Malaria surveillance–United States, 1994. MMWR. CDC Surveill. Summ. 1997;Oct 17;46(5):1-18.

Kaewmongkol G, Kaewmongkol S, Fleming PA, Adams PJ, Ryan U, Irwin PJ, Fenwick SG. Zoonotic Bartonella Species in Fleas and Blood from Red Foxes in Australia. Vector Borne Zoonotic Dis. 2011 Sep 15. [Epub ahead of print]

Kaewmongkol G, Kaewmongkol S, McInnes LM, Burmej H, Bennett MD, Adams PJ, Ryan U, Irwin PJ, Fenwick SG. Genetic characterization of flea-derived Bartonella species from native animals in Australia suggests host-parasite co-evolution. Infect Genet Evol. 2011 Aug 12. [Epub ahead of print]

Kaewmongkol G, Kaewmongkol S, Owen H, Fleming PA, Adams PJ, Ryan U, Irwin PJ, Fenwick SG. Candidatus Bartonella antechini: a novel Bartonella species detected in fleas and ticks from the yellow-footed antechinus (Antechinus flavipes), an Australian marsupial. Vet Microbiol. 2011 May 5;149(3-4):517-21. Epub 2010 Dec 8.

Kager PA, Schultz MJ, Zijlstra EE, et al. Arteether administration in humans: preliminary studies of pharmacokinetics, safety, and tolerance. Transactions of the Royal Society of Tropical Medicine and Hygiene. 1994;88:53-54.

Kaiser PO, Riess T, O'Rourke F, Linke D, Kempf VA. Bartonella spp.: throwing light on uncommon human infections. Int J Med Microbiol. 2011 Jan;301(1):7-15. Epub 2010 Sep 15. Review.

Kaiser PO, Riess T, Wagner CL, Linke D, Lupas AN, Schwarz H, Raddatz G, Schäfer A, Kempf VA. The head of Bartonella adhesin A is crucial for host cell interaction of Bartonella henselae. Cell Microbiol. 2008 Nov;10(11):2223-34. Epub 2008 Jul 7.

Kakkilaya, BS. The Malaria Site. Malaria Risk in Africa. Available from: http://www.malariasite.com/malaria/ artemisinin.htm. Accessed August 12,13 & 26, 2006.

Kalina P, Decker A, Kornel E, Halperin JJ. Lyme disease of the brainstem. Neuroradiology. 2005 Dec;47(12):903-7.

Kalish RA, McHugh G, Granquist J, Shea B, Ruthazer R, Steere AC. Persistence of immunoglobulin M or immunoglobulin G antibody responses to Borrelia burgdorferi 10-20 years after active Lyme disease. Clin Infect Dis. 2001 Sep 15;33(6):780-5. Epub 2001 Aug 10.

Kalish RA, Kaplan RF, Taylor E, Jones-Woodward L, Workman K, Steere AC. Evaluation of study patients with Lyme disease, 10-20-year follow-up. J Infect Dis. 2001 Feb 1;183(3):453-60. Epub 2000 Dec 27.

Kalish RA, Leong JM, Steere AC. Early and late antibody responses to full-length and truncated constructs of outer surface protein A of Borrelia burgdorferi in Lyme disease. Infect Immun. 1995 Jun;63(6):2228-35.

Kalish RA, Leong JM, Steere AC. Association of treatment-resistant chronic Lyme arthritis with HLA-DR4 and antibody reactivity to OspA and OspB of Borrelia burgdorferi. Infect Immun. 1993 Jul;61(7):2774-9.

Kalogeropoulos C, Koumpoulis I, Mentis A, Pappa C, Zafeiropoulos P, Aspiotis M. Bartonella and intraocular inflammation: a series of cases and review of literature. Clinical Ophthalmology, June 2011 Volume 2011:5, pages 817-829.

Kaminsky P, Grignon Y, Deibener J, Maurer P, Duc M. Nervous system borreliosis with pseudo-lymphoma cells in cerebrospinal fluid. Rev Neurol (Paris). 154(2):170-2. 1998.

Kamoi K, Yoshida T, Takase H, Yokota M, Kawaguchi T, Mochizuki M. Seroprevalence of Bartonella henselae in patients with uveitis and healthy individuals in Tokyo. Jpn J Ophthalmol. 2009 Sep;53(5):490-3. Epub 2009 Oct 22.

Kämpfer P, Rosselló-Mora R, Scholz HC, Welinder-Olsson C, Falsen E, Busse HJ. Description of Pseudochrobactrum gen. nov., with the two species Pseudochrobactrum asaccharolyticum sp. nov. and Pseudochrobactrum saccharolyticum sp. nov. Int J Syst Evol Microbiol. 2006 Aug;56(Pt 8):1823-9.

Kamradt T, Lengl-Janssen B, Strauss AF, Bansal G, Steere AC. Dominant recognition of a Borrelia burgdorferi outer surface protein A peptide by T helper cells in patients with treatment-resistant Lyme arthritis. Infect Immun. 1996 Apr;64(4):1284-9.

Kan L, Sood SK, Maytal J. Pseudotumor cerebri in Lyme disease: a case report and literature review. Pediatr Neurol. 1998 May;18(5):439-41. Review.

Kannian P, Drouin EE, Glickstein L, Kwok WW, Nepom GT, Steere AC. Decline in the frequencies of Borrelia burgdorferi OspA161 175-specific T cells after antibiotic therapy in HLA-DRB1*0401-positive patients with antibiotic-responsive or antibiotic-refractory lyme arthritis. J Immunol. 2007 Nov 1;179(9):6336-42.

Kannian P, McHugh G, Johnson BJ, Bacon RM, Glickstein LJ, Steere AC. Antibody responses to Borrelia burgdorferi in patients with antibiotic-refractory, antibiotic-responsive, or non-antibiotic-treated Lyme arthritis. Arthritis Rheum. 2007 Dec;56(12):4216-25.

Kaplan RF, Jones-Woodward L, Workman K, Steere AC, Logigian EL, Meadows ME. Neuropsychological deficits in Lyme disease patients with and without other evidence of central nervous system pathology. Appl Neuropsychol. 1999;6(1):3-11.

Kaplan RF, Meadows ME, Vincent LC, Logigian EL, Steere AC. Memory impairment and depression in patients with Lyme encephalopathy: comparison with fibromyalgia and nonpsychotically depressed patients. Neurology. 1992 Jul;42(7):1263-7.

Kaplan RF, Trevino RP, Johnson GM, Levy L, Dornbush R, Hu LT, Evans J, Weinstein A, Schmid CH, Klempner MS. Cognitive function in post-treatment Lyme disease: Do additional antibiotics help? Neurology. 2003 Jun 24;60:1916-22.

Karan' LS, Koliasnikova NM, Toporkova MG, Makhneva MA, Nadezhdina MV, Esaulkova AIu, Romanenko VV, Arumova EA, Platonov AE, Maleev VV. [Usage of real time polymerase chain reaction for diagnostics of different tick-borne infections]. [Article in Russian]. Zh Mikrobiol Epidemiol Immunobiol. 2010 May-Jun;(3):72-7.

Kariu T, Coleman AS, Anderson JF, Pal U. Methods for rapid transfer and localization of lyme disease pathogens within the tick gut. J Vis Exp. 2011 Feb 14;(48). pii: 2544.

Karma A, Seppala I, Mikkila H, Kaakkola S, Viljanen M, Tarkkanen A. Diagnosis and clinical characteristics of ocular Lyme borreliosis. Am J Ophthalmol. 119(2):127-35. 1995.

Karna SL, Sanjuan E, Esteve-Gassent MD, Miller CL, Maruskova M, Seshu J. CsrA modulates levels of lipoproteins and key regulators of gene expression critical for pathogenic mechanisms of Borrelia burgdorferi. Infect Immun. 2011 Feb;79(2):732-44. Epub 2010 Nov 15.

Karolak J, Gotz-Wipckowska A. [Neuroretinitis in cat scratch disease].[Article in Polish]. Klin Oczna. 2010;112(4-6):131-4.

Karras A, Thervet E, Legendre C; Groupe Coopératif de transplantation d'Ile de France. Hemophagocytic syndrome in renal transplant recipients: report of 17 cases and review of literature. Transplantation. 2004 Jan 27;77(2):238-43. Review.

Kathiresan S, Kelsey PB, Steere AC, Foster CS, Curvelo MS, Stone JR. Case records of the Massachusetts General Hospital. Case 14-2005. A 38-year-old man with fever and blurred vision. N Engl J Med. 2005 May 12;352(19):2003-12.

Katzel, J., Is there a consensus in treatment of Lyme Borreliosis?, in Lyme Disease 1991 Patient/Physician Perspectives from the U.S. & Canada, L. Mermin, Editor. 1992.

Kauffmann DJ, Wormser GP. Ocular Lyme disease: case report and review of the literature. Br J Ophthalmol. 1990 Jun;74(6):325-7. Review.

Kaufman LD, Gruber BL, Phillips ME, Benach JL. Late cutaneous Lyme disease: acrodermatitis chronica atrophicans. Am J Med, 86(6 Pt 2):828-30. 1989.

Kawagishi N, Takahashi H, Hashimoto Y, Miyamoto K, Iizuka H. A case of Lyme disease with parotitis. Dermatology. 1998;197(4):386-7.

Kazakoff MA, Sinusas K, Macchia C. Liver function test abnormalities in early Lyme disease. Arch Fam Med. 2(4):409-13. 1993.

Kazragis RJ, Dever LL, Jorgensen JH, Barbour AG. In vivo activities of ceftriaxone and vancomycin against Borrelia spp. in the mouse brain and other sites. Antimicrobial Agents & Chemotherapy, Nov;40(11):2632-6. 1996.

Keilp JG, Corbera K, Slavov I, Taylor MJ, Sackeim HA, Fallon BA. WAIS-III and WMS-III performance in chronic Lyme disease. J Int Neuropsychol Soc. 2006 Jan;12(1):119-29.

Keirans JE, Hutcheson HJ, Durden LA, Klompen JS. Ixodes (Ixodes) scapularis (Acari:Ixodidae): redescription of all active stages, distribution, hosts, geographical variation, and medical and veterinary importance. J Med Entomol. 1996 May;33(3):297-318.

Kelly B, Finnegan P, Cormican M, Calllaghan J. Lyme disease and glomerulonephritis. Irish Med J, 92(5):372-373. 1999.

Kelly P, Rolain JM, Maggi R, Sontakke S, Keene B, Hunter S, Lepidi H, Breitschwerdt KT, Breitschwerdt EB. Bartonella quintana endocarditis in dogs. Emerg Infect Dis. 2006 Dec;12(12):1869-72.

Kelly P, Rolain JM, Raoult D. Prevalence of human pathogens in cat and dog fleas in New Zealand. N Z Med J. 2005 Nov 25;118(1226):U1754.

Kelly PJ, Eoghain GN, Raoult D. Antibodies reactive with Bartonella henselae and Ehrlichia canis in dogs from the communal lands of Zimbabwe. J S Afr Vet Assoc. 2004 Sep;75(3):116-20.

Kelly PJ, Matthewman LA, Hayter D, Downey S, Wray K, Bryson NR, Raoult D. Bartonella (Rochalimaea) henselae in southern Africa--evidence for infections in domestic cats and implications for veterinarians. J S Afr Vet Assoc. 1996 Dec;67(4):182-7.

Kelly PJ, Meads N, Theobald A, Fournier PE, Raoult D. Rickettsia felis, Bartonella henselae, and B. clarridgeiae, New Zealand. Emerg Infect Dis. 2004 May;10(5):967-8.

Kelly PJ, Midwinter A, Rolain JM, Raoult D. Polymerase chain reaction (PCR) survey for rickettsias and bartonellas in ticks from New Zealand. N Z Vet J. 2005 Dec;53(6):468-9.

Kelly PJ, Moura L, Miller T, Thurk J, Perreault N, Weil A, Maggio R, Lucas H, Breitschwerdt E. Feline immunodeficiency virus, feline leukemia virus and Bartonella species in stray cats on St Kitts, West Indies. J Feline Med Surg. 2010 Jun;12(6):447-50. Epub 2010 Feb 6.

Kenedy MR, Akins DR. The OspE-related proteins inhibit complement deposition and enhance serum resistance of Borrelia burgdorferi, the lyme disease spirochete. Infect Immun. 2011 Apr;79(4):1451-7. Epub 2011 Jan 31.

Kern A, Collin E, Barthel C, Michel C, Jaulhac B, Boulanger N. Tick saliva represses innate immunity and cutaneous inflammation in a murine model of lyme disease. Vector Borne Zoonotic Dis. 2011 Oct;11(10):1343-50. Epub 2011 May 25.

Kernif T, Aissi M, Doumandji SE, Chomel BB, Raoult D, Bitam I. Molecular evidence of Bartonella infection in domestic dogs from Algeria, North Africa, by polymerase chain reaction (PCR). Am J Trop Med Hyg. 2010 Aug;83(2):298-300.

Kernif T, Parola P, Davoust B, Plaire L, Cabre O, Raoult D, Rolain JM. Bartonella clarridgeiae in Fleas, Tahiti, French Polynesia. Emerg Infect Dis. 2011 Sep;17(9):1773-5.

Kernif T, Parola P, Ricci JC, Raoult D, Rolain JM. Molecular detection of Bartonella alsatica in rabbit fleas, France. Emerg Infect Dis. 2010 Dec;16(12):2013-4.

Kersten A, Poitschek C, Rauch S, Aberer E. Effects of penicillin, ceftriaxone, and doxycycline on the morphology of Borrelia burgdorferi. Antimicrobial Agents & Chemotherapy, 39(5):1127-33. 1995.

Kessler RJ, Rankin S, Young S, O'Shea K, Calabrese M, Guldin A, Lipson N, Oakley DA, Giger U. Pseudomonas fluorescens contamination of a feline packed red blood cell unit and studies of canine units. Vet Clin Pathol. 2010 March; 39(1): 29–38. Published online 2009 October 15.

Kesteman T, Rossi C, Bastien P, Brouillard J, Avesani V, Olive N, Martin P, Delmée M. Prevalence and genetic heterogeneity of Borrelia burgdorferi sensu lato in Ixodes ticks in Belgium. Acta Clin Belg. 2010 Sep-Oct;65(5):319-22.

Keynan Y, Yakirevitch E, Shusterman T, Alter-Migdal E, Avidor B, Weber G, Giladi M. Bone marrow and skin granulomatosis in a patient with Bartonella infection. J Med Microbiol. 2007 Jan;56(Pt 1):133-5.

Khoudri I, Frémont G, Flageul B, Brière J, Dubertret L, Viguier M. [Bilateral inguinal lymphadenopathy and erythema nodosum: an uncommon presentation of cat scratch disease].[Article in French]. Rev Med Interne. 2011 Mar;32(3):e34-6. Epub 2010 Jun 19.

Kielian T. Toll-Like Receptors in Central Nervous System Glial Inflammation and Homeostasis. J Neurosci Res. 2006 April; 83(5): 711–730.

Kielich M, Fiedler A, Driever PH, Weis R, Schwabe D, Jacobi G. Lyme borreliosis mimicking central nervous system malignancy: the diagnostic pitfall of cerebrospinal fluid cytology. Brain Dev, 22(6):403-6. 2000.

Kim DM, Yu KD, Lee JH, Kim HK, Lee SH. Controlled trial of a 5-day course of telithromycin versus doxycycline for treatment of mild to moderate scrub typhus. Antimicrob Agents Chemother. 2007 Jun;51(6):2011-5. Epub 2007 Apr 2.

Kim JY, Cho SH, Joo HN, Tsuji M, Cho SR, Park IJ, Chung GT, Ju JW, Cheun HI, Lee HW, Lee YH, Kim TS. First case of human babesiosis in Korea: detection and characterization of a novel type of Babesia sp. (KO1) similar to ovine babesia. J Clin Microbiol. 2007 Jun;45(6):2084-7. Epub 2007 Mar 28.

Kim SJ, Kim MS, Lee JW, Lee CH, Yoo H, Shin SH, Park MJ, Lee SH. Dihydroartemisinin enhances radiosensitivity of human glioma cells in vitro. J Cancer Res Clin Oncol. 2006 Feb;132(2):129-35. [Epub 2005 Nov. 5]

Kirby JE. In Vitro Model of Bartonella henselae-Induced Angiogenesis. Infect Immun. 2004 December; 72(12): 7315–7317.

Kirby JE, Nekorchuk DM. Bartonella-associated endothelial proliferation depends on inhibition of apoptosis. Proc Natl Acad Sci U S A. 2002 April 2; 99(7): 4656–4661. Published online 2002 March 19.

Kirchner M, Brunner A, Edelhofer R, Joachim A. [Vector-borne parasites of dogs on the Islands of Cabo Verde]. [Article in German]. Wien Klin Wochenschr. 2008;120(19-20 Suppl 4):49-53.

Kirmizis D, Efstratiadis G, Economidou D, Diza-Mataftsi E, Leontsini M, Memmos D. MPGN secondary to Lyme disease. [MPGN = Mesangiocapillary Glomerulonephritis]. Am J Kidney Dis, 43:544-551. 2004.

Kirsch M, Ruben FL, Steere AC, Duray PH, Norden CW, Winkelstein A. Fatal adult respiratory distress syndrome in a patient with Lyme disease. JAMA. 1988 May 13;259(18):2737-9.

Kiss T, Cadar D, Krupaci AF, Bordeanu A, Brudaşcǎ GF, Mihalca AD, Mircean V, Gliga L, Dumitrache MO, Spînu M. Serological Reactivity to Borrelia burgdorferi Sensu Lato in Dogs and Horses from Distinct Areas in Romania. Vector Borne Zoonotic Dis. 2011 Sep;11(9):1259-62. Epub 2011 May 25.

Kitchell BE, Fan TM, Kordick D, Breitschwerdt EB, Wollenberg G, Lichtensteiger CA. Peliosis hepatis in a dog infected with Bartonella henselae. J Am Vet Med Assoc. 2000 Feb 15;216(4):519-23, 517.

Kitchen LW, Vaughn DW, Skillman DR. Role of US military research programs in the development of US food and drug administration-approved antimaleria drugs. Reviews of anti-infective agents. Clin Infect Dis. 2006 Jul 1;43(1):67-71. Epub 2006 May 24

Kjelland V, Stuen S, Skarpaas T, Slettan A. Borrelia burgdorferi sensu lato in Ixodes ricinus ticks collected from migratory birds in Southern Norway. Acta Vet Scand. 2010 Nov 6;52:59.

Kjelland V, Ytrehus B, Vikørren T, Stuen S, Skarpaas T, Slettan A. Borrelia burgdorferi sensu lato detected in skin of Norwegian mountain hares (Lepus timidus) without signs of dissemination. J Wildl Dis. 2011 Apr;47(2):293-9.

Kjemtrup AM, Lee B, Fritz CL, Evans C, Chervenak M, Conrad PA. Investigation of transfusion transmission of a WA1-type babesial parasite to a premature infant in California. Transfusion. 2002;42:1482-7.

Klayman D. Qinghaosu (Artemisinin): Antimalarial Drug from China. Science, 1985, May 31;238:p.1049.

Klayman DL, Ager AL Jr, Fleckenstein L, Lin AJ. Transdermal artelinic acid: an effective treatment for Plasmodium berghei-infected mice. Am J Trop Med Hyg. 1991 Nov;45(5):602-7.

Klempner MS, Hu LT, Evans J, Schmid CH, Johnson GM, Trevino RP, Norton D, Levy L, Wall D, McCall J, Kosinski M, Weinstein A. Two controlled trials of antibiotic treatment in patients with persistent symptoms and a history of Lyme disease. N Engl J Med. 2001 Jul 12;345:85-92.

Klempner MS, Noring R, Rogers RA. Invasion of Human Skin Fibroblasts by the Lyme Disease Spirochete, Borrelia burgdorferi. J Infect Diseases 1993;67:1074-81.

Klempner MS, Schmid CH, Hu L, Steere AC, Johnson G, McCloud B, Noring R, Weinstein A. Intralaboratory reliability of serologic and urine testing for Lyme disease. Am J Med. 2001 Feb 15;110(3):217-9.

Klempner MS, Wormser GH, Wade K, Trevino RP, Tang J, Kaslow RA, Schmid C. A case-control study to examine HLA haplotype associations in patients with posttreatment chronic Lyme disease. J Infect Dis. 2005 Sep 15;192(6):1010-3. Epub 2005 Aug 4.

Klieneberger-Nobel E. The filterable forms of bacteria. Bacteriol Rev, 15:77-103. 1951.

Klingebiel R, Benndorf G, Schmitt M, von Moers A, Lehmann R. Large cerebral vessel occlusive disease in Lyme neuroborreliosis. Neuropediatrics, 33(1):37-40. 2002.

Klotz SA, Ianas V, Elliott SP. Cat-scratch Disease. Am Fam Physician. 2011 Jan 15;83(2):152-5. Review.

Knauer J, Krupka I, Fueldner C, Lehmann J, Straubinger RK. Evaluation of the preventive capacities of a topically applied azithromycin formulation against Lyme borreliosis in a murine model. J Antimicrob Chemother. 2011 Sep 15. [Epub ahead of print]

Kobayashi K, Mizukoshi C, Aoki T, Muramori F, Hayashi M, et al. Borrelia burgdoferi-seropositive chronic encephalomyelopathy: Lyme neuroborreliosis? An autopsied report. Dement Geriatr Cogn Disord, 8(6):384-90. 1997.

Kodama Y, Maeno N, Nishi J, Imuta N, Oda H, Tanaka S, Kono Y, Kawano Y. Multifocal osteomyelitis due to Bartonella henselae in a child without focal pain. J Infect Chemother. 2007 Oct;13(5):350-2. Epub 2007 Oct 30.

Koening CL, Miller JC, Nelson JM, Ward DM, Kushner JP, Bockenstedt LK, Weis JJ, Kaplan J, De Domenico I. Toll-like receptors mediate induction of hepcidin in mice infected with Borrelia burgdorferi. Blood. 2009 August 27; 114(9): 1913–1918. Prepublished online 2009 July 8.

Koesling J, Aebischer T, Falch C, Schulein R, Dehio C. Cutting edge: antibody-mediated cessation of hemotropic infection by the intraerythrocytic mouse pathogen Bartonella grahamii. J Immunol. 2001;167(1):11-14.

Koga T, Taguchi J, Suzuki M, Higa Y, Kamimura T, Nishimura M, Arakawa M. Cat scratch disease presenting with a retroperitoneal abscess in a patient without animal contacts. J Infect Chemother. 2009 Dec;15(6):414-6. Epub .

Koga T, Taguchi J, Suzuki M, Higa Y, Kamimura T, Nishimura M, Arakawa M. A "silent culture-negative" abdominal aortic mycotic aneurysm: Rapid detection of Bartonella species using PCR and high-throughput mass spectrometry. Hawaii Med J. 2010 Mar;69(3):68-9.

Kohler J. Lyme borreliosis: a case of transverse myelitis with syrinx cavity. Neurology, 39(11):1553-4. 1989.

Kohler J, Kern U, Kasper J, Rhese-Kupper B, Thoden U. Chronic central nervous system involvement in Lyme borreliosis. Neurology, 38(6):863-7. 1988.

Kohler J, Schneider H, Vogt A. High-dose intravenous penicillin G does not prevent further progression in early neurological manifestation of Lyme borreliosis. 1989. Infection, 17(4):216-7.

Köhler W. Killed in action: microbiologists and clinicians as victims of their occupation. Part 2: Yellow fever and bartonellosis. Int J Med Microbiol. 2005 Aug;295(4):193-200.

Köllisch G, Kalali BN, Voelcker V, Wallich R, Behrendt H, Ring J, Bauer S, Jakob T, Mempel M, Ollert M. Various members of the Toll-like receptor family contribute to the innate immune response of human epidermal keratinocytes. Immunology. 2005 April; 114(4): 531–541.

Kolören Z, Avşar C, Şekeroğlu ZA. [Diagnosis of protozoa by loop-mediated isothermal amplification: (LAMP)].[Article in Turkish]. Turkiye Parazitol Derg. 2010;34(4):207-11.

Kon Y. Über die Silberreaktion der Zellen. Jena, Gustav Fischer. 1933.

Koranda FC. Antimalarials. J Am Acad Dermatol. 1981 Jun;4(6):650-5.

Kordick DL, Breitschwerdt EB. Intraerythrocytic presence of Bartonella henselae. J Clin Microbiol. 1995;33(6):1655-1656.

Kordick DL, Breitschwerdt EB. Relapsing bacteremia after blood transmission of Bartonella henselae to cats. Am J Vet Res. 1997 May;58(5):492-7.

Kordick DL, Breitschwerdt EB. Persistent infection of pets within a household with three Bartonella species. Emerg Infect Dis. 1998 Apr-Jun;4(2):325-8.

Kordick DL, Brown TT, Shin K, Breitschwerdt EB. Clinical and pathologic evaluation of chronic Bartonella henselae or Bartonella clarridgeiae infection in cats. J Clin Microbiol. 1999 May;37(5):1536-47.

Kordick DL, Hilyard EJ, Hadfield TL, Wilson KH, Steigerwalt AG, Brenner DJ, Breitschwerdt EB. Bartonella clarridgeiae, a newly recognized zoonotic pathogen causing inoculation papules, fever, and lymphadenopathy (cat scratch disease). J Clin Microbiol. 1997 Jul;35(7):1813-8.

Kordick DL, Papich MG, Breitschwerdt EB. Efficacy of enrofloxacin or doxycycline for treatment of Bartonella henselae or Bartonella clarridgeiae infection in cats. Antimicrob Agents Chemother. 1997 Nov;41(11):2448-55.

Kordick DL, Swaminathan B, Greene CE, Wilson KH, Whitney AM, O'Connor S, Hollis DG, Matar GM, Steigerwalt AG, Malcolm GB, Hayes PS, Hadfield TL, Breitschwerdt EB, Brenner DJ. Bartonella vinsonii subsp. berkhoffii subsp. nov., isolated from dogs; Bartonella vinsonii subsp. vinsonii; and emended description of Bartonella vinsonii. Int J Syst Bacteriol. 1996 Jul;46(3):704-9.

Kordick DL, Wilson KH, Sexton DJ, Hadfield TL, Berkhoff HA, Breitschwerdt EB. Prolonged Bartonella bacteremia in cats associated with cat-scratch disease patients. J Clin Microbiol. 1995 Dec;33(12):3245-51.

Kordick SK, Breitschwerdt EB, Hegarty BC, Southwick KL, Colitz CM, Hancock SI, Bradley JM, Rumbough R, Mcpherson JT, MacCormack JN. Coinfection with multiple tick-borne pathogens in a Walker Hound kennel in North Carolina. J Clin Microbiol. 1999 Aug;37(8):2631-8.

Koren G. Antimalarial drugs for rheumatoid disease during pregnancy. Can Fam Physician. 1999 Dec;45:2869-70.

Korenberg EI. Problems in the study and prophylaxis of mixed infections transmitted by ixodid ticks. Int J Med Microbiol. 2004;293 Suppl 37:80-5.

Kornblatt AN, Steere AC, Brownstein DG. Infection in rabbits with the Lyme disease spirochete. Yale J Biol Med. 1984 Jul-Aug;57(4):613-6.

Kornblatt AN, Urband PH, Steere AC. Arthritis caused by Borrelia burgdorferi in dogs. J Am Vet Med Assoc. 1985 May 1;186(9):960-4.

Kornblatt AN, Steere AC, Brownstein DG. Experimental Lyme disease in rabbits: spirochetes found in erythema migrans and blood. Infect Immun. 1984 Oct;46(1):220-3.

Kornmehl EW, Lesser RL, Jaros P, Rocco E, Steere AC. Bilateral keratitis in Lyme disease. Ophthalmology. 1989 Aug;96(8):1194-7.

Korotkov IuS, Kislenko GS, Burenkova LA, Rudnikova NA, Karan' LS. [Spatial and temporal variability of Ixodes ricinus and Ixodes persulcatus infection with the Lyme disease agent in Moscow Region]. [Article in Russian]. Parazitologiia. 2008 Nov-Dec;42(6):441-51.

Koryzna K, Skomro P, Leśniewski S, Szych Z. [Oral cavity health condition of HIV carriers].[Article in Polish]. Ann Acad Med Stetin. 2008;54(3):77-80.

Kosoy M, Bai Y, Lynch T, Kuzmin IV, Niezgoda M, Franka R, Agwanda B, Breiman RF, Rupprecht CE. Bartonella spp. in bats, Kenya. Emerg Infect Dis. 2010 Dec;16(12):1875-81.

Kosoy M, Bai Y, Sheff K, Morway C, Baggett H, Maloney SA, Boonmar S, Bhengsri S, Dowell SF, Sitdhirasdr A, Lerdthusnee K, Richardson J, Peruski LF. Identification of Bartonella infections in febrile human patients from Thailand and their potential animal reservoirs. Am J Trop Med Hyg. 2010 Jun;82(6):1140-5.

Kosoy M, Morway C, Sheff KW, Bai Y, Colborn J, Chalcraft L, Dowell SF, Peruski LF, Maloney SA, Baggett H, Sutthirattana S, Sidhirat A, Maruyama S, Kabeya H, Chomel BB, Kasten R, Popov V, Robinson J, Kruglov A, Petersen LR. Bartonella tamiae sp. nov., a newly recognized pathogen isolated from three human patients from Thailand. J Clin Microbiol. 2008 Feb;46(2):772-5. Epub 2007 Dec 12.

Köster LS, Van Schoor M, Goddard A, Thompson PN, Matjila PT, Kjelgaard-Hansen M. C-reactive protein in canine babesiosis caused by Babesia rossi and its association with outcome. J S Afr Vet Assoc. 2009 Jun;80(2):87-91.

Kostick JL, Szkotnicki LT, Rogers EA, Bocci P, Raffaelli N, Marconi RT. The diguanylate cyclase, Rrp1, regulates critical steps in the enzootic cycle of the Lyme disease spirochetes. Mol Microbiol. 2011 Jul;81(1):219-31. Epub 2011 Jun 5.

Kotilainen P, Heiro M, Jalava J, Rantakokko V, Nikoskelainen J, Nikkari S, Rantakokko-Jalava K. Aetiological diagnosis of infective endocarditis by direct amplification of rRNA genes from surgically removed valve tissue. An 11-year experience in a Finnish teaching hospital. Ann Med. 2006;38(4):263-73.

Kotsyfakis M, Horka H, Salat J, Andersen JF. The crystal structures of two salivary cystatins from the tick Ixodes scapularis and the effect of these inhibitors on the establishment of Borrelia burgdorferi infection in a murine model. Mol Microbiol. 2010 July; 77(2): 456–470. Published online 2010 June 1.

Krakowetz CN, Lindsay LR, Chilton NB. Genetic diversity in Ixodes scapularis (Acari: Ixodidae) from six established populations in Canada. Ticks Tick Borne Dis. 2011 Sep;2(3):143-50. Epub 2011 Jul 28.

Krause PJ, Gewurz BE, Hill D, Marty FM, Vannier E, Foppa IM, Furman RR, Neuhaus E, Skowron G, Gupta S, McCalla C, Pesanti EL, Young M, Heiman D, Hsue G, Gelfand JA, Wormser GP, Dickason J, Bia FJ, Hartman B, Telford SR 3rd, Christianson D, Dardick K, Coleman M, Girotto JE, Spielman A. Persistent and relapsing babesiosis in immunocompromised patients. Clin Infect Dis. 2008 Feb 1;46(3):370-6.

Krause PJ, Grant-Kels JM, Tahan SR, Dardick KR, Alarcon-Chaidez F, Bouchard K, Visini C, Deriso C, Foppa IM, Wikel S. Dermatologic Changes Induced by Repeated Ixodes scapularis Bites and Implications for Prevention of Tick-Borne Infection. Vector Borne Zoonotic Dis. 2009 December; 9(6): 603–610.

Krause, PJ. Spielman, A, Telford, SR et al. Persistent parasitemia after acute Babesiosis. N. Engl. J. Med. 1998; 339:160.

Krause, PJ, Telford, SR, Spielman, A, Sikand V, Ryan R, Christianson D, Burke G, Brassard P, Pollack R, Peck J, Persing DH. Concurrent Lyme disease and Babesiosis. JAMA. 1996;275 (21):1657.

Krause PJ, Lepore T, Sikand VK, Gadbaw J Jr, Burke G, Telford SR III, Brassard P, Pearl D, Azlanzadeh J, Christianson D, McGrath D, Spielman A. Atovaquone and azithromycin for the treatment of babesiosis. New England Journal of Medicine. 2000;343:1454-8.

Krause PJ. Babesiosis. Medical Clinics of North America. March 2002;Vol. 86. [cited 2006 Aug]. Available from: http://home. mdconsult.com.

Krause R, Piswanger-Soelkner C, Lipp RW, Daxböck F, Schnedl WJ, Hoier S, Reisinger EC. Somatostatin receptor scintigraphy in patients with cat-scratch disease. Nuklearmedizin. 2006;45(4):160-2. Erratum in: Nuklearmedizin. 2006;45(5):234.

Kreisel D, Pasque MK, Damiano RJ Jr, Medoff G, Kates A, Kreisel FH, Lawton JS. Bartonella species-induced prosthetic valve endocarditis associated with rapid progression of valvular stenosis. J Thorac Cardiovasc Surg. 2005 Aug;130(2):567-8.

Kreuziger LM, Tafur AJ, Thompson RL. 79-Year-Old Man With Fever, Malaise, and Jaundice. Mayo Clin Proc. 2009 March; 84(3): 281–284.

Krimer PM, Miller AD, Li Q, Grosenbaugh DA, Susta L, Schatzberg SJ. Molecular and pathological investigations of the central nervous system in Borrelia burgdorferi-infected dogs. J Vet Diagn Invest. 2011 Jul;23(4):757-63. Epub 2011 Jun 13.

Krishnamurthy KB, Liu GT, Logigian EL. Acute Lyme neuropathy presenting with polyradicular pain, abdominal protrusion, and cranial neuropathy. Muscle Nerve, 16(11):1261-4. 1993.

Krist D, Wenkel H. Posterior scleritis associated with Borrelia burgdorferi (Lyme disease) infection. Ophthalmology, 109(1):143-5. 2002.

Krüger H, Reuss K, Pulz M, et al. Meningoradiculitis and encephalo-myelitis due to Borrelia burgdorferi: A follow-up study of 72 patients over 27 years. J Neurol, 236:322-328. 1989.

Krungkrai SR, Yuthavong. The antimalarial action of Plasmodium falciparum of qinghaosu and artesunate in combination with agents which modulate oxidant stress. Trans. R Soc. Trop. Med Hyg. 1987;81:710-4.

Krupka M, Zachova K, Weigl E, Raska M. Prevention of lyme disease: promising research or sisyphean task? Arch Immunol Ther Exp (Warsz). 2011 Aug;59(4):261-75. Epub 2011 Jun 3.

Krupp LB, Masur D, Schwartz J, Coyle PK, Langenbach LJ, Fernquist SK, Jandorf L, Halperin JJ. Cognitive functioning in late Lyme borreliosis. Arch Neurol, 48(11):1125-9. 1991.

Krupp LB, Hyman LG, Grimson R, Coyle PK, Melville P, Ahnn S, Dattwyler R, Chandler B. Study and treatment of post Lyme disease. A randomized double masked clinical trial. Neurology. June 4, 2003. 60(12):1923-30.

Kubo N, Arashima Y, Kawabata M, Kawano K, Nakao M, Miyamoto K. [Study of the anti Borrelia burgdorferi antibody of hunters in Hokkaido].[Article in Japanese]. Kansenshogaku Zasshi. 1992 Jan;66(1):45-50.

Kubo N, Arashima Y, Yoshida M, Kawabata M, Nishinarita S, Hayama T, Sawada S, Horie T, Nakao M, Miyamoto K, et al. Questionnaire surveys of cases of tick bite and Lyme borreliosis in hunters in Hokkaido with reference to detection of anti-Borrelia burgdorferi antibody. Intern Med. 1992 Oct;31(10):1163-8.

Kubo N, Iimori H, Kanemaru M, Shinodo T, Okubo S, Nakao M, Miyamoto K, Arashima Y, Kawabata M, Kawano K. [Prevalence of Borrelia on tick collected in Yamanashi Prefecture].[Article in Japanese]. Kansenshogaku Zasshi. 1994 Jan;68(1):168-9.

Kufko IT, Mel'nikov VG, Andreeva EA, Sokolova ZI, Lesniak OM, Beikin IaB. Comparative study of results of serological diagnosis of Lyme borreliosis by indirect immunofluorescence and immunoenzyme analysis. 1999. Klin Lab Diagn, 3:34-7.

Kugeler KJ, Griffith KS, Gould LH, Kochanek K, Delorey MJ, Biggerstaff BJ, Mead PS. A review of death certificates listing Lyme disease as a cause of death in the United States. Clin Infect Dis. 2011 Feb 1;52(3):364-7. Epub 2010 Dec 28.

Kujala GA, Steere AC, Davis JS 4th. IgM rheumatoid factor in Lyme disease: correlation with disease activity, total serum IgM, and IgM antibody to Borrelia burgdorferi. J Rheumatol. 1987 Aug;14(4):772-6.

Kułakowska A, Zajkowska JM, Ciccarelli NJ, Mroczko B, Drozdowski W, Bucki R. Depletion of plasma gelsolin in patients with tick-borne encephalitis and Lyme neuroborreliosis. Neurodegener Dis. 2011;8(5):375-80. Epub 2011 Mar 10.

Kumar M, Kaur S, Kariu T, Yang X, Bossis I, Anderson JF, Pal U. Borrelia burgdorferi BBA52 is a potential target for transmission blocking Lyme disease vaccine. Vaccine. 2011 Sep 21. [Epub ahead of print]

Kumar S, Kumar R, Sugimoto C. A perspective on Theileria equi infections in donkeys. Jpn J Vet Res. 2009 Feb;56(4):171-80. Review.

Kumar T, Epstein M, Markovskaya Y, Narasimhan M, Rosen M, Talwar A. Bronchoscopy and endobronchial disease in patients with human immunodeficiency virus infection. Indian J Chest Dis Allied Sci. 2011 Apr-Jun;53(2):99-105. Review.

Kumru OS, Schulze RJ, Rodnin MV, Ladokhin AS, Zückert WR. Surface localization determinants of Borrelia OspC/Vsp family lipoproteins. J Bacteriol. 2011 Jun;193(11):2814-25. Epub 2011 Mar 25.

Kuntzer T, Bogousslavsky J, Miklossy J, Steck AJ, Janzer R, Regli F. Borrelia rhombencephalomyelopathy. Arch Neurol. 1991 Aug;48(8):832-6.

Kunz S, Oberle K, Sander A, Bogdan C, Schleicher U. Lymphadenopathy in a novel mouse model of Bartonella-induced cat scratch disease results from lymphocyte immigration and proliferation and is regulated by interferon-alpha/beta. Am J Pathol. 2008 Apr;172(4):1005-18. Epub 2008 Feb 21.

Kuo J, Nardelli DT, Warner TF, Callister SM, Schell RF. Interleukin-35 enhances Lyme arthritis in Borrelia-vaccinated and -infected mice. Clin Vaccine Immunol. 2011 Jul;18(7):1125-32. Epub 2011 May 25.

Kurtti TJ, Munderloh UG, Johnson RC, Ahlstrand GG. Colony formation and morphology in Borrelia burgdorferi. Journal of Clinical Microbiology, 25:2054-2058. 1987.

Kusuhara K, Nakao F, Saito M, Nakamura K, Ieiri S, Taguchi T, Hara T. Pyogenic splenic abscess in an infant with serological evidence of cat scratch disease. Eur J Pediatr. 2007 Dec;166(12):1289-91. Epub 2006 Dec 22.

Kuwayama DP, Briones RJ. Spontaneous splenic rupture caused by Babesia microti infection. Clin Infect Dis. 2008 May 1;46(9):e92-5.

Kvasnicka HM, Thiele J, Ahmadi T. Bone marrow manifestation of Lyme disease (Lyme borreliosis). British Journal of Haematology, 120(5):723. 2003.

Kyme PA, Haas A, Schaller M, Peschel A, Iredell J, Kempf VA. Unusual trafficking pattern of Bartonella henselae -containing vacuoles in macrophages and endothelial cells. Cell Microbiol. 2005 Jul;7(7):1019-34.

La VD, Clavel B, Lepetz S, Aboudharam G, Raoult D, Drancourt M. Molecular detection of Bartonella henselae DNA in the dental pulp of 800-year-old French cats. Clin Infect Dis. 2004 Nov 1;39(9):1391-4. Epub 2004 Oct 12.

La VD, Tran-Hung L, Aboudharam G, Raoult D, Drancourt M. Bartonella quintana in domestic cat. Emerg Infect Dis. 2005 Aug;11(8):1287-9.

La Scola B, Davoust B, Boni M, Raoult D. Lack of correlation between Bartonella DNA detection within fleas, serological results, and results of blood culture in a Bartonella-infected stray cat population. Clin Microbiol Infect. 2002 Jun;8(6):345-51.

La Scola B, Fournier PE, Brouqui P, Raoult D. Detection and culture of Bartonella quintana, Serratia marcescens, and Acinetobacter spp. from decontaminated human body lice. J Clin Microbiol. 2001 May;39(5):1707-9.

La Scola B, Holmberg M, Raoult D. Lack of Bartonella sp. in 167 Ixodes ricinus ticks collected in central Sweden. Scand J Infect Dis. 2004;36(4):305-6.

La Scola B, Liang Z, Zeaiter Z, Houpikian P, Grimont PA, Raoult D. Genotypic characteristics of two serotypes of Bartonella henselae. J Clin Microbiol. 2002 Jun;40(6):2002-8.

La Scola B, Raoult D. Culture of Bartonella quintana and Bartonella henselae from human samples: a 5-year experience (1993 to 1998). J Clin Microbiol. 1999 Jun;37(6):1899-905.

La Scola B, Raoult D. Acinetobacter baumannii in human body louse. Emerg Infect Dis. 2004 Sep;10(9):1671-3.

La Scola B, Zeaiter Z, Khamis A, Raoult D. Gene-sequence-based criteria for species definition in bacteriology: the Bartonella paradigm. Trends Microbiol. 2003 Jul;11(7):318-21. Review.

Lacy, LL Armstrong, MP Goldman, LL Lance. Drug Information Handbook. 14th edition. Hudson, Ohio: Lexi-Comp; 2006. p. 175-176, 795-796, 1315-1316, 1366-1367.

Ladbury GAF, Stuen S, Thomas R, Bown KJ, Woldehiwet Z, Granquist EG, Bergström K, Birtles RJ. Dynamic Transmission of Numerous Anaplasma phagocytophilum Genotypes among Lambs in an Infected Sheep Flock in an Area of Anaplasmosis Endemicity. J Clin Microbiol. 2008 May; 46(5): 1686–1691. Published online 2008 March 26.

Lader E. Lyme disease misdiagnosed as a temporomandibular joint disorder. J Prosthet Dent, 63(1):82-5. 1990.

LaFrance ME, Pierce JV, Antonara S, Coburn J. The Borrelia burgdorferi integrin ligand P66 affects gene expression by human cells in culture. Infect Immun. 2011 Aug;79(8):3249-61. Epub 2011 May 16.

Laham FR, Kaplan SL. Hepatosplenic cat-scratch fever. Lancet Infect Dis. 2008 Feb;8(2):140.

Lai. H, Singh, NP. Selective cancer cell cytotoxicity from exposure to dihydroartemisinin and holotransferrin. Cancer Letters. 1995;91:41-46.

Lai H, Singh NP. Oral artemisinin prevents and delays the development of 7,12-dimethylbenz[a]anthracene (DMBA)-induced breast cancer in the rat. Cancer Lett. 2006;231:43-8.

Lamas C, Curi A, Bóia M, Lemos E. Human bartonellosis: seroepidemiological and clinical features with an emphasis on data from Brazil - a review. Mem Inst Oswaldo Cruz. 2008 May;103(3):221-35. Review.

Lamas C, Favacho A, Ramos RG, Santos MS, Ferravoli GI, Weksler C, Rozental T, Bóia MN, Lemos ER. Bartonella native valve endocarditis: the first Brazilian case alive and well. Braz J Infect Dis. 2007 Dec;11(6):591-4.

Lamas CC, Mares-Guia MA, Rozental T, Moreira N, Favacho AR, Barreira J, Guterres A, Bóia MN, de Lemos ER. Bartonella spp. infection in HIV positive individuals, their pets and ectoparasites in Rio de Janeiro, Brazil: serological and molecular study. Acta Trop. 2010 Jul-Aug;115(1-2):137-41. Epub 2010 Mar 3.

Lamps LW, Scott MA. Cat-scratch disease: historic, clinical, and pathologic perspectives. Am J Clin Pathol. 2004;121 Suppl:S71-80.

Lane R, Baldwin D. Selective serotonin reuptake inhibitor-induced serotonin syndrome: review. J Clin Psychopharmacol. 1997;17(3):208-221.

Lane RS, Mun J, Peribáñez MA, Fedorova N. Differences in prevalence of Borrelia burgdorferi and Anaplasma spp. infection among host-seeking Dermacentor occidentalis, Ixodes pacificus, and Ornithodoros coriaceus ticks in northwestern California. Ticks Tick Borne Dis. 2010 Dec;1(4):159-67.

Lane RS, Moss RB, Hsu YP, Wei T, Mesirow ML, Kuo MM. Anti-arthropod saliva antibodies among residents of a community at high risk for Lyme disease in California. Am J Trop Med Hyg. 1999;61:850-9.

Lange D, Oeder C, Waltermann K, Mueller A, Oehme A, Rohrberg R, Marsch W, Fischer M. Bacillary angiomatosis. J Dtsch Dermatol Ges. 2009 Sep;7(9):767-69.

Lantos PM. Chronic Lyme disease: the controversies and the science. Expert Rev Anti Infect Ther. 2011 Jul;9(7):787-97.

Lappin MR, Breitschwerdt E, Brewer M, Hawley J, Hegarty B, Radecki S. Prevalence of Bartonella species antibodies and Bartonella species DNA in the blood of cats with and without fever. J Feline Med Surg. 2009 Feb;11(2):141-8. Epub 2008 Aug 29.

Lappin MR, Kordick DL, Breitschwerdt EB. Bartonella spp antibodies and DNA in aqueous humour of cats. J Feline Med Surg. 2000 Mar;2(1):61-8.

LaRocca TJ, Holthausen DJ, Hsieh C, Renken C, Mannella CA, Benach JL. The bactericidal effect of a complement-independent antibody is osmolytic and specific to Borrelia. Proc Natl Acad Sci U S A. 2009 June 30; 106(26): 10752–10757. Published online 2009 June 19.

Lastres JB. [Encephalopathies in verruga peruana (Carrion's disease)].[Article in Spanish]. An Fac Med Lima. 1956;39(1):73-104.

Lau AO. An overview of the Babesia, Plasmodium and Theileria genomes: a comparative perspective. Mol Biochem Parasitol. 2009 Mar;164(1):1-8. Epub 2008 Dec 6. Review.

Lauderdale V, Goldman JN. Serial ultrathin sectioning demonstrating the intracellularity of T. pallidum. British Journal of Venereal Diseases, 48:87. 1972.

Laudisoit A, Iverson J, Neerinckx S, Shako JC, Nsabimana JM, Kersh G, Kosoy M, Zeidner N. Human seroreactivity against Bartonella species in the Democratic Republic of Congo. Asian Pac J Trop Med. 2011 Apr;4(4):320-2. Epub 2011 May 29.

Laumbacher B, Fellerhoff B, Herzberger B, Wank R. Do dogs harbour risk factors for human breast cancer? Med Hypotheses. 2006;67(1):21-6. Epub 2006 Mar 3.

LaValle JA, Krinsky DL, Hawkin EB, Pelton R and A Ashbrook Willlis. Natural Therapeutics Pocket Guide 2000-2001. Hudson, OH;Lexi-Comp. 518,531.

Lavoie PE, Lattner BP, Duray PH, Barbour AG, Johnson HC. Culture positive seronegative transplacental Lyme borreliosis infant mortality. Arthritis Rheum, 30(4), 3(Suppl):S50. 1987.

Lawrence C, Lipton RB, Lowy FD, Coyle PK. Seronegative chronic relapsing neuroborreliosis. 1995. European Neurology, 35(2):113-7.

Lawrenz MB, Hardham JM, Owens RT, Nowakowski J, Steere AC, Wormser GP, Norris SJ. Human antibody responses to VlsE antigenic variation protein of Borrelia burgdorferi. J Clin Microbiol. 1999 Dec;37(12):3997-4004.

Lawson JP, Steere AC. Lyme arthritis: radiologic findings. Radiology. 1985 Jan;154(1):37-43.

Lazarus JJ, Kay MA, McCarter AL, Wooten RM. Viable Borrelia burgdorferi Enhances Interleukin-10 Production and Suppresses Activation of Murine Macrophages. Infect Immun. 2008 March; 76(3): 1153–1162. Published online 2007 December 17.

Lazri T, Duscher G, Edelhofer R, Bytyci B, Gjino P, Joachim A. [Arthropod-borne parasites of dogs, especially Leishmania, in the Kosovo and Albania].[Article in German]. Wien Klin Wochenschr. 2008;120(19-20 Suppl 4):54-8.

Le NH, Na-Bangchang K, Le TD, Thrinh KA, Karbwang J. Phamacokinetics of a single oral dose of dihydroartemisinin in Vietnamese healthy volunteers. Southeast Asian J Trop Med Public Health. 1999 Mar;30(1):11-6.

Le Nouën C, Munir S, Losq S, Winter CC, McCarty T, Stephany DA, Holmes KL, Bukreyev A, Rabin RL, Collins PL, Buchholz UJ. Infection and maturation of monocyte-derived human dendritic cells by human respiratory syncytial virus, human metapneumovirus, and human parainfluenza virus type 3. Virology. 2009 March 1; 385(1): 169–182. Published online 2009 January 6.

Lee CH, Hong H, Shin J, Jung M, Shin I, Yoon J, Lee W. NMR studies on novel antitumor drug candidates, deoxoartemisinin and carboxypropyldeoxoartemisinin. Biochem Biophys Res Commun. 2000;274:359-69.

Lee J, Wormser GP. Pharmacodynamics of doxycycline for chemoprophylaxis of Lyme disease: preliminary findings and possible implications for other antimicrobials. Int J Antimicrob Agents. 2008 Mar;31(3):235-9. Epub 2008 Jan 15.

Lee J, Zhou HJ, Wu XH. Dihydroartemisinin downregulates vascular endothelial growth factor expression and induces apoptosis in chronic myeloid leukemia K562 cells. Cancer Chemother Pharmacol. 2006 Jan;57(2):213-220. [Epub 2005 Aug 2]

Leeflang P, Oomen JMV, Zwart D, Meuwissen JH. The prevalence of Babesia antibodies in Nigerians. Int J Parasitol. 1976;6(2):156-161.

Leeper T, Zhang S, Van Voorhis WC, Myler PJ, Varani G. Comparative analysis of glutaredoxin domains from bacterial opportunistic pathogens. Acta Crystallogr Sect F Struct Biol Cryst Commun. 2011 Sep 1;67(Pt 9):1141-7. Epub 2011 Aug 16.

Leggat PA. Trends in antimalarial prescriptions in Australia from 1998 to 2002. J Travel Med. 2005 Nov-Dec;12(6):338-42.

Leibovitz K, Pearce L, Brewer M, Lappin MR. Bartonella species antibodies and DNA in cerebral spinal fluid of cats with central nervous system disease. J Feline Med Surg. 2008 Aug;10(4):332-7. Epub 2008 Apr 8.

Leiby DA. Transfusion-transmitted Babesia spp.: bull's-eye on Babesia microti. Clin Microbiol Rev. 2011 Jan;24(1):14-28. Review.

Leishman WB. The Horace Dobell lecture on an experimental investigation of Spirochaeta duttoni, the parasite of tick fever. Lancet, 2:1237-1244. 1920.

Leishman WB. A note on the "granule clumps" found in Ornithodorus moubata and their relation to the spirochaetes of African relapsing fever (tick fever). Annales de l'Institut Pasteur, 32:49-59. 1918.

Lejko-Zupanc T, Slemenik-Pusnik C, Kozelj M, Klokocovnik T, Avsic-Zupanc T, Dolenc-Strazar Z, Benko D, Duh D, Rojko T. Native valve endocarditis due to Bartonella henselae in an immunocompetent man. Wien Klin Wochenschr. 2008;120(7-8):246-9.

Lemos ER, Mares-Guia MA, Almeida DN, Silva RG, Silva CM, Britto C, Lamas CC. [Traveler's fever associated with cervical adenomegaly and antibodies for Bartonella sp in a Brazilian patient returning from South Africa].[Article in Portuguese]. Rev Soc Bras Med Trop. 2010 Jul-Aug;43(4):472-3.

Lenčáková DH, Schulte-Spechtel U, Fingerle V, Pet'ko B, Wilske B. Detection of a large linear plasmid in Borrelia spielmanii isolate. Can J Microbiol. 2011 Apr;57(4):343-6.

Lengl-Janssen B, Strauss AF, Steere AC, Kamradt T. The T helper cell response in Lyme arthritis: differential recognition of Borrelia burgdorferi outer surface protein A in patients with treatment-resistant or treatment-responsive Lyme arthritis. J Exp Med. 1994 Dec 1;180(6):2069-78.

Lennhoff C. Spirochaetes in aetiologically obscure diseases. Acta Dermato-Venereologica, Vol 28 Fasc 3:295-324. 1948.

Lepidi H, Coulibaly B, Casalta JP, Raoult D. Autoimmunohistochemistry: a new method for the histologic diagnosis of infective endocarditis. J Infect Dis. 2006 Jun 15;193(12):1711-7. Epub 2006 May 12.

Lepidi H, Fournier PE, Raoult D. Quantitative analysis of valvular lesions during Bartonella endocarditis. Am J Clin Pathol. 2000 Dec;114(6):880-9.

Lesage AD, Stip E, Grunberg F. ["What's up, doc?" The context, limitations, and issues for clinicians in evidence-based medicine]. [Article in French]. Can J Psychiatry. 2001 Jun;46(5):396-402.

Levander OA, Ager AL, Morris VC. Qinghaosu, dietary vitamin E, selenium and cod liver oil: effect on susceptibility of mice to the malarial parasite Plasmodium yoelii. Am. J. Clin. Nutr. 1989;5:346-52.

Levin ML, des Vignes F, Fish D. Disparity in the natural cycles of Borrelia burgdorferi and the agent of Human Granulocytic Ehrlichiosis. Emerg Infect Dis. 1999;Vol 5(2):204-8.

Levine ND. Taxonomy of the piroplasms. Trans. Am. Microsc. Soc. 90:2-33.

Levy I, Rolain JM, Lepidi H, Raoult D, Feinmesser M, Lapidoth M, Ben-Amitai D. Is pyogenic granuloma associated with Bartonella infection? J Am Acad Dermatol. 2005 Dec;53(6):1065-6.

Levy JK, Crawford PC, Lappin MR, Dubovi EJ, Levy MG, Alleman R, Tucker SJ, Clifford EL. Infectious diseases of dogs and cats on Isabela Island, Galapagos. J Vet Intern Med. 2008 Jan-Feb;22(1):60-5.

Levy M, Buskila D, Gladman DD, Urowitz MB, Koren G. Pregnancy outcome following first trimester exposure to chloroquine. Am J Perinatol. 1991 May;8 (3):174-8.

Levy PY, Corey R, Berger P, Habib G, Bonnet JL, Levy S, Messana T, Djiane P, Frances Y, Botta C, DeMicco P, Dumon H, Mundler O, Chomel JJ, Raoult D. Etiologic diagnosis of 204 pericardial effusions. Medicine (Baltimore). 2003 Nov;82(6):385-91.

Levy PY, Fournier PE, Carta M, Raoult D. Pericardial effusion in a homeless man due to Bartonella quintana. J Clin Microbiol. 2003 Nov;41(11):5291-3.

Lewis DW, Tucker SH. Central nervous system involvement in cat scratch disease. Pediatrics. 1986 May;77(5):714-21.

Leyfer OT, Ruberg JL, Woodruff-Borden J. Examination of the utility of the Beck Anxiety Inventory and its factors as a screener for anxiety disorders. J Anxiety Disord. 2006;20(4):444-458.

Li CW, Yin J, Zhang XL. [Cat scratch disease: report of a case]. [Article in Chinese]. Zhonghua Er Ke Za Zhi. 2007 Aug;45(8):573.

Li DM, Liu QY, Zhao F, Hu Y, Xiao D, Gu YX, Song XP, Zhang JZ. Proteomic and bioinformatic analysis of outer membrane proteins of the protobacterium Bartonella henselae (Bartonellaceae). Genet Mol Res. 2011 Aug 26;10(3):1789-818.

Li DM, Meng FX, Song XP, Qin ZJ, Yang XR, Wu HX, Ren DS, Liu QY. [Study on Bartonella vinsonii berkhoffii isolated from blood of native dogs in China].[Article in Chinese]. Zhonghua Liu Xing Bing Xue Za Zhi. 2006 Apr;27(4):333-8.

Li DM, Yu DZ, Liu QY, Gong ZD. [Study on the prevalence of Bartonella species in rodent hosts from different environmental areas in Yunnan].[Article in Chinese]. Zhonghua Liu Xing Bing Xue Za Zhi. 2004 Nov;25(11):934-7.

Li QG, Brueckner RP, Peggins JO, Trotman KM, Brewer TG. Arteether toxicokinetics and pharmacokinetics in rats after 25 mg/kg/day single and multiple doses. Eur J Drug Metab Pharmacokinet. 1999 Jul-Sept;24(3):213-23.

Li QG, Mog SR, Si YZ, Kyle DE, Gettayacamin M, Milhous WK. Neurotoxicity and efficacy of arteether related to its exposure times and exposure levels in rodents. Am J Trop Med Hyg. 2002 May;66(5):516-25.

Li W, Chomel BB, Maruyama S, Guptil L, Sander A, Raoult D, Fournier PE. Multispacer typing to study the genotypic distribution of Bartonella henselae populations. J Clin Microbiol. 2006 Jul;44(7):2499-506.

Li W, Raoult D, Fournier PE. Genetic diversity of Bartonella henselae in human infection detected with multispacer typing. Emerg Infect Dis. 2007 Aug;13(8):1178-83.

Li X, McHugh GA, Damle N, Sikand VK, Glickstein L, Steere AC. Burden and viability of Borrelia burgdorferi in skin and joints of patients with erythema migrans or lyme arthritis. Arthritis Rheum. 2011 Aug;63(8):2238-47.

Liang FT, Steere AC, Marques AR, Johnson BJ, Miller JN, Philipp MT. Sensitive and specific serodiagnosis of Lyme disease by enzyme-linked immunosorbent assay with a peptide based on an immunodominant conserved region of Borrelia burgdorferi vlsE. J Clin Microbiol. 1999 Dec;37(12):3990-6.

Liang Z, La Scola B, Lepidi H, Raoult D. Production of Bartonella genus-specific monoclonal antibodies. Clin Diagn Lab Immunol. 2001 Jul;8(4):847-9.

Liang Z, Raoult D. Species-specific monoclonal antibodies for rapid identification of Bartonella quintana. Clin Diagn Lab Immunol. 2000 Jan;7(1):21-4.

Liang Z, Raoult D. Differentiation of Bartonella species by a microimmunofluorescence assay, sodium dodecyl sulfate-polyacrylamide gel electrophoresis, and Western immunoblotting. Clin Diagn Lab Immunol. 2000 Jul;7(4):617-24.

Liao HM, Huang FY, Chi H, Wang NL, Chen BF. Systemic cat scratch disease. J Formos Med Assoc. 2006 Aug;105(8):674-9.

Liao M, Hatta T, Umemiya R, Huang P, Jia H, Gong H, Zhou J, Nishikawa Y, Xuan X, Fujisaki K. Identification of three protein disulfide isomerase members from Haemaphysalis longicornis tick. Insect Biochem Mol Biol. 2007 Jul;37(7):641-54. Epub 2007 Apr 5.

Liberto MC, Matera G, Lamberti AG, Barreca GS, Quirino A, Focà A. In vitro Bartonella quintana infection modulates the programmed cell death and inflammatory reaction of endothelial cells. Diagn Microbiol Infect Dis. 2003 Feb;45(2):107-15.

Lienhardt B, Irani S, Gaspert A, Weishaupt D, Boehler A. Disseminated infection with Bartonella henselae in a lung transplant recipient. J Heart Lung Transplant. 2009 Jul;28(7):736-9.

Liesenfeld O, Parvanova I, Zerrahn J, Han SJ, Heinrich F, Muñoz M, Kaiser F, Aebischer T, Buch T, Waisman A, Reichmann G, Utermöhlen O, von Stebut E, von Loewenich FD, Bogdan C, Specht S, Saeftel M, Hoerauf A, Mota MM, Könen-Waisman S, Kaufmann SH, Howard JC. The IFN-Inducible GTPase, Irga6, Protects Mice against Toxoplasma gondii but Not against Plasmodium berghei and Some Other Intracellular Pathogens. PLoS One. 2011; 6(6): e20568. Published online 2011 June 17.

Lightfoot RW Jr, Luft BJ, Rahn DW, Steere AC, Sigal LH, Zoschke DC, Gardner P, Britton MC, Kaufman RL. Empiric parenteral antibiotic treatment of patients with fibromyalgia and fatigue and a positive serologic result for Lyme disease. A cost-effectiveness analysis. Ann Intern Med. 1993 Sep 15;119(6):503-9.

Lin AJ, Ager AL Jr, Klayman DL. Antimalarial activity of dihydroartemisinin derivatives by transdermal application. Am J Trop Med Hyg. 1994 Jun;50(6):777-83.

Lin B, Kidder JM, Noring R, Steere AC, Klempner MS, Hu LT. Differences in synovial fluid levels of matrix metalloproteinases suggest separate mechanisms of pathogenesis in Lyme arthritis before and after antibiotic treatment. J Infect Dis. 2001 Jul 15;184(2):174-80. Epub 2001 Jun 25.

Lin B, Noring R, Steere AC, Klempner MS, Hu LT. Soluble CD14 levels in the serum, synovial fluid, and cerebrospinal fluid of patients with various stages of Lyme disease. J Infect Dis. 2000 Mar;181(3):1185-8.

Lin EY, Tsigrelis C, Baddour LM, Lepidi H, Rolain JM, Patel R, Raoult D. Candidatus Bartonella mayotimonensis and endocarditis. Emerg Infect Dis. 2010 Mar;16(3):500-3.

Lin JW, Chen CY, Chen WC, Chomel BB, Chang CC. Isolation of Bartonella species from rodents in Taiwan including a strain closely related to 'Bartonella rochalimae' from Rattus norvegicus. J Med Microbiol. 2008 Dec;57(Pt 12):1496-501.

Lindroos H, Vinnere O, Mira A, Repsilber D, Näslund K, Andersson SG. Genome rearrangements, deletions, and amplifications in the natural population of Bartonella henselae. J Bacteriol. 2006 Nov;188(21):7426-39. Epub 2006 Aug 25.

Lininger SW, Gaby AR, Austin S, Brown DR, Wright JV, Duncan A. The Natural Pharmacy. 2nd edition. Rocklin CA; Prima Publishing, 1999;p.470-471.

Lindsey J, Patel S. PCR for bacterial 16S ribosomal DNA in multiple sclerosis cerebrospinal fluid. Mult Scler. 2008 Mar;14(2):147-52. Epub 2007 Nov 6. Review.

Lipińiska-Ojrzanowska A, Wittczak T, Krzyczmanik D, Pałczyński C, Walusiak-Skorupa J. [Invasion by trichinae in the patient hospitalized with suspicion of occupational borreliosis: a case report].[Article in Polish]. Med Pr. 2011;62(1):73-6.

Litwin CM, Rawlins ML, Swenson EM. Characterization of an immunogenic outer membrane autotransporter protein, Arp, of Bartonella henselae. Infect Immun. 2007 Nov;75(11):5255-63. Epub 2007 Sep 4.

Livey I, O'Rourke M, Traweger A, Savidis-Dacho H, Crowe BA, Barrett PN, Yang X, Dunn JJ, Luft BJ. A new approach to a Lyme disease vaccine. Clin Infect Dis. 2011 Feb;52 Suppl 3:s266-70.

Listgarten MA, Loesche WJ, Socransky SS. Morphology of Treponema microdentium as revealed by electron microscopy of ultrathin sections. Journal of Bacteriology, 85:932-939. 1963.

Liu AN. Lyme disease in China and its ocular manifestations. 1993. Chung Hua Yen Ko Tsa Chih, 5:271-3.

Liu Q, Sun J, Lu L, Fu G, Ding G, Song X, Meng F, Wu H, Yang T, Ren Z, Chen E, Lin J, Lv H, Chai C. Detection of bartonella species in small mammals from Zhejiang Province, China. J Wildl Dis. 2010 Jan;46(1):179-85.

Liu Y, Wong VK, Ko BC, Wong MK, Che CM. Synthesis and cytotoxicity studies of artemisinin derivatives containing lipophilic alkyl carbon chains. Org Lett. 2005;7:1561-4.

Liveris D, Schwartz I, McKenna D, Nowakowski J, Nadelman RB, Demarco J, Iyer R, Cox ME, Holmgren D, Wormser GP. Quantitation of cell-associated borrelial DNA in the blood of Lyme disease patients with erythema migrans. Eur J Clin Microbiol Infect Dis. 2011 Aug 16. [Epub ahead of print]

Liveris D, Schwartz I, Bittker S, Cooper D, Iyer R, Cox ME, Wormser GP. Improving the yield of blood cultures from patients with early Lyme disease. J Clin Microbiol. 2011 Jun;49(6):2166-8. Epub 2011 Apr 13.

Liveris D, Varde S, Iyer R, Koenig S, Bittker S, Cooper D, McKenna D, Nowakowski J, Nadelman RB, Wormser GP, Schwartz I. Genetic diversity of Borrelia burgdorferi in lyme disease patients as determined by culture versus direct PCR with clinical specimens. J Clin Microbiol. 1999 Mar;37(3):565-9.

Liveris D, Wang G, Girao G, Byrne DW, Nowakowski J, McKenna D, Nadelman R, Wormser GP, Schwartz I. Quantitative detection of Borrelia burgdorferi in 2-millimeter skin samples of erythema migrans lesions: correlation of results with clinical and laboratory findings. J Clin Microbiol. 2002 Apr;40(4):1249-53.

Liveris D, Wormser GP, Nowakowski J, Nadelman R, Bittker S, Cooper D, Varde S, Moy FH, Forseter G, Pavia CS, Schwartz I. Molecular typing of Borrelia burgdorferi from Lyme disease patients by PCR-restriction fragment length polymorphism analysis. J Clin Microbiol. 1996 May;34(5):1306-9.

Ljøstad U, Skarpaas T, Mygland A. Clinical usefulness of intrathecal antibody testing in acute Lyme neuroborreliosis. Eur J Neurol. 2007 Aug;14(8):873-6.

Ljøstad U, Skogvoll E, Eikeland R, Midgard R, Skarpaas T, Berg A, Mygland A. Oral doxycycline versus intravenous ceftriaxone for European Lyme neuroborreliosis: a multicentre, non-inferiority, double-blind, randomised trial. Lancet Neurol. 2008 Aug;7(8):690-5. Epub 2008 Jun 21. Erratum in: Lancet Neurol. 2008 Aug;7(8):675.

Lledó L, Giménez-Pardo C, Domínguez-Peñafiel G, Sousa R, Gegúndez MI, Casado N, Criado A. Molecular detection of hemoprotozoa and Rickettsia species in arthropods collected from wild animals in the Burgos Province, Spain. Vector Borne Zoonotic Dis. 2010 Oct;10(8):735-8. Epub 2010 Jan 7.

Lo R, Menzies DJ, Archer H, Cohen TJ. Complete heart block due to Lyme carditis. Journal of Invasive Cardiology, 15(6):367-9. 2003.

Loa CC, Mordechai E, Tilton RC, Adelson ME. Production of recombinant Bartonella henselae 17-kDa protein for antibody-capture enzyme-linked immunosorbent assay. Diagn Microbiol Infect Dis. 2006 May;55(1):1-7. Epub 2006 Feb 20.

Lobato E, Pearce-Duvet J, Staszewski V, Gómez-Díaz E, González-Solís J, Kitaysky A, McCoy KD, Boulinier T. Seabirds and the Circulation of Lyme Borreliosis Bacteria in the North Pacific. Vector Borne Zoonotic Dis. 2011 Sep 15. [Epub ahead of print]

Loeckx I, Tuerlinckx D, Jespers S, Marchant AS, Bodart E. [A clinical case of spontaneous involution of systemic cat scratch disease].[Article in French]. Rev Med Liege. 2010 Feb;65(2):78-80.

Loftis AD, Reeves WK, Szumlas DE, Abbassy MM, Helmy IM, Moriarity JR, Dasch GA. Surveillance of Egyptian fleas for agents of public health significance: Anaplasma, Bartonella, Coxiella, Ehrlichia, Rickettsia, and Yersinia pestis. Am J Trop Med Hyg. 2006 Jul;75(1):41-8.

Logigian EL, Kaplan RF, Steere AC. Successful treatment of Lyme encephalopathy with intravenous ceftriaxone. J Infect Dis. 1999 Aug;180(2):377-83.

Logigian EL, Steere AC. Clinical and electrophysiologic findings in chronic neuropathy of Lyme disease. Neurology. 1992 Feb;42(2):303-11.

Logigian EL, Johnson KA, Kijewski MF, Kaplan RF, Becker JA, Jones KJ, Garada BM, Holman BL, Steere AC. Reversible cerebral hypoperfusion in Lyme encephalopathy. Neurology. 1997 Dec;49(6):1661-70.

Logigian EL, Kaplan RF, Steere AC. Chronic neurologic manifestations of Lyme disease. N Engl J Med. 1990 Nov 22;323(21):1438-44.

Londoño D, Cadavid D. Bacterial Lipoproteins Can Disseminate from the Periphery to Inflame the Brain. Am J Pathol. 2010 June; 176(6): 2848–2857.

Long SR, Whitfeld MJ, Eades C, Koehler JE, Korn AP, Zaloudek CJ. Bacillary angiomatosis of the cervix and vulva in a patient with AIDS. Obstet Gynecol. 1996 Oct;88(4 Pt 2):709-11.

Looaresuwan S, Wilairatana P, Vanijanonta S, et al. Treatment of acute, uncomplicated, falciparum malaria with oral dihydroartemisinin. Ann Trop Med Parasitol. 1996;90:21-28.

Looringh van Beeck FA, Reinink P, Hermsen R, Zajonc DM, Laven MJ, Fun A, Troskie M, Schoemaker NJ, Morar D, Lenstra JA, Vervelde L, Rutten VP, van Eden W, Van Rhijn I. Functional CD1d and/or NKT cell invariant chain transcript in horse, pig, African elephant and guinea pig, but not in ruminants. Mol Immunol. 2009 April; 46(7): 1424–1431.

Lopez-Andreu JA, Ferris J, Canosa CA, Sala-Lizarraga JA. Treatment of late Lyme disease: a challenge to accept. 1994. Journal of Clinical Microbiology, 32:1415-16.

Loss J, Nagel E. [Does evidence-based surgery harm autonomy in clinical decision making?].[Article in German]. Zentralbl Chir. 2005 Feb;130(1):1-6.

Loughlin M. Reason, reality and objectivity--shared dogmas and distortions in the way both 'scientistic' and 'postmodern' commentators frame the EBM debate. J Eval Clin Pract. 2008 Oct;14(5):665-71.

Lovrich SD, Jobe DA, Kowalski TJ, Policepatil SM, Callister SM. Expansion of the Midwestern Focus for Human Granulocytic Anaplasmosis into the Region Surrounding La Crosse, Wisconsin. J Clin Microbiol. 2011 Sep 14. [Epub ahead of print]

Luce-Fedrow A, Von Ohlen T, Chapes SK. Ehrlichia chaffeensis Infections in Drosophila melanogaster. Infect Immun. 2009 November; 77(11): 4815–4826. Published online 2009 August 17.

Luft BJ, Dattwyler RJ. Invasion of the central nervous system by Borrelia burgdorferi in acute disseminated infection. JAMA, 267:1364-67. 1992.

Luft BJ, Dattwyler RJ, Johnson RC, Luger SW, Bosler EM, Rahn DW, et al. Azithromycin compared with amoxicillin in the treatment of erythema migrans. A double-blind, randomized, controlled trial. 1996. Annals of Internal Medicine, 124(9):785-91.

Luger SW, Paparone P, Wormser GP, Nadelman RB, Grunwaldt E, Gomez G, Wisniewski M, Collins JJ. Comparison of cefuroxime axetil and doxycycline in treatment of patients with early Lyme disease associated with erythema migrans. Antimicrob Agents Chemother. 1995 Mar;39(3):661-7.

Luo Y, Jia H, Terkawi MA, Goo YK, Kawano S, Ooka H, Li Y, Yu L, Cao S, Yamagishi J, Fujisaki K, Nishikawa Y, Saito-Ito A, Igarashi I, Xuan X. Identification and characterization of a novel secreted antigen 1 of Babesia microti and evaluation of its potential use in enzyme-linked immunosorbent assay and immunochromatographic test. Parasitol Int. 2011 Jun;60(2):119-25. Epub 2010 Nov 8.

Luria BJ, Levy JK, Lappin MR, Breitschwerdt EB, Legendre AM, Hernandez JA, Gorman SP, Lee IT. Prevalence of infectious diseases in feral cats in Northern Florida. J Feline Med Surg. 2004 Oct;6(5):287-96.

Lydy SL, Eremeeva ME, Asnis D, Paddock CD, Nicholson WL, Silverman DJ, Dasch GA. Isolation and characterization of Bartonella bacilliformis from an expatriate Ecuadorian. J Clin Microbiol. 2008 Feb;46(2):627-37. Epub 2007 Dec 19.

Lynch T, Iverson J, Kosoy M. Combining culture techniques for Bartonella: the best of both worlds. J Clin Microbiol. 2011 Apr;49(4):1363-8. Epub 2011 Feb 2.

Lyon LW. Neurologic manifestations of cat-scratch disease. Report of a case and review of the literature. Arch Neurol. 1971 Jul;25(1):23-7.

Ma Y, A Sturrock A, Weis JJ. Intracellular localization of Borrelia burgdorferi within human endothelial cells. Infect Immun. 1991 February; 59(2): 671–678.

Maamun JM, Suleman MA, Akinyi M, Ozwara H, Kariuki T, Carlsson HE. Prevalence of Babesia microti in free-ranging baboons and African green monkeys. J Parasitol. 2011 Feb;97(1):63-7. Epub 2010 Sep 28.

Macauda MM, Erickson P, Miller J, Mann P, Closter L, Krause PJ. Long-term Lyme disease antibiotic therapy beliefs among New England residents. Vector Borne Zoonotic Dis. 2011 Jul;11(7):857-62. Epub 2011 Mar 21.

MacDonald A. Borrelia in the brains of patients dying with dementia. Journal of the American Medical Association, 256(16):2195-6. 1986.

MacDonald A. Human fetal borreliosis, toxemia of pregnancy, and fetal death. Zbl. Bakt. Hyg. A, 263:189-200. 1986.

MacDonald AB. Concurrent neocortical borreliosis and Alzheimer's disease: Demonstration of a spirochetal cyst form. Annals NY Academy of Sciences, 539:468-470. 1988.

MacDonald AB. Gestational Lyme borreliosis: implications for the fetus. Rheumatic Diseases Clinics of North America, 15(4):657-677. 1989.

MacDonald AB, Berger BW, Schwan TG. Clinical implications of delayed growth of the Lyme borreliosis spirochete, Borrelia burgdorferi. 1990. Acta Trop, Dec;48(2):89-94.

MacDonald KA, Chomel BB, Kittleson MD, Kasten RW, Thomas WP, Pesavento P. A prospective study of canine infective endocarditis in northern California (1999-2001): emergence of Bartonella as a prevalent etiologic agent. J Vet Intern Med. 2004 Jan-Feb;18(1):56-64.

MacKichan JK, Gerns HL, Chen YT, Zhang P, Koehler JE. A SacB mutagenesis strategy reveals that the Bartonella quintana variably expressed outer membrane proteins are required for bloodstream infection of the host. Infect Immun. 2008 Feb;76(2):788-95. Epub 2007 Dec 10.

Mackworth-Young CG, Harris EN, Steere AC, Rizvi F, Malawista SE, Hughes GR, Gharavi AE. Anticardiolipin antibodies in Lyme disease. Arthritis Rheum. 1988 Aug;31(8):1052-6.

Madagi S, Patil VM, Sadegh S, Singh AK, Garwal B, Banerjee A, Talambedu U, Bhattacharjee B. Identification of membrane associated drug targets in Borrelia burgdorferi ZS7- subtractive genomics approach. Bioinformation. 2011;6(9):356-9. Epub 2011 Jul 19.

Magalhães RF, Cintra ML, Barjas-Castro ML, Del Negro GM, Okay TS, Velho PE. Blood donor infected with Bartonella henselae. Transfus Med. 2010 Aug 1;20(4):280-2. Epub 2010 Mar 24.

Magalhães RF, Pitassi LH, Salvadego M, de Moraes AM, Barjas-Castro ML, Velho PE. Bartonella henselae survives after the storage period of red blood cell units: is it transmissible by transfusion? Transfus Med. 2008 Oct;18(5):287-91.

Magalhães RF, Urso Pitassi LH, Lania BG, Barjas-Castro ML, Neves Ferreira Velho PE. Bartonellosis as cause of death after red blood cell unit transfusion. Ultrastruct Pathol. 2009 Jul-Aug;33(4):151-4.

Magand F, Frésard A, Manoli P, Cazorla C, Lucht F. [Stellar neuroretinitis and Bartonella henselae infection. A case report without exposure to cats].[Article in French]. Med Mal Infect. 2008 May;38(5):275-7. Epub 2008 Jan 9.

Maggi RG, Breitschwerdt EB. Isolation of bacteriophages from Bartonella vinsonii subsp. berkhoffii and the characterization of Pap31 gene sequences from bacterial and phage DNA. J Mol Microbiol Biotechnol. 2005;9(1):44-51.

Maggi RG, Breitschwerdt EB. Potential limitations of the 16S-23S rRNA intergenic region for molecular detection of Bartonella species. J Clin Microbiol. 2005 Mar;43(3):1171-6.

Maggi RG, Chomel B, Hegarty BC, Henn J, Breitschwerdt EB. A Bartonella vinsonii berkhoffii typing scheme based upon 16S-23S ITS and Pap31 sequences from dog, coyote, gray fox, and human isolates. Mol Cell Probes. 2006 Apr;20(2):128-34. Epub 2006 Feb 7.

Maggi RG, Duncan AW, Breitschwerdt EB. Novel chemically modified liquid medium that will support the growth of seven bartonella species. J Clin Microbiol. 2005 Jun;43(6):2651-5.

Maggi RG, Harms CA, Hohn AA, Pabst DA, McLellan WA, Walton WJ, Rotstein DS, Breitschwerdt EB. Bartonella henselae in porpoise blood. Emerg Infect Dis. 2005 Dec;11(12):1894-8.

Maggi RG, Kosoy M, Mintzer M, Breitschwerdt EB. Isolation of Candidatus Bartonella melophagi from human blood. Emerg Infect Dis. 2009 Jan;15(1):66-8.

Maggi RG, Mascarelli PE, Pultorak EL, Hegarty BC, Bradley JM, Mozayeni BR, Breitschwerdt EB. Bartonella spp. bacteremia in high-risk immunocompetent patients. Diagn Microbiol Infect Dis. 2011 Oct 11. [Epub ahead of print]

Maggi RG, Raverty SA, Lester SJ, Huff DG, Haulena M, Ford SL, Nielsen O, Robinson JH, Breitschwerdt EB. Bartonella henselae in captive and hunter-harvested beluga (Delphinapterus leucas). J Wildl Dis. 2008 Oct;44(4):871-7.

Maggi RG, Reichelt S, Toliver M, Engber B. Borrelia species in Ixodes affinis and Ixodes scapularis ticks collected from the coastal plain of North Carolina. Ticks Tick Borne Dis. 2010 Dec;1(4):168-71. Epub 2010 Oct 20.

Magnarelli LA, Anderson JF, Johnson RC, Nadelman RB, Wormser GP. Comparison of different strains of Borrelia burgdorferi sensu lato used as antigens in enzyme-linked immunosorbent assays. J Clin Microbiol. 1994 May;32(5):1154-8.

Maguiña C, Guerra H, Ventosilla P. Bartonellosis. Clin Dermatol. 2009 May-Jun;27(3):271-80. Review.

Mainardi JL, Figliolini C, Goldstein FW, Blanche P, Baret-Rigoulet M, Galezowski N, Fournier PE, Raoult D. Cat scratch disease due to Bartonella henselae serotype Marseille (Swiss cat) in a seronegative patient. J Clin Microbiol. 1998 Sep;36(9):2800.

Majláthová V, Hurníková Z, Majláth I, Petko B. Hepatozoon canis infection in Slovakia: imported or autochthonous? Vector Borne Zoonotic Dis. 2007 Summer;7(2):199-202.

Malandrin L, Jouglin M, Sun Y, Brisseau N, Chauvin A. Redescription of Babesia capreoli (Enigk and Friedhoff, 1962) from roe deer (Capreolus capreolus): isolation, cultivation, host specificity, molecular characterisation and differentiation from Babesia divergens. Int J Parasitol. 2010 Mar 1;40(3):277-84. Epub 2009 Sep 4.

Malane MS, Grant-Kels JM, Feder HM, Luger SW. Diagnosis of Lyme disease based on dermatologic manifestations. Annals of Internal Medicine, 114:490-8. 1991.

Malawista SE, Steere AC, Hardin JA. Lyme disease: a unique human model for an infectious etiology of rheumatic disease. Yale J Biol Med. 1984 Jul-Aug;57(4):473-7.

Malawista SE, Steere AC. Lyme disease: infectious in origin, rheumatic in expression. Adv Intern Med. 1986;31:147-66. Review.

Malawista SE, Barthold SW, Persing DH. Fate of Borrelia burgdorferi DNA in tissues of infected mice after antibiotic treatment. 1994. Journal of Infectious Diseases, 170:1312-1316.

Mallecourt J, Landureau M, Wirth AM. [Lyme's disease. A clinical case observed in Western France (author's transl)]. Nouv Presse Med. 1982 Jan 9;11(1):39-41. [Article in French].

Maman E, Bickels J, Ephros M, Paran D, Comaneshter D, Metzkor-Cotter E, Avidor B, Varon-Graidy M, Wientroub S, Giladi M. Musculoskeletal manifestations of cat scratch disease. Clin Infect Dis. 2007 Dec 15;45(12):1535-40.

Mancino P, Ucciferri C, Falasca K, Racciatti D, Di Girolamo A, Vecchiet J, Pizzigallo E. Inguinal lymphadenopathy due to Bartonella henselae. Infez Med. 2008 Jun;16(2):91-3.

Mandell H, Steere AC, Reinhardt BN, Yoshinari N, Munsat TL, Brod SA, Clapshaw PA. Lack of antibodies to Borrelia burgdorferi in patients with amyotrophic lateral sclerosis. N Engl J Med. 1989 Jan 26;320(4):255-6.

Mandle T, Einsele H, Schaller M, et al. Infection of human CD34+ progenitor cells with Bartonella henselae results in intraerythrocytic presence of B. henselae. Blood. 2005;106(4):1215-1222.

Manfredi R, Sabbatani S. Bartonellosis: suggestive case reports in adult and pediatric patients and therapeutic issues. Braz J Infect Dis. 2006 Dec;10(6):411-5.

Mansueto P, Vitale G, Cascio A, Seidita A, Pepe I, Carroccio A, di Rosa S, Rini GB, Cillari E, Walker DH. New Insight into Immunity and Immunopathology of Rickettsial Diseases. Clin Dev Immunol. 2012; 2012: 967852. Published online 2011 September 6.

Mantadakis E, Spanaki AM, Psaroulaki A, Fitrolaki D, Minadakis G, Michaeloudi E, Tselentis Y, Briassoulis G. Encephalopathy complicated by Guillain-Barre syndrome and hydrocephalus and associated with acute Bartonella quintana infection. Pediatr Infect Dis J. 2007 Sep;26(9):860-2.

Marano N, Rupprecht C, Regnery R. Vaccines for emerging infections. Rev Sci Tech. 2007 Apr;26(1):203-15. Review.

Maraspin V, Ogrinc K, Ružić-Sabljić E, Lotrič-Furlan S, Strle F. Isolation of Borrelia burgdorferi sensu lato from blood of adult patients with borrelial lymphocytoma, Lyme neuroborreliosis, Lyme arthritis and acrodermatitis chronica atrophicans. Infection. 2011 Feb;39(1):35-40. Epub 2010 Dec 10.

Marchal C, Schramm F, Kern A, Luft BJ, Yang X, Schuijt T, Hovius J, Jaulhac B, Boulanger N. Antialarmin effect of tick saliva during the transmission of Lyme disease. Infect Immun. 2011 Feb;79(2):774-85. Epub 2010 Dec 6.

Marcus LC, Steere AC, Duray PH, Anderson AE, Mahoney EB. Fatal pancarditis in a patient with coexistent Lyme disease and babesiosis. Demonstration of spirochetes in the myocardium. Ann Intern Med. 1985 Sep;103(3):374-6.

Margileth AM. Cat scratch disease: nonbacterial regional lymphadenitis. The study of 145 patients and a review of the literature. Pediatrics. 1968 Nov;42(5):803-18.

Margos G, Gatewood AG, Aanensen DM, Hanincová K, Terekhova D, Vollmer SA, Cornet M, Piesman J, Donaghy M, Bormane A, Hurn MA, Feil EJ, Fish D, Casjens S, Wormser GP, Schwartz I, Kurtenbach K. MLST of housekeeping genes captures geographic population structure and suggests a European origin of Borrelia burgdorferi. Proc Natl Acad Sci U S A. 2008 Jun 24;105(25):8730-5. Epub 2008 Jun 23.

Margos G, Vollmer SA, Ogden NH, Fish D. Population genetics, taxonomy, phylogeny and evolution of Borrelia burgdorferi sensu lato. Infect Genet Evol. 2011 Aug 5. [Epub ahead of print]

Marié JL, Fournier PE, Rolain JM, Briolant S, Davoust B, Raoult D. Molecular detection of Bartonella quintana, B. Elizabethae, B. Koehlerae, B. Doshiae, B. Taylorii, and Rickettsia felis in rodent fleas collected in Kabul, Afghanistan. Am J Trop Med Hyg. 2006 Mar;74(3):436-9.

Marienfeld CB, Dicapua DB, Sze GK, Goldstein JM. Expressive aphasia as a presentation of encephalitis with Bartonella henselae infection in an immunocompetent adult. Yale J Biol Med. 2010 Jun;83(2):67-71.

Marignac G, Barrat F, Chomel B, Vayssier-Taussat M, Gandoin C, Bouillin C, Boulouis HJ. Murine model for Bartonella birtlesii infection: New aspects. Comp Immunol Microbiol Infect Dis. 2010 Mar;33(2):95-107. Epub 2010 Jan 25.

Marín M, Muñoz P, Sánchez M, del Rosal M, Alcalá L, Rodríguez-Créixems M, Bouza E; Group for the Management of Infective Endocarditis of the Gregorio Marañón Hospital. Molecular diagnosis of infective endocarditis by real-time broad-range polymerase chain reaction (PCR) and sequencing directly from heart valve tissue. Medicine (Baltimore). 2007 Jul;86(4):195-202.

Marinella MA. Jarisch-Herxheimer reaction. West J Med. 1996 Sep;165(3):161-2.

Markeljević J, Sarac H, Rados M. Tremor, seizures and psychosis as presenting symptoms in a patient with chronic lyme neuroborreliosis (LNB). Coll Antropol. 2011 Jan;35 Suppl 1:313-8.

Markowitz LE, Steere AC, Benach JL, Slade JD, Broome CV. Lyme disease during pregnancy. JAMA. 1986 Jun 27;255(24):3394-6.

Marley SE, Eberhard ML, Steurer FJ, Ellis WL, McGreevy PB, Ruebush TK 2nd. Evaluation of selected antiprotozoal drugs in the Babesia microti-hamster model. Antimicrob Agents Chemother. 1997 Jan;41(1):91-4.

Marquardt WC, Demaree RS, Grieve R. Piroplasmea and Piroplasmosis. In: Parasitology & Vector Biology, 2nd edition. San Diego, CA Harcourt Press. 2000; p.221-224.

Marques A, Shaw P, Schmid CH, Steere A, Kaplan RF, Hassett A, Shapiro E, Wormser GP. Re: A randomized, placebo-controlled trial of repeated IV antibiotic therapy for Lyme encephalopathy. Prolonged Lyme disease treatment: enough is enough. Neurology. 2009 Jan 27;72(4):383-4; author reply 384.

Márquez FJ. Molecular detection of Bartonella alsatica in European wild rabbits (Oryctolagus cuniculus) in Andalusia (Spain). Vector Borne Zoonotic Dis. 2010 Oct;10(8):731-4. Epub 2010 Jan 8.

Márquez FJ, Millán J, Rodríguez-Liébana JJ, García-Egea I, Muniain MA. Detection and identification of Bartonella sp. in fleas from carnivorous mammals in Andalusia, Spain. Med Vet Entomol. 2009 Dec;23(4):393-8.

Marra CM. Neurologic complications of Bartonella henselae infection. Curr Opin Neurol. 1995;8(3):164-169.

Marre ML, Darcy CT, Yinh J, Akira S, Uematsu S, Steere AC, Hu LT. Role of adrenomedullin in Lyme disease. Infect Immun. 2010 Dec;78(12):5307-13. Epub 2010 Oct 4.

Marsch WC, Mayet A, Wolter M. Cutaneous fibroses induced by Borrelia burgdorferi. Br J Dermatol, 128(6):674-8. 1993.

Marsilia GM, La Mura A, Galdiero R, Galdiero E, Aloj G, Ragozzino A. Isolated hepatic involvement of cat scratch disease in immunocompetent adults: Enhanced magnetic resonance imaging, pathological findings, and molecular analysis--two cases. Int J Surg Pathol. 2006 Oct;14(4):349-54.

Marsot M, Sigaud M, Chapuis JL, Ferquel E, Cornet M, Vourc'h G. Introduced Siberian chipmunks (Tamias sibiricus barberi) harbor more-diverse Borrelia burgdorferi sensu lato genospecies than native bank voles (Myodes glareolus). Appl Environ Microbiol. 2011 Aug 15;77(16):5716-21. Epub 2011 Jun 24.

Martín L, Vidal L, Campins A, Salvá F, Riera M, Carrillo A, Sáez de Ibarra JI. Bartonella as a cause of blood culture-negative endocarditis. Description of five cases. Rev Esp Cardiol. 2009 Jun;62(6):694-7.

Martinez-Diaz GJ, Kim J, Bruckner AL. A toddler with facial nodules: a case of idiopathic facial aseptic granuloma. Dermatol Online J. 2010 Jan 15;16(1):9.

Martínez-Girón R, Esteban JG, Ribas A, Doganci L. Protozoa in respiratory pathology: a review. Eur Respir J. 2008 Nov;32(5):1354-70. Review.

Martinot M, Zadeh MM, Hansmann Y, Grawey I, Christmann D, Aguillon S, Jouglin M, Chauvin A, De Briel D. Babesiosis in immunocompetent patients, Europe. Emerg Infect Dis. 2011 Jan;17(1):114-6.

Maruyama S. [Cat-scratch disease].[Article in Japanese]. Nihon Rinsho. 2010 Jun;68 Suppl 6:244-7.

Mascarelli PE, Iredell JR, Maggi RG, Weinberg G, Breitschwerdt EB. Bartonella species bacteremia in two patients with epitheliod hemangioendothelioma. J Clin Microbiol. 2011 Sep 14. [Epub ahead of print]

Massarotti EM, Luger SW, Rahn DW, Messner RP, Wong JB, Johnson RC, Steere AC. Treatment of early Lyme disease. Am J Med. 1992 Apr;92(4):396-403.

Massei F, Gori L, Macchia P, Maggiore G. The expanded spectrum of bartonellosis in children. Infect Dis Clin North Am. 2005;19(3):691-711.

Massei F, Gori L, Taddeucci G, Macchia P, Maggiore G. Bartonella henselae infection associated with Guillain-Barre syndrome. Pediatr Infect Dis J. 2006 Jan;25(1):90-1.

Massei F, Messina F, Talini I, Massimetti M, Palla G, Macchia P, Maggiore G. Widening of the clinical spectrum of Bartonella henselae infection as recognized through serodiagnostics. Eur J Pediatr. 2000;159(6):416-419.

Massung RF, Mather TN, Levin ML. Reservoir Competency of Goats for the Ap-Variant 1 Strain of Anaplasma phagocytophilum. Infect Immun. 2006 February; 74(2): 1373–1375.

Mastrandrea S, Simonetta Taras M, Capitta P, Tola S, Marras V, Strusi G, Masala G. Detection of Bartonella henselae--DNA in macronodular hepatic lesions of an immunocompetent woman. Clin Microbiol Infect. 2009 Dec;15 Suppl 2:116-7. Epub 2009 Sep 28.

Masuzawa T, Iwaki A, Sato Y, Miyamoto K, Korenberg EI, Yanagihara Y. Genetic diversity of Borrelia burgdorferi sensu lato isolated in far eastern Russia. Microbiol Immunol. 1997;41(8):595-600.

Masuzawa T, Kawabata H, Beppu Y, Miyamoto K, Nakao M, Sato N, Muramatsu K, Sato N, Johnson RC, Yanagihara Y. Characterization of monoclonal antibodies for identification of Borrelia japonica, isolates from Ixodes ovatus. Microbiol Immunol. 1994;38(5):393-8.

Matera G, Liberto MC, Joosten LA, Vinci M, Quirino A, Pulicari MC, Kullberg BJ, Van der Meer JW, Netea MG, Focà A. The Janus face of Bartonella quintana recognition by Toll-like receptors (TLRs): a review. Eur Cytokine Netw. 2008 Sep;19(3):113-8. Epub 2008 Sep 8. Review.

Matera G, Muto V, Vinci M, Zicca E, Abdollahi-Roodsaz S, van de Veerdonk FL, Kullberg BJ, Liberto MC, van der Meer JW, Focà A, Netea MG, Joosten LA. Receptor recognition of and immune intracellular pathways for Veillonella parvula lipopolysaccharide. Clin Vaccine Immunol. 2009 Dec;16(12):1804-9. Epub 2009 Oct 14.

Mathers A, Smith RP, Cahill B, Lubelczyk C, Elias SP, Lacombe E, Morris SR, Vary CP, Parent CE, Rand PW. Strain diversity of Borrelia burgdorferi in ticks dispersed in North America by migratory birds. J Vector Ecol. 2011 Jun;36(1):24-9.

Mathiesen DH, Glaser C, Lane RS, TelfordIII SR, Thomford JW, Mathieson D, Krause PJ, Phillip DF, and Conrad PA. Infection with a Babesia-like organism in north California. N Engl J Med. 1995;332:298-303.

Mathieu S, Vellin JF, Poujol D, Ristori JM, Soubrier M. Cat scratch disease during etanercept therapy. Joint Bone Spine. 2007 Mar;74(2):184-6. Epub 2007 Feb 5.

Mathis A, Hilpertshauser H, Deplazes P. [Piroplasms of ruminants in Switzerland and zoonotic significance of Babesia]. [Article in German]. Schweiz Arch Tierheilkd. 2006;148:151-9.

Matsuo T, Notohara K. Bartonella henselae bacilli detected in vitrectomy aspirates in a patient with massive vitreous opacity with total retinal detachment. Ocul Immunol Inflamm. 2006 Feb;14(1):47-9.

Matthee S, Horak IG, Beaucournu JC, Durden LA, Ueckermann EA, McGeoch MA. Epifaunistic arthropod parasites of the four-striped mouse, Rhabdomys pumilio, in the Western Cape Province, South Africa. J Parasitol. 2007 Feb;93(1):47-59.

Mattman LH. Cell wall deficient forms: stealth pathogens. CRC Press, Inc., Boca Raton, Fla., 2nd ed. 1993.

Maurin M, Birtles R, Raoult D. Current knowledge of Bartonella species. Eur J Clin Microbiol Infect Dis. 1997 Jul;16(7):487-506. Review.

Maurin M, Eb F, Etienne J, Raoult D. Serological cross-reactions between Bartonella and Chlamydia species: implications for diagnosis. J Clin Microbiol. 1997 Sep;35(9):2283-7.

Maurin M, Raoult D. Bartonella infections: diagnostic and management issues. Curr Opin Infect Dis. 1998 Apr;11(2):189-193.

Maurin M, Raoult D. Isolation in endothelial cell cultures of chlamydia trachomatis LGV (Serovar L2) from a lymph node of a patient with suspected cat scratch disease. J Clin Microbiol. 2000 Jun;38(6):2062-4.

Maurin M, Rolain JM, Raoult D. Comparison of in-house and commercial slides for detection by immunofluorescence of immunoglobulins G and M against Bartonella henselae and Bartonella quintana. Clin Diagn Lab Immunol. 2002 Sep;9(5):1004-9.

Mavin S, McDonagh S, Evans R, Milner RM, Chatterton JM, Ho-Yen DO. Interpretation criteria in Western blot diagnosis of Lyme borreliosis. Br J Biomed Sci. 2011;68(1):5-10.

May WS Jr, Cuatrecasas P. Transferrin receptor: its biological significance. J Membr Biol. 1985;88(3):205-15. Review.

Mazyad SA, Shoukry NM, El-Alfy NM. Efficacy of Ixodes ricinus as a vector of zoonotic babesiosis in Sinai Peninsula, Egypt. J Egypt Soc Parasitol. 2010 Aug;40(2):499-514.

Mba PA, Marié JL, Rolain JM, Davoust B, Beaucournu JC, Raoult D, Parola P. Rickettsia felis and Bartonella henselae in fleas from Lebanon. Vector Borne Zoonotic Dis. 2011 Jul;11(7):991-2. Epub 2011 Feb 1.

McAuliffe P, Brassard MR, Fallon B. Memory and executive functions in adolescents with posttreatment Lyme disease. Appl Neuropsychol. 2008;15(3):208-19.

McCarthy, JS. Malaria Chemoprophylaxis in War and Peace. [Editorial]. MJA vol. 182 No. 4, 2005 Feb. 21. Available from: http://www.mja.com.au/public/issues/182_04_210205/mcc10925_fm.pdf.

McCool TL, Hoey JG, Montileone F, Goldenberg HB, Mordechai E, Adelson ME. Discovery and analysis of Bartonella henselae antigens for use in clinical serologic assays. Diagn Microbiol Infect Dis. 2008 Jan;60(1):17-23. Epub 2007 Sep 21.

McCord AM, Burgess AW, Whaley MJ, Anderson BE. Interaction of Bartonella henselae with Endothelial Cells Promotes Monocyte/Macrophage Chemoattractant Protein 1 Gene Expression and Protein Production and Triggers Monocyte Migration. Infect Immun. 2005 September; 73(9): 5735–5742.

McCord AM, Cuevas J, Anderson BE. Bartonella-induced endothelial cell proliferation is mediated by release of calcium from intracellular stores. DNA Cell Biol. 2007 Sep;26(9):657-63.

McCord AM, Resto-Ruiz SI, Anderson BE. Autocrine role for interleukin-8 in Bartonella henselae-induced angiogenesis. Infect Immun. 2006 Sep;74(9):5185-90.

McCord G, Smucker WD, Selius BA, Hannan S, Davidson E, Schrop SL, Rao V, Albrecht P. Answering questions at the point of care: do residents practice EBM or manage information sources? Acad Med. 2007 Mar;82(3):298-303.

McDonagh JER. The life cycle of the organism of syphilis. Lancet, 2:1011. 1912.

McDonagh JER. The complete life history of the organism of syphilis. British Medical Journal of Dermatology & Syphilis, 25:1-14. 1913.

McDonagh JER. The nature of disease. Heinemann, London. 1924.

McElroy KM, Blagburn BL, Breitschwerdt EB, Mead PS, McQuiston JH. Flea-associated zoonotic diseases of cats in the USA: bartonellosis, flea-borne rickettsioses, and plague. Trends Parasitol. 2010 Apr;26(4):197-204. Epub 2010 Feb 23. Review.

McFadden JP, Greaves MW. Urticarial lesions and Lyme disease. J Am Acad Dermatol, 25(1 Pt 1):131-2. 1991.

McGill S, Rajs J, Hjelm E, Lindquist O, Friman G. A study on forensic samples of Bartonella spp antibodies in Swedish intravenous heroin addicts. APMIS. 2003;111(4):507-513.

McGill S, Wesslen L, Hjelm E, Holmberg M, Rolf C, Friman G. Serological and epidemiological analysis of the prevalence of Bartonella spp. antibodies in Swedish elite orienteers 1992-93. Scand J Infect Dis. 2001;33(6):423-428.

McGrath N, Wallis W. Cat-scratch encephalopathy. Neurology. 1998;51(4):1239.

McKenna D, Faustini Y, Nowakowski J, Wormser GP. Factors influencing the utilization of Lyme disease-prevention behaviors in a high-risk population. J Am Acad Nurse Pract. 2004 Jan;16(1):24-30.

McNeil DG Jr. Plant shortage leaves campaigns against malaria at risk. New York Times. 2004 Nov 14. [cited 2006 Jul]. Available from: http://www.nytimes.com/ 2004/11/14/international/ asia/14malaria.html?ex=11344 50000&en=7ce7c3af52873986& ei=5070.

Mead P, Goel R, Kugeler K. Canine serology as adjunct to human lyme disease surveillance. Emerg Infect Dis. 2011 Sep;17(9):1710-2.

Mediannikov O, Cabre O, Qu F, Socolovschi C, Davoust B, Marié JL, Parola P, Raoult D. Rickettsia felis and Bartonella clarridgeiae in fleas from New Caledonia. Vector Borne Zoonotic Dis. 2011 Feb;11(2):181-3. Epub 2010 Jun 23.

Mediannikov O, Diatta G, Fenollar F, Sokhna C, Trape JF, Raoult D. Tick-Borne Rickettsioses, Neglected Emerging Diseases in Rural Senegal. PLoS Negl Trop Dis. 2010 September; 4(9): e821. Published online 2010 September 14.

Mediannikov O, Ivanov L, Zdanovskaya N, Vysochina N, Fournier PE, Tarasevich I, Raoult D. Molecular screening of Bartonella species in rodents from the Russian Far East. Ann N Y Acad Sci. 2005 Dec;1063:308-11.

Mediannikov OIu, Melikian AL. [A case of cat scratch disease in a patient with diabetes mellitus and chronic renal failure].[Article in Russian]. Klin Med (Mosk). 2006;84(7):61-3.

Medical Diagnostic Laboratories L.L.C., 133 Gaither Dr., Suite C, Mt. Laurel, NJ 08054, USA. PCR analysis of Ixodes scapularis ticks collected in New Jersey identified infections with Borrelia burgdorferi (33.6%), Babesia microti (8.4%), Anaplasma phagocytophila (1.9%), and Bartonella spp. (34.5%). The I. Scapularis tick is a potential pathogen vector that can cause coinfection and contribute to the variety of clinical responses noted in some tick-borne disease patients. Cited in PubMed.

Medical News Today. [Monograph on the Internet]. Available from: http://www.medicalnewstoday.com/medicalnews. php?newsid=3518. Accessed 2006 Aug 13.

MedicineNet.com. Definition of Artemisinin. Available from: http://www.medterms.com/script/main/ art.asp?article key=24010. Accessed 2006 Aug 10.

Medkova Z. Bartonelloses. Klin Mikrobiol Infekc Lek. 2004;10(5): 207-213.

Medline Plus: Drugs and Supplements. "Hydroxychloroquine". [Monograph on the Internet]. Available from: http://www.nlm.nih. gov/medlineplus/ druginfo/medmaster/a601240.html

Medlock JM, Barrass I, Kerrod E, Taylor MA, Leach S. Analysis of climatic predictions for extrinsic incubation of Dirofilaria in the United kingdom. Vector Borne Zoonotic Dis. 2007 Spring;7(1):4-14.

Meer-Scherrer L, Chang Loa C, Adelson ME, Mordechai E, Lobrinus JA, Fallon BA, Tilton RC. Lyme disease associated with Alzheimer's disease. Curr Microbiol. 2006 Apr;52(4):330-2. Epub 2006 Mar 9.

Meeusen ENT, Walker J, Peters A, Pastoret P, Jungersen G. Current Status of Veterinary Vaccines. Clin Microbiol Rev. 2007 July; 20(3): 489–510.

Meghari S, Rolain JM, Grau GE, Platt E, Barrassi L, Mege JL, Raoult D. Antiangiogenic effect of erythromycin: an in vitro model of Bartonella quintana infection. J Infect Dis. 2006 Feb 1;193(3):380-6. Epub 2005 Dec 27.

Mehock JR, Greene CE, Gherardini FC, Hahn TW, Krause DC. Bartonella henselae invasion of feline erythrocytes in vitro. Infect Immun. 1998;66(7):3462-3466.

Mehmi M, Lim SP, Tan CY. An unusual cutaneous presentation of cat-scratch disease. Clin Exp Dermatol. 2007 Mar;32(2):219-20. Epub 2006 Dec 14.

Meier C, Reulen HJ, Huber P, Mumenthaler M. Meningo-radiculoneuritis mimicking vertebral disc herniation. A "neurosurgical" complication of Lyme-borreliosis. Acta Neurochir (Wien), 98(1-2):42-6. 1989.

Meier P, Blatz R, Gau M, Spencker FB, Wiedemann P. Pars plana vitrectomy in Borrelia burgdorferi endophthalmitis. 1998. Klin Monatsbl Augenheilkd, 213(6):351-4.

Meimoun P, Sayah S, Benali T, Bore AL, Bailly J, Beausoleil J, Jeleff C, Maitre B. [Lyme disease presenting as infarction pain. A case report]. [Article in French]. Arch Mal Coeur Vaiss, 94(12):1419-22. 2001.

Meininger GR, Nadasdy T, Hruban RH, Bollinger RC, Baughman KL, Hare JM. Chronic active myocarditis following acute Bartonella henselae infection (cat scratch disease). Am J Surg Pathol. 2001;25(9):1211-1214.

Meirelles Richer L, Aroso M, Contente-Cuomo T, Ivanova L, Gomes-Solecki M. Reservoir Targeted Vaccine for Lyme Borreliosis Induces a Year Long, Neutralizing Antibody Response to OspA in White-footed Mice. Clin Vaccine Immunol. 2011 Sep 14. [Epub ahead of print]

Meirowsky E. (Abstract by Dr. H. C. Semon) On t he biological position of the Spirochaeta pallida and its development. British Journal of Dermatology, 26:185. 1914.

Melet M, Gerard A, Voiriot P, Gayet S, May T, et al. [Fatal meningoradiculoneuritis in Lyme disease]. [Article in French]. Presse Med, 15(41):2075. 1986.

Meliani P, Khatibi S, Randazzo S, Gorenflot A, Marchou B. [Human babesiosis].[Article in French]. Med Mal Infect. 2006 Oct;36(10):499-504. Epub 2006 Oct 4. Review.

Melikian AL, Mediannikov OIu, Kaplanskaia IB, Komarova AI, Tarasevich IV. [Bartonella infection in hematological practice]. [Article in Russian]. Ter Arkh. 2007;79(4):58-62.

Mellor PJ, Fetz K, Maggi RG, Haugland S, Dunning M, Villiers EJ, Mellanby RJ, Williams D, Breitschwerdt E, Herrtage ME. Alpha1-proteinase inhibitor deficiency and Bartonella infection in association with panniculitis, polyarthritis, and meningitis in a dog. J Vet Intern Med. 2006 Jul-Aug;20(4):1023-8.

Menichetti F, Bindi ML, Tascini C, Urbani L, Biancofiore G, Doria R, Esposito M, Mozzo R, Catalano G, Filipponi F. Fever, mental impairment, acute anemia, and renal failure in patient undergoing orthotopic liver transplantation: posttransplantation malaria. Liver Transpl. 2006 Apr;12(4):674-6.

Mennel S, Meyer CH, Schroeder FM. [Multifocal chorioretinitis, papillitis, and recurrent optic neuritis in cat-scratch disease]. [Article in French]. J Fr Ophtalmol. 2005 Dec;28(10):e10.

Merle De Boever C, Mura F, Brun M, Reynes J. [Ocular bartonellosis in an HIV-HVC coinfected patient].[Article in French]. Med Mal Infect. 2008 Sep;38(9):504-6. Epub 2008 Aug 15.

Mermin J, Ekwaru JP, Liechty CA, Were W, Downing R, Ransom R, Weidle P, Lule J, Coutinho A, Solberg P. Effect of co-trimoxazole prophylaxis, antiretroviral therapy, and insecticide-treated bednets on the frequency of malaria in HIV-1-infected adults in Uganda: a prospective cohort study. Lancet. 2006 Apr 15;367(9518):1256-61.

Merrell DS, Falkow S. Frontal and stealth attack strategies in microbial pathogenesis. Nature. 2004 Jul 8;430(6996):250-6. Review.

Messori L, Gabbiani C, Casini A, Siragusa M, Vincieri FF, Bilia AR. The reaction of artemisinins with hemoglobin: a unified picture. Bioorg Med Chem. 2006 May 1;14(9):2972-7. [Epub 2006 Jan 10].

Metz CH, Buer J, Bornfeld N, Lipski A. Bilateral Bartonella henselae neuroretinitis with stellate maculopathy in a 6-year-old boy. Infection. 2011 Aug 9. [Epub ahead of print]

Metzkor-Cotter E, Kletter Y, Avidor B, et al. Long-term serological analysis and clinical follow-up of patients with cat scratch disease. Clin Infect Dis. 2003;37(9):1149-1154.

Mexas AM, Hancock SI, Breitschwerdt EB. Bartonella henselae and Bartonella elizabethae as potential canine pathogens. J Clin Microbiol. 2002 Dec;40(12):4670-4.

Meyer AL, Trollmo C, Crawford F, Marrack P, Steere AC, Huber BT, Kappler J, Hafler DA. Direct enumeration of Borrelia-reactive CD4 T cells ex vivo by using MHC class II tetramers. Proc Natl Acad Sci U S A. 2000 Oct 10;97(21):11433-8.

Meyniel C, Wiertlewski S. [Optic neuritis].[Article in French]. Rev Med Interne. 2010 Jul;31(7):481-5.

Michau TM, Breitschwerdt EB, Gilger BC, Davidson MG. Bartonella vinsonii subspecies berkhoffi as a possible cause of anterior uveitis and choroiditis in a dog. Vet Ophthalmol. 2003 Dec;6(4):299-304.

Michos A, Dessypris N, Pourtsidis A, Moschovi M, Polychronopoulou S, Athanasiadou-Piperopoulou F, Kalmanti M, Syriopoulou VP, Mavrouli MD, Petridou ET. Delayed exposure to infections and childhood lymphomas: a case-control study. Cancer Causes Control. 2009 Jul;20(5):795-802. Epub 2009 Jan 25.

Miettinen OS. Rationality in medicine. J Eval Clin Pract. 2009. Dec;15(6):960-3.

Mietze A, Morick D, Köhler H, Harrus S, Dehio C, Nolte I, Goethe R. Combined MLST and AFLP typing of Bartonella henselae isolated from cats reveals new sequence types and suggests clonal evolution. Vet Microbiol. 2011 Mar 24;148(2-4):238-45. Epub 2010 Sep 21.

Mietze A, Strube C, Beyerbach M, Schnieder T, Goethe R. Occurrence of Bartonella henselae and Borrelia burgdorferi sensu lato co-infections in ticks collected from humans in Germany. Clin Microbiol Infect. 2011 Jun;17(6):918-20.

Mihalca AD, Gherman CM, Cozma V. Coendangered hard-ticks: threatened or threatening? Parasit Vectors. 2011; 4: 71. Published online 2011 May 9.

Mikkila H, Seppala I, Leirisalo-Repo M, Immonen I, Karma A. The etiology of uveitis: the role of infections with special reference to Lyme borreliosis. Acta Ophthalmol Scand, 75(6):716-9. 1997.

Mikkila HO, Seppala IJ, Viljanen MK, Peltomaa MP, Karma A. The expanding clinical spectrum of ocular Lyme borreliosis. Ophthalmology, 107(3):581-7. 2000.

Miklossy J. Alzheimer's disease--a spirochetosis? Neuroreport. 1993. July;4(7):841-8.

Miklossy J. Biology and neuropathology of dementia in syphilis and Lyme disease. Handb Clin Neurol. 2008;89:825-44.

Miklossy J. Chronic inflammation and amyloidogenesis in Alzheimer's disease -- role of Spirochetes. J Alzheimers Dis. 2008 May;13(4):381-91. Review.

Miklossy J, Kasas S, Zurn AD, McCall S, Yu S, McGeer PL. Persisting atypical and cystic forms of Borrelia burgdorferi and local inflammation in Lyme neuroborreliosis. J Neuroinflammation. 2008 Sep 25;5:40.

Miklossy J, Khalili K, Gern L, Ericson RL, Darekar P, Bolle L, Hurlimann J, Paster BJ. Borrelia burgdorferi persists in the brain in chronic lyme neuroborreliosis and may be associated with Alzheimer disease. J Alzheimers Dis. 2004 Dec;6(6):639-49; discussion 673-81.

Miklossy J, Kis A, Radenovic A, Miller L, Forro L, Martins R, Reiss K, Darbinian N, Darekar P, Mihaly L, Khalili K. Beta-amyloid deposition and Alzheimer's type changes induced by Borrelia spirochetes. Neurobiol Aging. May, 2005.

Miklossy J, Kuntzer T, Bogousslavsky J, Regli F, Janzer RC. Meningovascular form of neuroborreliosis: similarities between neuropathological findings in a case of Lyme disease and those occurring in tertiary neurosyphilis. Acta Neuropathol. 1990;80(5):568-72.

Mikolajczyk MG, O'Reilly KL. Clinical disease in kittens inoculated with a pathogenic strain of Bartonella henselae. Am J Vet Res. 2000;61(4):375-379.

Miles RW. Cognitive bias and planning error: nullification of evidence-based medicine in the nursing home. J Am Med Dir Assoc. 2010 Mar;11(3):194-203.

Millán J. Comments on the manuscript by Bitam et al., 'Fleas and flea-borne diseases'. Int J Infect Dis. 2011 Mar;15(3):e219. Epub 2010 Dec 28.

Millar B, Moore J, Mallon P, Xu J, Crowe M, Mcclurg R, Raoult D, Earle J, Hone R, Murphy P. Molecular diagnosis of infective endocarditis--a new Duke's criterion. Scand J Infect Dis. 2001;33(9):673-80.

Millar BC, Moore JE. Emerging issues in infective endocarditis. Emerg Infect Dis. 2004 Jun;10(6):1110-6.

Miller DS, Sauther ML, Hunter-Ishikawa M, Fish K, Culbertson H, Cuozzo PF, Campbell TW, Andrews GA, Chavey PS, Nachreiner R, Rumbeiha W, Stacewicz-Sapuntzakis M, Lappin MR. Biomedical evaluation of free-ranging ring-tailed lemurs (Lemur catta) in three habitats at the Beza Mahafaly Special Reserve, Madagascar. J Zoo Wildl Med. 2007 Jun;38(2):201-16.

Miller JC, Ma Y, Bian J, Sheehan KC, Zachary JF, Weis JH, Schreiber RD, Weis JJ. A critical role for Type I IFN in arthritis development following Borrelia burgdorferi infection of mice. J Immunol. 2008 December 15; 181(12): 8492–8503.

Miller JC, Maylor-Hagen H, Ma Y, Weis JH, Weis JJ. The Lyme Disease Spirochete Borrelia burgdorferi Utilizes Multiple Ligands, Including RNA, for Interferon Regulatory Factor 3-Dependent Induction of Type I Interferon-Responsive Genes. Infect Immun. 2010 July; 78(7): 3144–3153. Published online 2010 April 19.

Miller LC, Lynch EA, Isa S, Logan JW, Dinarello CA, Steere AC. Balance of synovial fluid IL-1 beta and IL-1 receptor antagonist and recovery from Lyme arthritis. Lancet. 1993 Jan 16;341(8838):146-8.

Miller LC, Isa S, Vannier E, Georgilis K, Steere AC, Dinarello CA. Live Borrelia burgdorferi preferentially activate interleukin-1 beta gene expression and protein synthesis over the interleukin-1 receptor antagonist. J Clin Invest. 1992 Sep;90(3):906-12.

Miller RS, Wongsrichanalai C, Buathong N, McDaniel P, Walsh DS, Knirsch C, Ohrt C. Effective treatment of uncomplicated Plasmodium falciparum malaria with azithromycin-quinine combinations: a randomized, dose-ranging study. Am J Trop Med Hyg. 2006 Mar;74(3):401-6.

Minadakis G, Chochlakis D, Kokkini S, Gikas A, Tselentis Y, Psaroulaki A. Seroprevalence of Bartonella henselae antibodies in blood donors in Crete. Scand J Infect Dis. 2008;40(10):846-7.

Minnick MF, Anderson BE. Bartonella interactions with host cells. Subcell Biochem. 2000;33:97-123. Review.

Minnick MF, Battisti JM. Pestilence, persistence and pathogenicity: infection strategies of Bartonella. Future Microbiol. 2009 Aug;4(6):743-58. Review.

Minnick MF, Smitherman LS, Samuels DS. Mitogenic Effect of Bartonella bacilliformis on Human Vascular Endothelial Cells and Involvement of GroEL. Infect Immun. 2003 December; 71(12): 6933–6942.

Mischoulon D, Fava M. Role of S-adenosyl-L-methionine in the treatment of depression: a review of the evidence. Am J Clin Nutr. 2002;76(5):1158S-61S.

Mitchell BM, Font RL. Molecular detection of Bartonella henselae for the diagnosis of cat scratch disease and bacillary angiomatosis of the conjunctiva. Cornea. 2011 Jul;30(7):807-14.

Mitchell PD, Reed KD, Hofkes JM. Immunoserologic evidence of coinfection with Borrelia burgdorferi, Babesia microti, and human granulocytic Ehrlichia species in residents of Wisconsin and Minnesota. J Clin Microbiol. 1996 Mar;34(3):724-7.

Miura K, Rikihisa Y. Virulence Potential of Ehrlichia chaffeensis Strains of Distinct Genome Sequences. Infect Immun. 2007 July; 75(7): 3604–3613. Published online 2007 April 16.

Miyamoto K, Hashimoto Y. [Prevention of Lyme borreliosis infection after tick bites].[Article in Japanese]. Kansenshogaku Zasshi. 1998 May;72(5):512-6.

Miyamoto K, Nakao M, Sato N, Mori M. Isolation of Lyme disease spirochetes from an ixodid tick in Hokkaido, Japan. Acta Trop. 1991 Apr;49(1):65-8.

Miyamoto K, Nakao M, Uchikawa K, Fujita H. Prevalence of Lyme borreliosis spirochetes in ixodid ticks of Japan, with special reference to a new potential vector, Ixodes ovatus (Acari: Ixodidae). J Med Entomol. 1992 Mar;29(2):216-20.

Miyamoto K, Sato Y, Okada K, Fukunaga M, Sato F. Competence of a migratory bird, red-bellied thrush (Turdus chrysolaus), as an avian reservoir for the Lyme disease spirochetes in Japan. Acta Trop. 1997 Apr 30;65(1):43-51.

Miyamoto S, Takemura Y, Hanba Y, Kitani A, Ishizuka T, Suzuki K, Sekiguchi S. [Comparable evaluation of serological diagnostic tests (ELISA, IFA and PA methods) for the detection of anti-Borrelia burgdorferi antibody].[Article in Japanese]. Rinsho Byori. 1992 Nov;40(11):1204-9.

Miyashiro MJ, Yee RW, Patel G, Ruiz RS Lyme disease associated with unilateral interstitial keratitis. Cornea, 18(1):115-6. 1999.

Mofenson LM, Brady MT, Danner SP, Dominguez KL, Hazra R, Handelsman E, Havens P, Nesheim S, Read JS, Serchuck L, Van Dyke R; Centers for Disease Control and Prevention; National Institutes of Health; HIV Medicine Association of the Infectious Diseases Society of America; Pediatric Infectious Diseases Society; American Academy of Pediatrics. Guidelines for the Prevention and Treatment of Opportunistic Infections among HIV-exposed and HIV-infected children: recommendations from CDC, the National Institutes of Health, the HIV Medicine Association of the Infectious Diseases Society of America, the Pediatric Infectious Diseases Society, and the American Academy of Pediatrics. MMWR Recomm Rep. 2009 Sep 4;58(RR-11):1-166.

Moffat CM, Sigal LH, Steere AC, Freeman DH, Dwyer JM. Cellular immune findings in Lyme disease. Correlation with serum IgM and disease activity. Am J Med. 1984 Oct;77(4):625-32.

Mogollon-Pasapera E, Otvos L Jr, Giordano A, Cassone M. Bartonella: emerging pathogen or emerging awareness? Int J Infect Dis. 2009 Jan;13(1):3-8. Epub 2008 Jul 14. Review.

Mokry M, Flaschka G, Kleinert G, Kleinert R, Fazekas F, Kopp W. Chronic Lyme disease with an expansive granulomatous lesion in the cerebellopontine angle. Neurosurgery, 27(3):446-51. 1990.

Möller HJ, Maier W. Evidence-based medicine in psycho-pharmacotherapy: possibilities, problems and limitations. Eur Arch Psychiatry Clin Neurosci. 2010 Feb;260(1):25-39.

Moniuszko A, Gińdzieńska-Sieśkiewicz E, Pancewicz SA, Czupryna P, Zajkowska J, Sierakowski S. Evaluation of skin thickness lesions in patients with Lyme disease measured by modified Rodnan total skin score. Rheumatol Int. 2011 Sep 30. [Epub ahead of print]

Montcriol A, Benard F, Fenollar F, Ribeiri A, Bonnet M, Collart F, Guidon C. Fatal myocarditis-associated Bartonella quintana endocarditis: a case report. J Med Case Reports. 2009 Jul 17;3:7325.

Monteil M, Durand B, Bouchouicha R, Petit E, Chomel B, Arvand M, Boulouis HJ, Haddad N. Development of discriminatory multiple-locus variable number tandem repeat analysis for Bartonella henselae. Microbiology. 2007 Apr;153(Pt 4):1141-8.

Monteil RA, Michiels JF, Hofman P, Saint-Paul MC, Hitzig C, Perrin C, Santini J. Histological and ultrastructural study of one case of oral bacillary angiomatosis in HIV disease and review of the literature. Eur J Cancer B Oral Oncol. 1994 Jan;30B(1):65-71. Review.

Montero E, Rafiq S, Heck S, Lobo CA. Inhibition of human erythrocyte invasion by Babesia divergens using serine protease inhibitors. Mol Biochem Parasitol. 2007 May;153(1):80-4. Epub 2007 Jan 26.

Montero E, Rodriguez M, Oksov Y, Lobo CA. Babesia divergens apical membrane antigen 1 and its interaction with the human red blood cell. Infect Immun. 2009 Nov;77(11):4783-93. Epub 2009 Aug 31.

Moore JC, Lai H, Li JR, Ren RL, McDougall JA, Singh NP, Chou CK. Oral administration of dihydroartemisinin and ferrous sulfate retarded implanted fibrosarcoma growth in the rat. Cancer Lett. 1995 Nov;98(1):83-7.

Moore MW, Cruz AR, LaVake CJ, Marzo AL, Eggers CH, Salazar JC, Radolf JD. Phagocytosis of Borrelia burgdorferi and Treponema pallidum Potentiates Innate Immune Activation and Induces Gamma Interferon Production. Infect Immun. 2007 April; 75(4): 2046–2062. Published online 2007 January 12.

Moore TA, Tomayko JF Jr, Wierman AM, Rensimer ER, White AC Jr. Imported malaria in the 1990s. A report of 59 cases from Houston, Tex. Arch Fam Med. 1994 Feb;3(2):130-6.

Morales SC, Breitschwerdt EB, Washabau RJ, Matise I, Maggi RG, Duncan AW. Detection of Bartonella henselae DNA in two dogs with pyogranulomatous lymphadenitis. J Am Vet Med Assoc. 2007 Mar 1;230(5):681-5.

Moreno MA. Advice for patients. Lyme disease in children and adolescents. Arch Pediatr Adolesc Med. 2011 Jan;165(1):96.

Morick D, Krasnov BR, Khokhlova IS, Gottlieb Y, Harrus S. Investigation of Bartonella acquisition and transmission in Xenopsylla ramesis fleas (Siphonaptera: Pulicidae). Mol Ecol. 2011 Jul;20(13):2864-70. Epub 2011 Feb 24.

Moro MH, Zegarra-Moro OL, Bjornsson J, Hofmeister EK, Bruinsma E, Germer JJ, Persing DH. Increased arthritis severity in mice coinfected with Borrelia burgdorferi and Babesia microti. J Infec Dis. 2002 Aug 1;186(3):428-31. Epub 2002 Jul 5.

Mormont E, Esselinckx W, De Ronde T, Hanson P, Deltombe T, Laloux P. Abdominal wall weakness and lumboabdominal pain revealing neuroborreliosis: a report of three cases. Clin Rheumatol, 20(6):447-50. 2001.

Morway C, Kosoy M, Eisen R, Montenieri J, Sheff K, Reynolds PJ, Powers N. A longitudinal study of Bartonella infection in populations of woodrats and their fleas. J Vector Ecol. 2008 Dec;33(2):353-64.

Mosbacher M, Elliott SP, Shehab Z, Pinnas JL, Klotz JH, Klotz SA. Cat scratch disease and arthropod vectors: more to it than a scratch? J Am Board Fam Med. 2010 Sep-Oct;23(5):685-6.

Mosbacher ME, Klotz S, Klotz J, Pinnas JL. Bartonella henselae and the potential for arthropod vector-borne transmission. Vector Borne Zoonotic Dis. 2011 May;11(5):471-7. Epub 2010 Oct 25.

Moscatello AL, Worden DL, Nadelman RB, Wormser G, Lucente F. Otolaryngologic aspects of Lyme disease. Laryngoscope. 1991 Jun;101(6 Pt 1):592-5.

Motaleb MA, Pitzer JE, Sultan SZ, Liu J. A novel gene inactivation system reveals altered periplasmic flagellar orientation in a Borrelia burgdorferi fliL mutant. J Bacteriol. 2011 Jul;193(13):3324-31. Epub 2011 Mar 25.

Motaleb MA, Sultan SZ, Miller MR, Li C, Charon NW. CheY3 of Borrelia burgdorferi is the key response regulator essential for chemotaxis and forms a long-lived phosphorylated intermediate. J Bacteriol. 2011 Jul;193(13):3332-41. Epub 2011 Apr 29.

Mourin S, Bonnier C, Bigaignon G, Lyon G. Epilepsy disclosing neuroborreliosis. Rev Neurol (Paris), 149(8-9):489-91. 1993.

Movila A, Reye AL, Dubinina HV, Tolstenkov OO, Toderas I, Hübschen JM, Muller CP, Alekseev AN. Detection of Babesia Sp. EU1 and members of spotted fever group rickettsiae in ticks collected from migratory birds at Curonian Spit, North-Western Russia. Vector Borne Zoonotic Dis. 2011 Jan;11(1):89-91. Epub 2010 Jun 16.

Mudd S, Polevitsky K, Anderson TF. Bacterial morphology as shown by the electron microscope; V. Treponema pallidum, Treponema macrodentium and Treponema microdentium. Journal of Bacteriology, 46:15-24. 1943.

Muenzel D, Duetsch S, Fauser C, Slotta-Huspenina J, Gaa J, Rummeny EJ, Holzapfel K. Diffusion-weighted magnetic resonance imaging in cervical lymphadenopathy: report of three cases of patients with Bartonella henselae infection mimicking malignant disease. Acta Radiol. 2009 Oct;50(8):914-6.

Müllegger RR, Means TK, Shin JJ, Lee M, Jones KL, Glickstein LJ, Luster AD, Steere AC. Chemokine signatures in the skin disorders of Lyme borreliosis in Europe: predominance of CXCL9 and CXCL10 in erythema migrans and acrodermatitis and CXCL13 in lymphocytoma. Infect Immun. 2007 Sep;75(9):4621-8. Epub 2007 Jul 2.

Müllegger RR, McHugh G, Ruthazer R, Binder B, Kerl H, Steere AC. Differential expression of cytokine mRNA in skin specimens from patients with erythema migrans or acrodermatitis chronica atrophicans. J Invest Dermatol. 2000 Dec;115(6):1115-23.

Müller NF, Kaiser PO, Linke D, Schwarz H, Riess T, Schäfer A, Eble JA, Kempf VA. Trimeric autotransporter adhesin-dependent adherence of Bartonella henselae, Bartonella quintana, and Yersinia enterocolitica to matrix components and endothelial cells under static and dynamic flow conditions. Infect Immun. 2011 Jul;79(7):2544-53. Epub 2011 May 2.

Mun J, Eisen RJ, Eisen L, Lane RS. Detection of a Borrelia miyamotoi sensu lato relapsing-fever group spirochete from Ixodes pacificus in California. J Med Entomol. 2006 Jan;43(1):120-3.

Muñana KR, Vitek SM, Hegarty BC, Kordick DL, Breitschwerdt EB. Infection of fetal feline brain cells in culture with Bartonella henselae. Infect Immun. 2001 Jan;69(1):564-9.

Munderloh UG, Park YJ, Dioh JM, Fallon AM, Kurtti TJ. Plasmid modifications in a tick-borne pathogen, Borrelia burgdorferi, cocultured with tick cells. Insect Mol Biol. 1993;1(4):195-203.

Munford R, Lu M, Varley A. Kill the Bacteria … and Also Their Messengers? Adv Immunol. 2009; 103: 29.

Munoz J, Velasco M, Alonso D, Valls ME, Corachan M, Gascon J. [How much primaquine is needed to eradicate Plasmodium vivax hypnozoites?] Enferm Infecc Microbiol Clin. 2006 Jan;24(1):29-30. [Article in Spanish].

Munro JB, Silva JC. Ribonucleotide Reductase as a Target to Control Apicomplexan Diseases. Curr Issues Mol Biol. 2011 Jul 26;14(1):9-26. [Epub ahead of print]

Munson PD, Boyce TG, Salomao DR, Orvidas LJ. Cat-scratch disease of the head and neck in a pediatric population: surgical indications and outcomes. Otolaryngol Head Neck Surg. 2008 Sep;139(3):358-63.

Munter S, Way M, Frischknecht F. Signaling during pathogen infection. Sci STKE. 2006;2006(335):re5.

Murakami K, Tsukahara M, Tsuneoka H, et al. Cat scratch disease: analysis of 130 seropositive cases. J Infect Chemother. 2002;8(4):349-352.

Murray MA, Zamecki KJ, Paskowski J, Lelli GJ Jr. Ocular bacillary angiomatosis in an immunocompromised man. Ophthal Plast Reconstr Surg. 2010 Sep-Oct;26(5):371-2.

Murray MT. Encyclopedia of Nutritional Supplements. Prima; Rocklin, CA 1996;p.208-13.

Murray R, Morawetz R, Kepes J, el Gammal T, LeDoux M. Lyme neuroborreliosis manifesting as an intracranial mass lesion. Neurosurgery, 30(5):769-73. 1992.

Murray TS, Shapiro ED. Lyme disease. Clin Lab Med. 2010 Mar;30(1):311-28. Review.

Mursic VP, Wanner G, Reinhardt S, Wilske B, Busch U, Marget W. Formation and cultivation of Borrelia burgdorferi spheroplast L-form variants. 1996. Infection, 24(3):218-26.

Murthy SN, Faden HS, Cohen ME, Bakshi R. Acute disseminated encephalomyelitis in children. Pediatrics. 2002 Aug;110(2 Pt 1):e21.

Musto P, Falcone A, Sanpaolo G, et al. Heterogeneity of response to imatinib-mesylate (glivec) in patients with hypereosinophilic syndrome: implications for dosing and pathogenesis. Leuk Lymphoma. 2004;45(6):1219-1222.

Myers TA, Kaushal D, Philipp MT. Microglia Are Mediators of Borrelia burgdorferi–Induced Apoptosis in SH-SY5Y Neuronal Cells. PLoS Pathog. 2009 Nov;5(11):e1000659. Epub 2009 Nov 13.

Mygland A, Skarpaas T, Ljøstad U. Chronic polyneuropathy and Lyme disease. Eur J Neurol. 2006 Nov;13(11):1213-5.

Myint KS, Gibbons RV, Iverson J, Shrestha SK, Pavlin JA, Mongkolsirichaikul D, Kosoy MY. Serological response to Bartonella species in febrile patients from Nepal. Trans R Soc Trop Med Hyg. 2011 Sep 26. [Epub ahead of print]

Mylonakis, E. When to suspect and how to monitor babesiosis. American Family Physician. 2001;63:1969-74.

Mylonakis ME, Koutinas AF, Breitschwerdt EB, Hegarty BC, Billinis CD, Leontides LS, Kontos VS. Chronic canine ehrlichiosis (Ehrlichia canis): a retrospective study of 19 natural cases. J Am Anim Hosp Assoc. 2004 May-Jun;40(3):174-84.

Na-Bangchang K, Krudsood S, Silachamroon U, Molunto P, Tasanor O, Chalermrut K, Tangpukdee N, Matangkasombut O, Kano S, Looareesuwan S. The pharmacokinetics of oral dihydroartemisinin and artesunate in healthy Thai volunteers. Southeast Asian J Trop Med Public Health. 2004 Sept;35(3):575-82.

Naber CK, Erbel R. Infective endocarditis with negative blood cultures. Int J Antimicrob Agents. 2007 Nov;30 Suppl 1:S32-6. Epub 2007 Sep 24. Review.

Nadelman RB, Arlin Z, Wormser GP. Life-threatening complications of empiric ceftriaxone therapy for 'seronegative Lyme disease'. South Med J. 1991 Oct;84(10):1263-5.

Nadelman RB, Herman E, Wormser GP. Screening for Lyme disease in hospitalized psychiatric patients: prospective serosurvey in an endemic area. Mt Sinai J Med. 1997 Nov;64(6):409-12.

Nadelman RB, Horowitz HW, Hsieh TC, Wu JM, Aguero-Rosenfeld ME, Schwartz I, Nowakowski J, Varde S, Wormser GP. Simultaneous human granulocytic ehrlichiosis and Lyme borreliosis. N Engl J Med. 1997 Jul 3;337(1):27-30.

Nadelman RB, Luger SW, Frank E, Wisniewski M, Collins JJ, Wormser GP. Comparison of cefuroxime axetil and doxycycline in the treatment of early Lyme disease. Ann Intern Med. 1992 Aug 15;117(4):273-80.

Nadelman RB, Nowakowski J, Fish D, Falco RC, Freeman K, McKenna D, Welch P, Marcus R, Agüero-Rosenfeld ME, Dennis DT, Wormser GP; Tick Bite Study Group. Prophylaxis with single-dose doxycycline for the prevention of Lyme disease after an Ixodes scapularis tick bite. N Engl J Med. 2001 Jul 12;345(2):79-84.

Nadelman RB, Nowakowski J, Forseter G, Bittker S, Cooper D, Goldberg N, McKenna D, Wormser GP. Failure to isolate Borrelia burgdorferi after antimicrobial therapy in culture-documented Lyme borreliosis associated with erythema migrans: report of a prospective study. Am J Med. 1993 Jun;94(6):583-8.

Nadelman RB, Nowakowski J, Forseter G, Goldberg NS, Bittker S, Cooper D, Aguero-Rosenfeld M, Wormser GP. The clinical spectrum of early Lyme borreliosis in patients with culture-confirmed erythema migrans. Am J Med. 1996 May;100(5):502-8.

Nadelman RB, Nowakowski J, Horowitz HW, Strle F, Wormser GP. Thrombocytopenia and Borrelia burgdorferi: an association remains unproven. Clin Infect Dis. 1999 Dec;29(6):1603-5.

Nadelman RD, Nowakowski J, Wormser GP. Can Lyme borreliosis be prevented after tick bite? Lancet. 1993 Oct 23;342(8878):1052.

Nadelman RB, Nowakowski J, Wormser GP. A Lyme disease controversy: duration of treatment. Arch Intern Med. 1997 Mar 24;157(6):697, 700.

Nadelman RB, Nowakowski J, Wormser GP, Schwartz I. How should viability of Borrelia burgdorferi be demonstrated? Am J Med. 1999 Apr;106(4):491-2.

Nadelman RB, Pavia CS, Magnarelli LA, Wormser GP. Isolation of Borrelia burgdorferi from the blood of seven patients with Lyme disease. Am J Med. 1990 Jan;88(1):21-6.

Nadelman RB, Schwartz I, Wormser GP. Detecting Borrelia burgdorferi in blood from patients with Lyme disease. J Infect Dis. 1994 Jun;169(6):1410-1.

Nadelman RB, Sherer C, Mack L, Pavia CS, Wormser GP. Survival of Borrelia burgdorferi in human blood stored under blood banking conditions. Transfusion. 1990 May;30(4):298-301.

Nadelman RB, Sivak S, Wormser GP. Prevention of Lyme disease after tick bites. N Engl J Med. 1993 Jan 14;328(2):137; author reply 138-9.

Nadelman RB, Strle F, Horowitz HW, Agger WA, Wormser GP. Leukopenia, thrombocytopenia, and Lyme borreliosis: is there an association? Clin Infect Dis. 1997 May;24(5):1027-9.

Nadelman RB, Wormser GP. A clinical approach to Lyme disease. Mt Sinai J Med. 1990 May;57(3):144-56. Review.

Nadelman RB, Wormser GP. Erythema migrans and early Lyme disease. Am J Med. 1995 Apr 24;98(4A):15S-23S; discussion 23S-24S. Review.

Nadelman RB, Wormser GP. Lyme borreliosis. Lancet. 1998 Aug 15;352(9127):557-65. Review.

Nadelman RB, Wormser GP. Recognition and treatment of erythema migrans: are we off target? Ann Intern Med. 2002 Mar 19;136(6):477-9.

Nadelman RB, Wormser GP. Poly-ticks: Blue State versus Red State for Lyme disease. Lancet. 2005 Jan 22-28;365(9456):280.

Nadelman RB, Wormser GP. Reinfection in patients with Lyme disease. Clin Infect Dis. 2007 Oct 15;45(8):1032-8. Epub 2007 Sep 11. Review.

Nagao E, Arie T, Dorward DW, Fairhurst RM, Dvorak JA. The avian malaria parasite Plasmodium gallinaceum causes marked structural changes on the surface of its host erythrocyte. J Struct Biol. 2008 Jun;162(3):460-7. Epub 2008 Mar 21.

Nagi KS, Joshi R, Thakur RK. Cardiac manifestations of Lyme disease: a review. Can J Cardiol., 12(5):503-6. 1996.

Naik RS, Krishnegowda G, Gowda DC. Glucosamine inhibits inosital acylation of the glycosylphosphatidylinositol anchors in itraerythrocytic Plasmodium falciparum. J Biol Chem. 2003;278:2036-42.

Nakajima R, Tsuji M, Oda K, Zamoto-Niikura A, Wei Q, Kawabuchi-Kurata T, Nishida A, Ishihara C. Babesia microti-group parasites compared phylogenetically by complete sequencing of the CCTeta gene in 36 isolates. J Vet Med Sci. 2009 Jan;71(1):55-68.

Nakao M, Miyamoto K. Susceptibility of Ixodes persulcatus and I. ovatus (Acari: Ixodidae) to Lyme disease spirochetes isolated from humans in Japan. J Med Entomol. 1994 May;31(3):467-73.

Nakao M, Miyamoto K. Mixed infection of different Borrelia species among Apodemus speciosus mice in Hokkaido, Japan. J Clin Microbiol. 1995 Feb;33(2):490-2.

Nakao M, Miyamoto K, Fukunaga M. Lyme disease spirochetes in Japan: enzootic transmission cycles in birds, rodents, and Ixodes persulcatus ticks. J Infect Dis. 1994 Oct;170(4):878-82.

Nakao M, Miyamoto K, Fukunaga M. Borrelia japonica in nature: genotypic identification of spirochetes isolated from Japanese small mammals. Microbiol Immunol. 1994;38(10):805-8.

Nakao M, Miyamoto K, Fukunaga M, Hashimoto Y, Takahashi H. Comparative studies on Borrelia afzelii isolated from a patient of Lyme disease, Ixodes persulcatus ticks, and Apodemus speciosus rodents in Japan. Microbiol Immunol. 1994;38(6):413-20.

Nakao M, Miyamoto K, Kawagishi N, Hashimoto Y, Iizuka H. Comparison of Borrelia burgdorferi isolated from humans and ixodid ticks in Hokkaido, Japan. Microbiol Immunol. 1992;36(11):1189-93.

Nakao M, Miyamoto K, Uchikawa K, Fujita H. Characterization of Borrelia burgdorferi isolated from Ixodes persulcatus and Ixodes ovatus ticks in Japan. Am J Trop Med Hyg. 1992 Oct;47(4):505-11.

Nanagara R, Duray PH, Schumacher HR Jr. Ultrastructural demonstration of spirochetal antigens in synovial fluid and synovial membrane in chronic Lyme disease: possible factors contributing to persistence of organisms. Human Pathology, 27(10):1025-34. 1996.

Nandakumar DN, Nagaraj VA, Vathsala PG, Rangarajan P, Padmanaban G. Curcumin-artemisinin combination therapy for malaria. Antimicrob Agents Chemother. 2006 May;50(5):1859-60.

Nasveld P, Kitchener S. Treatment of acute vivax malaria with tafenoquine. Trans R Soc Trop Med Hyg. 2005 Jan;99(1):2-5.

Nealon C, Dzeing A, Muller-Romer U, Planche T, Sinou V, Kombila M, Kremsner PG, Parzy D, Krishna S. Intramuscular bioavailability and clinical efficacy of artesunate in gabonese children with severe malaria. Antimicrob Agents Chemother. 2002 Dec;46(12):3933-9.

Neelakanta G, Sultana H, Fish D, Anderson JF, Fikrig E. Anaplasma phagocytophilum induces Ixodes scapularis ticks to express an antifreeze glycoprotein gene that enhances their survival in the cold. J Clin Invest. 2010 September 1; 120(9): 3179–3190. Published online 2010 August 25.

Nelder MP, Reeves WK, Adler PH, Wozniak A, Wills W. Ectoparasites and associated pathogens of free-roaming and captive animals in zoos of South Carolina. Vector Borne Zoonotic Dis. 2009 Oct;9(5):469-77.

Nghiem PP, Schatzberg SJ. Conventional and molecular diagnostic testing for the acute neurologic patient. J Vet Emerg Crit Care (San Antonio). 2010 Feb;20(1):46-61. Review. Erratum in: J Vet Emerg Crit Care (San Antonio). 2010 Oct;20(5):538.

Ngo V, Civen R. Babesiosis acquired through blood transfusion, California, USA. Emerg Infect Dis. 2009 May;15(5):785-7.

Nicolas X, Granier H, Zagnoli F, Bellard S. Lyme borreliosis hepatitis. Presse Med, 23;31(7):319. 2002.

Nichol G, Dennis DT, Steere AC, Lightfoot R, Wells G, Shea B, Tugwell P. Test-treatment strategies for patients suspected of having Lyme disease: a cost-effectiveness analysis. Ann Intern Med. 1998 Jan 1;128(1):37-48.

Nicholson GT, Walsh CA, Madan RP. Transfusion-associated babesiosis in a 7-month-old infant after bidirectional Glenn procedure. Congenit Heart Dis. 2010 Nov-Dec;5(6):607-13.

Nields JA, Fallon BA, Jastreboff PJ. Carbamazepine in the treatment of Lyme disease-induced hyperacusis. J Neuropsychiatry Clin Neurosci. 1999 Winter;11(1):97-9.

Nishio N, Kubota T, Nakao Y, Hidaka H. Cat scratch disease with encephalopathy in a 9-year-old girl. Pediatr Int. 2008 Dec;50(6):823-4. Erratum in: Pediatr Int. 2009 Apr;51(2):318. Kubuta, Toshiko [corrected to Kubota, Toshiko].

Niu Q, Guan G, Yang J, Fu Y, Xu Z, Li Y, Ma M, Liu Z, Liu J, Liu A, Ren Q, Jorgensen W, Luo J, Yin H. Detection and differentiation of Borrelia burgdorferi sensu lato in ticks collected from sheep and cattle in China. BMC Vet Res. 2011 Apr 29;7:17.

Nocton JJ, Bloom BJ, Rutledge BJ, Persing DH, Logigian EL, Schmid CH, Steere AC. Detection of Borrelia burgdorferi DNA by polymerase chain reaction in cerebrospinal fluid in Lyme neuroborreliosis. J Infect Dis. 1996 Sep;174(3):623-7.

Nocton JJ, Dressler F, Rutledge BJ, Rys PN, Persing DH, Steere AC. Detection of Borrelia burgdorferi DNA by polymerase chain reaction in synovial fluid from patients with Lyme arthritis. N Engl J Med. 1994 Jan 27;330(4):229-34.

Nocton JJ, Steere AC. Lyme disease.Adv Intern Med. 1995;40:69-117. Review.

Noguchi H. A method for the pure cultivation of pathogenic Treponema pallidum. Journal of Experimental Medicine, XIV:99-112. 1911.

Nontprasert A, Pukrittayakamee S, Prakongpan S, Supanaranond W, Looareesuwan S, White NJ. Assessment of the neurotoxicity of oral dihydroartemisinin in mice. Trans R Soc Trop Med Hyg. 2002 Jan-Feb;96(1):99-101.

Nord JA, Karter D. Lyme disease complicated with pseudotumor cerebri. Clinical Infectious Diseases, 37(2):E25-6. 2003.

Norgard MV, Arndt LL, Akins DR, Curetty LL, Harrich DA, Radolf JD. Activation of human monocytic cells by Treponema pallidum and Borrelia burgdorferi lipoproteins and synthetic lipopeptides proceeds via a pathway distinct from that of lipopolysaccharide but involves the transcriptional activator NF-kappa B. Infect Immun. 1996 Sep;64(9):3845-52.

Norris SJ, Howell JK, Odeh EA, Lin T, Gao L, Edmondson DG. High-throughput plasmid content analysis of Borrelia burgdorferi B31 by using Luminex multiplex technology. Appl Environ Microbiol. 2011 Feb;77(4):1483-92. Epub 2010 Dec 17.

Nowakowski J, McKenna D, Nadelman RB, Bittker S, Cooper D, Pavia C, Holmgren D, Visintainer P, Wormser GP. Blood cultures for patients with extracutaneous manifestations of Lyme disease in the United States. Clin Infect Dis. 2009 Dec 1;49(11):1733-5.

Nowakowski J, McKenna D, Nadelman RB, Cooper D, Bittker S, Holmgren D, Pavia C, Johnson RC, Wormser GP. Failure of treatment with cephalexin for Lyme disease. Arch Fam Med. 2000 Jun;9(6):563-7.

Nowakowski J, Nadelman RB, Forseter G, McKenna D, Wormser GP. Doxycycline versus tetracycline therapy for Lyme disease associated with erythema migrans. J Am Acad Dermatol. 1995 Feb;32(2 Pt 1):223-7.

Nowakowski J, Nadelman RB, Sell R, McKenna D, Cavaliere LF, Holmgren D, Gaidici A, Wormser GP. Long-term follow-up of patients with culture-confirmed Lyme disease. Am J Med. 2003 Aug 1;115(2):91-6.

Nowakowski J, Schwartz I, Liveris D, Wang G, Aguero-Rosenfeld ME, Girao G, McKenna D, Nadelman RB, Cavaliere LF, Wormser GP; Lyme Disease Study Group. Laboratory diagnostic techniques for patients with early Lyme disease associated with erythema migrans: a comparison of different techniques. Clin Infect Dis. 2001 Dec 15;33(12):2023-7. Epub 2001 Nov 7.

Nowakowski J, Schwartz I, Nadelman RB, Liveris D, Aguero-Rosenfeld M, Wormser GP. Culture-confirmed infection and reinfection with Borrelia burgdorferi. Ann Intern Med. 1997 Jul 15;127(2):130-2.

Ntchobo H, Rothermel H, Chege W, Steere AC, Coburn J. Recognition of multiple antibody epitopes throughout Borrelia burgdorferi p66, a candidate adhesin, in patients with early or late manifestations of Lyme disease. Infect Immun. 2001 Mar;69(3):1953-6.

Nussbaum G, Ben-Adi S, Genzler T, Sela M, Rosen G. Involvement of Toll-Like Receptors 2 and 4 in the Innate Immune Response to Treponema denticola and Its Outer Sheath Components. Infect Immun. 2009 September; 77(9): 3939–3947. Published online 2009 July 13.

Nutter FB, Dubey JP, Levine JF, Breitschwerdt EB, Ford RB, Stoskopf MK. Seroprevalences of antibodies against Bartonella henselae and Toxoplasma gondii and fecal shedding of Cryptosporidium spp, Giardia spp, and Toxocara cati in feral and pet domestic cats. J Am Vet Med Assoc. 2004 Nov 1;225(9):1394-8.

Odenthal M, Koenig S, Farbrother P, Drebber U, Bury Y, Dienes HP, Eichinger L. Detection of opportunistic infections by low-density microarrays: a diagnostic approach for granulomatous lymphadenitis. Diagn Mol Pathol. 2007 Mar;16(1):18-26.

Ogden NH, Margos G, Aanensen DM, Drebot MA, Feil EJ, Hanincová K, Schwartz I, Tyler S, Lindsay LR. Investigation of genotypes of Borrelia burgdorferi in Ixodes scapularis ticks collected during surveillance in Canada. Appl Environ Microbiol. 2011 May;77(10):3244-54. Epub 2011 Mar 18.

Ogden NH, St-Onge L, Barker IK, Brazeau S, Bigras-Poulin M, Charron DF, Francis CM, Heagy A, Lindsay LR, Maarouf A, Michel P, Milord F, O'Callaghan CJ, Trudel L, Thompson RA. Risk maps for range expansion of the Lyme disease vector, Ixodes scapularis, in Canada now and with climate change. Int J Health Geogr. 2008; 7: 24. Published online 2008 May 22.

Ogura K, Hara Y, Tsukahara H, Maeda M, Tsukahara M, Mayumi M. MR signal changes in a child with cat scratch disease encephalopathy and status epilepticus. Eur Neurol. 2004;51(2):109-10. Epub 2004 Feb 11.

Ohad DG, Morick D, Avidor B, Harrus S. Molecular detection of Bartonella henselae and Bartonella koehlerae from aortic valves of Boxer dogs with infective endocarditis. Vet Microbiol. 2010 Feb 24;141(1-2):182-5. Epub 2009 Aug 8.

Ohmori S, Kawai A, Takada N, Saito-Ito A. Development of real-time PCR assay for differential detection and quantification for multiple Babesia microti-genotypes. Parasitol Int. 2011 Jun 25. [Epub ahead of print]

Ohnishi K, Murata M. Malaria–eight years of experience in a Tokyo metropolitan hospital. Intern Med. 1996 Feb;35(2):111-4.

Ohrt C, Purnomo, Sutamihardja MA, Tang D, Kain KC. Impact of microscopy error on estimates of protective efficacy in malaria-prevention trials. J Infect Dis. 2002 Aug;15;186(4):540-6. [Epub. 2002 Aug 2].

Ohrt C, Willingmyre GD, Lee P, Knirsch C, Milhous W. Assessment of azithromycin in combination with other antimalarial drugs against Plasmodium falciparum in vitro. Antimicrob Agents Chemother. 2002 Aug;46;(8):2518-24.

Oksi J, Kalimo H, Marttila RJ, Marjamaki M, Sonninen P, et al. Inflammatory brain changes in Lyme borreliosis: A report on three patients and review of literature. Brain, 119 (Pt 6):2143-54. 1996.

Oksi J, Kalimo H, Marttila RJ, Marjamaki M, Sonninen P, Nikoskelainen J, Viljanen MK. Intracranial aneurysms in three patients with disseminated Lyme borreliosis: cause or chance association? J Neurol Neurosurg Psychiatry, 64(5):636-42. 1998.

Oksi J, Marjamaki M, Nikoskelainen J, Viljanen MK. Borrelia burgdorferi detected by culture and PCR in clinical relapse of disseminated Lyme Borreliosis. Annals of Medicine, 31(3):225-32. 1999.

Oksi J, Marttila H, Soini H, Aho H, et al. Early dissemination of Borrelia burgdorferi without generalized symptoms in patients with erythema migrans. APMIS, 109(9):581-8. 2001.

Oksi J, Mertsola J, Reunanen M, Marjamaki M, Viljanen MK. Subacute multiple-site osteomyelitis caused by Borrelia burgdorferi. Clin Infect Dis, 19(5):891-6. 1994.

Oksi J, Nikoskelainen J, Viljanen MK. Comparison of oral cefixime and intravenous ceftriaxone followed by oral amoxicillin in disseminated Lyme borreliosis. Eur J Clin Microbiol Infec Dis 17:715-19, 1998.

Oksi J, Viljanen MK, Kalimo H, Peltonen R, Marttia R, et al. Fatal encephalitis caused by concomitant infection with tick-borne encephalitis virus and Borrelia burgdorferi. Clinical Infectious Diseases, 16(3):392-6. 1993.

Oksi J, Voipio-Pulkki L-M, Uksila J, Pulkki K, Laippala P, Viljanen MK. Borrelia burgdorferi infection in patients with suspected acute myocardial infarction. Lancet, 350(9089):1447-8. 1997.

Oleson CV, Sivalingam JJ, O'Neill BJ, Staas WE Jr. Transverse myelitis secondary to coexistent Lyme disease and babesiosis. J Spinal Cord Med, 26(2):168-71. 2003.

Olivares JP, Pallas F, Ceccaldi M, Viton JM, Raoult D, Planche D, Delarque A. Lyme disease presenting as isolated acute urinary retention caused by transverse myelitis: an electrophysiological and urodynamical study. Arch Phys Med Rehabil, 76(12):1171-2. 1995.

Oliveira AM, Maggi RG, Woods CW, Breitschwerdt EB. Suspected needle stick transmission of Bartonella vinsonii subspecies berkhoffii to a veterinarian. J Vet Intern Med. 2010 Sep-Oct;24(5):1229-32. Epub 2010 Jul 28.

Oliveira TM, Furuta PI, de Carvalho D, Machado RZ. A study of cross-reactivity in serum samples from dogs positive for Leishmania sp., Babesia canis and Ehrlichia canis in enzyme-linked immunosorbent assay and indirect fluorescent antibody test. Rev Bras Parasitol Vet. 2008 Jan-Mar;17(1):7-11.

Olliaro PL, Nair NK, Sathasivam K, Mansor SM, Navaratnam V. Pharmacokinetics of artesunate after single oral administration to rats. BMC Pharmacol. 2001;1:12. [Epub. 2001 Dec 20].

Olsen A, Nawiri J, Magnussen P, Krarup H, Friis H. Failure of twice-weekly iron supplementation to increase blood haemoglobin and serum ferritin concentrations: results of a randomized controlled trial. Ann Trop Med Parasitol. 2006 Apr;100(3):251-63.

Olson J, Esterly NB. Urticarial vasculitis and Lyme disease. J Am Acad Dermatol, 22(6), Part 1:1114-1116. 1990.

Onk G, Acun C, Kalayci M, Cagavi F, et al. Gestational Lyme disease as a rare cause of congenital hydrocephalus. J Turkish German Gynecology Association Artemis, 6(2):156-157. 2005.

Ooka H, Terkawi MA, Goo YK, Luo Y, Li Y, Yamagishi J, Nishikawa Y, Igarashi I, Xuan X. Babesia microti: molecular and antigenic characterizations of a novel 94-kDa protein (BmP94). Exp Parasitol. 2011 Jan;127(1):287-93. Epub 2010 Jun 25.

Oosting M, Ter Hofstede H, Sturm P, Adema GJ, Kullberg BJ, van der Meer JW, Netea MG, Joosten LA. TLR1/TLR2 Heterodimers Play an Important Role in the Recognition of Borrelia Spirochetes. PLoS One. 2011; 6(10): e25998. Published online 2011 October 5.

Oosting M, Ter Hofstede H, van de Veerdonk FL, Sturm P, Kullberg BJ, van der Meer JW, Netea MG, Joosten LA. Role of the IL-23 receptor signaling for IL-17 responses in human Lyme disease. Infect Immun. 2011 Sep 6. [Epub ahead of print]

Oosting M, van de Veerdonk FL, Kanneganti TD, Sturm P, Verschueren I, Berende A, van der Meer JW, Kullberg BJ, Netea MG, Joosten LA. Borrelia species induce inflammasome activation and IL-17 production through a caspase-1-dependent mechanism. Eur J Immunol. 2011 Jan;41(1):172-81. Epub 2010 Dec 9.

Orinda GO, Waltisbuhl DJ, Young AS, Wright IG. Low doses of natural human interferon alpha inhibit the development of Babesia microti infection in BALB/c mice. Vet Parasitol. 1994;53(1-2):53-58.

O'Rourke LG, Pitulle C, Hegarty BC, Kraycirik S, Killary KA, Grosenstein P, Brown JW, Breitschwerdt EB. Bartonella quintana in cynomolgus monkey (Macaca fascicularis). Emerg Infect Dis. 2005 Dec;11(12):1931-4.

O'Rourke F, Schmidgen T, Kaiser PO, Linke D, Kempf VA. Adhesins of Bartonella spp. Adv Exp Med Biol. 2011;715:51-70. Review.

Oscarsson J, Karched M, Thay B, Chen C, Asikainen S. Proinflammatory effect in whole blood by free soluble bacterial components released from planktonic and biofilm cells. BMC Microbiol. 2008; 8: 206. Published online 2008 November 27.

Osorno BM, Vega C, Ristic M, et al. Isolation of Babesia spp. from asymptomatic human beings. Vet. Parasitol. 1976;2:111-120.

Osterhoudt KC, Zaoutis T, Zorc JJ. Lyme disease masquerading as brown recluse spider bite. Annals of Emergency Medicine, 39(5):558-561. 2002.

Oteo JA, Castilla A, Arosey A, Blanco JR, Ibarra V, Morano LE. [Endocarditis due to Bartonella spp. Three new clinical cases and Spanish literature review].[Article in Spanish]. Enferm Infecc Microbiol Clin. 2006 May;24(5):297-301. Review.

Otranto D, de Caprariis D, Lia RP, Tarallo V, Lorusso V, Testini G, Dantas-Torres F, Latrofa S, Diniz PP, Mencke N, Maggi RG, Breitschwerdt E, Capelli G, Stanneck D. Prevention of endemic canine vector-borne diseases using imidacloprid 10% and permethrin 50% in young dogs: a longitudinal field study. Vet Parasitol. 2010 Sep 20;172(3-4):323-32. Epub 2010 May 25.

Ouyang Z, Deka RK, Norgard MV. BosR (BB0647) controls the RpoN-RpoS regulatory pathway and virulence expression in Borrelia burgdorferi by a novel DNA-binding mechanism. PLoS Pathog. 2011 Feb 10;7(2):e1001272.

Ovcinnikov NM, Delectorsku VV. Current concepts of the morphology and biology of Treponema pallidum based on electron microscopy. British Journal of Venereal Diseases, 47:315-328. 1971.

Ovcinnikov NM, Delectorsku VV. Further studies of the morphology of Treponema pallidum under the electron microscope. British Journal of Venereal Diseases, Jun;45(2):87-116. 1969.

Ovcinnikov NM, Delectorsku VV. Further study of ultrathin sections of Treponema pallidum under the electron microscope. British Journal of Venereal Diseases, 44:1-34. 1968.

Ovcinnikov NM, Delectorsku VV. Morphology of Treponema pallidum. British Journal of Venereal Diseases, 35:223-229. 1966.

Pachner AR. Early disseminated Lyme disease. American Journal of Medicine 1995;98 (suppl):4A-30S-43S.

Pachner AR, Steere AC, Sigal LH, Johnson CJ. Antigen-specific proliferation of CSF lymphocytes in Lyme disease. Neurology. 1985 Nov;35(11):1642-4.

Pachner AR, Steere AC. The triad of neurologic manifestations of Lyme disease: meningitis, cranial neuritis, and radiculoneuritis. Neurology. 1985 Jan;35(1):47-53.

Pachner AR, Steere AC. Neurological findings of Lyme disease. Yale J Biol Med. 1984 Jul-Aug;57(4):481-3.

Pachner AR, Steere AC. CNS manifestations of third stage Lyme disease. Zentralbl Bakteriol Mikrobiol Hyg A. 1987 Feb;263(3):301-6.

Pachner AR, Duray P, Steere AC. Central nervous system manifestations of Lyme disease. Arch Neurol. 1989 Jul;46(7):790-5.

Pachner AR, Steere AC. Neurologic involvement in the third stage of Lyme disease: CNS manifestations can mimic multiple sclerosis and psychiatric illness. [poster presentation] Neurology, 36(suppl 1):286. 1986.

Pachner AR. Neurologic manifestations of Lyme disease, the new "Great Imitator." Rev Inf Dis 1989;Vol. 11(Suppl 6):S1482-6.

Pachner AR. Borrelia burgdorferi in the nervous system: the new "great imitator". Annals of the New York Academy of Sciences, 539:56-64. 1988.

Pachner AR, Delaney E, O'Neill T. Neuroborreliosis in the nonhuman primate: Borrelia burgdorferi persists in the central nervous system. Annals of Neurology, 38:667-9. 1995.

Paik IH, Xie S, Shapiro TA, Labonte T, Narducci Sarjeant AA, Baege AC, Posner GH. Second generation, orally active, antimalarial, artemisinin-derived trioxane dimers with high stability, efficacy, and anticancer activity. J Med Chem. 2006;49:2731-4.

Paitoonpong L, Chitsomkasem A, Chantrakooptungool S, Kanjanahareutai S, Tribuddharat C, Srifuengfung S. Bartonella henselae: first reported isolate in a human in Thailand. Southeast Asian J Trop Med Public Health. 2008 Jan;39(1):123-9.

Pal U, Wang P, Bao F, Yang X, Samanta S, Schoen R, Wormser GP, Schwartz I, Fikrig E. Borrelia burgdorferi basic membrane proteins A and B participate in the genesis of Lyme arthritis. J Exp Med. 2008 Jan 21;205(1):133-41. Epub 2007 Dec 31.

Palanivelu DV, Goepfert A, Meury M, Guye P, Dehio C, Schirmer T. Fic domain-catalyzed adenylylation: insight provided by the structural analysis of the type IV secretion system effector BepA. Protein Sci. 2011 Mar;20(3):492-9. Epub 2011 Feb 17.

Palumbo E, Sodini F, Boscarelli G, Nasca G, Branchi M, Pellegrini G. Immune thrombocytopenic purpura as a complication of Bartonella henselae infection. Infez Med. 2008 Jun;16(2):99-102.

Pancewicz S, Moniuszko A, Bieniarz E, Puciło K, Grygorczuk S, Zajkowska J, Czupryna P, Kondrusik M, Swierzbińska-Pijanowska R. Anti-Babesia microti antibodies in foresters highly exposed to tick bites in Poland. Scand J Infect Dis. 2011 Mar;43(3):197-201. Epub 2010 Dec 9.

Pandak N, Daković-Rode O, Cabraja I, Kristof Z, Kotarac S. Prevalence of Bartonella henselae antibodies in children and blood donors in Croatia. Infection. 2009 Apr;37(2):166-7. Epub 2009 Mar 9.

Panossian LA, Garga NI, Pelletier D. Toxic brainstem encephalopathy after artemisinin treatment for breast cancer. Ann. Neurol 2005;56;812-813.

Papadopouli E, Michailidi E, Papadopoulou E, Paspalaki P, Vlahakis I, Kalmanti M. Cervical lymphadenopathy in childhood epidemiology and management. Pediatr Hematol Oncol. 2009 Sep;26(6):454-60.

Papagrigorakis MJ, Yapijakis C, Synodinos PN, Baziotopoulou-Valavani E. DNA examination of ancient dental pulp incriminates typhoid fever as a probable cause of the Plague of Athens. Int J Infect Dis. 2006 May;10(3):206-14. Epub 2006 Jan 18.

Pape M, Kollaras P, Mandraveli K, Tsona A, Metallidis S, Nikolaidis P, Alexiou-Daniel S. Occurrence of Bartonella henselae and Bartonella quintana among human immunodeficiency virus-infected patients. Ann N Y Acad Sci. 2005 Dec;1063:299-301.

Pape M, Mandraveli K, Alexiou-Daniel S. Clinical aspects of Bartonella infection in northern Greece. Clin Microbiol Infect. 2009 Dec;15 Suppl 2:91-2. Epub 2009 May 18.

Pappalardo BL, Brown T, Gebhardt D, Sontakke S, Breitschwerdt EB. Cyclic CD8+ lymphopenia in dogs experimentally infected with Bartonella vinsonii subsp. berkhoffii. Vet Immunol Immunopathol. 2000 Jun 30;75(1-2):43-57.

Pappalardo BL, Brown T, Gookin JL, Morrill CL, Breitschwerdt EB. Granulomatous disease associated with Bartonella infection in 2 dogs. J Vet Intern Med. 2000 Jan-Feb;14(1):37-42.

Pappalardo BL, Brown TT, Tompkins M, Breitschwerdt EB. Immunopathology of Bartonella vinsonii (berkhoffii) in experimentally infected dogs. Vet Immunol Immunopathol. 2001 Dec;83(3-4):125-47.

Pappalardo BL, Correa MT, York CC, Peat CY, Breitschwerdt EB. Epidemiologic evaluation of the risk factors associated with exposure and seroreactivity to Bartonella vinsonii in dogs. Am J Vet Res. 1997 May;58(5):467-71.

Pappas CJ, Iyer R, Petzke MM, Caimano MJ, Radolf JD, Schwartz I. Borrelia burgdorferi requires glycerol for maximum fitness during the tick phase of the enzootic cycle. PLoS Pathog. 2011 Jul;7(7):e1002102. Epub 2011 Jul 7.

Parapini S, Basilico N, Mondani M, et al.Evidence that haem iron in the malaria parasite is not needed for the antimalarial effects of artemisinin. FEBS Lett. 2004;575:p.91-94.

Parkhomenko IuG, Tishkevich OA, Barkhina TG, Potekaev SN, Potekaev NS. [Bacillary generalized angiomatosis in HIV infection].[Article in Russian]. Arkh Patol. 1998 Sep-Oct;60(5):66-8.

Parkins MD, Deirdre L Church DL, Xiu Yan Jiang XY, Daniel B Gregson DB Human granulocytic anaplasmosis: First reported case in Canada. Can J Infect Dis Med Microbiol. 2009 Autumn; 20(3): e100–e102.

Parola P, Fournier PE, Raoult D. Bartonella quintana, lice, and molecular tools. J Med Entomol. 2006 Sep;43(5):787; author reply 788.

Parola P, Sanogo OY, Lerdthusnee K, Zeaiter Z, Chauvancy G, Gonzalez JP, Miller RS, Telford SR 3rd, Wongsrichanalai C, Raoult D. Identification of Rickettsia spp. and Bartonella spp. in ffrom the Thai-Myanmar border. Ann N Y Acad Sci. 2003 Jun;990:173-81.

Parola P, Shpynov S, Montoya M, Lopez M, Houpikian P, Zeaiter Z, Guerra H, Raoult D. First molecular evidence of new Bartonella spp. in fleas and a tick from Peru. Am J Trop Med Hyg. 2002 Aug;67(2):135-6.

Parrott JH, Dure L, Sullender W, Buraphacheep W, Frye TA, Galliani CA, Marston E, Jones D, Regnery R. Central nervous system infection associated with Bartonella quintana: a report of two cases. Pediatrics. 1997 Sep;100(3 Pt 1):403-8.

Parrow NL, Abbott J, Lockwood AR, Battisti JM, Minnick MF. Function, regulation, and transcriptional organization of the hemin utilization locus of Bartonella quintana. Infect Immun. 2009 Jan;77(1):307-16. Epub 2008 Nov 3.

Parveen N, Cornell KA. Methylthioadenosine/S-adenosyl-homocysteine nucleosidase, a critical enzyme for bacterial metabolism. Mol Microbiol. 2011 Jan;79(1):7-20. Epub 2010 Nov 18. Review.

Pasini EM, Kirkegaard M, Mortensen P, Mann M, Thomas AW. Deep-coverage rhesus red blood cell proteome: a first comparison with the human and mouse red blood cell. Blood Transfus. 2010 Jun;8 Suppl 3:s126-39.

Pasticci MB, Di Candilo F, Egidi MA, Lapalorcia LM, Marroni M, Tinca E, Sfara C, Stagni G. Bartonella henselae lymphadenitis progressing to hepatosplenic disease with slow clinical response despite early diagnosis and treatment. Int J Clin Pract. 2008 Dec;62(12):1956-7. Epub 2007 Mar 1.

Patel SJ, Petrarca R, Shah SM, Zimmer-Galler I, Janjua KA, Do DV, Nguyen QD. Atypical Bartonella hensalae chorioretinitis in an immunocompromised patient. Ocul Immunol Inflamm. 2008 Jan-Feb;16(1):45-9.

Patial RK, Kashyap S, Bansal SK, Sood A. Lyme disease in a Shimla boy. J Assoc Physicians India. 1990 Jul;38(7):503-4.

Patton TG, Dietrich G, Dolan MC, Piesman J, Carroll JA, Gilmore RD Jr. Functional analysis of the Borrelia burgdorferi bba64 gene product in murine infection via tick infestation. PLoS One. 2011 May 3;6(5):e19536.

Pavia C, Inchiosa MA Jr, Wormser GP. Efficacy of short-course ceftriaxone therapy for Borrelia burgdorferi infection in C3H mice. Antimicrob Agents Chemother. 2002 Jan;46(1):132-4.

Pavia CS, Wormser GP, Bittker S, Cooper D. An indirect hemagglutination antibody test to detect antibodies to Borrelia burgdorferi in patients with Lyme disease. J Microbiol Methods. 2000 Apr;40(2):163-73.

Pavia CS, Wormser GP, Norman GL. Activity of sera from patients with Lyme disease against Borrelia burgdorferi. Clin Infect Dis. 1997 Jul;25 Suppl 1:S25-30.

Pavia CS, Wormser GP, Nowakowski J, Cacciapuoti A. Efficacy of an evernimicin (SCH27899) in vitro and in an animal model of Lyme disease. Antimicrob Agents Chemother. 2001 Mar;45(3):936-7.

Pavlovic D, Levic Z, Dmitrovic R, Ocic G. Chronic encephalomyelitis caused by Borrelia burgdorferi. Case report. [Article in Serbian]. Glas Srp Akad Nauka [Med], (43):225-8. 1993.

Pedersen BK. Sudden cardiac death in Swedish orienteers--a mystery solved? Scand J Med Sci Sports. 2001;11(5):259.

Pedersen BK. [Bartonella bacterium is suspected as the cause of sudden death among Swedish cross-country runners].[Article in Danish]. Ugeskr Laeger. 2001 May 21;163(21):2951.

Peltomaa M, McHugh G, Steere AC. Persistence of the antibody response to the VlsE sixth invariant region (IR6) peptide of Borrelia burgdorferi after successful antibiotic treatment of Lyme disease. J Infect Dis. 2003 Apr 15;187(8):1178-86. Epub 2003 Apr 2.

Peltomaa M, McHugh G, Steere AC. The VlsE (IR6) peptide ELISA in the serodiagnosis of lyme facial paralysis. Otol Neurotol. 2004 Sep;25(5):838-41.

Peltomaa M, Pyykkö I, Seppälä I, Viljanen M. Lyme borreliosis--an unusual cause of vertigo. Auris Nasus Larynx, 25:233-242. 1998.

Pelton SI, Kim JY, Kradin RL. Case records of the Massachusetts General Hospital. Case 27-2006. A 17-year-old boy with fever and lesions in the liver and spleen. N Engl J Med. 2006 Aug 31;355(9):941-8.

Pendle S, Ginn A, Iredell J. Antimicrobial susceptibility of Bartonella henselae using Etest methodology. J Antimicrob Chemother. 2006 Apr;57(4):761-3. Epub 2006 Feb 7.

Pendse S, Bilyk JR, Lee MS. The ticking time bomb. Survey of Ophthalmology, 51(3):274-9. 2006.

Pennisi MG, La Camera E, Giacobbe L, Orlandella BM, Lentini V, Zummo S, Fera MT. Molecular detection of Bartonella henselae and Bartonella clarridgeiae in clinical samples of pet cats from Southern Italy. Res Vet Sci. 2010 Jun;88(3):379-84. Epub 2009 Dec 5.

Penzhorn BL, Lewis BD, Lopez-Rebollar LM, Swan GE. Screening of five drugs for efficacy against Babesia felis in experimentally infected cats. J S Afr Vet Assoc. 2000 Mar;71(1):53-7.

Penzhorn BL, Schoeman T, Jacobson LS. Feline babesiosis in South Africa: a review. Ann N Y Acad Sci. 2004 Oct;1026:183-6.

Pereyra-Rodríguez JJ, Bernabeu-Wittel J, Cañas E, Conejo-Mir J. [Slowly enlarging erythematous macule].[Article in Spanish]. Enferm Infecc Microbiol Clin. 2011 Jan;29(1):68-9. Epub 2010 Dec 30.

Perez C, Hummel JB, Keene BW, Maggi RG, Diniz PP, Breitschwerdt EB. Successful treatment of Bartonella henselae endocarditis in a cat. J Feline Med Surg. 2010 Jun;12(6):483-6. Epub 2010 Feb 6.

Pérez C, Maggi RG, Diniz PP, Breitschwerdt EB. Molecular and serological diagnosis of Bartonella infection in 61 dogs from the United States. J Vet Intern Med. 2011 Jul-Aug;25(4):805-10. Epub 2011 May 25.

Pérez D, Kneubühler Y, Rais O, Jouda F, Gern L. Borrelia afzelii ospC genotype diversity in Ixodes ricinus questing ticks and ticks from rodents in two Lyme borreliosis endemic areas: Contribution of co-feeding ticks. Ticks Tick Borne Dis. 2011 Sep;2(3):137-42. Epub 2011 Aug 19.

Pérez G J, Munita S JM, Araos B R, López G JP, Stevenson A R, González A P, Pérez C D, Noriega R LM. [Cat scratch disease associated neuroretinitis: clinical report and review of the literature].[Article in Spanish]. Rev Chilena Infectol. 2010 Oct;27(5):417-22. Review.

Pérez de León AA, Strickman DA, Knowles DP, Fish D, Thacker E, de la Fuente J, Krause PJ, Wikel SK, Miller RS, Wagner GG, Almazán C, Hillman R, Messenger MT, Ugstad PO, Duhaime RA, Teel PD, Ortega-Santos A, Hewitt DG, Bowers EJ, Bent SJ, Cochran MH, McElwain TF, Scoles GA, Suarez CE, Davey R, Howell Freeman JM, Lohmeyer K, Li AY, Guerrero FD, Kammlah DM, Phillips P, Pound JM; the Group for Emerging Babesioses and One Health Research and Development in the U.S. One Health approach to identify research needs in bovine and human babesioses: workshop report. Parasit Vectors. 2010 Apr 8;3(1):36.

Pérez-Irezábal J, Aguirrebengoa K, Cilla G. [Endocarditis due to Bartonella spp. Three new clinical cases and Spanish literature review].[Article in Spanish]. Enferm Infecc Microbiol Clin. 2006 Nov;24(9):597.

Pérez-Martínez L, Blanco JR, Oteo JA. [Treatment of human infections caused by Bartonella spp.].[Article in Spanish]. Rev Esp Quimioter. 2010 Sep;23(3):109-14. Review.

Pérez-Martínez L, Venzal JM, González-Acuña D, Portillo A, Blanco JR, Oteo JA. Bartonella rochalimae and other Bartonella spp. in fleas, Chile. Emerg Infect Dis. 2009 Jul;15(7):1150-2.

Perides G, Charness ME, Tanner LM, Péter O, Satz N, Steere AC, Klempner MS. Matrix metalloproteinases in the cerebrospinal fluid of patients with Lyme neuroborreliosis. J Infect Dis. 1998 Feb;177(2):401-8.

Persing DH, Herwaldt BL, Glaser C, Lane RS, Thomford JW, Mathiesen D, Krause PJ, Phillip DF, Conrad PA. Infection with a Babesia-like organism in northern California. N Engl J Med.1995. Feb;2;332(5): 298-303.

Petanides TA, Koutinas AF, Mylonakis ME, Day MJ, Saridomichelakis MN, Leontides LS, Mischke R, Diniz P, Breitschwerdt EB, Kritsepi M, Garipidou VA, Koutinas CK, Lekkas S. Factors associated with the occurrence of epistaxis in natural canine leishmaniasis (Leishmania infantum). J Vet Intern Med. 2008 Jul-Aug;22(4):866-72.

Petersen K, Earhart KC, Wallace MR. Bacillary angiomatosis in a patient with chronic lymphocytic leukemia. Infection. 2008 Oct;36(5):480-4. Epub 2007 Dec 28.

Petney TN, Hassler D, Bruckner M, Maiwald M. Comparison of urinary bladder and ear biopsy samples for determining prevalence of Borrelia burgdorferi in rodents in central Europe. J Clin Microbiol, 34(5):1310-2. 1996.

Petnicki-Ocwieja T, DeFrancesco AS, Chung E, Darcy CT, Bronson RT, Kobayashi KS, Hu LT. Nod2 suppresses Borrelia burgdorferi mediated murine Lyme arthritis and carditis through the induction of tolerance. PLoS One. 2011 Feb 28;6(2):e17414.

Petrogiannopoulos C, Valla K, Mikelis A, Kalogeropoulos SG, Karachalios G, Karachaliou I, Skandami I. Parotid mass due to cat scratch disease. Int J Clin Pract. 2006 Dec;60(12):1679-80. Epub 2006 Mar 27.

Petrovic M, Vogelaers D, Van Renterghern L, Carton D, et al. Lyme borreliosis-A review of the late stages and treatment of four cases. 1998. Acta Clinica Belgica, 53(3):178-83.

Peys E, Vandenkerckhove J, Van Hemel J, Sas B. Intermediate-term toxicity of repeated orally administered doses of the anti-malarial beta-artemether in dogs. Exp Toxicol Pathol. 2006 Mar;57(4):299-304. [Epub 2005 Dec 20].

Pfadenhauer K, Schonsteiner T, Stohr M. [Thoraco-abdominal manifestation of stage II Lyme neuroborreliosis] [Article in German].Nervenarzt, 69(4):296-9. 1998.

Pfister HW, Kristoferitsch W, Meier C. Early neurological involvement (Bannwarth's syndrome). In Aspects of Lyme Borreliosis, ed. Klaus Weber, M.D., Willy Burgdorfer, Ph.D., M.D. Berlin Heidelberg:Springer-Verlag:pp 152-167. 1993.

Pfister HW, Preac-Mursic V, Wilske B, Einhäupl KM, Weinberger K. Latent Lyme neuroborreliosis: presence of Borrelia burgdorferi in the cerebrospinal fluid without concurrent inflammatory signs. Neurology, 39(8):1118-20. 1989.

Pfister HW, Preac-Mursic V, Wilske B, Einhäupl KM. Cefotaxime vs penicillin F for acute neurologic manifestations in Lyme borreliosis. A prospective randomized study. Arch Neurol. 46:1190-4, 1989.

Pfister HW, Preac-Mursic V, Wilske B, Schielke E, Sorgel F, Einhaupl KM. Randomized comparison of ceftriaxone and cefotaxime in Lyme neuroborreliosis. 1991. Journal of Infectious Diseases, Feb;163(2):311-8.

Pfrommer S, Maier M, Mayer C, Erben A, Engelmann V, Lohmann CP. [Vasoproliferative retinal tumours].[Article in German]. Ophthalmologe. 2011 Mar;108(3):265-8.

Philipp MT, Masters E, Wormser GP, Hogrefe W, Martin D. Serologic evaluation of patients from Missouri with erythema migrans-like skin lesions with the C6 Lyme test. Clin Vaccine Immunol. 2006 Oct;13(10):1170-1.

Philipp MT, Wormser GP, Marques AR, Bittker S, Martin DS, Nowakowski J, Dally LG. A decline in C6 antibody titer occurs in successfully treated patients with culture-confirmed early localized or early disseminated Lyme Borreliosis. Clin Diagn Lab Immunol. 2005 Sep;12(9):1069-74.

Philippon A. [Bacterial zoonoses: emerging concepts].[Article in French]. Bull Acad Natl Med. 2006 Mar;190(3):579-94; discussion 595, 625-7. Review.

Phillips SE, Burrascano JJ, Harris NS, Horowitz R, Johnson L, Smith PV, Stricker RB. Rash decisions about southern tick-associated rash illness and Lyme disease. Clin Infect Dis. 2006 Jan 15;42(2):306-7; author reply 307-8.

Phillips SE, Burrascano JJ, Harris NS, Johnson L, Smith PV, Stricker RB. Chronic infection in 'post-Lyme borreliosis syndrome'. Int J Epidemiol. 2005 Dec;34(6):1439-40; author reply 1440-3. Epub 2005 Nov 30.

Phillips SE, Burrascano JJ, Horowitz R, Savely VR, Stricker RB. Lyme disease testing. Lancet Infect Dis. 2006 Mar;6(3):122.

Phillips SE, Harris NS, Horowitz R, Johnson L, Stricker RB. Lyme disease: scratching the surface. Lancet. 2005 Nov 19;366(9499):1771.

Phillips-Howard P. Regulation of the quality and use of artemesinin and its derivatives. In Artemesia, Wright, CW, Ed. Taylor & Francis, London. 2002;p.319-320.

Piccolo I, Thiella G, Sterzi R, Colombo N, Defanti CA. Chorea as a symptom of neuroborreliosis: a case study. Ital J Neurol Sci. 1998 Aug;19(4):235-9.

Piesman J, Mather TN, Dammin GJ,Telford SR III, Lastavica CC, Spielman A. Seasonal variation of transmission risk of Lyme disease and human babesiosis. Am J Epidemiol. 1987 Dec;126(6):1187-9.

Piérard-Franchimont C, Quatresooz P, Piérard GE. Skin diseases associated with Bartonella infection: facts and controversies. Clin Dermatol. 2010 Sep-Oct;28(5):483-8.

Pietrobelli M, Cancrini G, Moretti A, Tampieri MP. Animal babesiosis: an emerging zoonosis also in Italy? Parassitologia. 2007 May;49 Suppl 1:33-8.

Pinilla Moraza J, Labarga Echevarría P, Cachorro San Pedro I. [Inguinal mass as presentation of cat-scratch disease].[Article in Spanish]. An Med Interna. 2005 Aug;22(8):400-1.

Pinna A, Puglia E, Dore S. Unusual retinal manifestations of cat scratch disease. Int Ophthalmol. 2011 Apr;31(2):125-8. Epub 2011 Jan 26.

Pinto Jr VL, Curi AL, Pinto Ada S, Nunes EP, Teixeira Mde L, Rozental T, Favacho AR, Castro EL, Bóia MN. Cat scratch disease complicated with aseptic meningitis and neuroretinitis. Braz J Infect Dis. 2008 Apr;12(2):158-60.

Pipili C, Katsogridakis K, Cholongitas E. Myocarditis due to Bartonella henselae. South Med J. 2008 Nov;101(11):1186.

Pitassi LH, Cintra ML, Ferreira MR, Magalhães RF, Velho PE. Blood cell findings resembling Bartonella spp. Ultrastruct Pathol. 2010 Feb;34(1):2-6.

Pitassi LH, Magalhães RF, Barjas-Castro ML, de Paula EV, Ferreira MR, Velho PE. Bartonella henselae infects human erythrocytes. Ultrastruct Pathol. 2007 Nov-Dec;31(6):369-72.

Pitchford CW, Creech CB 2nd, Peters TR, Vnencak-Jones CL. Bartonella henselae endocarditis in a child. Pediatr Cardiol. 2006 Nov-Dec;27(6):769-71. Epub 2006 Nov 16.

Pitulle C, Strehse C, Brown JW, Breitschwerdt EB. Investigation of the phylogenetic relationships within the genus Bartonella based on comparative sequence analysis of the rnpB gene, 16S rDNA and 23S rDNA. Int J Syst Evol Microbiol. 2002 Nov;52(Pt 6):2075-80.

Pitzer JE, Sultan SZ, Hayakawa Y, Hobbs G, Miller MR, Motaleb MA. Analysis of the Borrelia burgdorferi cyclic-di-GMP-binding protein PlzA reveals a role in motility and virulence. Infect Immun. 2011 May;79(5):1815-25. Epub 2011 Feb 28. Erratum in: Infect Immun. 2011 Jun;79(6):2499.

Platonov AE, Karan LS, Kolyasnikova NM, Makhneva NA, Toporkova MG, Maleev VV, Fish D, Krause PJ. Humans Infected with Relapsing Fever Spirochete Borrelia miyamotoi, Russia. Emerg Infect Dis. 2011 Oct;17(10):1816-23.

Platonov AE, Maleev VV, Karan' LS. [Relapsing borrelioses fevers: forgotten and new ones]. [Article in Russian]. Ter Arkh. 2010;82(11):74-80.

Plotkin SA. Correcting a public health fiasco: The need for a new vaccine against Lyme disease. Clin Infect Dis. 2011 Feb;52 Suppl 3:s271-5.

Podsiadły E, Chmielewski T, Karbowiak G, Kędra E, Tylewska-Wierzbanowska S. The occurrence of spotted fever rickettsioses and other tick-borne infections in forest workers in Poland. Vector Borne Zoonotic Dis. 2011 Jul;11(7):985-9. Epub 2010 Nov 17.

Podsiadly E, Chmielewski T, Marczak R, Sochon E, Tylewska-Wierzbanowska S. Bartonella henselae in the human environment in Poland. Scand J Infect Dis. 2007;39(11-12):956-62. Epub 2007 Jun 1.

Podsiadly E, Chmielewski T, Sochon E, Tylewska-Wierzbanowska S. Bartonella henselae in Ixodes ricinus ticks removed from dogs. Vector Borne Zoonotic Dis. 2007 Summer;7(2):189-92.

Podsiadły E, Sapiejka E, Dabrowska-Bień J, Majkowski J, Tylewska-Wierzbanowska S. [Diagnostics of cat scratch disease and present methods of bartonellosis recognition--a case report]. [Article in Polish]. Pol Merkur Lekarski. 2009 Feb;26(152):131-5.

Pohl-Koppe A, Logigian EL, Steere AC, Hafler DA. Cross-reactivity of Borrelia burgdorferi and myelin basic protein-specific T cells is not observed in borrelial encephalomyelitis. Cell Immunol. 1999 May 25;194(1):118-23.

Pohl-Koppe A, Balashov KE, Steere AC, Logigian EL, Hafler DA. Identification of a T cell subset capable of both IFN-gamma and IL-10 secretion in patients with chronic Borrelia burgdorferi infection. J Immunol. 1998 Feb 15;160(4):1804-10.

Poland GA. Vaccines against Lyme disease: What happened and what lessons can we learn? Clin Infect Dis. 2011 Feb;52 Suppl 3:s253-8. Review.

Pone EJ, Zan H, Zhang J, Al-Qahtani A, Xu Z, Casali P. Toll-like Receptors and B-cell Receptors Synergize to Induce Immunoglobulin Class Switch DNA Recombination: Relevance to Microbial Antibody Responses. Crit Rev Immunol. 2010; 30(1): 1–29.

Pons I, Sanfeliu I, Cardeñosa N, Nogueras MM, Font B, Segura F. Serological evidence of Bartonella henselae infection in healthy people in Catalonia, Spain. Epidemiol Infect. 2008 Dec;136(12):1712-6. Epub 2008 Feb 25.

Pons I, Sanfeliu I, Nogueras MM, Sala M, Cervantes M, Amengual MJ, Segura F. Seroprevalence of Bartonella spp. infection in HIV patients in Catalonia, Spain. BMC Infect Dis. 2008 May 1;8:58.

Popa C, Abdollahi-Roodsaz S, Joosten LA, Takahashi N, Sprong T, Matera G, Liberto MC, Foca A, van Deuren M, Kullberg BJ, van den Berg WB, van der Meer JW, Netea MG. Bartonella quintana lipopolysaccharide is a natural antagonist of Toll-like receptor 4. Infect Immun. 2007 Oct;75(10):4831-7. Epub 2007 Jul 2.

Popov A, Abdullah Z, Wickenhauser C, Saric T, Driesen J, Hanisch FG, Domann E, Raven EL, Dehus O, Hermann C, Eggle D, Debey S, Chakraborty T, Krönke M, Utermöhlen O, Schultze JL. Indoleamine 2,3-dioxygenase-expressing dendritic cells form suppurative granulomas following Listeria monocytogenes infection. J Clin Invest. 2006 Dec;116(12):3160-70. Epub 2006 Nov 16.

Porwancher RB, Hagerty CG, Fan J, Landsberg L, Johnson BJ, Kopnitsky M, Steere AC, Kulas K, Wong SJ. Multiplex immunoassay for Lyme disease using VlsE1-IgG and pepC10-IgM antibodies: improving test performance through bioinformatics. Clin Vaccine Immunol. 2011 May;18(5):851-9. Epub 2011 Mar 2.

Posey JE, Hardham JM, Norris SJ, Gherardini FC. Characterization of a manganese-dependent regulatory protein, TroR, from Treponema pallidum. Proc Natl Acad Sci U S A. 1999 Sep 14;96(19):10887-92.

Posfay Barbe K, Jaeggi E, Ninet B, et al. Bartonella quintana endocarditis in a child. N Engl J Med. 2000;342(24):1841-1842.

Posner GH, McRiner AJ, Paik IH, Sur S, Borstnik K, Xie S, Shapiro TA, Alagbala A, Foster B. Anticancer and antimalarial efficacy and safety of artemisinin-derived trioxane dimers in rodents. J Med Chem. 2004;47:1299-301.

Postma NS, Mommers EC, Eling WM, Zuidema J. Oxidative stress in malaria; implications for prevention and therapy. Pharm World Sci. 1996 Aug;18(4):121-9.

Potgieter FT. Chemotherapy of Babesia felis infection: efficacy of certain drugs. J S Afr Vet Assoc. 1981 Dec;52(4):289-93.

Poyraz O, Güneş T. [Seroprevalance of Babesia microti in humans living in rural areas of the Sinop region].[Article in Turkish]. Turkiye Parazitol Derg. 2010;34(2):81-5.

Pozsgay V, Kubler-Kielb J, Coxon B, Marques A, Robbins JB, Schneerson R. Synthesis and antigenicity of BBGL-2 glycolipids of Borrelia burgdorferi, the causative agent of Lyme disease. Carbohydr Res. 2011 Sep 6;346(12):1551-63. Epub 2011 May 3.

Pratt JW, Meyer DR, Wroblewski D, Carlson JA. Orbital inflammation and lyme disease. Ophthalmology. 2011 Sep;118(9):1892.e1-2.

Preac-Mursic V, Marget W, Busch U, Pleterski Rigler D, Hagl S. Kill kinetics of Borrelia burgdorferi and bacterial findings in relation to the treatment of Lyme borreliosis. 1996. Infection, 24(1):9-16.

Preac-Mursic V, Pfister HW, Spiegel H, Burk R, Wilske B, Reinhardt S, Bohmer R. First isolation of Borrelia burgdorferi from an iris biopsy. Journal of Clinical Neuroophthalmology, 13(3):155-61; discussion 162. 1993.

Preac-Mursic V, Weber K, Pfister HW, Wilske B, et al. Survival of Borrelia burgdorferi in antibiotically treated patients with Lyme borreliosis. 1989. Infection, 17(6):355-9.

Pretorius AM, Kelly PJ, Birtles RJ, Raoult D. Isolation of Bartonella henselae from a serologically negative cat in Bloemfontein, South Africa. J S Afr Vet Assoc. 1999 Dec;70(4):154-5.

Pretorius AM, Kelly PJ, Birtles RJ, Raoult D. Are Bartonella emerging and re-emerging pathogens in southern Africa? S Afr Med J. 2000 Jan;90(1):12.

Pretorius AM, Kelly PJ, Birtles RJ, Raoult D. Are Bartonella emerging and re-emerging pathogens in southern Africa? S Afr Med J. 2000 Jun;90(6):566.

Priem S, Burmester GR, Kamradt T, Wolbart K, Rittig MG, Krause A. Detection of Borrelia burgdorferi by polymerase chain reaction in synovial membrane, but not in synovial fluid from patients with persisting Lyme arthritis after antibiotic therapy. 1998. Annals of the Rheumatic Diseases, 57(2):118-21.

Prince HE, Lapé-Nixon M, Patel H, Yeh C. Comparison of the Babesia duncani (WA1) IgG detection rates among clinical sera submitted to a reference laboratory for WA1 IgG testing and blood donor specimens from diverse geographic areas of the United States. Clin Vaccine Immunol. 2010 Nov;17(11):1729-33. Epub 2010 Sep 22.

Probert W, Louie JK, Tucker JR, Longoria R, Hogue R, Moler S, Graves M, Palmer HJ, Cassady J, Fritz CL. Meningitis due to a "Bartonella washoensis"-like human pathogen. J Clin Microbiol. 2009 Jul;47(7):2332-5. Epub 2009 May 13.

Proceedings and abstracts from the 2nd Babesia World Summit, 4-5 May 2007, Palermo, Italy. Parassitologia. 2007 May;49 Suppl 1:1-109.

Psaroulaki A, Antoniou M, Toumazos P, Mazeris A, Ioannou I, Chochlakis D, Christophi N, Loukaides P, Patsias A, Moschandrea I, Tselentis Y. Rats as indicators of the presence and dispersal of six zoonotic microbial agents in Cyprus, an island ecosystem: a seroepidemiological study. Trans R Soc Trop Med Hyg. 2010 Nov;104(11):733-9. Epub 2010 Sep 25.

Pukhovskaia NM, Rar VA, Ivanov LI, Vysochina NP, Igolkina IaP, Fomenko NV, Zaraǐchenkova NV, Plashkova VV, Oreshkina SG, Mal'tseva IP, Chistov VA, Chechikova VA. [PCR detection of the causative agents of infections transmitted by ticks on the Kamchatka Peninsula].[Article in Russian]. Med Parazitol (Mosk). 2010 Oct-Dec;(4):36-9.

Pulliainen AT, Dehio C. Bartonella henselae: subversion of vascular endothelial cell functions by translocated bacterial effector proteins. Int J Biochem Cell Biol. 2009 Mar;41(3):507-10. Epub 2008 Oct 25. Review.

Puligheddu M, Giagheddu A, Genugu F, Giagheddu M, Marrosu F. Epilepsia partialis continua in cat scratch disease. Seizure. 2004 Apr;13(3):191-5. Erratum in: Seizure. 2006 Jul;15(5):357. Dosage error in article text.

Purcell, Katherine. Gates Foundation Invests $42.6 Million in Malaria Drug Research. From: HerbalGram. American Botanical Council. 2006;69:24-252. Available from: http://www.herbalgram. org/herbalgram/article-view.asp?a=2919. Accessed 2006 Aug 13.

Purcell, K. Gates Foundation Invests $42.6 Million in Malaria Drug Research. American Botanical Council. [homepage on the Internet]. HerbalGram. 2006;69:24-252. Available from: http://www.herbalgram.org/ herbalgram/articleview.asp?a=2919. Accessed August 10, 2006.

Puri SK, Dutta GP. Blood schizontocidal activity of WR 238605 (Tafenoquine) against Plasmodium cynomolgi and Plasmodium fragile infections in rhesus monkeys. Acta Trop. 2003 Apr;86(1):35-40.

Que YA, Moreillon P. Infective endocarditis. Nat Rev Cardiol. 2011 Jun;8(6):322-36. Epub 2011 Apr 12. Review.

Quebatte M, Dehio M, Tropel D, Basler A, Toller I, Raddatz G, Engel P, Huser S, Schein H, Lindroos HL, Andersson SG, Dehio C. The BatR/BatS two-component regulatory system controls the adaptive response of Bartonella henselae during human endothelial cell infection. J Bacteriol. 2010 Jul;192(13):3352-67. Epub 2010 Apr 23.

Qi C, Zhou D, Liu J, Cheng Z, Zhang L, Wang L, Wang Z, Yang D, Wang S, Chai T. Detection of Babesia divergens using molecular methods in anemic patients in Shandong Province, China. Parasitol Res. 2011 Jul;109(1):241-5. Epub 2011 Apr 19.

Quick RE, Herwaldt BL, Thomford JW, et al. Babesiosis in Washington State: a new species of Babesia? Ann Intern Med. 1993;119(4):284-290.

Quinn SJ, Boucher BJ, Booth JB. Reversible sensorineural hearing loss in Lyme disease. J Laryngol Otol, 111(6):562-4. 1997.

Quintão-Silva MG, Melo MN, Ribeiro MF. Comparison of duplex PCR and microscopic techniques for the identification of Babesia bigemina and Babesia bovis in engorged female ticks of Boophilus microplus. Zoonoses Public Health. 2007;54(3-4):147-51.

Radolf JD, Norgard MV, Brandt ME, Isaacs RD, Thompson PA, Beutler B. Lipoproteins of Borrelia burgdorferi and Treponema pallidum activate cachectin/tumor necrosis factor synthesis. Analysis using a CAT reporter construct. J Immunol. 1991 Sep 15;147(6):1968-74.

Rahimian J, Raoult D, Tang YW, Hanna BA. Bartonella quintana endocarditis with positive serology for Coxiella burnetii. J Infect. 2006 Sep;53(3):e151-3. Epub 2005 Dec 27.

Rahn DW, Steere AC, Grodzicki RL, Levine JH, Hardin JA. Evidence for Pseudomonas antigen in immune complexes in Pseudomonas osteomyelitis. Arthritis Rheum. 1982 Dec;25(12):1403-8.

Raju BV, Esteve-Gassent MD, Karna SL, Miller CL, Van Laar TA, Seshu J. Oligopeptide permease A5 modulates vertebrate host-specific adaptation of Borrelia burgdorferi. Infect Immun. 2011 Aug;79(8):3407-20. Epub 2011 May 31.

Raju M, Salazar JC, Leopold H, Krause PJ. Atovaquone and azithromycin treatment for babesiosis in an infant. Pediatr Infect Dis J. 2007 Feb;26(2):181-3.

Ramharter A, Kremser B. [Bilateral panuveitis with serous retinal detachment].[Article in German]. Ophthalmologe. 2009 Apr;106(4):351-5.

Ramharter M, Noedl H, Thimasarn K, Wiedermann G, Wernsdorfer G, Wernsdorfer WH. In vitro activity of tafenoquine alone and in combination with artemisinin against Plasmodium falciparum. Am J Trop Med Hyg. 2002 Jul;67(1):39-43.

Ramharter M, Walochnik J, Lagler H, Winkler S, Wernsdorfer WH, Stoiser B, Graninger W. Clinical and molecular characterization of a near fatal case of human babesiosis in Austria. J Travel Med. 2010 Nov-Dec;17(6):416-8.

Rand PW, Lacombe EH, Elias SP, Cahill BK, Lubelczyk CB, Smith RP Jr. Multitarget test for emerging Lyme disease and anaplasmosis in a serosurvey of dogs, Maine, USA. Emerg Infect Dis. 2011 May;17(5):899-902.

Randazzo JP, DiSpaltro FX, Cottrill C, Klainer AS, Steere AC, Bisaccia E. Successful treatment of a patient with chronic Lyme arthritis with extracorporeal photochemotherapy. J Am Acad Dermatol. 1994 May;30(5 Pt 2):908-10.

Randsborg PH, Naess CE. Ankle arthritis in a 6-year-old boy after a tick bite - a case report. Open Orthop J. 2011 May 2;5:165-7.

Rank EL, Dias SM, Hasson J, Duray PH, Johnson RC, Magnarelli LA, Fister RD. Human necrotizing splenitis caused by Borrelia burgdorferi. Am J Clin Pathol, 91(4):493-8. 1989.

Raoult D. [Emerging pathologies].[Article in French]. Med Trop (Mars). 1997;57(3 Suppl):5-6.

Raoult D. [Bartonella infection in humans].[Article in French]. Presse Med. 1999 Feb 27;28(8):429-34, 438. Review.

Raoult D. Etiological diagnosis of blood-culture-negative endocarditis. Enferm Infecc Microbiol Clin. 2006 May;24(5):295-6.

Raoult D. From Cat scratch disease to Bartonella henselae infection. Clin Infect Dis. 2007 Dec 15;45(12):1541-2.

Raoult D, Birtles RJ, Montoya M, Perez E, Tissot-Dupont H, Roux V, Guerra H. Survey of three bacterial louse-associated diseases among rural Andean communities in Peru: prevalence of epidemic typhus, trench fever, and relapsing fever. Clin Infect Dis. 1999 Aug;29(2):434-6.

Raoult D, Casalta JP, Richet H, Khan M, Bernit E, Rovery C, Branger S, Gouriet F, Imbert G, Bothello E, Collart F, Habib G. Contribution of systematic serological testing in diagnosis of infective endocarditis. J Clin Microbiol. 2005 Oct;43(10):5238-42.

Raoult D, Dutour O, Houhamdi L, Jankauskas R, Fournier PE, Ardagna Y, Drancourt M, Signoli M, La VD, Macia Y, Aboudharam G. Evidence for louse-transmitted diseases in soldiers of Napoleon's Grand Army in Vilnius. J Infect Dis. 2006 Jan 1;193(1):112-20. Epub 2005 Nov 18.

Raoult D, Foucault C, Brouqui P. Infections in the homeless. Lancet Infect Dis. 2001 Sep;1(2):77-84. Review.

Raoult D, Fournier PE, Drancourt M, Marrie TJ, Etienne J, Cosserat J, Cacoub P, Poinsignon Y, Leclercq P, Sefton AM. Diagnosis of 22 new cases of Bartonella endocarditis. Ann Intern Med. 1996 Oct 15;125(8):646-52. Erratum in: Ann Intern Med 1997 Aug 1;127(3):249.

Raoult D, Fournier PE, Vandenesch F, Mainardi JL, Eykyn SJ, Nash J, James E, Benoit-Lemercier C, Marrie TJ. Outcome and treatment of Bartonella endocarditis. Arch Intern Med. 2003 Jan 27;163(2):226-30.

Raoult D, La Scola B, Kelly PJ, Davoust B, Gomez J. Bartonella bovis in cattle in Africa. Vet Microbiol. 2005 Jan 31;105(2):155-6. Epub 2004 Dec 15.

Raoult D, Ndihokubwayo JB, Tissot-Dupont H, Roux V, Faugere B, Abegbinni R, Birtles RJ. Outbreak of epidemic typhus associated with trench fever in Burundi. Lancet. 1998 Aug 1;352(9125):353-8.

Raoult D, Roblot F, Rolain JM, Besnier JM, Loulergue J, Bastides F, Choutet P. First isolation of Bartonella alsatica from a valve of a patient with endocarditis. J Clin Microbiol. 2006 Jan;44(1):278-9.

Raoult D, Roux V. The body louse as a vector of reemerging human diseases. Clin Infect Dis. 1999 Oct;29(4):888-911. Review.

Rar VA, Epikhina TI, Livanova NN, Panov VV, Pukhovskaia NM, Vysochina NP, Ivanov LI. [Detection of Babesia spp. DNA in small mammals and ixodic ticks on the territory of north Ural, west Siberia and far east of Russia].[Article in Russian]. Mol Gen Mikrobiol Virusol. 2010;(3):26-30.

Ras NM, Lascola B, Postic D, Cutler SJ, Rodhain F, Baranton G, Raoult D. Phylogenesis of relapsing fever Borrelia spp. Int J Syst Bacteriol. 1996 Oct;46(4):859-65.

Raspe H. ["Clinical medicine will be a science or it will not be," Observations on evidence-based medicine and its critique by Rogler and Scholmerich (2000)].[Article in German]. Z Arztl Fortbild Qualitatssich. 2001 Jul;95(7):495-501.

Raucher HS, Kaufman DM, Goldfarb J, Jacobson RI, Roseman B, Wolff RR. Pseudotumor cerebri and Lyme disease: a new association. J Pediatr. 1985 Dec;107(6):931-3.

Ray A, Quade J, Carson CA, Ray BK. Calcium-dependent protein phosphorylation in Babesia bovis and its role in growth regulation. J Parasitol. 1990;76(2):153-161.

Ray M, Marwaha RK, Trehan A, Banerjee AK. Palatal nerve palsy and cervical adenopathy in a probable case with cat scratch disease. Indian Pediatr. 1999 Nov;36(11):1154-7.

Rebholz CE, Michel AJ, Maselli DA Dr, Saipphudin K Dr, Wyss K Dr. Frequency of malaria and glucose-6-phosphate dehydrogenase deficiency in Tajikistan. Malar J. 2006 Jun 16;5(1):51 [Epub ahead of print].

Reddy AK, Morriss MC, Ostrow GI, Stass-Isern M, Olitsky SE, Lowe LH. Utility of MR imaging in cat-scratch neuroretinitis. Pediatr Radiol. 2007 Aug;37(8):840-3. Epub 2007 Jun 22.

Rees P, Schoeman JP. Plasma insulin concentrations in hypoglycaemic dogs with Babesia canis rossi infection. Vet Parasitol. 2008 Mar 25;152(1-2):60-6. Epub 2007 Nov 22.

Reeves WK, Loftis AD, Gore JA, Dasch GA. Molecular evidence for novel bartonella species in Trichobius major (Diptera: Streblidae) and Cimex adjunctus (Hemiptera: Cimicidae) from two southeastern bat caves, U.S.A. J Vector Ecol. 2005 Dec;30(2):339-41.

Reeves WK, Loftis AD, Sanders F, Spinks MD, Wills W, Denison AM, Dasch GA. Borrelia, Coxiella, and Rickettsia in Carios capensis (Acari: Argasidae) from a brown pelican (Pelecanus occidentalis) rookery in South Carolina, USA. Exp Appl Acarol. 2006;39(3-4):321-9. Epub 2006 Jul 5.

Reeves WK, Loftis AD, Szumlas DE, Abbassy MM, Helmy IM, Hanafi HA, Dasch GA. Rickettsial pathogens in the tropical rat mite Ornithonyssus bacoti (Acari: Macronyssidae) from Egyptian rats (Rattus spp.). Exp Appl Acarol. 2007;41(1-2):101-7. Epub 2007 Jan 16.

Reeves WK, Nelder MP, Cobb KD, Dasch GA. Bartonella spp. in deer keds, Lipoptena mazamae (Diptera: Hippoboscidae), from Georgia and South Carolina, USA. J Wildl Dis. 2006 Apr;42(2):391-6.

Reeves WK, Nelder MP, Korecki JA. Bartonella and Rickettsia in fleas and lice from mammals in South Carolina, U.S.A. J Vector Ecol. 2005;30(2):310-315.

Reeves WK, Rogers TE, Durden LA, Dasch GA. Association of Bartonella with the fleas (Siphonaptera) of rodents and bats using molecular techniques. J Vector Ecol. 2007 Jun;32(1):118-22.

Reeves WK, Szumlas DE, Moriarity JR, Loftis AD, Abbassy MM, Helmy IM, Dasch GA. Louse-borne bacterial pathogens in lice (Phthiraptera) of rodents and cattle from Egypt. J Parasitol. 2006 Apr;92(2):313-8.

Rego RO, Bestor A, Rosa PA. Defining the plasmid-borne restriction-modification systems of the Lyme disease spirochete Borrelia burgdorferi. J Bacteriol. 2011 Mar;193(5):1161-71. Epub 2010 Dec 30.

Reik L Jr. Stroke due to Lyme disease. Neurology. 1993 Dec;43(12):2705-7.

Reik L Jr. Lyme Disease and the Nervous System. New York:Thieme Medical Publishers. 1991.

Reik L Jr. Neurologic aspects of North American Lyme disease. In Lyme Disease, ed. Patricia K. Coyle, M.D. St. Louis: Mosby-Year Book Inc. 1993, pp.101-112.

Reik L Jr, Burgdorfer W, Donaldson JO. Neurologic abnormalities in Lyme disease without erythema chronicum migrans. Am J Med. 1986 Jul;81(1):73-8.

Reik L Jr, Smith L, Khan A, Nelson W. Demyelinating encephalopathy in Lyme disease. Neurology. 1985 Feb;35(2):267-9.

Reik L, Steere AC, Bartenhagen NH, Shope RE, Malawista SE. Neurologic abnormalities of Lyme disease. Medicine (Baltimore). 1979 Jul;58(4):281-94.

Reimers CD, de Koning J, Neubert U, Preac-Mursic V, Koster JG, Müller-Felber W, Pongratz DE, Duray PH. Borrelia burgdorferi myositis: report of eight patients. J Neuro, 240(5):278-83. 1993.

Reis C, Cote M, Le Rhun D, Lecuelle B, Levin ML, Vayssier-Taussat M, Bonnet SI. Vector competence of the tick Ixodes ricinus for transmission of Bartonella birtlesii. PLoS Negl Trop Dis. 2011;5(5):e1186. Epub 2011 May 31.

Reis C, Cote M, Paul RE, Bonnet S. Questing ticks in suburban forest are infected by at least six tick-borne pathogens. Vector Borne Zoonotic Dis. 2011 Jul;11(7):907-16. Epub 2010 Dec 15.

Reis SP, Maddineni S, Rozenblit G, Allen D. Spontaneous splenic rupture secondary to Babesia microti infection: treatment with splenic artery embolization. J Vasc Interv Radiol. 2011 May;22(5):732-4.

Remy V. [Biologic diagnosis of Lyme borreliosis].[Article in French]. Med Mal Infect. 2007 Jul-Aug;37(7-8):410-21. Epub 2007 Mar 13.

Rencricca NJ, Cleman RM, Altschule MD, et al. Quantification of hyperbaric oxygen-induced toxicity utilizing a malarial system. Aviat space environ med. 1981;52:85-87.

Renesto P, Gautheret D, Drancourt M, Raoult D. Determination of the rpoB gene sequences of Bartonella henselae and Bartonella quintana for phylogenic analysis. Res Microbiol. 2000 Dec;151(10):831-6.

Renesto P, Gouvernet J, Drancourt M, Roux V, Raoult D. Use of rpoB gene analysis for detection and identification of Bartonella species. J Clin Microbiol. 2001 Feb;39(2):430-7.

Renou F, Raffray L, Gerber A, Moiton MP, Ferrandiz D, Yvin JL. [Hepatic localization of cat scratch disease in an immunocompetent patient].[Article in French]. Med Mal Infect. 2010 Mar;40(3):172-4. Epub 2009 Jul 17.

Resto-Ruiz SI, Schmiederer M, Sweger D, Newton C, Klein TW, Friedman H, Anderson BE. Induction of a Potential Paracrine Angiogenic Loop between Human THP-1 Macrophages and Human Microvascular Endothelial Cells during Bartonella henselae Infection. Infect Immun. 2002 August; 70(8): 4564–4570.

Reye AL, Hübschen JM, Sausy A, Muller CP. Prevalence and seasonality of tick-borne pathogens in questing Ixodes ricinus ticks from Luxembourg. Appl Environ Microbiol. 2010 May;76(9):2923-31. Epub 2010 Mar 12.

Reynolds MG, Holman RC, Curns AT, O'Reilly M, McQuiston JH, Steiner CA. Epidemiology of cat-scratch disease hospitalizations among children in the United States. Pediatr Infect Dis J. 2005;24(8):700-704.

Rheault MN, van Burik JA, Mauer M, Ingulli E, Ferrieri P, Jessurun J, Chavers BM. Cat-scratch disease relapse in a kidney transplant recipient. Pediatr Transplant. 2007 Feb;11(1):105-9.

Rhomberg TA, Truttmann MC, Guye P, Ellner Y, Dehio C. A translocated protein of Bartonella henselae interferes with endocytic uptake of individual bacteria and triggers uptake of large bacterial aggregates via the invasome. Cell Microbiol. 2009 Jun;11(6):927-45. Epub 2009 Feb 27.

Ricart JJ. [Infective endocarditis due to Bartonella quintana]. [Article in Spanish]. Medicina (B Aires). 2008;68(6):478.

Rich SM, Armstrong PM, Smith RD, Telford SR 3rd. Lone star tick-infecting borreliae are most closely related to the agent of bovine borreliosis. J Clin Microbiol. 2001 Feb;39(2):494-7.

Richardson H, Birchall JP, Hill J, McMaster T. Should we routinely screen for Lyme disease in patients with asymmetrical hearing loss? Br J Audiol, 28(2):59-61. 1994.

Richier E, Biagini GA, Wein S, Boudou F, Bray PG, Ward SA, Precigout E, Calas M, Dubremetz JF, Vial HJ. Potent antihematozoan activity of novel bisthiazolium drug T16: evidence for inhibition of phosphatidylcholine metabolism in erythrocytes infected with Babesia and Plasmodium spp. Antimicrob Agents Chemother. 2006 Oct;50(10):3381-8.

Richter D, Debski A, Hubalek Z, Matuschka FR. Absence of Lyme Disease Spirochetes in Larval Ixodes ricinus Ticks. Vector Borne Zoonotic Dis. 2011 Sep 16. [Epub ahead of print]

Richter D, Matuschka FR. Modulatory effect of cattle on risk for lyme disease. Emerg Infect Dis. 2006 Dec;12(12):1919-23.

Richter D, Matuschka FR. Elimination of lyme disease spirochetes from ticks feeding on domestic ruminants. Appl Environ Microbiol. 2010 Nov;76(22):7650-2. Epub 2010 Sep 24.

Richter D, Schlee DB, Matuschka FR. Reservoir competence of various rodents for the lyme disease Spirochete Borrelia spielmanii. Appl Environ Microbiol. 2011 Jun;77(11):3565-70. Epub 2011 Apr 1.

Ridder GJ, Boedeker CC, Technau-Ihling K, Sander A. Cat-scratch disease: Otolaryngologic manifestations and management. Otolaryngol Head Neck Surg. 2005;132(3):353-358.

Ridder-Schröter R, Marx A, Beer M, Tappe D, Kreth HW, Girschick HJ. Abscess-forming lymphadenopathy and osteomyelitis in children with Bartonella henselae infection. J Med Microbiol. 2008 Apr;57(Pt 4):519-24.

Riedel M, Straube A, Schwarz MJ, Wilske BM, Muller N. Lyme disease presenting as Tourette's syndrome. Lancet, 351(9100):418-419. 1998.

Riess T, Andersson SG, Lupas A, Schaller M, Schäfer A, Kyme P, Martin J, Wälzlein JH, Ehehalt U, Lindroos H, Schirle M, Nordheim A, Autenrieth IB, Kempf VA. Bartonella Adhesin A Mediates a Proangiogenic Host Cell Response. J Exp Med. 2004 November 15; 200(10): 1267–1278.

Riess T, Raddatz G, Linke D, Schäfer A, Kempf VA. Analysis of Bartonella Adhesin A Expression Reveals Differences between Various B. henselae Strains. Infect Immun. 2007 January; 75(1): 35–43. Published online 2006 October 23.

Riess T, Dietrich F, Schmidt KV, Kaiser PO, Schwarz H, Schäfer A, Kempf VA. Analysis of a novel insect cell culture medium-based growth medium for Bartonella species. Appl Environ Microbiol. 2008 Aug;74(16):5224-7. Epub 2008 Jun 20.

Ritchie AE. Morphology of leptospires. The Biology of Parasitic Spirochetes, Johnson RC, ed. NY Academy Press, pp. 19-37. 1976.

Ro DK, Paradise EM, Ouellet M, Fisher KJ, Newman KL, Ndungu JM, Ho KA, Eachus RA, Ham TS, Kirby J, Chang MC, Withers ST, Shiba Y, Sarpong R, Keasling JD. Production of the antimalarial drug precursor artemisinic acid in engineered yeast. Nature. 2006 Apr 13;440(7086):852-3 [and] 940-3. Accessed 2006 Aug 12.

Rocha JL, Pellegrino LN, Riella LV, Martins LT. Acute hemiplegia associated with cat-scratch disease. Braz J Infect Dis. 2004. Jun;8(3):263-266. Epub 2004 Sep 29.

Rocha JL, Pellegrino LN, Riella LV, Martins LT. Acute hemiplegia associated with cat-scratch disease. Braz J Infect Dis. 2004 Jun;8(3):263-6. Epub 2004 Sep 29.

Rodgers SE, Mather TN. Human Babesia microti incidence and Ixodes scapularis distribution, Rhode Island, 1998-2004. Emerg Infect Dis. 2007 Apr;13(4):633-5.

Rodriguez AC, Meyer WJ, Watrobka T. The Jarisch-Herxheimer reaction in pregnancy: a nursing perspective. J Obstet Gynecol Neonatal Nurs. 1996 Jun;25(5):383-6.

Rodríguez CM, Giachetto LG, Cuneo EA, Gutiérrez B Mdel C, Shimchack RM, Pírez G MC. [Cat-scratch disease with bone compromise: atypical manifestation].[Article in Spanish]. Rev Chilena Infectol. 2009 Aug;26(4):363-9. Epub 2009 Sep 23.

Roe RH, Michael Jumper J, Fu AD, Johnson RN, Richard McDonald H, Cunningham ET. Ocular bartonella infections. Int Ophthalmol Clin. 2008 Summer;48(3):93-105. Review.

Roebuck DJ. Cat-scratch disease with an extraaxial mass. AJNR Am J Neuroradiol. 1998 Aug;19(7):1294-5.

Roelcke U, Barnett W, Wilder-Smith E, Sigmund D, Hacke W. Untreated neuroborreliosis: Bannwarth's syndrome evolving into acute schizophrenia-like psychosis. A case report. J Neurol, 239(3):129-31. 1992.

Roggero E, Zucca E, Mainetti C, Bertoni F, Valsangiacomo C, Pedrinis E, et al. Eradication of Borrelia burgdorferi infection in primary marginal zone B-cell lymphoma of the skin. Hum Pathol, 31(2):263-8. 2000.

Rolain JM, Arnoux D, Parzy D, Sampol J, Raoult D. Experimental infection of human erythrocytes from alcoholic patients with Bartonella quintana. Ann N Y Acad Sci. 2003 Jun;990:605-11.

Rolain JM, Boureau-Voultoury A, Raoult D. Serological evidence of Bartonella vinsonii lymphadenopathies in a child bitten by a dog. Clin Microbiol Infect. 2009 Dec;15 Suppl 2:122-3. Epub 2009 Apr 3.

Rolain JM, Bourry O, Davoust B, Raoult D. Bartonella quintana and Rickettsia felis in Gabon. Emerg Infect Dis. 2005 Nov;11(11):1742-4.

Rolain JM, Brouqui P, Koehler JE, Maguina C, Dolan MJ, Raoult D. Recommendations for treatment of human infections caused by Bartonella species. Antimicrob Agents Chemother. 2004 Jun;48(6):1921-33. Review.

Rolain JM, Chanet V, Laurichesse H, Lepidi H, Beytout J, Raoult D. Cat scratch disease with lymphadenitis, vertebral osteomyelitis, and spleen abscesses. Ann N Y Acad Sci. 2003 Jun;990:397-403. Review.

Rolain JM, Foucault C, Brouqui P, Raoult D. Erythroblast cells as a target for Bartonella quintana in homeless people. Ann N Y Acad Sci. 2003 Jun;990:485-7.

Rolain JM, Foucault C, Guieu R, La Scola B, Brouqui P, Raoult D. Bartonella quintana in human erythrocytes. Lancet. 2002;360(9328):226-228.

Rolain JM, Fournier PE, Raoult D, Bonerandi JJ. First isolation and detection by immunofluorescence assay of Bartonella koehlerae in erythrocytes from a French cat. J Clin Microbiol. 2003 Aug;41(8):4001-2.

Rolain JM, Franc M, Davoust B, Raoult D. Molecular detection of Bartonella quintana, B. koehlerae, B. henselae, B. clarridgeiae, Rickettsia felis, and Wolbachia pipientis in cat fleas, France. Emerg Infect Dis. 2003 Mar;9(3):338-42.

Rolain JM, Gouriet F, Enea M, Aboud M, Raoult D. Detection by immunofluorescence assay of Bartonella henselae in lymph nodes from patients with cat scratch disease. Clin Diagn Lab Immunol. 2003 Jul;10(4):686-91.

Rolain JM, La Scola B, Liang Z, Davoust B, Raoult D. Immuno-fluorescent detection of intraerythrocytic Bartonella henselae in naturally infected cats. J Clin Microbiol. 2001 Aug;39(8):2978-80.

Rolain JM, Lecam C, Raoult D. Simplified serological diagnosis of endocarditis due to Coxiella burnetii and Bartonella. Clin Diagn Lab Immunol. 2003 Nov;10(6):1147-8.

Rolain JM, Lepidi H, Zanaret M, Triglia JM, Michel G, Thomas PA, Texereau M, Stein A, Romaru A, Eb F, Raoult D. Lymph node biopsy specimens and diagnosis of cat-scratch disease. Emerg Infect Dis. 2006 Sep;12(9):1338-44.

Rolain JM, Locatelli C, Chabanne L, Davoust B, Raoult D. Prevalence of Bartonella clarridgeiae and Bartonella henselae in domestic cats from France and detection of the organisms in erythrocytes by immunofluorescence. Clin Diagn Lab Immunol. 2004 Mar;11(2):423-425.

Rolain JM, Maurin M, Bryskier A, Raoult D. In vitro activities of telithromycin (HMR 3647) against Rickettsia rickettsii, Rickettsia conorii, Rickettsia africae, Rickettsia typhi, Rickettsia prowazekii, Coxiella burnetii, Bartonella henselae, Bartonella quintana, Bartonella bacilliformis, and Ehrlichia chaffeensis. Antimicrob Agents Chemother. 2000 May;44(5):1391-3.

Rolain JM, Maurin M, Mallet MN, Parzy D, Raoult D. Culture and antibiotic susceptibility of Bartonella quintana in human erythrocytes. Antimicrob Agents Chemother. 2003 Feb;47(2):614-9.

Rolain JM, Maurin M, Raoult D. Bactericidal effect of antibiotics on Bartonella and Brucella spp.: clinical implications. J Antimicrob Chemother. 2000 Nov;46(5):811-4.

Rolain JM, Novelli S, Ventosilla P, Maguina C, Guerra H, Raoult D. Immunofluorescence detection of Bartonella bacilliformis flagella in vitro and in vivo in human red blood cells as viewed by laser confocal microscopy. Ann N Y Acad Sci. 2003 Jun;990:581-4.

Rolain JM, Rousset E, La Scola B, Duquesnel R, Raoult D. Bartonella schoenbuchensis isolated from the blood of a French cow. Ann N Y Acad Sci. 2003 Jun;990:236-8.

Romanelli F, Smith KM, Hoven AD. Chloroquine and hydroxy-chloroquine as inhibitors of human immunodeficiency virus (HIV-1) activity. Curr Pharm Des. 2004;10(21):2643-8.

Rosenblatt JE. Laboratory diagnosis of infections due to blood and tissue parasites. Clin Infect Dis. 2009 Oct 1;49(7):1103-8. Review.

Rosenhall U, Hanner P, Kaijser B. Borrelia infection and vertigo. Acta Otolaryngol, 106(1-2):111-6. 1988.

Rothermel H, Hedges TR 3rd, Steere AC. Optic neuropathy in children with Lyme disease. Pediatrics. 2001 Aug;108(2):477-81.

Rotily M, Obadia Y, Tissot-Dupont H, Cavailler P, Raoult D. [The epidemiology of trench fever: a pilot study in homeless people in Marseilles].[Article in French]. Sante. 1996 Sep-Oct;6(5):275-8.

Rotily M, Obadia Y, Tissot-Dupont H, Raoult D. Trench fever among homeless people in Marseille, France: a seroprevalence survey. J Epidemiol Community Health. 1997 Apr;51(2):205.

Roubaud-Baudron C, Fortineau N, Goujard C, Le Bras P, Lambotte O. [Cat scratch disease with bone involvement: a case report and literature review].[Article in French]. Rev Med Interne. 2009 Jul;30(7):602-8. Epub 2009 Mar 19. Review.

Rouqui P, Bodiga S and Raoult D. Eucarytic cells protect Borrelia burgdorferi from the action of penicillin and ceftriaxone but not from the action of doxycycline and erythromycin. Antimicrob Agents Chemother. 1996;40:1552-1554.

Rousseau JJ, Lust C, Zangerle PF, Bizgaignon G. Acute transverse myelitis as presenting neurological feature of Lyme disease. Lancet, 2(8517):1222-3. 1986.

Roux V, Eykyn SJ, Wyllie S, Raoult D. Bartonella vinsonii subsp. berkhoffii as an agent of afebrile blood culture-negative endocarditis in a human. J Clin Microbiol. 2000 Apr;38(4):1698-700.

Roux V, Raoult D. Body lice as tools for diagnosis and surveillance of reemerging diseases. J Clin Microbiol. 1999 Mar;37(3):596-9.

Rovery C, Greub G, Lepidi H, Casalta JP, Habib G, Collart F, Raoult D. PCR detection of bacteria on cardiac valves of patients with treated bacterial endocarditis. J Clin Microbiol. 2005 Jan;43(1):163-7.

Rovery C, Rolain JM, Lepidi H, Zandotti C, Moreau J, Brouqui P. Bartonella quintana coinfection with Mycobacterium avium complex and CMV in an AIDS patient: case presentation. BMC Infect Dis. 2006 May 29;6:89.

Rowen, Robert Jay. Artemisinin: From Malaria to Cancer Treatment. Townsend Letter for Doctors & Patients, 2002 Dec.

Rozmanic V, Banac S, Miletic D, Manestar K, Kamber S, Paparic S. Role of magnetic resonance imaging and scintigraphy in the diagnosis and follow-up of osteomyelitis in cat-scratch disease. J Paediatr Child Health. 2007 Jul-Aug;43(7-8):568-70.

Rubaire-Akiiki C, Okello-Onen J, Nasinyama GW, Vaarst M, Kabagambe EK, Mwayi W, Musunga D, Wandukwa W. The prevalence of serum antibodies to tick-borne infections in Mbale District, Uganda: The effect of agro-ecological zone, grazing management and age of cattle. J Insect Sci. 2004; 4: 8. Published online 2004 March 25.

Ruberti G, Begovich AB, Steere AC, Klitz W, Erlich HA, Fathman CG. Molecular analysis of the role of the HLA class II genes DRB1, DQA1, DQB1, and DPB1 in susceptibility to Lyme arthritis. Hum Immunol. 1991 May;31(1):20-7.

Rubin DA, Sorbera C, Nikitin P, McAllister A, Wormser GP, Nadelman RB. Prospective evaluation of heart block complicating early Lyme disease. Pacing Clin Electrophysiol. 1992 Mar;15(3):252-5.

Rudenko N, Golovchenko M, Grubhoffer L, Oliver JH Jr. Updates on Borrelia burgdorferi sensu lato complex with respect to public health. Ticks Tick Borne Dis. 2011 Sep;2(3):123-8. Epub 2011 May 27.

Rudnik-Szalaj I, Poplawska R, Zajkowska J, Szulc A, Pancewicz SA, Gudel I. [Mental disorders in Lyme disease.] [Article in Polish]. Pol Merkuriusz Lek, 11(65):460-2. 2001.

Ruef C. Borrelia burgdorferi bacteremia. Infection. 2011 Feb;39(1):1.

Rupprecht TA, Kirschning CJ, Popp B, Kastenbauer S, Fingerle V, Pfister HW, Koedel U. Borrelia garinii Induces CXCL13 Production in Human Monocytes through Toll-Like Receptor 2. Infect Immun. 2007 September; 75(9): 4351–4356. Published online 2007 June 11.

RXList. [Monograph on the Internet]. Available from: http://www.rxlist.com/cgi/generic2/clindam_cp.htm.

Rydkina EB, Roux V, Gagua EM, Predtechenski AB, Tarasevich IV, Raoult D. Bartonella quintana in body lice collected from homeless persons in Russia. Emerg Infect Dis. 1999 Jan-Feb;5(1):176-8.

Rydzewski J, Mateus-Pinilla N, Warner RE, Hamer S, Weng HY. Ixodes scapularis and Borrelia burgdorferi Among Diverse Habitats Within a Natural Area in East-Central Illinois. Vector Borne Zoonotic Dis. 2011 Oct;11(10):1351-8. Epub 2011 Jun 20.

Sabarinath SN, Asthana OP, Puri SK, Srivastava K, Madhusudanan KP, Gupta RC. Clinical pharmacokinetics of the diastereomers of arteether in healthy volunteers. Clin Pharmacokinet. 2005;44(11):1191-203.

Sabarinath S, Madhusudanan KP, Gupta RC. Pharmacokinetics of the diastereomers of arteether, a potent antimalarial drug, in rats. Biopharm Drug Dispos. 2005 Sept;26(6):211-23.

Sabine Bork, Naoaki Yokoyama, Yuzuru Ikehara, Sanjay Kumar, Chihiro Sugimoto, and Ikuo Igarashi. Growth-Inhibitory Effect of Heparin on Babesia Parasites. Antimicrobial Agents and Chemotherapy. 2004 Jan;48:1:236–41.

Sabino GJ, Hwang SJ, McAllister SC, Mena P, Furie MB. Interferon-γ Influences the Composition of Leukocytic Infiltrates in Murine Lyme Carditis. Am J Pathol. 2011 Oct;179(4):1917-28. Epub 2011 Aug 5.

Sackal C, Laudisoit A, Kosoy M, Massung R, Eremeeva ME, Karpathy SE, Van Wyk K, Gabitzsch E, Zeidner NS. Bartonella spp. and Rickettsia felis in fleas, Democratic Republic of Congo. Emerg Infect Dis. 2008 Dec;14(12):1972-4.

Sadava D, Phillips T, Lin C, Kane SE. Transferrin overcomes drug resistance to artemisinin in human small-cell lung carcinoma cells. Cancer Lett. 2002;179:151-6.

Sadziene A, Jonsson M, Bergstrom S, Bright RK, Kennedy RC, Barbour AG. A bactericidal antibody to Borrelia burgdorferi is directed against a variable region of the OspB protein. Infect Immun. 1994 May;62(5):2037-45.

Sahay B, Singh A, Gnanamani A, Patsey RL, Blalock JE, Sellati TJ. CD14 signaling reciprocally controls collagen deposition and turnover to regulate the development of lyme arthritis. Am J Pathol. 2011 Feb;178(2):724-34.

Şahın İ, Yaman O, Hamamci B, Çetınkaya Ü. [The molecular mechanisms of erythrocyte invasion of Plasmodium spp. as a model organism of apicomplexan protozoa].[Article in Turkish]. Turkiye Parazitol Derg. 2010;34(4):203-6.

Saisongkorh W, Barrassi L, Davoust B, de Broucker CA, Raoult D, Rolain JM. First isolation of Bartonella bovis from animals in French Guyana, South America. Clin Microbiol Infect. 2009 Dec;15 Suppl 2:124-6. Epub 2009 May 18.

Saisongkorh W, Kowalczewska M, Azza S, Decloquement P, Rolain JM, Raoult D. Identification of candidate proteins for the diagnosis of Bartonella henselae infections using an immunoproteomic approach. FEMS Microbiol Lett. 2010 Sep 1;310(2):158-67. Epub 2010 Jul 9.

Saisongkorh W, Robert C, La Scola B, Raoult D, Rolain JM. Evidence of transfer by conjugation of type IV secretion system genes between Bartonella species and Rhizobium radiobacter in amoeba. PLoS One. 2010 Sep 13;5(9):e12666.

Saisongkorh W, Rolain JM, Suputtamongkol Y, Raoult D. Emerging Bartonella in humans and animals in Asia and Australia. J Med Assoc Thai. 2009 May;92(5):707-31. Review.

Saisongkorh W, Wootta W, Sawanpanyalert P, Raoult D, Rolain JM. "Candidatus Bartonella thailandensis": a new genotype of Bartonella identified from rodents. Vet Microbiol. 2009 Oct 20;139(1-2):197-201. Epub 2009 Jun 6.

Saito Y, Tomita K, Nozaki H, Kobayashi S, Kubo M, Inomata I. [A case of cat scratch disease complicated by reversible encephalopathy].[Article in Japanese]. Kansenshogaku Zasshi. 1991 Nov;65(11):1464-9. Review.

Saito-Ito A, Kasahara M, Kasai M, Dantrakool A, Kawai A, Fujita H, Yano Y, Kawabata H, Takada N. Survey of Babesia microti infection in field rodents in Japan: records of the Kobe-type in new foci and findings of a new type related to the Otsu-type. Microbiol Immunol. 2007;51(1):15-24.

Saito-Ito A, Takada N, Ishiguro F, Fujita H, Yano Y, Ma XH, Chen ER. Detection of Kobe-type Babesia microti associated with Japanese human babesiosis in field rodents in central Taiwan and southeastern mainland China. Parasitology. 2008 May;135(6):691-9. Epub 2008 Apr 16.

Sala E, Lipiec A, Zygmunt A, Burdzel Z, Ogórek M, Chyla M. [Cat scratch disease--course, diagnosis].[Article in Polish]. Przegl Epidemiol. 2006;60(2):307-13.

Sala M, Font B, Sanfeliu I, Quesada M, Ponts I, Segura F. Bacillary angiomatosis caused by Bartonella quintana. Ann N Y Acad Sci. 2005 Dec;1063:302-7.

Salazar CA, Rothemich M, Drouin EE, Glickstein L, Steere AC. Human Lyme arthritis and the immunoglobulin G antibody response to the 37-kilodalton arthritis-related protein of Borrelia burgdorferi. Infect Immun. 2005 May;73(5):2951-7.

Salazar JC, Duhnam-Ems S, La Vake C, Cruz AR, Moore MW, Caimano MJ, Velez-Climent L, Shupe J, Krueger W, Radolf JD. Activation of Human Monocytes by Live Borrelia burgdorferi Generates TLR2-Dependent and -Independent Responses Which Include Induction of IFN-β. PLoS Pathog. 2009 May;5(5):e1000444. Published online 2009 May 22.

Salcido RS. Evidence-based medicine: inherent limitations. Adv Skin Wound Care. 2010 Dec;23(12):535-6.

Salehi N, Custodio H, Rathore MH. Renal microabscesses due to Bartonella infection. Pediatr Infect Dis J. 2010 May;29(5):472-3.

Salem Z, Zalloua PA, Chehal A, et al. Effective treatment of hypereosinophilic syndrome with imatinib mesylate. Hematol J. 2003;4(6):410-412.

Salman-Dilgimen A, Hardy PO, Dresser AR, Chaconas G. HrpA, a DEAH-box RNA helicase, is involved in global gene regulation in the Lyme disease spirochete. PLoS One. 2011;6(7):e22168. Epub 2011 Jul 26.

Salo J, Loimaranta V, Lahdenne P, Viljanen MK, Hytönen J. Decorin binding by DbpA and B of Borrelia garinii, Borrelia afzelii, and Borrelia burgdorferi sensu Stricto. J Infect Dis. 2011 Jul;204(1):65-73.

Salvatore P, Casamassimi A, Sommese L, Fiorito C, Ciccodicola A, Rossiello R, Avallone B, Grimaldi V, Costa V, Rienzo M, Colicchio R, Williams-Ignarro S, Pagliarulo C, Prudente ME, Abbondanza C, Lamberti F, Baroni A, Buommino E, Farzati B, Tufano MA, Ignarro LJ, Napoli C. Detrimental effects of Bartonella henselae are counteracted by L-arginine and nitric oxide in human endothelial progenitor cells. Proc Natl Acad Sci U S A. 2008 Jul 8;105(27):9427-32. Epub 2008 Jun 30.

Salzman MB, Rubin LG, Sood SK. Prevention of Lyme disease after tick bites. N Engl J Med. 1993 Jan 14;328(2):137; author reply 138-9.

Samimi S, Salah S, Bonicel P. [Acquired nystagmus in a 12-year-old boy as initial presentation of Lyme disease].[Article in French]. J Fr Ophtalmol. 2011 May;34(5):325.e1-3. Epub 2011 Apr 14.

Samson L, Drancourt M, Casalta JP, Raoult D. Corpuscular antigenic microarray for the serodiagnosis of blood culture-negative endocarditis. Ann N Y Acad Sci. 2006 Oct;1078:595-6.

Samuels DS. Gene Regulation in Borrelia burgdorferi. Annu Rev Microbiol. 2011 Oct 13;65:479-99.

Sanders ML, Glass GE, Nadelman RB, Wormser GP, Scott AL, Raha S, Ritchie BC, Jaworski DC, Schwartz BS. Antibody levels to recombinant tick calreticulin increase in humans after exposure to Ixodes scapularis (Say) and are correlated with tick engorgement indices. Am J Epidemiol. 1999 Apr 15;149(8):777-84.

Sanfeliu I, Antón E, Pineda V, Pons I, Perez J, Font B, Segura F. Description of Bartonella spp. infections in a general hospital of Catalonia, Spain. Clin Microbiol Infect. 2009 Dec;15 Suppl 2:130-1. Epub 2009 May 18.

Sanguinetti-Morelli D, Angelakis E, Richet H, Davoust B, Rolain JM, Raoult D. Seasonality of cat-scratch disease, France, 1999-2009. Emerg Infect Dis. 2011 Apr;17(4):705-7.

Sankatsing SU, Kolader ME, Bouma BJ, Bennink RJ, Verberne HJ, Ansink TM, Visser CE, van der Meer JT. 18F-fluoro-2-deoxyglucose positron emission tomography-negative endocarditis lenta caused by Bartonella henselae. J Heart Valve Dis. 2011 Jan;20(1):100-2.

Sanofi-Synthelabo: Prescribing Information. [Monograph on the Internet]. Available from: http://products.sanofiaventis.us/plaquenil/plaquenil.html.

Sanogo YO, Zeaiter Z, Caruso G, Merola F, Shpynov S, Brouqui P, Raoult D. Bartonella henselae in Ixodes ricinus ticks (Acari: Ixodida) removed from humans, Belluno province, Italy. Emerg Infect Dis. 2003 Mar;9(3):329-32.

Santino I, Longobardi V. Clinical and serological features of patients with suspected Lyme borreliosis. Int J Immunopathol Pharmacol. 2011 Jul-Sep;24(3):797-801.

Santos M, Haddad Júnior V, Ribeiro-Rodrigues R, Talhari S. [Lyme borreliosis].[Article in English and Portuguese]. An Bras Dermatol. 2010 Dec;85(6):930-8.

Sá-Nunes A, Bafica A, Antonelli LR, Choi EY, Francischetti IM, Andersen JF, Shi GP, Chavakis T, Ribeiro JM, Kotsyfakis M. The immunomodulatory action of sialostatin L on dendritic cells reveals its potential to interfere with autoimmunity. J Immunol. 2009 Jun 15;182(12):7422-9.

Sapi E, Kaur N, Anyanwu S, Luecke DF, Datar A, Patel S, Rossi M, Stricker RB. Evaluation of in-vitro antibiotic susceptibility of different morphological forms of Borrelia burgdorferi. Infect Drug Resist. 2011;4:97-113. Epub 2011 May 3.

Sarkar A, Hayes BM, Dulebohn DP, Rosa PA. Regulation of the Virulence Determinant OspC by bbd18 on Linear Plasmid lp17 of Borrelia burgdorferi. J Bacteriol. 2011 Oct;193(19):5365-73. Epub 2011 Jul 22.

Sasaki T, Poudel SK, Isawa H, Hayashi T, Seki N, Tomita T, Sawabe K, Kobayashi M. First molecular evidence of Bartonella quintana in Pediculus humanus capitis (Phthiraptera: Pediculidae), collected from Nepalese children. J Med Entomol. 2006 Jan;43(1):110-2.

Sasseigne G, Herbert A, Larvol L, Damade R, Cartry O. [Fever and abdominal pain in a 56-year-old woman].[Article in French]. Rev Med Interne. 2009 Dec;30(12):1049-53. Epub 2009 Oct 7.

Sato Y, Miyamoto K, Iwaki A, Masuzawa T, Yanagihara Y, Korenberg EI, Gorelova NB, Volkov VI, Ivanov LI, Liberova RN. Prevalence of Lyme disease spirochetes in Ixodes persulcatus and wild rodents in far eastern Russia. Appl Environ Microbiol. 1996 Oct;62(10):3887-9.

Savely VR, Leitao MM, Stricker RB. The mystery of Morgellons disease: infection or delusion? Am J Clin Dermatol. 2006;7(1):1-5. Review.

Savely VR, Stricker RB. Morgellons disease: Analysis of a population with clinically confirmed microscopic subcutaneous fibers of unknown etiology. Clin Cosmet Investig Dermatol. 2010 May 13;3:67-78.

Savić S, Vidić B, Lazić S, Lako B, Potkonjak A, Lepsanović Z. Borrelia burgdorferi in ticks and dogs in the province of Vojvodina, Serbia. Parasite. 2010 Dec;17(4):357-61.

Sawczuk M. [Cattle babesiosis].[Article in Polish]. Wiad Parazytol. 2007;53(2):73-9. Review.

Scelsa SN, Lipton RB, Sander H, Herskovitz S. Headache characteristics in hospitalized patients with Lyme disease. Headache. 1995 Mar;35(3):125-30.

Schafley, Andrew. Presentation at the 2005 American Association of Physicians and Surgeons.

Schaller J. A Laboratory Guide to Human Babesia Hematology Forms. Tampa, FL:Hope Academic Press. 2008.

Schaller J. The Diagnosis, Treatment and Prevention of Bartonella: Atypical Bartonella Treatment Failures and 40 Hypothetical Physical Exam Findings – Full Color Edition. Volume I-II. Tampa, FL:Hope Academic Press. 2008.

Schaller J. Babesia. in Encyclopedia of Plagues, Pestilence and Pandemics. Ed. J. Bryre. Westport, CT: Greenwood Press; 2008.

Schaller J. Bartonella. in Encyclopedia of Plagues, Pestilence and Pandemics. Ed. J. Bryre, Westport, CT: Greenwood Press; 2008.

Schaller J. Lyme Disease. in Encyclopedia of Plagues, Pestilence and Pandemics. Ed. J. Bryre. Westport, CT: Greenwood Press; 2008.

Schaller J. Babesia 2009 Supplement and Update. Tampa, FL:Hope Academic Press. 2009.

Schaller JA. Personal regular monthly communications. 1996-2011.

Schaller JL. Artemisin, Artesunate, Artemisinic Acid and Other Derivatives of Artemisia Used for Malaria, Babesia and Cancer. Tampa, FL: Hope Academic Press. 2006.

Schaller JL. The Health Care Professional's Guide to the Treatment and Diagnosis of Human Babesiosis, An Extensive Review of New Human Species and Advanced Treatments. Tampa, FL: Hope Academic Press. 2006.

Schaller JL, Burkland GA. Case report: rapid and complete control of idiopathic hypereosinophilia with imatinib mesylate. MedGenMed. 2001;3(5):9.

Schaller JL, Burkland GA, Langhoff PJ. Are various Babesia species a missed cause for hypereosinophilia? A follow-up on the first reported case of imatinib mesylate for idiopathic hypereosinophilia. MedGenMed. 2007 Feb 27;9(1):38.

Schaller JL, Burkland GA, Langhoff PJ. Do bartonella infections cause agitation, panic disorder, and treatment-resistant depression? MedGenMed. 2007 Sep 13;9(3):54.

Schaller M, Neubert U. Ultrastructure of Borrelia burgdorferi after exposure to benzylpenicillin. Infection. 1994 Nov-Dec;22(6):401-406.

Schechter SL. Lyme disease associated with optic neuropathy. Am J Med. 1986 Jul;81(1):143-5.

Scheid R, Hund-Georgiadis M, von Cramon DY. Intracerebral haemorrhage as a manifestation of Lyme neuroborreliosis? Eur J Neurol. 2003 ;10(1):99-101.

Scheidegger F, Ellner Y, Guye P, Rhomberg TA, Weber H, Augustin HG, Dehio C. Distinct activities of Bartonella henselae type IV secretion effector proteins modulate capillary-like sprout formation. Cell Microbiol. 2009 Jul;11(7):1088-101. Epub 2009 Mar 12.

Scheidegger F, Quebatte M, Mistl C, Dehio C. The Bartonella henselae VirB/Bep system interferes with vascular endothelial growth factor (VEGF) signalling in human vascular endothelial cells. Cell Microbiol. 2011 Mar;13(3):419-31. Epub 2010 Dec 3.

Schicht S, Junge S, Schnieder T, Strube C. Prevalence of Anaplasma phagocytophilum and Coinfection with Borrelia burgdorferi Sensu Lato in the Hard Tick Ixodes ricinus in the City of Hanover (Germany). Vector Borne Zoonotic Dis. 2011 Sep 15. [Epub ahead of print]

Schiellerup P, Dyhr T, Rolain JM, Christensen M, Damsgaard R, Ethelberg S, Fisker N, Frost Andersen N, Raoult D, Krogfelt KA. Low seroprevalence of bartonella species in danish elite orienteers. Scand J Infect Dis. 2004;36(8):604-6.

Schlesinger PA, Duray PH, Burke BA, Steere AC, Stillman MT. Maternal-fetal transmission of the Lyme disease spirochete, Borrelia burgdorferi. Ann Intern Med. 1985 Jul;103(1):67-8.

Schmid GP, Steere AC, Kornblatt AN, Kaufmann AF, Moss CW, Johnson RC, Hovind-Hougen K, Brenner DJ. Newly recognized Leptospira species ("Leptospira inadai" serovar lyme) isolated from human skin. J Clin Microbiol. 1986 Sep;24(3):484-6.

Schmid GP, Steigerwalt AG, Johnson SE, Barbour AG, Steere AC, Robinson IM, Brenner DJ. DNA characterization of the spirochete that causes Lyme disease. J Clin Microbiol. 1984 Aug;20(2):155-8.

Schmid GP, Steigerwalt AG, Johnson S, Barbour AG, Steere AC, Robinson IM, Brenner DJ. DNA characterization of Lyme disease spirochetes. Yale J Biol Med. 1984 Jul-Aug;57(4):539-42.

Schmid GP, Horsley R, Steere AC, Hanrahan JP, Davis JP, Bowen GS, Osterholm MT, Weisfeld JS, Hightower AW, Broome CV. Surveillance of Lyme disease in the United States, 1982. J Infect Dis. 1985 Jun;151(6):1144-9.

Schmid GP, Centers for Disease Control. Epidemiology and clinical similarities of human spirochetal diseases. Rev Infect Dis. 1989;11(Suppl 6):S1460-9.

Schmid MC, Scheidegger F, Dehio M, Balmelle-Devaux N, Schulein R, Guye P, Chennakesava CS, Biedermann B, Dehio C. A translocated bacterial protein protects vascular endothelial cells from apoptosis. PLoS Pathog. 2006 Nov;2(11):e115.

Schmid MC, Schulein R, Dehio M, Denecker G, Carena I, Dehio C. The VirB type IV secretion system of Bartonella henselae mediates invasion, proinflammatory activation and antiapoptotic protection of endothelial cells. Mol Microbiol. 2004;52(1):81-92.

Schmidli J, Hunziker T, Moesli P, Schaad UB. Cultivation of Borrelia burgdorferi from joint fluid three months after treatment of facial palsy due to Lyme borreliosis. J Infect Dis. 1988 Oct;158(4):905-6.

Schmidt BL, Aberer E, Stockenhuber C, Klade H, Breier F, Luger A. Detection of Borrelia burgdorferi DNA by polymerase chain reaction in the urine and breast milk of patients with Lyme borreliosis. Diagn Microbiol Infect Dis. 1995 Mar;21(3):121-8.

Schmidt C, Plate A, Angele B, Pfister HW, Wick M, Koedel U, Rupprecht TA. A prospective study on the role of CXCL13 in Lyme neuroborreliosis. Neurology. 2011 Mar 22;76(12):1051-8.

Schmit VL, Patton TG, Gilmore RD Jr. Analysis of Borrelia burgdorferi Surface Proteins as Determinants in Establishing Host Cell Interactions. Front Microbiol. 2011;2:141. Epub 2011 Jul 1.

Schneer S, Marcoviciu D, Beilin V, Goffman M, Dicker D. [Stroke as a manifestation of acute Bartonella henselae endocarditis]. [Article in Hebrew]. Harefuah. 2007 Nov;146(11):902-4, 908.

Schoeman JP. Canine babesiosis. Onderstepoort J Vet Res. 2009 Mar;76(1):59-66. Review.

Schoeman JP, Herrtage ME. Adrenal response to the low dose ACTH stimulation test and the cortisol-to-adrenocorticotrophic hormone ratio in canine babesiosis. Vet Parasitol. 2008 Jul 4;154(3-4):205-13. Epub 2008 Apr 7.

Schoen RT. Relapsing or reinfectious Lyme hepatitis. Hepatology. 1989 Feb;9(2):335-6.

Schoen RT. A case revealing the natural history of untreated Lyme disease. Nat Rev Rheumatol. 2011 Mar;7(3):179-84. Epub 2010 Dec 21.

Schoen RT. Treatment of Lyme disease. Conn Med. 1989 Jun;53(6):335-7.

Schoen RT, Aversa JM, Rahn DW, Steere AC. Treatment of refractory chronic Lyme arthritis with arthroscopic synovectomy. Arthritis Rheum. 1991 Aug;34(8):1056-60.

Schönherr U, Strle F. In Aspects of Lyme Borreliosis, Ed. Klaus Weber, M.D., Willy Burgdorfer, Ph.D., M.D. Berlin Heidelberg:Springer-Verlag. 1993. pp 248-258.

Scholz HC, Al Dahouk S, Tomaso H, Neubauer H, Witte A, Schloter M, Kämpfer P, Falsen E, Pfeffer M, Engel M. Genetic diversity and phylogenetic relationships of bacteria belonging to the Ochrobactrum-Brucella group by recA and 16S rRNA gene-based comparative sequence analysis. Syst Appl Microbiol. 2008 Mar;31(1):1-16. Epub 2008 Jan 28.

Schorn S, Pfister K, Reulen H, Mahling M, Silaghi C. Occurrence of Babesia spp., Rickettsia spp. and Bartonella spp. in Ixodes ricinus in Bavarian public parks, Germany. Parasit Vectors. 2011 Jul 15;4:135.

Schraga ED. Cat scratch disease in Emergency Medicine. http://www.emedicine.com/emerg/topic84.htm. Accessed September 6, 2007.

Schröder G, Schuelein R, Quebatte M, Dehio C. Conjugative DNA transfer into human cells by the VirB/VirD4 type IV secretion system of the bacterial pathogen Bartonella henselae. Proc Natl Acad Sci U S A. 2011 Aug 30;108(35):14643-8. Epub 2011 Aug 15.

Schroeter V, Belz GG, Blenk H. Paralysis of recurrent laryngeal nerve in Lyme disease. Lancet. 1988 Nov 26;2(8622):1245.

Schroff S. Update on emerging infections: news from the Centers for Disease Control and Prevention. Bartonella quintana in body lice and head lice from homeless persons, San Francisco, California, USA. Ann Emerg Med. 2010 Mar;55(3):280-2; discussion 282-3.

Schuijt TJ, Coumou J, Narasimhan S, Dai J, Deponte K, Wouters D, Brouwer M, Oei A, Roelofs JJ, van Dam AP, van der Poll T, Van't Veer C, Hovius JW, Fikrig E. A tick mannose-binding lectin inhibitor interferes with the vertebrate complement cascade to enhance transmission of the lyme disease agent. Cell Host Microbe. 2011 Aug 18;10(2):136-46.

Schulein R, Dehio C. The VirB/VirD4 type IV secretion system of Bartonella is essential for establishing intraerythrocytic infection. Mol Microbiol. 2002;46(4):1053-67.

Schulein R, Seubert A, Gille C, et al. Invasion and persistent intracellular colonization of erythrocytes. A unique parasitic strategy of the emerging pathogen Bartonella. J Exp Med. 2001 May 7;193(9):1077-86.

Schulte B, Linke D, Klumpp S, Schaller M, Riess T, Autenrieth IB, Kempf VA. Bartonella quintana Variably Expressed Outer Membrane Proteins Mediate Vascular Endothelial Growth Factor Secretion but Not Host Cell Adherence. Infect Immun. 2006 Sep;74(9):5003-13.

Schultz MG. Who is this man? Emerg Infect Dis. 2010 Jun;16(6):1025-7.

Schulze TL,Jordan RA,Hung RW,Puelle RS,Markowski D,Chomsky MS. Prevalence of Borrelia burgdorferi in Ixodes scapularis adults in New Jersey, 2000-2001. J Med Entomol. 2003;40(4):555-8.

Schutzer SE, Angel TE, Liu T, Schepmoes AA, Clauss TR, Adkins JN, Camp DG, Holland BK, Bergquist J, Coyle PK, Smith RD, Fallon BA, Natelson BH. Distinct cerebrospinal fluid proteomes differentiate post-treatment lyme disease from chronic fatigue syndrome. PLoS One. 2011 Feb 23;6(2):e17287.

Schwartz BS, Nadelman RB, Fish D, Childs JE, Forseter G, Wormser GP. Entomologic and demographic correlates of anti-tick saliva antibody in a prospective study of tick bite subjects in Westchester County, New York. Am J Trop Med Hyg. 1993 Jan;48(1):50-7.

Schwartz E. Regev-Yochay G. Primaquine as prophylaxis for malaria for nonimmune travelers: A comparison with mefloquine and doxycycline. Clin Infect Dis. 1999 Dec;29(6):1502-6.

Schwartz I, Bittker S, Bowen SL, Cooper D, Pavia C, Wormser GP. Polymerase chain reaction amplification of culture supernatants for rapid detection of Borrelia burgdorferi. Eur J Clin Microbiol Infect Dis. 1993 Nov;12(11):879-82.

Schwartz I, Varde S, Nadelman RB, Wormser GP, Fish D. Inhibition of efficient polymerase chain reaction amplification of Borrelia burgdorferi DNA in blood-fed ticks. Am J Trop Med Hyg. 1997 Mar;56(3):339-42.

Schwartz I, Wormser GP, Schwartz JJ, Cooper D, Weissensee P, Gazumyan A, Zimmermann E, Goldberg NS, Bittker S, Campbell GL, Pavia CS. Diagnosis of early Lyme disease by polymerase chain reaction amplification and culture of skin biopsies from erythema migrans lesions. J Clin Microbiol. 1992 Dec;30(12):3082-8.

Schweyer S, Fayyazi A. Activation and apoptosis of macrophages in cat scratch disease. J Pathol. 2002 Dec;198(4):534-40.

Scoles GA, Papero M, Beati L, Fish D. A relapsing fever group spirochete transmitted by Ixodes scapularis ticks. Vector Borne Zoonotic Dis. 2001 Spring;1(1):21-34.

Scolfaro C, Leunga GG, Bezzio S, Chiapello N, Riva C, Balbo L, Bertaina C, Tovo PA. Prolonged follow up of seven patients affected by hepatosplenic granulomata due to cat-scratch disease. Eur J Pediatr. 2008 Apr;167(4):471-3. Epub 2007 Jun 1.

Scolfaro C, Mignone F, Gennari F, Alfarano A, Veltri A, Romagnoli R, Salizzoni M. Possible donor-recipient bartonellosis transmission in a pediatric liver transplant. Transpl Infect Dis. 2008 Dec;10(6):431-3. Epub 2008 Jul 22.

Scott C, Azwa A, Cohen C, McIntyre M, Desmond N. Cat scratch disease: a diagnostic conundrum. Int J STD AIDS. 2009 Aug;20(8):585-6.

Scott JD, Anderson JF, Durden LA. Widespread dispersal of Borrelia burgdorferi-infected ticks collected from songbirds across Canada. J Parasitol. 2011 Aug 24. [Epub ahead of print]

Scott MC, Rosen ME, Hamer SA, Baker E, Edwards H, Crowder C, Tsao JI, Hickling GJ. High-prevalence Borrelia miyamotoi infection among [corrected] wild turkeys (Meleagris gallopavo) in Tennessee. J Med Entomol. 2010 Nov;47(6):1238-42. Erratum in J Med Entomol. 2011 May;48(3):iv.

Scrimenti RJ. Erythema migrans. Arch Dermatol. 1970;102:104-5.

Seah AB, Azran MS, Newman NJ. Cat-scratch encephalopathy. Arch Neurol. 2004 Jan;61(1):145-7.

Seah AB, Azran MS, Rucker JC, Biousse V, Martin DF, Newman NJ. Magnetic resonance imaging abnormalities in cat-scratch disease encephalopathy. J Neuroophthalmol. 2003 Mar;23(1):16-21.

Seals JE, Oken HA. Cat scratch encephalopathy. Md Med J. 1999 Jul-Aug;48(4):176-8.

Sedláčková L, Bartosová D, Vydrzalová P, Crhová K, Zarosská E, Holcíková A, Habanec T, Janecek D. [Abscessing lymphadenitis in a 1.5-year-old boy].[Article in Czech]. Klin Mikrobiol Infekc Lek. 2007 Jun;13(3):119-21.

Seemanapalli SV, Xu Q, McShan K, Liang FT. Outer surface protein C is a dissemination-facilitating factor of Borrelia burgdorferi during mammalian infection. PLoS One. 2010 Dec 31;5(12):e15830.

Seijo MM, Grandes IJ, Sanchez HJ, Garcia-Monco JC. Spontaneous brain hemorrhage associated with Lyme neuroborreliosis. Neurologia. 2001 Jan;16(1):43-5.

Seinost G, Dykhuizen DE, Dattwyler RJ, Golde WT, Dunn JJ, Wang IN, Wormser GP, Schriefer ME, Luft BJ. Four clones of Borrelia burgdorferi sensu stricto cause invasive infection in humans. Infect Immun. 1999 Jul;67(7):3518-24.

Seki N, Sasaki T, Sawabe K, Sasaki T, Matsuoka M, Arakawa Y, Marui E, Kobayashi M. Epidemiological studies on Bartonella quintana infections among homeless people in Tokyo, Japan. Jpn J Infect Dis. 2006 Feb;59(1):31-5.

Sellati TJ, Bouis DA, Kitchens RL, Darveau RP, Pugin J, Ulevitch RJ, Gangloff SC, Goyert SM, Norgard MV, Radolf JD. Treponema pallidum and Borrelia burgdorferi lipoproteins and synthetic lipopeptides activate monocytic cells via a CD14-dependent pathway distinct from that used by lipopolysaccharide. J Immunol. 1998 Jun 1;160(11):5455-64.

Selmani Z, Pyykko I, Ishizaki H, Ashammakhi N. Use of electro-cochleography for assessing endolymphatic hydrops in patients with Lyme disease and Meniere's disease. Acta Otolaryngol. 2002;122(2):173-8.

Selmeczi K, Robert A, Claparols C, Meunier B. Alkylation of human hemoglobin by the antimalarial drug artemisinin. FEBS Lett. 2004 Jan 2;(1-3):245-48,556.

Seltzer EG, Shapiro ED. Misdiagnosis of Lyme disease: when not to order serologic tests. Pediatr Infect Dis J. 1996 Sep;15(9):762-3.

Seltzer EG, Shapiro ED, Gerber MA. Long-term outcomes of lyme disease. JAMA. 2000 Jun 21;283(23):3068-9.

Seltzer EG, Gerber MA, Cartter ML, Freudigman K, Shapiro ED. Long-term outcomes of persons with Lyme disease. JAMA. 2000 Feb 2;283(5):609-16.

Semel ME, Tavakkolizadeh A, Gates JD. Babesiosis in the immediate postoperative period after splenectomy for trauma. Surg Infect (Larchmt). 2009 Dec;10(6):553-6. Review.

Sen E, Uchishima Y, Okamoto Y, Fukui T, Kadosaka T, Ohashi N, Masuzawa T. Molecular detection of Anaplasma phagocytophilum and Borrelia burgdorferi in Ixodes ricinus ticks from Istanbul metropolitan area and rural Trakya (Thrace) region of north-western Turkey. Ticks Tick Borne Dis. 2011 Jun;2(2):94-8. Epub 2011 May 25.

Sereda MJ. Purines 2010: Adenine Nucleosides and Nucleotides in Biomedicine. IDrugs. 2010 Aug;13(8):534-8.

Serratrice J, Rolain JM, Granel B, Ene N, Conrath J, Avierinos JF, Disdier P, Raoult D, Weiller PJ. [Bilateral retinal artery branch occlusions revealing Bartonella grahamii infection].[Article in French]. Rev Med Interne. 2003 Sep;24(9):629-30.

Sethi S, Alcid D, Kesarwala H, Tolan RW Jr. Probable congenital babesiosis in infant, New Jersey, USA. Emerg Infect Dis. 2009 May;15(5):788-91.

Setty S, Khalil Z, Schori P, Azar M, Ferrieri P. Babesiosis. Two atypical cases from Minnesota and a review. Am J Clin Pathol. 2003 Oct;120(4):554-9.

Seubert A, Hiestand R, de la Cruz F, Dehio C. A bacterial conjugation machinery recruited for pathogenesis. Mol Microbiol. 2003;49(5):1253-66.

Sève P, Turner R, Stankovic K, Perard L, Broussolle C. Transient monoclonal gammopathy in a patient with Bartonella quintana endocarditis. Am J Hematol. 2006 Feb;81(2):115-7.

Seward RJ, Drouin EE, Steere AC, Costello CE. Peptides presented by HLA-DR molecules in synovia of patients with rheumatoid arthritis or antibiotic-refractory Lyme arthritis. Mol Cell Proteomics. 2011 Mar;10(3):M110.002477. Epub 2010 Nov 16.

Shadick NA, Phillips CB, Logigian EL, Steere AC, Kaplan RF, Berardi VP, Duray PH, Larson MG, Wright EA, Ginsburg KS, Katz JN, Liang MH. The long-term clinical outcomes of Lyme disease. A population-based retrospective cohort study. Ann Intern Med. 1994 Oct 15;121(8):560-7.

Shah SI. Viewpoint: pancakes and medical statistics. Acad Med. 2005. May;80(5):452-4.

Shamim EA, Shamim SA, Liss G, Nylen E, Pincus JH, Yepes M. Constipation heralding neuroborreliosis: an atypical tale of 2 patients. Arch Neurol. 2005 ;62(4):671-3.

Shanks GD, Edstein MD. Modern malaria chemoprophylaxis. Drugs. 2005;65(15):2091-110.

Shapiro ED. Lyme disease in children. Am J Med. 1995 Apr 24;98(4A):69S-73S. Review.

Shapiro ED. Tick-borne diseases. Adv Pediatr Infect Dis. 1997;13:187-218. Review.

Shapiro ED. Lyme disease. Pediatr Rev. 1998 May;19(5):147-54. Review.

Shapiro ED. Doxycycline for tick bites--not for everyone. N Engl J Med. 2001 Jul 12;345(2):133-4.

Shapiro ED. Long-term outcomes of persons with Lyme disease. Vector Borne Zoonotic Dis. 2002 Winter;2(4):279-81.

Shapiro ED. Lyme disease. Adv Exp Med Biol. 2008;609:185-95. Review.

Shapiro ED, Dattwyler R, Nadelman RB, Wormser GP. Response to meta-analysis of Lyme borreliosis symptoms. Int J Epidemiol. 2005 Dec;34(6):1437-9; author reply 1440-3. Epub 2005 Nov 30.

Shapiro ED, Gerber MA. Lyme disease and facial nerve palsy. Arch Pediatr Adolesc Med. 1997 Dec;151(12):1183-4.

Shapiro ED, Gerber MA. Lyme disease: fact versus fiction. Pediatr Ann. 2002 Mar;31(3):170-7. Review.

Shapiro ED, Gerber MA. Lyme disease. Clin Infect Dis. 2000 Aug;31(2):533-42. Epub 2000 Sep 14. Review.

Shapiro ED, Gerber MA, Holabird NB, Berg AT, Feder HM Jr, Bell GL, Rys PN, Persing DH. A controlled trial of antimicrobial prophylaxis for Lyme disease after deer-tick bites. N Engl J Med. 1992 Dec 17;327(25):1769-73.

Shapiro ED, Seltzer EG. Lyme disease in children. Semin Neurol. 1997 Mar;17(1):39-44. Review.

Shen AK, Mead PS, Beard CB. The Lyme disease vaccine--a public health perspective. Clin Infect Dis. 2011 Feb;52 Suppl 3:s247-52. Review.

Shen S, Shin JJ, Strle K, McHugh G, Li X, Glickstein LJ, Drouin EE, Steere AC. Treg cell numbers and function in patients with antibiotic-refractory or antibiotic-responsive Lyme arthritis. Arthritis Rheum. 2010 Jul;62(7):2127-37.

Sherr VT. Long-term outcomes of Lyme disease. JAMA. 2000 Jun 21;283(23):3068-9

Sherr VT. Panic attacks may reveal previously unsuspected chronic disseminated Lyme disease. J Psychiatr Pract. 2000 Nov;6(6):352-6.

Sherr, VT. Human babesiosis - an unrecorded reality absence of formal registry undermines its detection, diagnosis and treatment, suggesting need for immediate mandatory reporting. Medical Hypotheses. 2004;63(4):609-15.

Sherr VT. Munchausen's syndrome by proxy and Lyme disease: medical misogyny or diagnostic mystery? Med Hypotheses. 2005;65(3):440-7.

Shin JJ, Strle K, Glickstein LJ, Luster AD, Steere AC. Borrelia burgdorferi stimulation of chemokine secretion by cells of monocyte lineage in patients with Lyme arthritis. Arthritis Res Ther. 2010;12(5):R168. Epub 2010 Sep 9.

Shin JJ, Glickstein LJ, Steere AC. High levels of inflammatory chemokines and cytokines in joint fluid and synovial tissue throughout the course of antibiotic-refractory lyme arthritis. Arthritis Rheum. 2007 Apr;56(4):1325-35.

Shin OS, Isberg RR, Akira S, Uematsu S, Behera AK, Hu LT. Distinct Roles for MyD88 and Toll-Like Receptors 2, 5, and 9 in Phagocytosis of Borrelia burgdorferi and Cytokine Induction. Infect Immun. 2008 Jun;76(6):2341-51. Published online 2008 March 31.

Shoemaker RC, Hudnell HK, House DE, Van Kempen A, Pakes GE; COL40155 Study Team. Atovaquone plus cholestyramine in patients coinfected with Babesia microti and Borrelia burgdorferi refractory to other treatment. Adv Ther. 2006 Jan-Feb;23(1):1-11.

Shrestha M, Grodzicki RL, Steere AC. Diagnosing early Lyme disease. Am J Med. 1985 Feb;78(2):235-40.

Shulman ST. Attention: attention-deficit/ hyperactivity disorder. Pediatr Ann. 2008 Jan;37(1):5-6.

Siciliano RF, Strabelli TM, Zeigler R, Rodrigues C, Castelli JB, Grinberg M, Colombo S, da Silva LJ, Mendes do Nascimento EM, Pereira dos Santos FC, Uip DE. Infective endocarditis due to Bartonella spp. and Coxiella burnetii: experience at a cardiology hospital in Sao Paulo, Brazil. Ann N Y Acad Sci. 2006 Oct;1078:215-22.

Sigal LH. Musculoskeletal features of Lyme disease: understanding the pathogenesis of clinical findings helps make appropriate therapeutic choices. J Clin Rheumatol. 2011 Aug;17(5):256-65.

Sigal LH, Steere AC, Niederman JC. Symmetric polyarthritis associated with heterophile-negative infectious mononucleosis. Arthritis Rheum. 1983 Apr;26(4):553-6.

Sigal LH, Steere AC, Dwyer JM. In vivo and in vitro evidence of B cell hyperactivity during Lyme disease. J Rheumatol. 1988 Apr;15(4):648-54.

Sigal LH, Moffat CM, Steere AC, Dwyer JM. Cellular immune findings in Lyme disease. Yale J Biol Med. 1984 Jul-Aug;57(4):595-8.

Sigal LH, Steere AC, Freeman DH, Dwyer JM. Proliferative responses of mononuclear cells in Lyme disease. Reactivity to Borrelia burgdorferi antigens is greater in joint fluid than in blood. Arthritis Rheum. 1986 Jun;29(6):761-9.

Sigal LH. Summary of the first 100 patients seen at a Lyme disease referral center. Am J Med. 1990 Jun;88(6):577-81.

Sigal L. Clinical manifestations of Lyme disease. N J Med. 1990 Jul;87(7):549-55.

Sigler S, Kershaw P, Scheuch R, Sklarek H, Halperin J.
Respiratory failure due to Lyme meningopolyradiculitis. Am J
Med.
1997;103:544-7.

Sigurdsson MI, Gudnason T, Thorgrímsson S. [Case of the
month: A boy with a notable skin rash].[Article in Icelandic].
Laeknabladid. 2011 Jan;97(1):35-6.

Sikand VK, Halsey N, Krause PJ, Sood SK, Geller R, Van Hoecke
C, Buscarino C, Parenti D; Pediatric Lyme Vaccine Study Group.
Safety and immunogenicity of a recombinant Borrelia burgdorferi
outer surface protein A vaccine against lyme disease in healthy
children and adolescents: a randomized controlled trial. Pediatrics.
2001 Jul;108(1):123-8.

Sillanpää H, Lahdenne P, Sarvas H, Arnez M, Steere A, Peltomaa
M, Seppälä I. Immune responses to borrelial VlsE IR6 peptide
variants. Int J Med Microbiol. 2007 Feb;297(1):45-52. Epub 2007
Jan 17.

Silva MT, Sophar M, Howard RS, Spencer GT. Neuroborreliosis as
a cause of respiratory failure. J Neurol. 1995 ;242(9):604-7.

Silveira Cancela M. [Cat scratch disease].[Article in Spanish]. An
Pediatr (Barc). 2007 Apr;66(4):419-20.

Simonsson US, Jansson B, Hai TN, Huong DX, Tybring G,
Ashton M. Artemisinin autoinduction is caused by involvement
of cytochrome P450 2B6 but not 2C9. Clin Pharmacol Ther.
2003;74:32-43.

Sindhava V, Woodman ME, Stevenson B, Bondada S.
Interleukin-10 Mediated Autoregulation of Murine B-1 B-Cells
and Its Role in Borrelia hermsii Infection. PLoS One. 2010; 5(7):
e11445. Published online 2010 July 6.

Singh NP, Lai H. Selective toxicity of dihydroartemisinin and holotransferrin toward human breast cancer cells. Life Sci. 2001;70(1):49-56.

Singh NP, Lai HC. Artemisinin induces apoptosis in human cancer cells. Anticancer Res. 2004 Jul-Aug;24(4):2277-80.

Singh NP, Lai HC. Synergistic cytotoxicity of artemisinin and sodium butyrate on human cancer cells. Anticancer Res. 2005 Nov-Dec;25(6B):4325-31.

Singhal AB, Newstein MC, Budzik R, Cha JH, Rordorf G, Buonanno FS, Panzara MA. Diffusion-weighted magnetic resonance imaging abnormalities in Bartonella encephalopathy. J Neuroimaging. 2003 Jan;13(1):79-82.

Siński E. [Effect of coinfections in Ixodidae ticks on transmission of blood microparasites].[Article in Polish]. Wiad Parazytol. 2009;55(4):341-7. Review.

Siński E. [Enzootic reservoir for new Ixodes ricinus-transmitted infections].[Article in Polish]. Wiad Parazytol. 1999;45(2):135-42. Review.

Siński E, Welc-Faleciak R, Pogłód R. Babesia spp. infections transmitted through blood transfusion. Wiad Parazytol. 2011;57(2):77-81.

Sivak SL, Aguero-Rosenfeld ME, Nowakowski J, Nadelman RB, Wormser GP. Accuracy of IgM immunoblotting to confirm the clinical diagnosis of early Lyme disease. Arch Intern Med. 1996 Oct 14;156(18):2105-9.

Siwula JM, Mathieu G. Acute onset of facial nerve palsy associated with Lyme disease in a 6 year-old child. Pediatr Dent. 2002 Nov-Dec;24(6):572-4.

Sjöwall J, Carlsson A, Vaarala O, Bergström S, Ernerudh J, Forsberg P, Ekerfelt C. Innate immune responses in Lyme borreliosis: enhanced tumour necrosis factor-α and interleukin-12 in asymptomatic individuals in response to live spirochetes. Clin Exp Immunol. 2005 Jul;141(1):89–98.

Sjöwall J, Fryland L, Nordberg M, Sjögren F, Garpmo U, Jansson C, Carlsson SA, Bergström S, Ernerudh J, Nyman D, Forsberg P, Ekerfelt C. Decreased Th1-type inflammatory cytokine expression in the skin is associated with persisting symptoms after treatment of erythema migrans. PLoS One. 2011 Mar 31;6(3):e18220.

Skarpaas T, Ljøstad U, Søbye M, Mygland A. Sensitivity and specificity of a commercial C6 peptide enzyme immuno assay in diagnosis of acute Lyme neuroborreliosis. Eur J Clin Microbiol Infect Dis. 2007 Sep;26(9):675-7.

Skotarczak B. [Babesiosis of human and domestic dog; ethiology, pathogenesis, diagnostics].[Article in Polish]. Wiad Parazytol. 2007;53(4):271-80. Review.

Skotarczak B, Sawczuk M. [Occurrence of Babesia microti in ticks Ixodes ricinus on selected areas of western Pomerania].[Article in Polish]. Wiad Parazytol. 2003;49(3):273-80.

Skrabalo Z, Deanovic Z. Piroplasmosis in man; report of a case. Doc Med Geogr Trop. 1957 Mar;9(1):11-6.

Slack GS, Mavin S, Yirrell D, Ho-Yen DO. Is Tayside becoming a Scottish hotspot for Lyme borreliosis? J R Coll Physicians Edinb. 2011 Mar;41(1):5-8.

Slatko BE, Taylor MJ, Foster JM. The Wolbachia endosymbiont as an anti-filarial nematode target. Symbiosis. 2010 Jul;51(1):55–65. Published online 2010 June 5.

Smajlovic F, Ibralic M. Color Doppler pseudolymphomatous manifestations of the cat scratch disease. Med Arh. 2009;63(5):297-9.

Smismans A, Goossens VJ, Nulens E, Bruggeman CA. Comparison of five different immunoassays for the detection of Borrelia burgdorferi IgM and IgG antibodies. Clin Microbiol Infect. 2006 Jul;12(7):648-55.

Smith BE, Tompkins MB, Breitschwerdt EB. Antinuclear antibodies can be detected in dog sera reactive to Bartonella vinsonii subsp. berkhoffii, Ehrlichia canis, or Leishmania infantum antigens. J Vet Intern Med. 2004 Jan-Feb;18(1):47-51.

Smith BG, Cruz AI Jr, Milewski MD, Shapiro ED. Lyme disease and the orthopaedic implications of lyme arthritis. J Am Acad Orthop Surg. 2011 Feb;19(2):91-100. Review.

Smith JL, Israel CW. The presence of spirochetes in late seronegative syphilis. JAMA. 1967 Mar 27;199(13):126-30.

Smith JL, Israel CW. Spirochetes in the aqueous humor in seronegative ocular syphilis. Persistence after penicillin therapy. Arch Ophthalmol. 1967 Apr;77(4):474-7.

Smith JL, Winward KE, Nicholson DF, Albert DW Retinal vasculitis in Lyme borreliosis. J Clin Neuroophthalmol. 1991 Mar;11(1):7-15.

Smith RA, Scott B, Beverley DW, Lyon F, Taylor R. Encephalopathy with retinitis due to cat-scratch disease. Dev Med Child Neurol. 2007 Dec;49(12):931-4.

Smith RE, Darling RM. Encephalopathy of cat-scratch disease. AMA J Dis Child. 1960 Jan;99:107-8.

Smith RP, Schoen RT, Rahn DW, Sikand VK, Nowakowski J, Parenti DL, Holman MS, Persing DH, Steere AC. Clinical characteristics and treatment outcome of early Lyme disease in patients with microbiologically confirmed erythema migrans. Ann Intern Med. 2002 Mar 19;136(6):421-8.

Smith SL, Fishwick L, McLean WG, Edwards G, Ward SA. Enhanced in vitro neurotoxicity of artemisinin derivatives in the presence of haemin. Biochem Pharmacol. 1997 Jan 10;53(1):5-10.

Smith SL, Sadler CJ, Dodd CC, Edwards G, Ward SA, Park BK, McLean WG. The role of glutathione in the neurotoxicity of artemisinin derivatives in vitro. Biochem Pharmacol. 2001 Feb 15;61(4):409-16.

Smitherman LS, Minnick MF. Bartonella bacilliformis GroEL: effect on growth of human vascular endothelial cells in infected cocultures. Ann N Y Acad Sci. 2005 Dec;1063:286-98.

Snydman DR, Schenkein DP, Berardi VP, Lastavica CC, Pariser KM. Borrelia burgdorferi in joint fluid in chronic Lyme arthritis. Ann Intern Med. 1986 Jun;104(6):798-800.

Sobraquès M, Maurin M, Birtles RJ, Raoult D. In vitro susceptibilities of four Bartonella bacilliformis strains to 30 antibiotic compounds. Antimicrob Agents Chemother. 1999 Aug;43(8):2090-2.

Socolovschi C, Mediannikov O, Raoult D, Parola P. The relationship between spotted fever group Rickettsiae and Ixodid ticks. Vet Res. 2009 Mar-Apr;40(2):34. Published online 2009 April 10.

Solano-Gallego L, Bradley J, Hegarty B, Sigmon B, Breitschwerdt E. Bartonella henselae IgG antibodies are prevalent in dogs from southeastern USA. Vet Res. 2004 Sep-Oct;35(5):585-95.

Solano-Gallego L, Hegarty B, Espada Y, Llull J, Breitschwerdt E. Serological and molecular evidence of exposure to arthropod-borne organisms in cats from northeastern Spain. Vet Microbiol. 2006 Dec 20;118(3-4):274-7. Epub 2006 Aug 17.

Solano-Gallego L, Llull J, Osso M, Hegarty B, Breitschwerdt E. A serological study of exposure to arthropod-borne pathogens in dogs from northeastern Spain. Vet Res. 2006 Mar-Apr;37(2):231-44.

Sonenshine DE. The biology of tick vectors of human disease. In: Tick-bourne Diseases of Humans. Ed. JL Goodman, DT Dennis, and DE Sonenshine. Washington, DC:AMS Press. 2005;pp.22-23.

Song AT, Gory M, Roussi J, Salomon J, Cremieux AC, Perronne C, Bernard L. Familial occurrence of cat-scratch disease, with varying clinical expression. Scand J Infect Dis. 2007;39(8):728-30.

Sood A, Panush RS, Pinals RS. Case management study: polyarthritis with fever. Bull Rheum Dis. 1998 May;47(3):1-4.

Sood FH, Chaudhari MS. Bartonella bacilliformis or a similar organism and cardiovascular disease. Med Hypotheses. 1994 Sep;43(3):135-7.

Sood FH, Khatpe DS, Chaudhari MS, Phatak VD. Microbes and sequestered substances as mechanisms for disease: Bartonella and L-forms as common global etiological agents. Med Hypotheses. 1999 Apr;52(4):293-6.

Sood FH, Phatak VD, Chaudhari MS. Bartonellosis and human immunodeficiency disease (AIDS): L-forms as persisters, activating factors, and mechanism of disease. Med Hypotheses. 1997 Jun;48(6):511-5.

Sood SK. Lyme disease: recognition, management, and prevention in the primary care setting. Am J Manag Care. 1997 Jul;3(7):1063-6; quiz 1068, 1073.

Sood SK. Facial palsy in Lyme disease. Arch Pediatr Adolesc Med. 1998 Sep;152(9):928-9.

Sood SK. Lyme disease. Pediatr Infect Dis J. 1999 Oct;18(10):913-25. Review.

Sood SK. Lyme disease vaccine as a strategy for prevention. J Pediatr. 2001 Apr;138(4):609-10.

Sood SK. Effective retrieval of Lyme disease information on the Web. Clin Infect Dis. 2002 Aug 15;35(4):451-64. Epub 2002 Jul 19.

Sood SK. What we have learned about Lyme borreliosis from studies in children. Wien Klin Wochenschr. 2006 Nov;118(21-22):638-42. Review.

Sood SK, Ilowite NT. Lyme arthritis in children: is chronic arthritis a common complication? J Rheumatol. 2000 Aug;27(8):1836-8.

Sood SK, Rubin LG, Blader ME, Ilowite NT. Positive serology for Lyme borreliosis in patients with juvenile rheumatoid arthritis in a Lyme borreliosis endemic area: analysis by immunoblot. J Rheumatol. 1993 Apr;20(4):739-41.

Sood SK, Salzman MB, Johnson BJ, Happ CM, Feig K, Carmody L, Rubin LG, Hilton E, Piesman J. Duration of tick attachment as a predictor of the risk of Lyme disease in an area in which Lyme disease is endemic. J Infect Dis. 1997 Apr;175(4):996-9.

Sood SK, Zemel LS, Ilowite NT. Interpretation of immunoblot in pediatric Lyme arthritis. J Rheumatol. 1995 Apr;22(4):758-61.

Sowunmi A, Gbotosho GO, Fateye BA, Adedeji AA. Predictors of the failure of treatment with trimethoprimsulfamethoxazole in children with uncomplicated, Plasmodium falciparum malaria. Ann Trop Med Parasitol. 2006 Apr;100(3):205-11.

Spach DH, Panther LA, Thorning DR, Dunn JE, Plorde JJ, Miller RA. Intracerebral bacillary angiomatosis in a patient infected with human immunodeficiency virus. Ann Intern Med. 1992 May 1;116(9):740-2.

Spach DH, Shimada JK, Paauw DS. Localized alopecia at the site of erythema migrans. J Am Acad Dermatol. 1992 Dec;27(6 Pt 1):1023-4.

Spapen H, Zhang H, Demanet C, et al. Does N-acetyl-L-cysteine influence cytokine response during early human septic shock. Chest. 1998;113:1616-24.

Spielman A, Wilson ML, Levine JF, et al. Ecology of Ixodes dammini-borne human babesiosis and Lyme disease. Ann Rev Entomol. 1985;30:439-60.

Spirin NN, Baranova NS, Fadeeva OA, Shipova EG, Stepanov IO. [Differential aspects of multiple sclerosis and chronic borrelial encephalomyelitis].[Article in Russian]. Zh Nevrol Psikhiatr Im S S Korsakova. 2011;111(7):8-12.

Spolidorio MG, Labruna MB, Machado RZ, Moraes-Filho J, Zago AM, Donatele DM, Pinheiro SR, Silveira I, Caliari KM, Yoshinari NH. Survey for tick-borne zoonoses in the state of Espirito Santo, southeastern Brazil. Am J Trop Med Hyg. 2010 Jul;83(1):201-6.

Sreter-Lancz Z, Tornyai K, Szell Z, Sreter T, Marialigeti K. Bartonella infections in fleas (Siphonaptera: Pulicidae) and lack of bartonellae in ticks (Acari: Ixodidae) from Hungary. Folia Parasitol (Praha). 2006;53(4):313-6.

Stafford KC, Massung RF, Magnarelli LA, Ijdo JW, Anderson JF. Infection with the agents of human granulocytic ehrlichiosis, Lyme disease, and babaesiosis in white-footed mice (Peromyscus leucopus) in Connecticut. J Clin Microbiol. 1999 Sep;37(9):2887-92.

Staggemeier R, Venker CA, Klein DH, Petry M, Spilki FR, Cantarelli VV. Prevalence of Bartonella henselae and Bartonella clarridgeiae in cats in the south of Brazil: a molecular study. Mem Inst Oswaldo Cruz. 2010 Nov;105(7):873-8.

Stańczak J. The occurrence of Spotted Fever Group (SFG) Rickettsiae in Ixodes ricinus ticks (Acari: Ixodidae) in northern Poland. Ann N Y Acad Sci. 2006 Oct;1078:512-4.

Stańczak J, Myjak P, Bajer A, Siński E, Wedrychowicz H, Majewska AC, Gołab E, Budak A. [Usefulness of the molecular techniques for detecting and/or identifing of parasites and fungi in humans and animals or pathogens transmitted by ticks. Part III]. [Article in Polish]. Wiad Parazytol. 2001;47(3):465-75. Review.

Stanek G. [Pandora's Box: pathogens in Ixodes ricinus ticks in Central Europe].[Article in German]. Wien Klin Wochenschr. 2009;121(21-22):673-83.

Stanek G, Gray J, Strle F, Wormser G. Lyme borreliosis. Lancet Infect Dis. 2004 Apr;4(4):197-8; discussion 198-9.

Stanek G, Klein J, Bittner R, Glogar D. Isolation of Borrelia burgdorferi from the myocardium of a patient with longstanding cardiomyopathy. N Engl J Med. 1990 Jan 25;322(4):249-52.

Stanek G, Reiter M. The expanding Lyme Borrelia complex--clinical significance of genomic species? Clin Microbiol Infect. 2011 Apr;17(4):487-93. Review.

Stanek G, Wormser GP, Gray J, Strle F. Lyme borreliosis. Lancet. 2011 Sep 6. [Epub ahead of print]

Steere AC. Acute monocytic arthritis. Discussion. Arthritis Rheum. 1979 Mar;22(3):300-1.

Steere AC. [Lyme disease--a tick-transmitted spirochete infection]. [Article in Russian]. Ter Arkh. 1987;59(4):32-4.

Steere AC. Pathogenesis of Lyme arthritis. Implications for rheumatic disease. Ann N Y Acad Sci. 1988;539:87-92. Review.

Steere AC. Lyme disease. N Engl J Med. 1989 Aug 31;321(9):586-96. Review.

Steere AC. Clinical definitions and differential diagnosis of Lyme arthritis. Scand J Infect Dis Suppl. 1991;77:51-4. Review.

Steere AC. Lyme disease--1993. Bull Rheum Dis. 1993 Oct;42(6):4-7. Review.

Steere AC. Seronegative Lyme disease. JAMA. 1993 Sep 15;270(11): 1369.

Steere AC. Current understanding of Lyme disease. Hosp Pract (Off Ed). 1993 Apr 15;28(4):37-44. Review.

Steere AC. Lyme disease. Trans Am Acad Insur Med. 1993;76:73-81. Review.

Steere AC. Treatment of chronic Lyme disease. Science. 1996 Mar 1;271(5253):1216-8.

Steere AC. Musculoskeletal manifestations of Lyme disease. Am J Med. 1995 Apr 24;98(4A):44S-48S; discussion 48S-51S. Review.

Steere AC. [Lyme arthritis: the joint lesions in Lyme borreliosis in the USA].[Article in Russian]. Ter Arkh. 1995;67(11):43-5.

Steere AC. Diagnosis and treatment of Lyme arthritis. Med Clin North Am. 1997 Jan;81(1):179-94. Review.

Steere AC. Lyme disease. N Engl J Med. 2001 Jul 12;345(2):115-25. Review.

Steere AC. A 58-year-old man with a diagnosis of chronic lyme disease. JAMA. 2002 Aug 28;288(8):1002-10.

Steere AC. Duration of antibiotic therapy for Lyme disease. Ann Intern Med. 2003 May 6;138(9):761-2.

Steere AC. Lyme borreliosis in 2005, 30 years after initial observations in Lyme Connecticut. Wien Klin Wochenschr. 2006 Nov;118(21-22):625-33. Review.

Steere AC. Reply to letter by Volkman commenting on the possible onset of seronegative disease in Lyme arthritis. Arthritis Rheum. 2009 Jan;60(1):310.

Steere AC, Angelis SM. Therapy for Lyme arthritis: strategies for the treatment of antibiotic-refractory arthritis. Arthritis Rheum. 2006 Oct;54(10):3079-86. Review.

Steere AC, Bartenhagen NH, Craft JE, Hutchinson GJ, Newman JH, Pachner AR, Rahn DW, Sigal LH, Taylor E, Malawista SE. Clinical manifestations of Lyme disease. Zentralbl Bakteriol Mikrobiol Hyg A. 1986 Dec;263(1-2):201-5. Review.

Steere AC, Bartenhagen NH, Craft JE, Hutchinson GJ, Newman JH, Rahn DW, Sigal LH, Spieler PN, Stenn KS, Malawista SE. The early clinical manifestations of Lyme disease. Ann Intern Med. 1983 Jul;99(1):76-82.

Steere AC, Batsford WP, Weinberg M, Alexander J, Berger HJ, Wolfson S, Malawista SE. Lyme carditis: cardiac abnormalities of Lyme disease. Ann Intern Med. 1980 Jul;93(1):8-16.

Steere AC, Berardi VP, Weeks KE, Logigian EL, Ackermann R. Evaluation of the intrathecal antibody response to Borrelia burgdorferi as a diagnostic test for Lyme neuroborreliosis. J Infect Dis. 1990 Jun;161(6):1203-9.

Steere AC, Brinckerhoff CE, Miller DJ, Drinker H, Harris ED Jr, Malawista SE. Elevated levels of collagenase and prostaglandin E2 from synovium associated with erosion of cartilage and bone in a patient with chronic Lyme arthritis. Arthritis Rheum. 1980 May;23(5):591-9.

Steere AC, Broderick TF, Malawista SE. Erythema chronicum migrans and Lyme arthritis: epidemiologic evidence for a tick vector. Am J Epidemiol. 1978 Oct;108(4):312-21.

Steere AC, Coburn J, Glickstein L. The emergence of Lyme disease. J. Clin Invest. 2004 Apr;113(8):1093-101. Review.

Steere AC, Dhar A, Hernandez J, Fischer PA, Sikand VK, Schoen RT, Nowakowski J, McHugh G, Persing DH. Systemic symptoms without erythema migrans as the presenting picture of early Lyme disease. Am J Med. 2003 Jan;114(1):58-62.

Steere AC, Drouin EE, Glickstein LJ. Relationship between immunity to Borrelia burgdorferi outer-surface protein A (OspA) and Lyme arthritis. Clin Infect Dis. 2011 Feb;52 Suppl 3:s259-65. Review.

Steere AC, Duray PH, Butcher EC. Spirochetal antigens and lymphoid cell surface markers in Lyme synovitis. Comparison with rheumatoid synovium and tonsillar lymphoid tissue. Arthritis Rheum. 1988 Apr;31(4):487-95.

Steere AC, Duray PH, Kauffmann DJ, Wormser GP. Unilateral blindness caused by infection with the Lyme disease spirochete, Borrelia burgdorferi. Ann Intern Med. 1985 Sep;103(3):382-4.

Steere AC, Dwyer E, Winchester R. Association of chronic Lyme arthritis with HLA-DR4 and HLA-DR2 alleles. N Engl J Med. 1990 Jul 26;323(4):219-23. Erratum in: N Engl J Med. 1991 Jan 10;324(2):129.

Steere AC, Falk B, Drouin EE, Baxter-Lowe LA, Hammer J, Nepom GT. Binding of outer surface protein A and human lymphocyte function-associated antigen 1 peptides to HLA-DR molecules associated with antibiotic treatment-resistant Lyme arthritis. Arthritis Rheum. 2003 Feb;48(2):534-40.

Steere AC, Gibofsky A, Patarroyo ME, Winchester RJ, Hardin JA, Malawista SE. Chronic Lyme arthritis. Clinical and immunogenetic differentiation from rheumatoid arthritis. Ann Intern Med. 1979 Jun;90(6):896-901.

Steere AC, Glickstein L. Elucidation of Lyme arthritis. Nat Rev Immunol. 2004 Feb;4(2):143-52. Review.

Steere AC, Green J, Hutchinson GJ, Rahn DW, Pachner AR, Schoen RT, Sigal LH, Taylor E, Malawista SE. Treatment of Lyme disease. Zentralbl Bakteriol Mikrobiol Hyg A. 1987 Feb;263(3):352-6.

Steere AC, Green J, Schoen RT, Taylor E, Hutchinson GJ, Rahn DW, Malawista SE. Successful parenteral penicillin therapy of established Lyme arthritis. N Engl J Med. 1985 Apr 4;312(14):869-74.

Steere AC, Grodzicki RL, Craft JE, Shrestha M, Kornblatt AN, Malawista SE. Recovery of Lyme disease spirochetes from patients. Yale J Biol Med. 1984 Jul-Aug;57(4):557-60.

Steere AC, Grodzicki RL, Kornblatt AN, Craft JE, Barbour AG, Burgdorfer W, Schmid GP, Johnson E, Malawista SE. The spirochetal etiology of Lyme disease. N Engl J Med. 1983 Mar 31;308(13):733-40.

Steere AC, Gross D, Meyer AL, Huber BT. Autoimmune mechanisms in antibiotic treatment-resistant lyme arthritis. J Autoimmun. 2001 May;16(3):263-8. Review.

Steere AC, Hardin JA, Malawista SE. Erythema chronicum migrans and Lyme arthritis: cryoimmunoglobulins and clinical activity of skin and joints. Science. 1977 Jun 3;196(4294):1121-2.

Steere AC, Hardin JA, Malawista SE. Lyme arthritis: a new clinical entity. Hosp Pract. 1978 Apr;13(4):143-58.

Steere AC, Hardin JA, Malawista SE. Erythema chronicum migrans and Lyme arthritis: related problems recently recognized in Connecticut. Conn Med. 1978 Jun;42(6):353-7.

Steere AC, Hardin JA, Ruddy S, Mummaw JG, Malawista SE. Lyme arthritis: correlation of serum and cryoglobulin IgM with activity, and serum IgG with remission. Arthritis Rheum. 1979 May;22(5):471-83.

Steere AC, Hutchinson GJ, Rahn DW, Sigal LH, Craft JE, DeSanna ET, Malawista SE. Treatment of the early manifestations of Lyme disease. Ann Intern Med. 1983 Jul;99(1):22-6.

Steere AC, Klitz W, Drouin EE, Falk BA, Kwok WW, Nepom GT, Baxter-Lowe LA. Antibiotic-refractory Lyme arthritis is associated with HLA-DR molecules that bind a Borrelia burgdorferi peptide. J Exp Med. 2006 Apr 17;203(4):961-71. Epub 2006 Apr 3.

Steere AC, Levin RE, Molloy PJ, Kalish RA, Abraham JH 3rd, Liu NY, Schmid CH. Treatment of Lyme arthritis. Arthritis Rheum. 1994 Jun;37(6):878-88.

Steere AC, Malawista SE. Cases of Lyme disease in the United States: locations correlated with distribution of Ixodes dammini. Ann Intern Med. 1979 Nov;91(5):730-3.

Steere AC, Malawista SE, Bartenhagen NH, Spieler PN, Newman JH, Rahn DW, Hutchinson GJ, Green J, Snydman DR, Taylor E. The clinical spectrum and treatment of Lyme disease. Yale J Biol Med. 1984 Jul-Aug;57(4):453-61.

Steere AC, Malawista SE, Hardin JA, Ruddy S, Askenase W, Andiman WA. Erythema chronicum migrans and Lyme arthritis. The enlarging clinical spectrum. Ann Intern Med. 1977 Jun;86(6):685-98.

Steere AC, Malawista SE, Newman JH, Spieler PN, Bartenhagen NH. Antibiotic therapy in Lyme disease. Ann Intern Med. 1980 Jul;93(1):1-8.

Steere AC, Malawista SE, Syndman DR. Shope RE, Andiman WA, Ross MR, Steele FM. Lyme arthritis: an epidemic of oligoarticular arthritis in children and adults in three Connecticut communities. Arthritis Rheum. 1977;Jan-Feb;20(1):7-17.

Steere AC, McHugh G, Damle N, Sikand VK. Prospective study of serologic tests for lyme disease. Clin Infect Dis. 2008 Jul 15;47(2):188-95.

Steere AC, McHugh G, Suarez C, Hoitt J, Damle N, Sikand VK. Prospective study of coinfection in patients with erythema migrans. Clin Infect Dis. 2003 Apr 15;36(8):1078-81. Epub 2003 Mar 31.

Steere AC, Pachner AR, Malawista SE. Neurologic abnormalities of Lyme disease: successful treatment with high-dose intravenous penicillin. Ann Intern Med. 1983 Dec;99(6):767-72.

Steere AC, Schoen RT, Taylor E. The clinical evolution of Lyme arthritis. Ann Intern Med. 1987 Nov;107(5):725-31.

Steere AC, Sikand VK. The presenting manifestations of Lyme disease and the outcomes of treatment. N Engl J Med. 2003 Jun 12;348(24):2472-4.

Steere AC, Sikand VK, Schoen RT, Nowakowski J. Asymptomatic infection with Borrelia burgdorferi. Clin Infect Dis. 2003 Aug 15;37(4):528-32. Epub 2003 Jul 30.

Steere AC, Sikand VK, Meurice F, Parenti DL, Fikrig E, Schoen RT, Nowakowski J, Schmid CH, Laukamp S, Buscarino C, Krause DS. Vaccination against Lyme disease with recombinant Borrelia burgdorferi outer-surface lipoprotein A with adjuvant. Lyme Disease Vaccine Study Group. N Engl J Med. 1998 Jul 23;339(4):209-15.

Steere AC, Snydman D, Murray P, Mensch J, Main AJ Jr, Wallis RC, Shope RE, Malawista SE. Historical perspective of Lyme disease. Zentralbl Bakteriol Mikrobiol Hyg A. 1986 Dec;263(1-2):3-6.

Steere AC, Taylor E, McHugh GL, Logigian EL. The overdiagnosis of Lyme disease. JAMA. 1993 Apr 14;269(14):1812-6.

Steere AC, Taylor E, Wilson ML, Levine JF, Spielman A. Longitudinal assessment of the clinical and epidemiological features of Lyme disease in a defined population. J Infect Dis. 1986 Aug;154(2):295-300.

Stein SL, Solvason HB, Biggart E, Spiegel D. A 25-year-old woman with hallucinations, hypersexuality, nightmares, and a rash. Am J Psychiatry. 1996 Apr;153(4):545-51.

Steiner FE, Pinger RR, Vann CN, Abley MJ, Sullivan B, Grindle N, Clay K, Fuqua C. Detection of Anaplasma phagocytophilum and Babesia odocoilei DNA in Ixodes scapularis (Acari: Ixodidae) collected in Indiana. J Med Entomol. 2006;43:437-42.

Steiner FE, Pinger RR, Vann CN, Grindle N, Civitello D, Clay K, Fuqua C. Infection and co-infection rates of Anaplasma phagocytophilum variants, Babesia spp., Borrelia burgdorferi, and the rickettsial endosymbiont in Ixodes scapularis (Acari: Ixodidae) from sites in Indiana, Maine, Pennsylvania, and Wisconsin. J Med Entomol. 2008 Mar;45(2):289-97.

Steiner G. Morphology of spirochaeta myelophthora in multiple sclerosis. J Neuropathol Exp Neurol. 1954 Jan;13(1):221-9.

Steiner G. Acute plaques in multiple sclerosis, their pathogenic significance and the role of spirochaetes as etiological factor. J Neuropathol Exp Neurol. 1952 Oct;11(4):343-72.

Steiner G. Morphologic appearances of spirochetal reproduction in tissues. Archives of Pathology: 189-199. 1940.

Steiner G. Krankheitserreger und Gewebsbefund bei multipler Sklerose: Vergleichend-histologisch-parasitologische Untersuchungen bei multipler Sklerose und anderen Spirochatosen. Ergebn. d. Hyg., Bakt., Immunitatsforsch. u. exper. Therap. 1931;12:269-464.

Steiner RD. Evidence based medicine in inborn errors of metabolism: is there any and how to find it. Am J Med Genet A. 2005 Apr 15;134A(2):192-7.

Stek CJ, van Eijk JJ, Jacobs BC, Enting RH, Sprenger HG, van Alfen N, van Assen S. Neuralgic amyotrophy associated with Bartonella henselae infection. J Neurol Neurosurg Psychiatry. 2011 Jun;82(6):707-8. Epub 2010 Aug 14.

Stevenson HL, Estes MD, Thirumalapura NR, Walker DH, Ismail N. Natural Killer Cells Promote Tissue Injury and Systemic Inflammatory Responses During Fatal Ehrlichia-Induced Toxic Shock-Like Syndrome. Am J Pathol. 2010 Aug;177(2):766-76. Epub 2010 Jul 8.

Stevenson HL, Jordan JM, Peerwani Z, Wang HQ, Walker DH, Ismail N. An Intradermal Environment Promotes a Protective Type-1 Response against Lethal Systemic Monocytotropic Ehrlichial Infection. Infect Immun. 2006 Aug;74(8):4856-64.

Stiernstedt G, Eriksson G, Enfors W, Jörbeck H, Svenungsson B, Sköldenberg B, Granström M. Erythema chronicum migrans in Sweden: clinical manifestations and antibodies to Ixodes ricinus spirochete measured by indirect immunofluorescence and enzyme-linked immunosorbent assay. Scand J Infect Dis. 1986;18(3):217-24.

Stiernstedt G, Gustafsson R, Karlsson M, Svenungsson B, Skoldenberg B. Clinical manifestations and diagnosis of neuroborreliosis. Ann N Y Acad Sci. 1988;539:46-55.

Stiernstedt GT, Sköldenberg BR, Vandvik B, Hederstedt B, Gårde A, Kolmodin G, Jörbäck H, Svenungsson B. Chronic meningitis and Lyme disease in Sweden. Yale J Biol Med. 1984 Jul-Aug;57(4):491-7.

Stiles J. Bartonellosis in cats: a role in uveitis? Vet Ophthalmol. 2011 Sep;14 Suppl 1:9-14.

Stockmeyer B, Schoerner C, Frangou P, Moriabadi T, Heuss D, Harrer T. Chronic vasculitis and polyneuropathy due to infection with Bartonella henselae. Infection. 2007 Apr;35(2):107-9.

Stramer SL, Hollinger FB, Katz LM, Kleinman S, Metzel PS, Gregory KR, Dodd RY. Emerging infectious disease agents and their potential threat to transfusion safety. Transfusion. 2009 Aug;49 Suppl 2:1S-29S.

Straubinger RK. PCR-based quantification of Borrelia burgdorferi organisms in canine tissues over a 500-day postinfection period. J Clin Microbiol. 2000 Jun;38(6):2191-9.

Straubinger RK, Straubinger AF, Jacobson RH, Chang Y, Summer BA, Hollis N, Appel M. Two lessons from the canine model of Lyme Disease: migration of Borrelia burgdorferi in tissues and persistence after antibiotic treatment. 1997. Journal of Spirochetal & Tick-borne Diseases, Vol. 4, No. 1/2.

Straubinger RK, Straubinger AF, Summers BA, Jacobson RH. Status of Borrelia burgdorferi Infection after antibiotic treatment and the effects of corticosteroids: an experimental study. Journal of Infectious Diseases, 2000. 181(3):1069-1081.

Straubinger RK, Straubinger AF, Summers BA, Jacobson RH, Erb HN. Clinical manifestations, pathogenesis, and effect of antibiotic treatment on Lyme borreliosis in dogs. 1998. Wien Klin Wochenschr, 110(24):874-81.

Straubinger RK, Summers BA, Chang YF, Appel MJ. Persistence of Borrelia burgdorferi in experimentally infected dogs after antibiotic treatment. J Clin Microbiol. 1997 Jan;35(1):111-6.

Stricker RB. Counterpoint: long-term antibiotic therapy improves persistent symptoms associated with lyme disease. Clin Infect Dis. 2007 Jul 15;45(2):149-57. Epub 2007 Jun 5. Review.

Stricker RB. Lyme disease controversy: use and misuse of language. Ann Intern Med. 2002 Nov 5;137(9):775-7; author reply 775-7.

Stricker RB. Counterpoint: long-term antibiotic therapy improves persistent symptoms associated with lyme disease. Clin Infect Dis. 2007 Jul 15;45(2):149-57. Epub 2007 Jun 5. Review.

Stricker RB, Brewer JH, Burrascano JJ, Horowitz R, Johnson L, Phillips SE, Savely VR, Sherr VT. Possible role of tick-borne infection in "cat-scratch disease": comment on the article by Giladi et al. Arthritis Rheum. 2006 Jul;54(7):2347-8.

Stricker RB, Burrascano JJ, Harris NS, Horowitz R, Johnson L, Smith PV, Phillips SE. Coinfection with Borrelia burgdorferi and Babesia microti: bad or worse? J Infect Dis. 2006 Mar 15;193(6):901-2; author reply 902.

Stricker RB, Burrascano J, Winger E. Longterm decrease in the CD57 lymphocyte subset in a patient with chronic Lyme disease. Ann Agric Environ Med. 2002;9(1):111-3.

Stricker RB, Corson AF, Johnson L. Reinfection versus relapse in patients with lyme disease: not enough evidence. Clin Infect Dis. 2008 Mar 15;46(6):950; author reply 950-1.

Stricker RB, Delong AK, Green CL, Savely VR, Chamallas SN, Johnson L. Benefit of intravenous antibiotic therapy in patients referred for treatment of neurologic Lyme disease. Int J Gen Med. 2011;4:639-46. Epub 2011 Sep 6.

Stricker RB, Gaito A, Harris NS, Burrascano JJ. Coinfection in patients with lyme disease: how big a risk? Clin Infect Dis. 2003 Nov 1;37(9):1277-8; author reply 1278-9.

Stricker RB, Gaito A, Harris NS, Burrascano JJ. Treatment of early Lyme disease. Ann Intern Med. 2004 Apr 6;140(7):577; author reply 577-8.

Stricker RB, Johnson L. Lyme disease: a turning point. Expert Rev Anti Infect Ther. 2007 Oct;5(5):759-62.

Stricker RB, Johnson L. Lyme wars: let's tackle the testing. BMJ. 2007 Nov 17;335(7628):1008.

Stricker RB, Johnson L. Persistent Borrelia burgdorferi infection after treatment with antibiotics and anti-tumor necrosis factor-alpha. J Infect Dis. 2008 May 1;197(9):1352-3.

Stricker RB, Johnson L. Searching for autoimmunity in "antibiotic-refractory" Lyme arthritis. Mol Immunol. 2008 Jun;45(11):3023-4. Epub 2008 Apr 18.

Stricker RB, Johnson L. Re: Practice parameter: treatment of nervous system Lyme disease (an evidence-based review): report of the Quality Standards Subcommittee of the American Academy of Neurology. Neurology. 2008 May 6;70(19):1719; author reply 1719-20.

Stricker RB, Johnson L. Serologic tests for lyme disease: more smoke and mirrors. Clin Infect Dis. 2008 Oct 15;47(8):1111-2; author reply 1112-3.

Stricker RB, Johnson L. Re: Prolonged Lyme disease treatment: enough is enough. Neurology. 2008 Oct 21;71(17):1380; author reply 1380-1.

Stricker RB, Johnson L. Chronic Lyme disease and the 'Axis of Evil'. Future Microbiol. 2008 Dec;3(6):621-4. Review.

Stricker RB, Johnson L. The Infectious Diseases Society of America Lyme guidelines: poster child for guidelines reform. South Med J. 2009 Jun;102(6):565-6.

Stricker RB, Johnson L. Gender bias in chronic lyme disease. J Womens Health (Larchmt). 2009 Oct;18(10):1717-8; author reply 1719-20.

Stricker RB, Johnson L. Long-term outcomes in patients with early lyme disease: more false hope? Clin Infect Dis. 2010 Jun 15;50(12):1683-4; author reply 1684.

Stricker RB, Johnson L. Letter to the editor re "Anti-neural antibody reactivity in patients with a history of Lyme borreliosis and persistent symptoms" by Chandra et al. Brain Behav Immun. 2010 Aug;24(6):1025; author reply 1026. Epub 2010 Apr 24.

Stricker RB, Johnson L. Persistent symptoms following treatment of early Lyme disease: false hope? Am J Med. 2010 Aug;123(8):e25; author reply e27-8.

Stricker RB, Johnson L. Lyme disease diagnosis and treatment: lessons from the AIDS epidemic. Minerva Med. 2010 Dec;101(6):419-25. Review.

Stricker RB, Johnson L. The Lyme disease chronicles, continued. Chronic Lyme disease: in defense of the patient enterprise. FASEB J. 2010 Dec;24(12):4632-3; author reply 4633-4.

Stricker RB, Johnson L. Lyme disease: the next decade. Infect Drug Resist. 2011;4:1-9. Epub 2011 Jan 7.

Stricker RB, Johnson L. "Lyme literacy" and physicians in Connecticut. J Pediatr. 2011 Mar;158(3):518-9; author reply 519-20. Epub 2011 Jan 13.

Stricker RB, Johnson L. 'Rare' infections mimicking multiple sclerosis: consider Lyme disease. Clin Neurol Neurosurg. 2011 Apr;113(3):259-60. Epub 2010 Dec 18.

Stricker RB, Johnson L, Harris N, Burrascano JJ. Inaccurate information about lyme disease on the internet. Pediatr Infect Dis J. 2005 Jun;24(6):577-8; author reply 578-9.

Stricker RB, Lautin A. The Lyme Wars: time to listen. Expert Opin Investig Drugs. 2003 Oct;12(10):1609-14.

Stricker RB, Lautin A. Lyme disease and optic neuritis: long-term follow-up of seropositive patients. Neurology. 2003 Oct 28;61(8):1162; author reply 1162-3.

Stricker RB, Lautin A, Burrascano JJ. Lyme disease: the quest for magic bullets. Chemotherapy. 2006;52(2):53-9. Epub 2006 Feb 22. Review.

Stricker RB, Lautin A, Burrascano JJ. Lyme disease: point/counterpoint. Expert Rev Anti Infect Ther. 2005 Apr;3(2):155-65. Review.

Stricker RB, Maloney EL. Acute infection with human monocytic ehrlichiosis: the tip of the iceberg? South Med J. 2008 Feb;101(2):214-5.

Stricker RB, McNeil EL. Duration of antibiotic therapy for Lyme disease. Ann Intern Med. 2004 Feb 17;140(4):W6; author reply W7.

Stricker RB, Phillips SE. Lyme disease without erythema migrans: cause for concern? Am J Med. 2003 Jul;115(1):72-3; author reply 73-4.

Stricker RB, Savely VR, Motanya NC, Giclas PC. Complement split products c3a and c4a in chronic lyme disease. Scand J Immunol. 2009 Jan;69(1):64-9.

Stricker RB, Winger EE. Decreased CD57 lymphocyte subset in patients with chronic Lyme disease. Immunol Lett. 2001 Feb 1;76(1):43-8.

Stricker RB, Winger EE. Holmes-Adie syndrome and Lyme disease. Lancet. 2001 Mar 10;357(9258):805.

Stricker RB, Winger EE. Musical hallucinations in patients with Lyme disease. South Med J. 2003 Jul;96(7):711-5.

Stricker RB, Winger EE. Natural killer cells in chronic Lyme disease. Clin Vaccine Immunol. 2009 Nov;16(11):1704; author reply 1704-6.

Strle F, Cheng Y, Cimperman J, Maraspin V, Lotric-Furlan S, Nelson JA, et al. Persistence of Borrelia burgdorferi sensu lato in resolved erythema migrans lesions. Clin Infect Dis. 1995 Aug;21(2):380-389.

Strle F, Nadelman RB, Cimperman J, Nowakowski J, Picken RN, Schwartz I, Maraspin V, Aguero-Rosenfeld ME, Varde S, Lotric-Furlan S, Wormser GP. Comparison of culture-confirmed erythema migrans caused by Borrelia burgdorferi sensu stricto in New York State and by Borrelia afzelii in Slovenia. Ann Intern Med. 1999 Jan 5;130(1):32-6.

Strle K, Drouin EE, Shen S, Khoury JE, McHugh G, Ruzic-Sabljic E, Strle F, Steere AC. Borrelia burgdorferi stimulates macrophages to secrete higher levels of cytokines and chemokines than Borrelia afzelii or Borrelia garinii. J Infect Dis. 2009 Dec 15;200(12):1936-43.

Strle K, Jones KL, Drouin EE, Li X, Steere AC. Borrelia burgdorferi RST1 (OspC type A) genotype is associated with greater inflammation and more severe Lyme disease. Am J Pathol. 2011 Jun;178(6):2726-39.

Stübs G, Fingerle V, Zähringer U, Schumann RR, Rademann J, Schröder NW. Acylated cholesteryl galactosides are ubiquitous glycolipid antigens among Borrelia burgdorferi sensu lato. FEMS Immunol Med Microbiol. 2011 Oct;63(1):140-3. Epub 2011 Jun 27.

Stupica D, Lusa L, Cerar T, Ružić-Sabljić E, Strle F. Comparison of post-Lyme Borreliosis symptoms in erythema migrans patients with positive and negative Borrelia burgdorferi sensu lato skin culture. Vector Borne Zoonotic Dis. 2011 Jul;11(7):883-9. Epub 2010 Nov 17.

Subeki, Nomura S, Matsuura H, Yamasaki M, Yamato O, Maede Y, Katakura K, Suzuki M, Trimurningsih, Chairul, Yoshihara T. Anti-babesial activity of some central kalimantan plant extracts and active oligostilbenoids from Shorea balangeran. Planta Med. 2005 May;71(5):420-3.

Sugerman HJ, Kral JG. Evidence-based medicine reports on obesity surgery: a critique. Int J Obes (Lond). 2005 Jul;29(7):735-45.

Sugiyama H, Sahara M, Imai Y, Ono M, Okamoto K, Kikuchi K, Nagai R. Infective endocarditis by Bartonella quintana masquerading as antineutrophil cytoplasmic antibody-associated small vessel vasculitis. Cardiology. 2009;114(3):208-11. Epub 2009 Jul 15.

Suh B, Chun JK, Yong D, Lee YS, Jeong SH, Yang WI, Kim DS. A report of cat scratch disease in Korea confirmed by PCR amplification of the 16S-23S rRNA intergenic region of Bartonella henselae. Korean J Lab Med. 2010 Feb;30(1):34-7.

Suksawat J, Xuejie Y, Hancock SI, Hegarty BC, Nilkumhang P, Breitschwerdt EB. Serologic and molecular evidence of coinfection with multiple vector-borne pathogens in dogs from Thailand. J Vet Intern Med. 2001 Sep-Oct;15(5):453-62.

Sultan SZ, Pitzer JE, Boquoi T, Hobbs G, Miller MR, Motaleb MA. Analysis of the HD-GYP domain cyclic dimeric GMP phosphodiesterase reveals a role in motility and the enzootic life cycle of Borrelia burgdorferi. Infect Immun. 2011 Aug;79(8):3273-83. Epub 2011 Jun 13.

Sun J, Fu G, Lin J, Song X, Lu L, Liu Q. Seroprevalence of Bartonella in Eastern China and analysis of risk factors. BMC Infect Dis. 2010 May 20;10:121.

Sun WC, Han JX, Yang WY, Deng DA, Yue XF. [Antitumor activities of 4 derivatives of artemisic acid and artemisinin B in vitro]. [Article in Chinese]. Zhongguo Yao Li Xue Bao. 1992 Nov;13(6):541-3. Erratum in: Chung Kuo Yao Li Hsueh Pao 1993;14:192.

Sun Y, Liu G, Yang L, Xu R, Cao W. Babesia microti-like rodent parasites isolated from Ixodes persulcatus (Acari: Ixodidae) in Heilongjiang Province, China. Vet Parasitol. 2008 Oct 1;156(3-4):333-9. Epub 2008 May 23.

Suputtamongkol Y, Newton PN, Angus B, Teja-Isavadharm P, Keeratithakul D, Rasameesoraj M, Pukrittayakamee S, White NJ. A comparison of oral artesunate and artemether antimalarial bioactivities in acute falciparum malaria. Br J Clin Pharmacol. 2001 Dec;52(6):655-61.

Sureda A, García D, Loma-Osorio P. [Embolic stroke as the first manifestation of Bartonella henselae endocarditis in an immunocompetent patient].[Article in Spanish]. Enferm Infecc Microbiol Clin. 2010 Jan;28(1):64-5. Epub 2009 May 1.

Svensson US, Ashton M. Identification of the human cytochrome P450 enzymes involved in the in vitro metabolism of artemisinin. Br J Clin Pharmacol. 1999 Oct;48:528-35.

Svensson US, Sandstrom R, Carlborg O, Lennernas H, Ashton M. High in situ rat intestinal permeability of artemisinin unaffected by multiple dosing and with no evidence of P-glycoprotein involvement. Drug Metab Dispos. 1999 Feb;27(2):227-32.

Sweeney CJ, Ghassemi M, Agger WA, Persing DH. Coinfection with Babesia microti and Borrelia burgdorferi in a western Wisconsin resident. Mayo Clinic Proc. 1998 Apr;73(4):338-41.

Swei A, Meentemeyer R, Briggs CJ. Influence of abiotic and environmental factors on the density and infection prevalence of Ixodes pacificus (Acari:Ixodidae) with Borrelia burgdorferi. J Med Entomol. 2011 Jan;48(1):20-8.

Swei A, Ostfeld RS, Lane RS, Briggs CJ. Impact of the experimental removal of lizards on Lyme disease risk. Proc Biol Sci. 2011 Oct 7;278(1720):2970-8. Epub 2011 Feb 16.

Sykes JE. Feline hemotropic mycoplasmas. J Vet Emerg Crit Care (San Antonio). 2010 Feb;20(1):62-9. Review.

Sykes JE, Lindsay LL, Maggi RG, Breitschwerdt EB. Human coinfection with Bartonella henselae and two hemotropic mycoplasma variants resembling Mycoplasma ovis. J Clin Microbiol. 2010 Oct;48(10):3782-5. Epub 2010 Aug 11.

Szajewska H. Advances and limitations of evidence-based medicine--impact for probiotics. Ann Nutr Metab. 2010;57 Suppl:6-9. Epub 2010 Sep 8. Review.

Szaleniec J, Oleś K, Składzień J, Strek P. [Cat scratch disease--an underestimated diagnosis].[Article in Polish]. Otolaryngol Pol. 2009 May-Jun;63(3):271-3.

Sze CW, Li C. Inactivation of bb0184, which encodes carbon storage regulator A, represses the infectivity of Borrelia burgdorferi. Infect Immun. 2011 Mar;79(3):1270-9. Epub 2010 Dec 20.

Szer IS, Taylor E, Steere AC. The long-term course of Lyme arthritis in children. N Engl J Med. 1991 Jul 18;325(3):159-63.

Szyfelbein WM, Ross JS. Lyme disease meningopolyneuritis simulating malignant lymphoma. Mod Pathology. 1988 Nov;1(6):464-8.

Tabara K, Arai S, Kawabuchi T, Itagaki A, Ishihara C, Satoh H, Okabe N, Tsuji M. Molecular survey of Babesia microti, Ehrlichia species and Candidatus neoehrlichia mikurensis in wild rodents from Shimane Prefecture, Japan. Microbiol Immunol. 2007;51(4):359-67.

Täger FM, Jahnsen KJ, Mediavilla RM, Burgos LR. [Ocular bartonellosis: report of three clinical cases]. [Article in Spanish]. Rev Chilena Infectol. 2008 Feb;25(1):58-63. Epub 2008 Feb 8.

Tager FA, Fallon BA, Keilp J, Rissenberg M, Jones CR, Liebowitz MR. A controlled study of cognitive deficits in children with chronic Lyme disease. J Neuropsychiatry Clin Neurosci. 2001 Fall;13(4):500-7.

Taiwo B, Lee C, Venkat D, Tambar S, Sutton SH. Can tumor necrosis factor alpha blockade predispose to severe babesiosis? Arthritis Rheum. 2007 Feb 15;57(1):179-81.

Takahashi Y, Fukunaga M. Physical mapping of the Borrelia miyamotoi HT31 chromosome in comparison with that of Borrelia turicatae, an etiological agent of tick-borne relapsing fever. Clin Diagn Lab Immunol. 1996 Sep;3(5):533-40.

Takahashi Y, Sohnaka M, Nakao M, Miyamoto K, Fukunaga M. Characterization of Borrelia species isolated from ixodid ticks, Ixodes ovatus. Microbiol Immunol. 1993;37(9):721-7.

Takano A, Nakao M, Masuzawa T, Takada N, Yano Y, Ishiguro F, Fujita H, Ito T, Ma X, Oikawa Y, Kawamori F, Kumagai K, Mikami T, Hanaoka N, Ando S, Honda N, Taylor K, Tsubota T, Konnai S, Watanabe H, Ohnishi M, Kawabata H. Multilocus sequence typing implicates rodents as the main reservoir host of human-pathogenic Borrelia garinii in Japan. J Clin Microbiol. 2011 May;49(5):2035-9. Epub 2011 Mar 16.

Takeda N, Ishiwada N, Fukasawa C, Furuya Y, Tsuneoka H, Tsukahara M, Kohno Y. [Pediatric pneumonia, pleural effusion, and pericarditis following cat scratch disease and serological cross-reactions among Bartonella henselae and Rickettsia japonica determined by indirect fluorescence antibodies].[Article in Japanese]. Kansenshogaku Zasshi. 2007 Mar;81(2):206-9.

Talour K, Karam A, Dreux N, Lemasson G, Gilbert D, Abasq C, Misery L. Incipiens linear IgA disease with IgA antibodies directed against 200-kDa epidermal antigens. Eur J Dermatol. 2011 May-Jun;21(3):411-2.

Tampieri MP, Galuppi R, Bonoli C, Cancrini G, Moretti A, Pietrobelli M. Wild ungulates as Babesia hosts in northern and central Italy. Vector Borne Zoonotic Dis. 2008 Oct;8(5):667-74.

Tan D, Hwang W, Ng HJ, Goh YT, Tan P. Successful treatment of idiopathic hypereosinophilic syndrome with imatinib mesylate: a case report. Int J Hematol. 2004;80(1):75-77.

Tang YW. Duplex PCR assay simultaneously detecting and differentiating Bartonella quintana, B. henselae, and Coxiella burnetii in surgical heart valve specimens. J Clin Microbiol. 2009 Aug;47(8):2647-50. Epub 2009 Jun 24.

Tangpukdee N, Krudsood S, Thanachartwet W, Chalermrut K, Pengruksa C, Srivilairit S, Silachamroon U, Wilairatana P, Phong-tananant S, Kano S, Looareesuwan S. An open randomized clinical trial of Artekin vs artesunate-mefloquine in the treatment of acute uncomplicated falciparum malaria. Southeast Asian J Trop Med Public Health. 2005 Sept;36(5):1085-91.

Tarasow E, Ustymowicz A, Zajkowska J, Hermanowska-Szpakowicz T. [Neuroborreliosis: CT and MRI findings in 14 cases]. [Article in Polish]. Neurol Neurochir Pol. 2001 Sep-Oct;35(5):803-13.

Tasato D, Tateyama M, Inamine M, Hibiya K, Tamaki Y, Haranaga S, Yara S, Higa F, Maruyama S, Fujita J. [Case report: a case of cat scratch disease in elderly patient needed to differentiate tuberculous lymphadenitis].[Article in Japanese]. Nihon Naika Gakkai Zasshi. 2011 Jul 10;100(7):1969-71.

Tasher D, Armarnik E, Mizrahi A, Liat BS, Constantini S, Grisaru-Soen G. Cat scratch disease with cervical vertebral osteomyelitis and spinal epidural abscess. Pediatr Infect Dis J. 2009 Sep;28(9):848-50.

Tatro JB, Romero LI, Beasley D, Steere AC, Reichlin S. Borrelia burgdorferi and Escherichia coli lipopolysaccharides induce nitric oxide and interleukin-6 production in cultured rat brain cells. J Infect Dis. 1994 May;169(5):1014-22.

Tauber SC, Ribes S, Ebert S, Heinz T, Fingerle V, Bunkowski S, Kugelstadt D, Spreer A, Jahn O, Eiffert H, Nau R. Long-term intrathecal infusion of outer surface protein C from Borrelia burgdorferi causes axonal damage. J Neuropathol Exp Neurol. 2011 Sep;70(9):748-57.

Tavakoli NP, Wang H, Dupuis M, Hull R, Ebel GD, Gilmore EJ, Faust PL. Fatal Case of Deer Tick Virus Encephalitis. N Engl J Med. 2009 May 14; 360(20): 2099–2107.

Tefferi A. Modern diagnosis and treatment of primary eosinophilia. Acta Haematol. 2005;114(1):52-60.

Telfer S, Birtles R, Bennett M, Lambin X, Paterson S, Begon M. Parasite interactions in natural populations: insights from longitudinal data. Parasitology. 2008 Jun;135(7):767-81. Epub 2008 May 12.

Telfer S, Lambin X, Birtles R, Beldomenico P, Burthe S, Paterson S, Begon M. Species interactions in a parasite community drive infection risk in a wildlife population. Science. 2010 Oct 8;330(6001):243-6.

Telford SR III, Gorenflot A, Brasseur P and Spielman A. Babesial infections in humans and wildlife. In: Parasitic protozoa. 2nd ed. JP Kreier (ed.). San Diego, CA:Academic Press.1993. pp.1-47.

Telford SR 3rd, Wormser GP. Bartonella spp. transmission by ticks not established. Emerg Infect Dis. 2010 Mar;16(3):379-84. Review.

ten Hove CH, Gubler FM, Kiezebrink-Lindenhovius HH. Back pain in a child caused by cat scratch disease. Pediatr Infect Dis J. 2009 Mar;28(3):258.

Terrada C, Bodaghi B, Conrath J, Raoult D, Drancourt M. Uveitis: an emerging clinical form of Bartonella infection. Clin Microbiol Infect. 2009 Dec;15 Suppl 2:132-3. Epub 2009 Jun 22.

Terekhova D, Iyer R, Wormser GP, Schwartz I. Comparative genome hybridization reveals substantial variation among clinical isolates of Borrelia burgdorferi sensu stricto with different pathogenic properties. J Bacteriol. 2006 Sep;188(17):6124-34.

Terekhova D, Sartakova ML, Wormser GP, Schwartz I, Cabello FC. Erythromycin resistance in Borrelia burgdorferi. Antimicrob Agents Chemother. 2002 Nov;46(11):3637-40.

Terkawi MA, Jia H, Zhou J, Lee EG, Igarashi I, Fujisaki K, Nishikawa Y, Xuan X. Babesia gibsoni ribosomal phosphoprotein P0 induces cross-protective immunity against B. microti infection in mice. Vaccine. 2007 Mar 1;25(11):2027-35. Epub 2006 Dec 8.

Thera MA, Sehdev PS, Coulibaly D, Traore K, Garba MN, Cissoko Y, Kone A, Guindo A, Dicko A, Beavogui AH, Djimde AA, Lyke KE, Diallo DA, Doumbo OK, Plowe CV. Impact of trimethoprim-sulfamethoxazole prophylaxis on falciparum malaria infection and disease. J Infect Dis. 2005 Nov 15;192(10):1823-9. Epub 2005 Oct 13.

Thirumalapura NR, Crossley EC, Walker DH, Ismail N. Persistent Infection Contributes to Heterologous Protective Immunity against Fatal Ehrlichiosis. Infect Immun. 2009 December; 77(12): 5682–5689. Published online 2009 October 5.

Thirumalapura NR, Stevenson HL, Walker DH, Ismail N. Protective Heterologous Immunity against Fatal Ehrlichiosis and Lack of Protection following Homologous Challenge. Infect Immun. 2008 May; 76(5): 1920–1930. Published online 2008 February 19.

Thomas, MJ. Occasional Newsletter from the Blood Care Foundation. 2003 Dec. 3. www.bloodcare.org.uk/ pdfs/ Newsletter%20No%2021.pdf Accessed 2006 Sept 1.

Thomas S, Thirumalapura NR, Crossley EC, Ismail N, Walker DH. Antigenic protein modifications in Ehrlichia. Parasite Immunol. 2009 June; 31(6): 296–303.

Thomford JW, Conrad PA, Telford SR, Mathiesen M, Bowman BH, Spielman A, Eberhard ML, Herwaldt BL, Quick RE, and DH Persing. Cultivation and Phylogenetic Characterization of a Newly Recognized Human Pathogenic Protozoan. J Infect Dis. 1994;169:1050-1056.

Thompson C, Spielman A, Krause PJ. Coinfecting deer-associated zoonoses: Lyme disease, babesiosis, and ehrlichiosis. Clinical Infectious Diseases 2001;33(5):676-85.

Thriemer K, Wernsdorfer G, Rojanawatsirivet C, Kollaritsch H, Sirichainsinthop J, Wernsdorfer WH. In vitro activity of artemisinin alone and in combination with retinol against Plasmodium falciparum. Wien Klin Wochenschr. 2005;117 Suppl 4:45-48.

Thudi KR, Kreikemeier JT, Phillips NJ, Salvalaggio PR, Kennedy DJ, Hayashi PH. Cat scratch disease causing hepatic masses after liver transplant. Liver Int. 2007 Feb;27(1):145-8.

Ticona E, Huaroto L, Garcia Y, Vargas L, Madariaga MG. The pathophysiology of the acute phase of human bartonellosis resembles AIDS. Med Hypotheses. 2010 Jan;74(1):45-9. Epub 2009 Aug 7.

Tijsse-Klasen E, Fonville M, Gassner F, Nijhof AM, Hovius EK, Jongejan F, Takken W, Reimerink JR, Overgaauw PA, Sprong H. Absence of zoonotic Bartonella species in questing ticks: first detection of Bartonella clarridgeiae and Rickettsia felis in cat fleas in the Netherlands. Parasit Vectors. 2011 Apr 18;4:61.

Tijsse-Klasen E, Jacobs JJ, Swart A, Fonville M, Reimerink JH, Brandenburg AH, van der Giessen JW, Hofhuis A, Sprong H. Small risk of developing symptomatic tick-borne diseases following a tick bite in The Netherlands. Parasit Vectors. 2011 Feb 10;4:17.

Tison F, Boulan P, Le Bail B, Catry-Thomas I, Ragnaud JM, Henry P. [Encephalopathy in cat scratch disease].[Article in French]. Presse Med. 1995 Nov 18;24(35):1664.

Tjernberg I, Henningsson AJ, Eliasson I, Forsberg P, Ernerudh J. Diagnostic performance of cerebrospinal fluid chemokine CXCL13 and antibodies to the C6-peptide in Lyme neuroborreliosis. J Infect. 2011 Feb;62(2):149-58. Epub 2010 Nov 16.

Todd S, Xu J, Millar BC, Moore JE, Crowe M, Raoult D, Harrison T, Hill C, Douglas J. Culture-negative Bartonella endocarditis in a patient with renal failure: the value of molecular methods in diagnosis. Br J Biomed Sci. 2004;61(4):190-3. Review.

Tokarz R, Jain K, Bennett A, Briese T, Lipkin WI. Assessment of polymicrobial infections in ticks in New York state. Vector Borne Zoonotic Dis. 2010 Apr;10(3):217-21.

Tokunaga H, Ohyagi Y, Furuya H, Araki T, Yamada T, Isogai E, Kira J. [A patient with neuroborreliosis presenting gadolinium-enhanced MRI lesions in bilateral facial nerves].[Article in Japanese]. Rinsho Shinkeigaku, 41(9):632-4. 2001.

Toledo A, Olmeda AS, Escudero R, Jado I, Valcárcel F, Casado-Nistal MA, Rodríguez-Vargas M, Gil H, Anda P. Tick-borne zoonotic bacteria in ticks collected from central Spain. Am J Trop Med Hyg. 2009 Jul;81(1):67-74.

Toledo Rdos S, Tamekuni K, Haydu VB, Vidotto O. [Seasonal dynamics of Amblyomma ticks (Acari:Ixodidae) in an urban Park of Londrina City, Parana, Brazil].[Article in Portuguese]. Rev Bras Parasitol Vet. 2008 Sep;17 Suppl 1:50-4.

Tonnetti L, Eder AF, Dy B, Kennedy J, Pisciotto P, Benjamin RJ, Leiby DA. Transfusion-transmitted Babesia microti identified through hemovigilance. Transfusion. 2009 Dec;49(12):2557-63. Epub 2009 Jul 16.

Tonnetti L, Proctor MC, Reddy HL, Goodrich RP, Leiby DA. Evaluation of the Mirasol pathogen [corrected] reduction technology system against Babesia microti in apheresis platelets and plasma. Transfusion. 2010 May;50(5):1019-27. Epub 2009 Dec 18. Erratum in: Transfusion. 2010 Jul;50(7):1594.

Toovey S, Jamieson A. Audiometric changes associated with the treatment of uncomplicated falciparum malaria with co-artemeter. Trans R Soc Trop Med Hyg. 2004;98:261-267.

Toovey S. Effects of weight, age, and time on artemether-lumefantrine associated ototoxicity and evidence of irreversibility. Travel Med Infect Dis. 2006;4:71-76.

Toovey S. Safety of Artemisinin Antimalarials. Clinical Infectious Diseases. 2006;42:1214-1215.

Torina A, Alongi A, Scimeca S, Vicente J, Caracappa S, de la Fuente J. Prevalence of tick-borne pathogens in ticks in Sicily. Transbound Emerg Dis. 2010 Apr;57(1-2):46-8.

Torina A, Caracappa S. Anaplasmosis in cattle in Italy. Vet Res Commun. 2007 Aug;31 Suppl 1:73-8.

Torina A, Vicente J, Alongi A, Scimeca S, Turlá R, Nicosia S, Di Marco V, Caracappa S, de la Fuente J. Observed prevalence of tick-borne pathogens in domestic animals in Sicily, Italy during 2003-2005. Zoonoses Public Health. 2007;54(1):8-15.

Torres JR, Sanders CV, Strub RL, Black FW. Cat-scratch disease causing reversible encephalopathy. JAMA. 1978 Oct 6;240(15):1628-9.

Torres L, Almazán C, Ayllón N, Galindo RC, Rosario-Cruz R, Quiroz-Romero H, de la Fuente J. Functional genomics of the horn fly, Haematobia irritans (Linnaeus, 1758). BMC Genomics. 2011; 12: 105. Published online 2011 February 10.

Touyama M, Uezu K, Nakamoto A, Shinzato T, Higa F, Tateyama M, Saito A, Nakamura M, Tsuneoka H, Tsukahara M. [A case of cat scratch disease with encephalopathy].[Article in Japanese]. Kansenshogaku Zasshi. 2002 Feb;76(2):113-7.

Tran TN, Forestier CL, Drancourt M, Raoult D, Aboudharam G. Brief communication: co-detection of Bartonella quintana and Yersinia pestis in an 11th-15th burial site in Bondy, France. Am J Phys Anthropol. 2011 Jul;145(3):489-94. Epub 2011 May 3.

Tran TN, Signoli M, Fozzati L, Aboudharam G, Raoult D, Drancourt M. High throughput, multiplexed pathogen detection authenticates plague waves in medieval Venice, Italy. PLoS One. 2011 Mar 10;6(3):e16735.

Treeprasertsuk S, Krudsood S, Tosukhowong T, Maek-A-Nantawat W, Vannaphan S, Saengnetswang T, Looareesuwan S, Kuhn WF, Brittenham G, Carroll J. N-acetylcysteine in severe falciparum malaria in Thailand. Southeast Asian J Trop Med Public Health. 2003 Mar;34(1):37-42.

Treib J, Fernandez A, Haass A, Grauer MT, Holzer G, Woessner R. Clinical and serologic follow-up in patients with neuroborreliosis. 1998. Neurology, Nov;51(5):1489-91.

Trock DH, Craft JE, Rahn DW. Clinical manifestations of Lyme disease in the United States. Conn Med. 1989 Jun;53(6):327-30.

Trollmo C, Meyer AL, Steere AC, Hafler DA, Huber BT. Molecular mimicry in Lyme arthritis demonstrated at the single cell level: LFA-1 alpha L is a partial agonist for outer surface protein A-reactive T cells. J Immunol. 2001 Apr 15;166(8):5286-91.

Trombert-Paolantoni S, Clairet V, Gaulier E, Figarella P. [Evaluation of a in house serology reagent for the diagnosis of cat-scratch disease defined by PCR].[Article in French]. Pathol Biol (Paris). 2007 Nov;55(8-9):441-5. Epub 2007 Oct 1.

Trout RT, Steelman CD, Szalanski AL. Phylogenetics and population genetics of the louse fly, Lipoptena mazamae, from Arkansas, USA. Med Vet Entomol. 2010 Sep;24(3):258-65. Epub 2010 Jun 1.

Truttmann MC, Rhomberg TA, Dehio C. Combined action of the type IV secretion effector proteins BepC and BepF promotes invasome formation of Bartonella henselae on endothelial and epithelial cells. Cell Microbiol. 2011 Feb;13(2):284-99. Epub 2010 Oct 22.

Tsai KH, Huang CG, Fang CT, Shu PY, Huang JH, Wu WJ. Prevalence of Rickettsia felis and the first identification of Bartonella henselae Fizz/CAL-1 in cat fleas (Siphonaptera: Pulicidae) from Taiwan. J Med Entomol. 2011 Mar;48(2):445-52.

Tsai YL, Chang CC, Chuang ST, Chomel BB. Bartonella species and their ectoparasites: selective host adaptation or strain selection between the vector and the mammalian host? Comp Immunol Microbiol Infect Dis. 2011 Jul;34(4):299-314. Epub 2011 May 25.

Tsai YL, Lin CC, Chomel BB, Chuang ST, Tsai KH, Wu WJ, Huang CG, Yu JC, Sung MH, Kass PH, Chang CC. Bartonella infection in shelter cats and dogs and their ectoparasites. Vector Borne Zoonotic Dis. 2011 Aug;11(8):1023-30. Epub 2010 Dec 13.

Tsao CY. Generalized tonic-clonic status epilepticus in a child with cat-scratch disease and encephalopathy. Clin Electroencephalogr. 1992 Apr;23(2):65-7.

Tsuji N, Miyoshi T, Battsetseg B, Matsuo T, Xuan X, Fujisaki K. A cysteine protease is critical for Babesia spp. transmission in Haemaphysalis ticks. PLoS Pathog. 2008 May 16;4(5):e1000062.

Tsuneoka H, Tsukahara M. Analysis of data in 30 patients with cat scratch disease without lymphadenopathy. J Infect Chemother. 2006 Aug;12(4):224-6.

Tsuneoka H, Yanagihara M, Nojima J, Ichihara K. Antimicrobial susceptibility by Etest of Bartonella henselae isolated from cats and human in Japan. J Infect Chemother. 2010 Dec;16(6):446-8. Epub 2010 Jun 22.

Tsuneoka H, Yanagihara M, Otani S, Katayama Y, Fujinami H, Nagafuji H, Asari S, Nojima J, Ichihara K. A first Japanese case of Bartonella henselae-induced endocarditis diagnosed by prolonged culture of a specimen from the excised valve. Diagn Microbiol Infect Dis. 2010 Oct;68(2):174-6.

Tucci E, Della Rocca C, Santilli F. Localized bacillary angiomatosis in the oral cavity: observations about a neoplasm with atypical behavior. Description of a case and review of the literature. Minerva Stomatol. 2006 Jan-Feb;55(1-2):67-75.

Tuerk M, Cheng LS, Konia T, Armstrong AW. Umbilicated erythematous papules in an immunocompromised patient. Lancet Infect Dis. 2011 Jun;11(6):488.

Tugwell P, Dennis DT, Weinstein A, Wells G, Shea B, Nichol G, Hayward R, Lightfoot R, Baker P, Steere AC. Laboratory evaluation in the diagnosis of Lyme disease. Ann Intern Med. 1997 Dec 15;127(12):1109-23.

Tunev SS, Hastey CJ, Hodzic E, Feng S, Barthold SW, Baumgarth N. Lymphoadenopathy during lyme borreliosis is caused by spirochete migration-induced specific B cell activation. PLoS Pathog. 2011 May;7(5):e1002066. Epub 2011 May 26.

Tuttle AD, Birkenheuer AJ, Juopperi T, Levy MG, Breitschwerdt EB. Concurrent bartonellosis and babesiosis in a dog with persistent thrombocytopenia. J Am Vet Med Assoc. 2003 Nov 1;223(9):1306-10, 1280-1.

Tuuminen T, Hedman K, Söderlund-Venermo M, Seppälä I. Acute parvovirus B19 infection causes nonspecificity frequently in Borrelia and less often in Salmonella and Campylobacter serology, posing a problem in diagnosis of infectious arthropathy. Clin Vaccine Immunol. 2011 Jan;18(1):167-72. Epub 2010 Nov 24.

Ullmann AJ, Gabitzsch ES, Schulze TL, Zeidner NS, Piesman J. Three multiplex assays for detection of Borrelia burgdorferi sensu lato and Borrelia miyamotoi sensu lato in field-collected Ixodes nymphs in North America. J Med Entomol. 2005 Nov;42(6):1057-62.

Umekoji A, Fukai K, Yanagihara S, Ono E, Sowa J, Ishii M. Rapid detection of Bartonella henselae heat shock protein DNA by nested polymerase chain reaction from swollen lymph nodes of a patient with cat-scratch disease. J Dermatol. 2009 Oct;36(10):548-50.

Umemoto T, Namikawa I, Yoshii Z, Konishi H. An internal view of the spherical body of Treponema macrodentium as revealed by scanning electron microscopy. Microbiol Immunol. 1982;26(3):191-8.

Umemoto T, Namikawa, I, Yamamoto M. Colonial morphology of treponemes observed by electron microscopy. Microbiol Immunol. 1984;28:11-22.

Umemoto T, Namikawa I. Electron microscopy of the spherical bodies of oral spirochetes in vitro. Microbiol Immunol. 1980;24:321-334.

United States of America Department of Health and Human Services Food and Drug Administration Center for Biologics Evaluation and Research Vaccines and Related Biological products Advisory Committee Meeting, May 26, 1998.

University of Virginia Health System. Hematology and Blood Disorders. What is G6PD Deficiency? [Monograph on the Internet]. Available from:

http://www.healthsystem.virginia.edu/uvahealth/adult_blood/glucose.cfm

Vaarala O. Binding profiles of anticardiolipin antibodies in sera from patients with SLE and infectious diseases. J Autoimmun. 1991 Oct;4(5):819-30.

Valentine KH, Harms CA, Cadenas MB, Birkenheuer AJ, Marr HS, Braun-McNeill J, Maggi RG, Breitschwerdt EB. Bartonella DNA in loggerhead sea turtles. Emerg Infect Dis. 2007 Jun;13(6):949-50.

Valesov H, Mailer J, Havlík J, Hulínská D, Hercogová J. Long-term results in patients with Lyme arthritis following treatment with ceftriaxone. Infection. 1996 Jan-Feb;24(1):98-102.

Valesova H, Mailer J, Havlik J, Hulinska D, Hercogova J. Long-term results in patients with Lyme arthritis following treatment with ceftriaxone. 1996. Infection, 24(1):98-102.

Valverde-Gubianas M, Ramos-López JF, López-Torres JA, Toribio-García M, Milla-Peñalver C, Gálvez Torres-Puchol J, Medialdea-Marcos S. [Neuroretinitis. Clinical cases].[Article in Spanish]. Arch Soc Esp Oftalmol. 2009 Aug;84(8):389-94.

Van Agtmael MA, Eggelte TA and CJ van Boxtel. Artmisinin drugs in the treatment of malaria: from medicinal herb to registered medication. Trends Pharmacol. Sci. 1999 May;20:199-205.

Van Agtmael MA, Gupta V, van der Wosten, et al. Grapefruit juice increases the bioavailability of artemether. Eur. J. Clin. Pharmacol. 1999;55:405-10.

Van der Linde MR, Ballmer PE. Lyme carditis. In Aspects of Lyme Borreliosis. Ed. Klaus Weber, M.D., Willy Burgdorfer, Ph.D., M.D. Berlin Heidelberg:Springer-Verlag. 1993. pp 131-151.

van der Veer-Meerkerk M, van Zaanen HC. Visceral involvement in an immunocompetent male: a rare presentation of cat scratch disease. Neth J Med. 2008 Apr;66(4):160-2.

van Duivenvoorde LM, Voorberg-van der Wel A, van der Werff NM, Braskamp G, Remarque EJ, Kondova I, Kocken CH, Thomas AW. Suppression of Plasmodium cynomolgi in rhesus macaques by coinfection with Babesia microti. Infect Immun. 2010 Mar;78(3):1032-9. Epub 2010 Jan 4.

Van Heerden J, Reyers F, Stewart CG. Treatment and thrombocyte levels in experimentally induced canine ehrlichiosis and canine babesiosis. Onderstepoort J Vet Res. 1983 Dec;50(4):267-70.

Vannier E, Gewurz BE, Krause PJ. Human babesiosis. Infect Dis Clin North Am. 2008 Sep;22(3):469-88, viii-ix. Review.

Vannier E, Krause PJ. Update on babesiosis. Interdiscip Perspect Infect Dis. 2009;2009:984568. Epub 2009 Aug 27.

Varagnol M, Parola P, Jouan R, Beaucournu JC, Rolain JM, Raoult D. First detection of Rickettsia felis and Bartonella clarridgeiae in fleas from Laos. Clin Microbiol Infect. 2009 Dec;15 Suppl 2:334-5. Epub 2009 May 2.

Varanat M, Broadhurst J, Linder KE, Maggi RG, Breitschwerdt EB. Identification of Bartonella henselae in 2 Cats With Pyogranulomatous Myocarditis and Diaphragmatic Myositis. Vet Pathol. 2011 Apr 13. [Epub ahead of print]

Varanat M, Maggi RG, Linder KE, Horton S, Breitschwerdt EB. Cross-contamination in the molecular detection of Bartonella from paraffin-embedded tissues. Vet Pathol. 2009 Sep;46(5):940-4. Epub 2009 May 9.

Varanat M, Travis A, Lee W, Maggi RG, Bissett SA, Linder KE, Breitschwerdt EB. Recurrent osteomyelitis in a cat due to infection with Bartonella vinsonii subsp. berkhoffii genotype II. J Vet Intern Med. 2009 Nov-Dec;23(6):1273-7. Epub 2009 Aug 26.

Varde S, Wormser GP, Nowakowski J, Nadelman RB, Bittker S, Cooper D, Schwartz I. Lyme disease: disparity between culture and polymerase chain reaction detection of Borrelia burgdorferi after exposure to ceftriaxone in vitro. Conn Med. 1999 Oct;63(10):589-91.

Vartiovaara I. Living with Lyme. 1995. Lancet, 345:842-4.

Varis A, Oksi J, Järveläinen H. [Central nervous system infection--tick-borne encephalitis, neuroborreliosis or both?].[Article in Finnish]. Duodecim. 2011;127(1):75-9.

Vasconcellos-Silva PR, Castiel LD. [Proliferation of paradigmatic ruptures: the case of evidence-based medicine].[Article in Portuguese]. Rev Saude Publica. 2005 Jun;39(3):498-506. Epub 2005 Jun 30.

Vasil'eva IS, Gutova VP, Ershova AS. [The parasitic system of human babesiasis].[Article in Russian]. Med Parazitol (Mosk). 2008 Jan-Mar;(1):36-40. Review.

Vassallo C, Ardigò M, Brazzelli V, Zecca M, Locatelli F, Alessandrino PE, Lazzarino M, Corona S, Lanzerini P, Benazzo M, Fabbi M, Borroni G. Bartonella-related pseudomembranous angiomatous papillomatosis of the oral cavity associated with allogeneic bone marrow transplantation and oral graft-versus-host disease. Br J Dermatol. 2007 Jul;157(1):174-8. Epub 2007 Jun 6.

Vásquez T P, Chanqueo C L, García C P, Poggi M H, Ferrés G M, Bustos M M, Piottante B A. [Bacillary angiomatosis caused by Bartonella quintana in an human immunodeficiency virus positive patient].[Article in Spanish]. Rev Chilena Infectol. 2007 Apr;24(2):155-9. Epub 2007 Apr 12.

Vayssier-Taussat M, Le Rhun D, Bonnet S, Cotté V. Insights in Bartonella host specificity. Ann N Y Acad Sci. 2009 May;1166:127-32. Review.

Vayssier-Taussat M, Le Rhun D, Deng HK, Biville F, Cescau S, Danchin A, Marignac G, Lenaour E, Boulouis HJ, Mavris M, Arnaud L, Yang H, Wang J, Quebatte M, Engel P, Saenz H, Dehio C. The Trw type IV secretion system of Bartonella mediates host-specific adhesion to erythrocytes. PLoS Pathog. 2010 Jun 10;6(6):e1000946.

Vaz A, Glickstein L, Field JA, McHugh G, Sikand VK, Damle N, Steere AC. Cellular and humoral immune responses to Borrelia burgdorferi antigens in patients with culture-positive early Lyme disease. Infect Immun. 2001 Dec;69(12):7437-44.

Vázquez M, Muehlenbein C, Cartter M, Hayes EB, Ertel S, Shapiro ED. Effectiveness of personal protective measures to prevent Lyme disease. Emerg Infect Dis. 2008 Feb;14(2):210-6.

Vázquez M, Sparrow SS, Shapiro ED. Long-term neuropsychologic and health outcomes of children with facial nerve palsy attributable to Lyme disease. Pediatrics. 2003 Aug;112(2):e93-7.

Vento A, Pätilä T, Vaara M, Larinkari U, Sipponen J. Bartonella quintana and Bartonella pediococcus Infection after Aortic Valve Replacement Heart Surg Forum. 2008;11(2):E94-5.

Velho PE. Blood transfusion as an alternative bartonellosis transmission in a pediatric liver transplant. Transpl Infect Dis. 2009 Oct;11(5):474.

Velho PE, Pimentel V, Del Negro GM, Okay TS, Diniz PP, Breitschwerdt EB. Severe anemia, panserositis, and cryptogenic hepatitis in an HIV patient infected with Bartonella henselae. Ultrastruct Pathol. 2007 Nov-Dec;31(6):373-7.

Vento A, Pätilä T, Vaara M, Larinkari U, Sipponen J. Bartonella quintana and Bartonella pediococcus Infection after Aortic Valve Replacement. Heart Surg Forum. 2008;11(2):E94-5.

Vermeulen MJ, Diederen BM, Verbakel H, Peeters MF. Low sensitivity of Bartonella henselae PCR in serum samples of patients with cat-scratch disease lymphadenitis. J Med Microbiol. 2008 Aug;57(Pt 8):1049-50.

Vermeulen MJ, Herremans M, Verbakel H, Bergmans AM, Roord JJ, van Dijken PJ, Peeters MF. Serological testing for Bartonella henselae infections in The Netherlands: clinical evaluation of immunofluorescence assay and ELISA. Clin Microbiol Infect. 2007 Jun;13(6):627-34. Epub 2007 Mar 22.

Vermeulen MJ, Peeters MF, Verbakel H, de Moor RA, Roord JJ, van Dijken PJ. No etiological role for Bartonella henselae infection in Henoch Schönlein purpura. Pediatr Infect Dis J. 2009 Dec;28(12):1142-3.

Vermeulen MJ, Rutten GJ, Verhagen I, Peeters MF, van Dijken PJ. Transient paresis associated with cat-scratch disease: case report and literature review of vertebral osteomyelitis caused by Bartonella henselae. Pediatr Infect Dis J. 2006 Dec;25(12):1177-81. Review.

Vermeulen MJ, Verbakel H, Notermans DW, Reimerink JH, Peeters MF. Evaluation of sensitivity, specificity and cross-reactivity in Bartonella henselae serology. J Med Microbiol. 2010 Jun;59(Pt 6):743-5. Epub 2010 Mar 11.

Veselinović D. [Bartonella henselae as a cause of optical nerve neuritis].[Article in Serbian]. Vojnosanit Pregl. 2006 Nov;63(11):971-4.

Viader F , Poncelet AM , Chapon F , Thenint JP , et al. Neurologic forms of Lyme disease. 12 cases. Rev Neurol (Paris), 145(5):362-8 1989.

Vial C, Petiot P, Latombe D, Ruel JH, Confavreux C, Trillet M, Bady B. [Paralysis of abdominal muscles caused by Lyme disease]. [Article in French]. Rev Neurol (Paris). 1993;149(12):810-2.

Vikram HR, Bacani AK, DeValeria PA, Cunningham SA, Cockerill FR 3rd. Bivalvular Bartonella henselae prosthetic valve endocarditis. J Clin Microbiol. 2007 Dec;45(12):4081-4. Epub 2007 Oct 17.

Vincent JL. Evidence-based medicine in the ICU: important advances and limitations. Chest. 2004 Aug;126(2):592-600.

Vincent JM, Demers DM, Bass JW. Infectious exanthems and unusual infections. Adolesc Med. 2000;11(2):327-358.

Vitale G, Incandela S, Incandela C, Micalizzi A, Mansueto P. Isolation and characterization of Bartonella quintana from the parotid gland of an immunocompetent man. J Clin Microbiol. 2009 Mar;47(3):862-4. Epub 2009 Jan 7.

Vitorino L, Margos G, Zé-Zé L, Kurtenbach K, Collares-Pereira M. Plasmid profile analysis of Portuguese Borrelia lusitaniae strains. Ticks Tick Borne Dis. 2010 Sep;1(3):125-8. Epub 2010 Aug 30.

von Felbert V, Meybehm M, Megahed M. [Cat scratch disease]. [Article in German]. Hautarzt. 2008 Jun;59(6):457-8.

von Loewenich FD, Geißdörfer W, Disqué C, Matten J, Schett G, Sakka SG, Bogdan C. Detection of "Candidatus Neoehrlichia mikurensis" in Two Patients with Severe Febrile Illnesses: Evidence for a European Sequence Variant. J Clin Microbiol. 2010 Jul;48(7):2630-5. Published online 2010 June 2.

Vorou RM, Papavassiliou VG, Tsiodras S. Emerging zoonoses and vector-borne infections affecting humans in Europe. Epidemiol Infect. 2007 Nov;135(8):1231-47. Epub 2007 Apr 20. Review.

Vrethem M, Hellblom L, Widlund M, Ahl M, Danielsson O, Ernerudh J, Forsberg P. Chronic symptoms are common in patients with neuroborreliosis – a questionnaire follow-up study. Acta Neurol Scand. 2002;106(4):205-8.

Vukelić D, Benić B, Bozinović D, Vuković B, Dakovic Rode O, Culig Z, Vuković J, Batinica S, Visnjić S, Puljiz I. An unusual outcome in a child with hepatosplenic cat-scratch disease. Wien Klin Wochenschr. 2006 Oct;118(19-20):615-8.

Vyas JM, Telford SR, Robbins GK. Treatment of refractory Babesia microti infection with atovaquone-proguanil in an HIV-infected patient: case report. Clin Infect Dis. 2007 Dec 15;45(12):1588-90.

Wackernagel A, Bergmann AR, Aberer E. Acute exacerbation of systemic scleroderma in Borrelia burgdorferi infection. J Eur Acad Dermatol Venereol. 2005 Jan;19(1):93-6.

Wagner B, Freer H, Rollins A, Erb HN. A fluorescent bead-based multiplex assay for the simultaneous detection of antibodies to B. burgdorferi outer surface proteins in canine serum. Vet Immunol Immunopathol. 2011 Apr 15;140(3-4):190-8. Epub 2010 Dec 10.

Wagner B, Freer H, Rollins A, Erb HN, Lu Z, Gröhn Y. Development of a multiplex assay for the detection of antibodies to Borrelia burgdorferi in horses and its validation using Bayesian and conventional statistical methods. Vet Immunol Immunopathol. 2011 Aug 17. [Epub ahead of print]

Wagner CL, Riess T, Linke D, Eberhardt C, Schäfer A, Reutter S, Maggi RG, Kempf VA. Use of Bartonella adhesin A (BadA) immunoblotting in the serodiagnosis of Bartonella henselae infections. Int J Med Microbiol. 2008 Oct;298(7-8):579-90. Epub 2008 May 22.

Wahlberg P, Granlund H, Nyman D, Panelius J, Seppala I. Treatment of Lyme borreliosis. J Infect. 1994 Nov;29(3):255-61.

Walk ST, Xu G, Stull JW, Rich SM. Correlation between tick density and pathogen endemicity, New Hampshire. Emerg Infect Dis. 2009 Apr;15(4):585-7.

Walker DH. Rickettsiae. In: Baron S, editor. Medical Microbiology. 4th edition. Galveston (TX): University of Texas Medical Branch at Galveston; 1996. Chapter 38.

Walker DH, Ismail N, Olano JP, McBride JW, Yu XJ, Feng HM. Ehrlichia chaffeensis: a prevalent, life-threatening, emerging pathogen. Trans Am Clin Climatol Assoc. 2004;115:375-84.

Walls T, Moshal K, Trounce J, Hartley J, Harris K, Davies G. Broad-range polymerase chain reaction for the diagnosis of Bartonella henselae endocarditis. J Paediatr Child Health. 2006 Jul-Aug;42(7-8):469-71.

Walsh DS, Wilairatana P, Tang DB, Heppner DG Jr, Brewer TG, Krudsood S, Silachamroon U, Phumratanaprapin W, Siriyanonda D, Looareesuwan S. Randomized trial of 3-dose regimens of tafenoquine (WR238605) versus low-dose primaquine for preventing Plasmodium vivax malaria relapse. Clin Infect Dis. 2004 Oct 15;39(8):1095-103. Epub 2004 Sep 24.

Walsh DS, Looareesuwan S, Wilairatana P, Heppner DG Jr, Tang DB, Brewer TG, Chokejindachai W, Viriyavejakul P, Kyle DE, Milhous WK, Schuster BG, Horton J, Braitman DJ, Brueckner RP. Randomized Dose-Ranging Study of the Safety and Efficacy of WR 238605 (Tafenoquine) in the Prevention of Relapse of Plasmodium vivax Malaria in Thailand. J Infect Dis. 1999 Oct;180(4):1282-7.

Walsh DS, Eamsila C, Sasiprapha T, Sangkharomya S, Khaewsathien P, Supakalin P, Tang DB, Jarasrumgsichol P, Cherdchu C, Edstein MD, Rieckmann KH, Brewer TG. Efficacy of monthly tafenoquine for prophylaxis of Plasmodium vivax and multidrug-resistant P. falciparum malaria. J Infect Dis. 2004 Oct 15;190(8):1456-63. Epub 2004 Sep 20.

Wang CW, Chang WC, Chao TK, Liu CC, Huang GS. Computed tomography and magnetic resonance imaging of cat-scratch disease: a report of two cases. Clin Imaging. 2009 Jul-Aug;33(4):318-21. Review.

Wang G, Iyer R, Bittker S, Cooper D, Small J, Wormser GP, Schwartz I. Variations in Barbour-Stoenner-Kelly culture medium modulate infectivity and pathogenicity of Borrelia burgdorferi clinical isolates. Infect Immun. 2004 Nov;72(11):6702-6.

Wang G, Ojaimi C, Iyer R, Saksenberg V, McClain SA, Wormser GP, Schwartz I. Impact of genotypic variation of Borrelia burgdorferi sensu stricto on kinetics of dissemination and severity of disease in C3H/HeJ mice. Infect Immun. 2001 Jul;69(7):4303-12.

Wang G, Ojaimi C, Wu H, Saksenberg V, Iyer R, Liveris D, McClain SA, Wormser GP, Schwartz I. Disease severity in a murine model of lyme borreliosis is associated with the genotype of the infecting Borrelia burgdorferi sensu stricto strain. J Infect Dis. 2002 Sep 15;186(6):782-91. Epub 2002 Aug 20.

Wang G, Petzke MM, Iyer R, Wu H, Schwartz I. Pattern of pro-inflammatory cytokine induction in RAW264.7 mouse macrophages is identical for virulent and attenuated Borrelia burgdorferi. J Immunol. 2008 Jun 15;180(12):83-15.

Waniek C, Prohovnik I, Kaufman MA, Dwork AJ. Rapidly progressive frontal-type dementia associated with Lyme disease. Journal of Neuropsychiatry Clin Neurosci. 1995;7(3):345-7.

Warhurst DC, Steele JC, Adagu IS, Craig JC, Cullander C. Hydroxychloroquine is much less active than chloroquine against chloroquine-resistant Plasmodium falciparum, in agreement with its physicochemical properties. J Antimicrob Chemother. 2003 Aug;52(2):188-93. Epub 2003 Jul 1.

Warner G, O'Connell S, Lawton N. Atypical features in three patients with florid neurological Lyme disease. J Neurol Neurosurg Psychiatry. 1999;67(2):275.

Warshafsky S, Lee DH, Francois LK, Nowakowski J, Nadelman RB, Wormser GP. Efficacy of antibiotic prophylaxis for the prevention of Lyme disease: an updated systematic review and meta-analysis. J Antimicrob Chemother. 2010 Jun;65(6):1137-44. Epub 2010 Apr 9.

Warshafsky S, Nowakowski J, Nadelman RB, Kamer RS, Peterson SJ, Wormser GP. Efficacy of antibiotic prophylaxis for prevention of Lyme disease. J Gen Intern Med. 1996 Jun;11(6):329-33.

Warthin AS, Olsen RE. The apparent sequence of spirochetes and granular forms in syphilitic buboes. American Journal of Syphilis, 15:145. 1931.

Warthin AS, Olson RE. The granular transformation of Spirochaeta pallida in aortic focal lesions. American Journal of Syphilis, 14:433-437. 1930.

Watt G, Jongsakul K, Ruangvirayuth R. A pilot study of N-acetylcysteine as adjunctive therapy for severe malaria. QJM. 2002 May;95(5):285-90.

Weber K. Treatment failure in erythema migrans: a review. Infection. 1996;24:73-5.

Weber K, Bratzke HJ, Neubert U, Wilske B, Duray PH. Borrelia burgdorferi in a newborn despite oral penicillin for Lyme borreliosis during pregnancy. Pediatr Infect Dis J. 1988 Apr;7(4):286-9.

Weber K, Neubert U. Clinical features of early erythema migrans disease and related disorders. Zentralbl Bakteriol Mikrobiol Hyg A. 1986 Dec;263(1-2):209-28.

Weber K, Neubert U, Büchner SA. Erythema migrans and early signs and symptoms. In Aspects of Lyme Borreliosis, ed. Klaus Weber, M.D., Willy Burgdorfer, Ph.D., M.D. Berlin Heidelberg:Springer-Verlag. 1993. pp 105-121.

Weber K, Pfister HW, Reimers CD. Clinical features of Lyme borreliosis. In Aspects of Lyme Borreliosis, ed. Klaus Weber, M.D., Willy Burgdorfer, Ph.D., M.D. Berlin Heidelberg:Springer-Verlag.1933. pp 93-104.

Weber K, Wilske B. Mini erythema migrans – a sign of early Lyme borreliosis. Dermatology. 2006 ;212(2): 113-116.

Weder B, Wiedersheim P, Matter L, Steck A, Otto F. Chronic progressive neurological involvement in Borrelia burgdorferi infection. J Neurology. 1987 ;234(1):40-3.

Wei LC, Chen SN, Ho CL, Kuo YH, Ho JD. Progression of hydroxychloroquine retinopathy after discontinuation of therapy: case report. Chang Gung Med J. 2001 May;24(5):329-34.

Weinspach S, Tenenbaum T, Schönberger S, Schaper J, Engers R, Rueggeberg J, Mackenzie CR, Wolf A, Mayatepek E, Schroten H. Cat scratch disease--heterogeneous in clinical presentation: five unusual cases of an infection caused by Bartonella henselae. Klin Padiatr. 2010 Mar;222(2):73-8. Epub 2009 Sep 29.

Weisinger HS, Pesudovs K, Collin HB. Management of patients undergoing hydroxychloroquine (Plaquenil) therapy. Clin Exp Optom. 2000 Jan;83(1):32-36.

Weiss LM. Babesiosis in humans: a treatment review. Expert Opin Pharmacother. 2002 Aug;3(8):1109-15.

Weissenbacher S, Ring J, Hofmann H. Gabapentin for the symptomatic treatment of chronic neuropathic pain in patients with late-stage lyme borreliosis: a pilot study. Dermatology. 2005;211(2):123-7.

Welc-Faleciak R. [Current state of the knowledge of Bartonella infections].[Article in Polish]. Przegl Epidemiol. 2009;63(1):11-7. Review.

Welc-Falęciak R, Hildebrandt A, Siński E. Co-infection with Borrelia species and other tick-borne pathogens in humans: two cases from Poland. Ann Agric Environ Med. 2010 Dec;17(2):309-13.

Welc-Faleciak R, Paziewska A, Bajer A, Behnke JM, Siński E. Bartonella spp. infection in rodents from different habitats in the Mazury Lake District, Northeast Poland. Vector Borne Zoonotic Dis. 2008 Aug;8(4):467-74.

Weld ED, Eimer KM, Saharia K, Orenstein A, Hess JR. Transfusion medicine illustrated. The expanding range and severity of babesiosis. Transfusion. 2010 Feb;50(2):290-1.

Welker RD, Narby GM, Legare EJ, Sweeney DM. Lyme disease acquired in Europe and presenting in CONUS. Mil Med. 1993 Oct;158(10):684-5.

Wennberg JE, Fisher ES, Skinner JS. Geography and the debate over Medicare reform. Health Aff (Millwood). 2002 Jul-Dec;Suppl Web Exclusives:W96-114.

Werner JA, Feng S, Chomel BB, Hodzic E, Kasten RW, Barthold SW. P26-based serodiagnosis for Bartonella spp. infection in cats. Comp Med. 2008 Aug;58(4):375-80.

Werner M, Fournier PE, Andersson R, Hogevik H, Raoult D. Bartonella and Coxiella antibodies in 334 prospectively studied episodes of infective endocarditis in Sweden. Scand J Infect Dis. 2003;35(10):724-7.

Wesslen L, Ehrenborg C, Holmberg M, McGill S, Hjelm E, Lindquist O, Henriksen E, Rolf C, Larsson E, Friman G. Subacute bartonella infection in Swedish orienteers succumbing to sudden unexpected cardiac death or having malignant arrhythmias. Scand J Infect Dis. 2001;33(6):429-38.

Westling K, Farra A, Jorup C, Nordenberg A, Settergren B, Hjelm E. Bartonella henselae antibodies after cat bite. Emerg Infect Dis. 2008 Dec;14(12):1943-4.

Westport Westin Health District. Available at: http:// www.wwhd. org.

Wheeler CM, Garcia Monco JC, Benach JL, Golightly MG, Habicht GS, Steere AC. Nonprotein antigens of Borrelia burgdorferi. J Infect Dis. 1993 Mar;167(3):665-74.

Wheeler SW, Wolf SM, Steinberg EA. Cat-scratch encephalopathy. Neurology. 1997 Sep;49(3):876-8.

Whitman BW, Krafte-Jacobs B. Cat-scratch disease associated with pleural effusions and encephalopathy in a child. Respiration. 1995;62(3):171-3.

Wielinga PR, Fonville M, Sprong H, Gaasenbeek C, Borgsteede F, Giessen JW. Persistent Detection of Babesia EU1 and Babesia microti in Ixodes ricinus in The Netherlands During a 5-Year Surveillance: 2003-2007. Vector Borne Zoonotic Dis. 2009 Feb;9(1):119-22. Epub 2008 Aug 30.

Wiesner J, Reichenberg A, Heinrich S, Schlitzer M, Jomaa H. The plastid-like organelle of apicomplexan parasites as drug target. Curr Pharm Des. 2008;14(9):855-71. Review.

Wikswo ME, Hu R, Metzger ME, Eremeeva ME. Detection of Rickettsia rickettsii and Bartonella henselae in Rhipicephalus sanguineus ticks from California. J Med Entomol. 2007 Jan;44(1):158-62.

Wilairatana P, Looaresuwan S. The clinical use of artemisinin and its derivatives in the treatment of malaria. In Artemesia, Ed. CW Wright. London:Taylor & Francis. 2002. pp.291-306.

Wile UJ, Picard RG, Kearny EB. The morphology of spirochaeta pallida in the electron microscope. JAMA. 1942;199:880-1.

Wilhelmsson P, Fryland L, Börjesson S, Nordgren J, Bergström S, Ernerudh J, Forsberg P, Lindgren PE. Prevalence and diversity of Borrelia species in ticks that have bitten humans in Sweden. J Clin Microbiol. 2010 Nov;48(11):4169-76. Epub 2010 Sep 15. Erratum in J Clin Microbiol. 2011 Jan;49(1):481.

Wilke M, Eiffert H, Christen HJ, Hanefeld F. Primarily chronic and cerebrovascular course of Lyme neuroborreliosis: case reports and literature review. Arch Dis Child. 2000;83(1):67-71.

Wilkins HJ, Crane MM, Copeland K, Williams WV. Hypereosinophilic syndrome: an update. Am J Hematol. 2005;80(2):148-157.

Willcox M, Bodeker G, Bourdy G et al. Artemesia annua as a traditional herbal antimalarial. In: Traditional Medicinal Plants and Malaria. Eds. M. Willcox, G. Bodeker, P. Rasoanaivo. New York: CRC Press. 2004. pp.46-52.

Willis AA, Widmann RF, Flynn JM, Green DW, Onel KB. Lyme arthritis presenting as acute septic arthritis in children. J Pediatr Orthop 2003;23(1):114-8.

Wilske B. Microbiological diagnosis in Lyme borreliosis. Int J Med Microbiol. 2002 Jun;291 Suppl 33:114-9.

Wimberly MC, Baer AD, Yabsley MJ. Enhanced spatial models for predicting the geographic distributions of tick-borne pathogens. Int J Health Geogr. 2008;7:15. Published online 2008 April 15.

Wimmersberger Y, Baglivo E. Bartonella henselae infection presenting as a unilateral acute maculopathy. Klin Monbl Augenheilkd. 2007 Apr;224(4):311-3.

Winoto IL, Goethert H, Ibrahim IN, Yuniherlina I, Stoops C, Susanti I, Kania W, Maguire JD, Bangs MJ, Telford SR 3rd, Wongsrichanalai C. Bartonella species in rodents and shrews in the greater Jakarta area. Southeast Asian J Trop Med Public Health. 2005 Nov;36(6):1523-9.

Winterberg DH. [Diagnostic imaging (257). A boy with a swollen inguinal gland].[Article in Dutch]. Ned Tijdschr Geneeskd. 2006 Jan 14;150(2):89.

Winterholler M, Erbguth FJ. Tick bite induced respiratory failure. Diaphragm palsy in Lyme disease. Intensive Care Med. 2001 Jun;27(6):1095.

Wodecka B. [Significance of red deer (Cervus elaphus) in the ecology of Borrelia burgdorferi sensu lato]. [Article in Polish]. Wiad Parazytol. 2007;53(3):231-7.

Wodecka B. flaB Gene as a Molecular Marker for Distinct Identification of Borrelia Species in Environmental Samples by the PCR-Restriction Fragment Length Polymorphism Method. Appl Environ Microbiol. 2011 Oct;77(19):7088-92. Epub 2011 Aug 12.

Wodecka B, Leońska A, Skotarczak B. A comparative analysis of molecular markers for the detection and identification of Borrelia spirochaetes in Ixodes ricinus. J Med Microbiol. 2010 Mar;59(Pt 3):309-14. Epub 2009 Dec 10.

Wojciechowska-Koszko I, Mączyńska I, Szych Z, Giedrys-Kalemba S. Serodiagnosis of borreliosis: indirect immunofluorescence assay, enzyme-linked immunosorbent assay and immunoblotting. Arch Immunol Ther Exp (Warsz). 2011 Feb;59(1):69-77. Epub 2011 Jan 22.

Wójcik-Fatla A, Cisak E, Chmielewska-Badora J, Zwoliński J, Buczek A, Dutkiewicz J. Prevalence of Babesia microti in Ixodes ricinus ticks from Lublin region (eastern Poland). Ann Agric Environ Med. 2006;13(2):319-22.

Wójcik-Fatla A, Szymańska J, Wdowiak L, Buczek A, Dutkiewicz J. Coincidence of three pathogens (Borrelia burgdorferi sensu lato, Anaplasma phagocytophilum and Babesia microti) in Ixodes ricinus ticks in the Lublin macroregion. Ann Agric Environ Med. 2009 Jun;16(1):151-8.

Wolańska-Klimkiewicz E, Szymańska J, Bachanek T. Orofacial symptoms related to boreliosis--case report. Ann Agric Environ Med. 2010 Dec;17(2):319-21.

Wolf V, Wecke J. Formation of multiple treponemes. Zbl Bakt, 280:297-303. 1994.

Wong SJ, Demarest VL, Boyle RH, Wang T, Ledizet M, Kar K, Kramer LD, Fikrig E, Koski RA. Detection of Human Anti-Flavivirus Antibodies with a West Nile Virus Recombinant Antigen Microsphere Immunoassay. J Clin Microbiol. 2004 January; 42(1): 65–72.

Wong JW, Yuen KH, Nagappan S, Shahul WS, Ho SS, Gan EK, Toh WT. Therapeutic equivalence of a low dose artemisinin formulation in falciparum malaria patients. J Pharm Pharmacol. 2003 Feb;55(2):193-8.

Wong M, Isaacs D, Dorney S. Fever, abdominal pain and an intracranial mass. Pediatr Infect Dis J. 1995 Aug;14(8):725-8. Review.

Wong WS, Chung JY, Wong KF. Images in haematology. Human babesiosis. Br J Haematol. 2008 Feb;140(4):364. Epub 2007 Nov 27.

Woo SB, Treister N. Ciclosporin-induced fibrovascular polyps vs. bacillary angiomatosis. Br J Dermatol. 2008 Mar;158(3):652-3. Epub 2008 Jan 17.

Woody HB, Woody NC. Encephalopathy with cat-scratch disease. Bull Tulane Univ Med Fac. 1961 Feb;20:83-7.

Woolley MW, Gordon DL, Wetherall BL. Analysis of the first Australian strains of Bartonella quintana reveals unique genotypes. J Clin Microbiol. 2007 Jun;45(6):2040-3. Epub 2007 Apr 11.

The World Health Organization. Roll Back Malaria Infosheet. Facts on ACTs (Artemisinin-based Combination Therapies), An Update on Recent Progress in Policy and Access to Treatment. Available from: http://www.rbm.who.int/cmc_upload/0/000/015/364/RBMInfosheet_9.htm. Accessed 2006 Aug 10.

WHO and UNICEF. Global Financing, Commodities and Service Delivery. World Malaria Report 2005. http://rbm.who.int/wmr2005/html/3-1.htm. Accessed February 9, 2007.

WHO and UNICEF. Global Financing, Commodities and Service Delivery. World Malaria Report 2005. [cited 2006 Jul]. Available from: http://rbm.who.int/wmr2005/ html/3-1.htm.

The use of artemisinin and its derivatives as anti-malarial drugs. WHO/MAL/98.1086. Malaria Unit, Division of Control of Tropical Diseases, WHO, Geneva. 1998.

Wormser GP. Duration of therapy for Lyme borreliosis. J Infect Dis. 1995 May;171(5):1379-80.

Wormser GP. Lyme disease: insights into the use of antimicrobials for prevention and treatment in the context of experience with other spirochetal infections. Mt Sinai J Med. 1995 May;62(3):188-95. Review.

Wormser GP. A vaccine against Lyme disease? Ann Intern Med. 1995 Oct 15;123(8):627-9.

Wormser GP. Prospects for a vaccine to prevent Lyme disease in humans. Clin Infect Dis. 1995 Nov;21(5):1267-74. Review.

Wormser GP. Controversies in the use of antimicrobials for the prevention and treatment of Lyme disease. Infection. 1996 Mar-Apr;24(2):178-81. Review.

Wormser GP. Lyme disease vaccine. Infection. 1996 Mar-Apr;24(2):203-7. Review.

Wormser GP. Treatment and prevention of Lyme disease, with emphasis on antimicrobial therapy for neuroborreliosis and vaccination. Semin Neurol. 1997 Mar;17(1):45-52. Review.

Wormser GP. Vaccination as a modality to prevent Lyme disease. A status report. Infect Dis Clin North Am. 1999 Mar;13(1):135-48, vii. Review.

Wormser GP. Impressions of the IX Conference on Lyme Borreliosis and Other Tick-Borne Diseases, August 18-22, 2002. Vector Borne Zoonotic Dis. 2002 Winter;2(4):201-7.

Wormser GP. Prevention of Lyme borreliosis. Wien Klin Wochenschr. 2005 Jun;117(11-12):385-91. Review.

Wormser GP. Clinical practice. Early Lyme disease. N Engl J Med. 2006 Jun 29;354(26):2794-801. Review.

Wormser GP. Hematogenous dissemination in early Lyme disease. Wien Klin Wochenschr. 2006 Nov;118(21-22):634-7. Review.

Wormser GP. Discovery of new infectious diseases - bartonella species. N Engl J Med. 2007 Jun 7;356(23):2346-7.

Wormser GP, Aguero-Rosenfeld ME, Nadelman RB. Lyme disease serology: problems and opportunities. JAMA. 1999 Jul 7;282(1):79-80.

Wormser GP, Barthold SW, Shapiro ED, Dattwyler RJ, Bakken JS, Steere AC, Bockenstedt LK, Radolf JD. Anti-tumor necrosis factor-alpha activation of Borrelia burgdorferi spirochetes in antibiotic-treated murine Lyme borreliosis: an unproven conclusion. J Infect Dis. 2007 Dec 15;196(12):1865-6; author reply 1866-7.

Wormser GP, Bittker S, Cooper D, Nowakowski J, Nadelman RB, Pavia C. Comparison of the yields of blood cultures using serum or plasma from patients with early Lyme disease. J Clin Microbiol. 2000 Apr;38(4):1648-50.

Wormser GP, Bittker S, Cooper D, Nowakowski J, Nadelman RB, Pavia C. Yield of large-volume blood cultures in patients with early Lyme disease. J Infect Dis. 2001 Oct 15;184(8):1070-2. Epub 2001 Aug 29.

Wormser GP, Brisson D, Liveris D, Hanincová K, Sandigursky S, Nowakowski J, Nadelman RB, Ludin S, Schwartz I. Borrelia burgdorferi genotype predicts the capacity for hematogenous dissemination during early Lyme disease. J Infect Dis. 2008 Nov 1;198(9):1358-64.

Wormser GP, Carbonaro C, Miller S, Nowakowski J, Nadelman RB, Sivak S, Aguero-Rosenfeld ME. A limitation of 2-stage serological testing for Lyme disease: enzyme immunoassay and immunoblot assay are not independent tests. Clin Infect Dis. 2000 Mar;30(3):545-8.

Wormser GP, Dattwyler RJ, Shapiro ED, Dumler JS, O'Connell S, Radolf JD, Nadelman RB. Single-dose prophylaxis against Lyme disease. Lancet Infect Dis. 2007 Jun;7(6):371-3.

Wormser GP, Dattwyler RJ, Shapiro ED, Halperin JJ, Steere AC, Klempner MS, Krause PJ, Bakken JS, Strle F, Stanek G, Bockenstedt L, Fish D, Dumler JS, Nadelman RB. The clinical assessment, treatment, and prevention of lyme disease, human granulocytic anaplasmosis, and babesiosis: clinical practice guidelines by the Infectious Diseases Society of America. Clin Infect Dis. 2006 Nov 1;43(9):1089-134. Epub 2006 Oct 2. Erratum in: Clin Infect Dis. 2007 Oct 1;45(7):941.

Wormser GP, Forseter G, Cooper D, Nowakowski J, Nadelman RB, Horowitz H, Schwartz I, Bowen SL, Campbell GL, Goldberg NS. Use of a novel technique of cutaneous lavage for diagnosis of Lyme disease associated with erythema migrans. JAMA. 1992 Sep 9;268(10):1311-3.

Wormser GP, Halperin JJ. Oral doxycycline for neuroborreliosis. Lancet Neurol. 2008 Aug;7(8):665-6. Epub 2008 Jun 21.

Wormser GP, Horowitz HW, Dumler JS, Schwartz I, Aguero-Rosenfeld M. False-positive Lyme disease serology in human granulocytic ehrlichiosis. Lancet. 1996 Apr 6;347(9006):981-2.

Wormser GP, Horowitz HW, Nowakowski J, McKenna D, Dumler JS, Varde S, Schwartz I, Carbonaro C, Aguero-Rosenfeld M. Positive Lyme disease serology in patients with clinical and laboratory evidence of human granulocytic ehrlichiosis. Am J Clin Pathol. 1997 Feb;107(2):142-7.

Wormser GP, Kaslow R, Tang J, Wade K, Liveris D, Schwartz I, Klempner M. Association between human leukocyte antigen class II alleles and genotype of Borrelia burgdorferi in patients with early lyme disease. J Infect Dis. 2005 Dec 1;192(11):2020-6. Epub 2005 Oct 28.

Wormser GP, Liveris D, Hanincová K, Brisson D, Ludin S, Stracuzzi VJ, Embers ME, Philipp MT, Levin A, Aguero-Rosenfeld M, Schwartz I. Effect of Borrelia burgdorferi genotype on the sensitivity of C6 and 2-tier testing in North American patients with culture-confirmed Lyme disease. Clin Infect Dis. 2008 Oct 1;47(7):910-4.

Wormser GP, Liveris D, Nowakowski J, Nadelman RB, Cavaliere LF, McKenna D, Holmgren D, Schwartz I. Association of specific subtypes of Borrelia burgdorferi with hematogenous dissemination in early Lyme disease. J Infect Dis. 1999 Sep;180(3):720-5.

Wormser GP, Lombardo G, Silverblatt F, El Khoury MY, Prasad A, Yelon JA, Sanda A, Karim S, Coku L, Savino JA. Babesiosis as a cause of fever in patients undergoing a splenectomy. Am Surg. 2011 Mar;77(3):345-7.

Wormser GP, Masters E, Liveris D, Nowakowski J, Nadelman RB, Holmgren D, Bittker S, Cooper D, Wang G, Schwartz I. Microbiologic evaluation of patients from Missouri with erythema migrans. Clin Infect Dis. 2005 Feb 1;40(3):423-8. Epub 2005 Jan 10.

Wormser GP, Masters E, Nowakowski J, McKenna D, Holmgren D, Ma K, Ihde L, Cavaliere LF, Nadelman RB. Prospective clinical evaluation of patients from Missouri and New York with erythema migrans-like skin lesions. Clin Infect Dis. 2005 Oct 1;41(7):958-65. Epub 2005 Aug 31.

Wormser GP, McKenna D, Carlin J, Nadelman RB, Cavaliere LF, Holmgren D, Byrne DW, Nowakowski J. Brief communication: hematogenous dissemination in early Lyme disease. Ann Intern Med. 2005 May 3;142(9):751-5.

Wormser GP, McKenna D, Nadelman RB, Nowakowski J, Weinstein A. Lyme disease in children. N Engl J Med. 1997 Apr 10;336(15):1107; author reply 1107-8.

Wormser GP, Nadelman RB, Dattwyler RJ, Dennis DT, Shapiro ED, Steere AC, Rush TJ, Rahn DW, Coyle PK, Persing DH, Fish D, Luft BJ. Practice guidelines for the treatment of Lyme disease. The Infectious Diseases Society of America. Clin Infect Dis. 2000 Jul;31 Suppl 1:1-14.

Wormser GP, Nadelman RB, Nowakowski J, Schwartz I. Asymptomatic Borrelia burgdorferi infection. Med Hypotheses. 2001 Oct;57(4):435-8.

Wormser GP, Nowakowski J, Nadelman RB. Duration of treatment for Lyme borreliosis: time for a critical reappraisal. Wien Klin Wochenschr. 2002 Jul 31;114(13-14):613-5. Review.

Wormser GP, Nowakowski J, Nadelman RB, Bittker S, Cooper D, Pavia C. Improving the yield of blood cultures for patients with early Lyme disease. J Clin Microbiol. 1998 Jan;36(1):296-8.

Wormser GP, Nowakowski J, Nadelman RB, Schwartz I, McKenna D, Holmgren D, Aguero-Rosenfeld M. Efficacy of an OspA vaccine preparation for prevention of Lyme disease in New York State. Infection. 1998 Jul-Aug;26(4):208-12.

Wormser GP, Nowakowski J, Nadelman RB, Visintainer P, Levin A, Aguero-Rosenfeld ME. Impact of clinical variables on Borrelia burgdorferi-specific antibody seropositivity in acute-phase sera from patients in North America with culture-confirmed early Lyme disease. Clin Vaccine Immunol. 2008 Oct;15(10):1519-22. Epub 2008 Aug 20.

Wormser GP, O'Connell S. Treatment of infection caused by Borrelia burgdorferi sensu lato. Expert Rev Anti Infect Ther. 2011 Feb;9(2):245-60. Review.

Wormser GP, Prasad A, Neuhaus E, Joshi S, Nowakowski J, Nelson J, Mittleman A, Aguero-Rosenfeld M, Topal J, Krause PJ. Emergence of resistance to azithromycin-atovaquone in immunocompromised patients with Babesia microti infection. Clin Infect Dis. 2010 Feb 1;50(3):381-6.

Wormser GP, Ramanathan R, Nowakowski J, McKenna D, Holmgren D, Visintainer P, Dornbush R, Singh B, Nadelman RB. Duration of antibiotic therapy for early Lyme disease. A randomized, double-blind, placebo-controlled trial. Ann Intern Med. 2003 May 6;138(9):697-704.

Wormser GP, Schwartz I. Antibiotic treatment of animals infected with Borrelia burgdorferi. Clin Microbiol Rev. 2009 Jul;22(3):387-95. Review.

Wormser GP, Shapiro ED. Implications of gender in chronic Lyme disease. J Womens Health (Larchmt). 2009 Jun;18(6):831-4.

Wormser GP, Shapiro ED, Halperin JJ, Porwancher RB, O'Connell S, Nadelman RB, Strle F, Radolf JD, Hovius JW, Baker PJ, Fingerle V, Dattwyler R. Analysis of a flawed double-blind, placebo-controlled, clinical trial of patients claimed to have persistent Lyme disease following treatment. Minerva Med. 2009 Apr;100(2):171-2.

Wormser GP, Stanek G, Strle F, Gray JS. Advances in the treatment and prevention of Lyme borreliosis. Wien Klin Wochenschr. 2005 Jun;117(11-12):381-4. Review.

Wright IG, Goodger BV, Clark IA. Immunopathophysiology of Babesia bovis and Plasmodium falciparum infections. Babesia. Malaria Treatment. Parasitol Today. 1988 Aug;4(8):214-8.

Wright SA, Lemenager DA, Tucker JR, Armijos MV, Yamamoto SA. An avian contribution to the presence of Ixodes pacificus (Acari: Ixodidae) and Borrelia burgdorferi on the sutter buttes of California. J Med Entomol. 2006 Mar;43(2):368-74.

Wright SA, Tucker JR, Donohue AM, Castro MB, Kelley KL, Novak MG, Macedo PA. Avian hosts of Ixodes pacificus (Acari: Ixodidae) and the detection of Borrelia burgdorferi in larvae feeding on the Oregon junco. J Med Entomol. 2011 Jul;48(4):852-9.

Wu J, Weening EH, Faske JB, Höök M, Skare JT. Invasion of eukaryotic cells by Borrelia burgdorferi requires β(1) integrins and Src kinase activity. Infect Immun. 2011 Mar;79(3):1338-48. Epub 2010 Dec 20.

Xiao S, Tanner M, N'Goran EK, Utzinger J, Chollet J, Bergquist R, Chen M, Zheng J. Recent investigations of artemether, a novel agent for the prevention of schistosomiasis japonica, mansoni and haematobia. Acta Trop. 2002 May;82(2):175-81.

Xiao SH, Yao JM, Utzinger J, Cai Y, Chollet J, Tanner M. Selection and reversal of Plasmodium berghei resistance in the mouse model following repeated high doses of artemether. Parasitol Res. 2004 Feb;92(3):215-9. [Epub 2003 Dec 16].

Xu C, Liu Q, Diao B, Kan B, Song X, Li D. Optimization of pulse-field gel electrophoresis for Bartonella subtyping. J Microbiol Methods. 2009 Jan;76(1):6-11. Epub 2008 Sep 5.

Xu H, Liew LN, Kuo IC, Huang CH, Goh DL, Chua KY. The modulatory effects of lipopolysaccharide-stimulated B cells on differential T-cell polarization. Immunology. 2008 October; 125(2): 218-28.

Xu H, Raddi G, Liu J, Charon NW, Li C. Chemoreceptors and flagellar motors are subterminally located in close proximity at the two cell poles in spirochetes. J Bacteriol. 2011 May;193(10):2652-6. Epub 2011 Mar 25.

Xu L, Winn BJ, Odel JG. Lyme-Associated Orbital Inflammation Presenting as Painless Subacute Unilateral Ptosis. J Neuroophthalmol. 2011 Sep 27. [Epub ahead of print]

Xu Q, McShan K, Liang FT. Essential protective role attributed to the surface lipoproteins of Borrelia burgdorferi against innate defenses. Mol Microbiol. 2008 Jul;69(1):15–29. Published online 2008 April 28.

Yabsley MJ, McKibben J, Macpherson CN, Cattan PF, Cherry NA, Hegarty BC, Breitschwerdt EB, O'Connor T, Chandrashekar R, Paterson T, Perea ML, Ball G, Friesen S, Goedde J, Henderson B, Sylvester W. Prevalence of Ehrlichia canis, Anaplasma platys, Babesia canis vogeli, Hepatozoon canis, Bartonella vinsonii berkhoffii, and Rickettsia spp. in dogs from Grenada. Vet Parasitol. 2008 Feb 14;151(2-4):279-85. Epub 2007 Nov 17.

Yager JA, Best SJ, Maggi RG, Varanat M, Znajda N, Breitschwerdt EB. Bacillary angiomatosis in an immunosuppressed dog. Vet Dermatol. 2010 Mar 31. [Epub ahead of print]

Yagupsky P, Sofer S. Cat-scratch encephalopathy presenting as status epilepticus and lymphadenitis. Pediatr Emerg Care. 1990 Mar;6(1):43-5.

Yakimchuk K, Roura-Mir C, Magalhaes KG, de Jong A, Kasmar AG, Granter SR, Budd R, Steere A, Pena-Cruz V, Kirschning C, Cheng TY, Moody DB. Borrelia burgdorferi infection regulates CD1 expression in human cells and tissues via IL1-β. Eur J Immunol. 2011 Mar;41(3):694-705. Epub 2011 Jan 18.

Yamachika E, Habte T, Oda D. Artemisinin: an alternative treatment for oral squamous cell carcinoma. Anticancer Res. 2004;24:2153-60.

Yamada Y, Ohkusu K, Yanagihara M, Tsuneoka H, Ezaki T, Tsuboi J, Okabayashi H, Suwabe A. Prosthetic valve endocarditis caused by Bartonella quintana in a patient during immunosuppressive therapies for collagen vascular diseases. Diagn Microbiol Infect Dis. 2011 Jul;70(3):395-8. Epub 2011 May 10.

Yamasaki M, Tajima M, Yamato O, Hwang SJ, Ohta H, Maede Y. Heat shock response of Babesia gibsoni heat shock protein 70. J Parasitol. 2008 Feb;94(1):119-24.

Yanagihara M, Tsuneoka H, Hoshide S, Ishido E, Umeda A, Tsukahara M, Nojima J, Ichihara K, Hino K, Hirai I, Yamamoto Y. Molecular typing of Bartonella henselae DNA extracted from human clinical specimens and cat isolates in Japan. FEMS Immunol Med Microbiol. 2010 Oct;60(1):44-8.

Yanagihara M, Tsuneoka H, Sugasaki M, Nojima J, Ichihara K. Multispacer typing of Bartonella henselae isolates from humans and cats, Japan. Emerg Infect Dis. 2010 Dec;16(12):1983-5.

Yang L, Weis JH, Eichwald E, Kolbert DP, Persing DH, Weis JJ. Heritable susceptibility to severe Borrelia burgdorferi-induced arthritis is dominant and is associated with persistence of large numbers of spirochetes in tissues. Infect. Immun. 1994;62(2):492-500.

Yang X, Izadi H, Coleman AS, Wang P, Ma Y, Fikrig E, Anguita J, Pal U. Borrelia burgdorferi lipoprotein BmpA activates pro-inflammatory responses in human synovial cells through a protein moiety. Microbes Infect. 2008 Oct;10(12-13):1300-8. Published online 2008 August 5.

Yang XR, Liu QY, Cui BY, Wang LX, Peng ZH, Ren DS. [Using direct enzyme linked immunosorbent assay for the detection of IgG antibody on Bartonella henselae among healthy people in Changping, Beijing].[Article in Chinese]. Zhonghua Liu Xing Bing Xue Za Zhi. 2007 Jul;28(7):688-91.

Yang Y, Li C. Transcription and genetic analyses of a putative N-acetylmuramyl-L-alanine amidase in Borrelia burgdorferi. FEMS Microbiol Lett. 2009 Jan;290(2):164-73. Published online 2008 November 18.

Yerebakan C, Westphal B, Aepinus C. Infective endocarditis due to Bartonella quintana: a challenging diagnostic entity. Acta Cardiol. 2008 Aug;63(4):519-21.

Yilmaz C, Ergin C, Kaleli I. [Investigation of Bartonella henselae seroprevalence and related risk factors in blood donors admitted to Pamukkale University Blood Center].[Article in Turkish]. Mikrobiyol Bul. 2009 Jul;43(3):391-401.

Yoda M, Hata M, Sezai A, Unosawa S, Furukawa N, Minami K. First report of Bartonella quintana endocarditis in Japan. Circ J. 2008 Jun;72(6):1022-4.

Yoon HJ, Lee WC, Choi YS, Cho S, Song YG, Choi JY, Kim CO, Kim EJ, Kim JM. Cervical lymphadenitis in a patient coinfected with Toxoplasma gondii and Bartonella henselae. Vector Borne Zoonotic Dis. 2010 May;10(4):415-9.

Yoshinari NH, Oyafuso LK, Monteiro FG, de Barros PJ, da Cruz FC, Ferreira LG, Bonasser F, Baggio D, Cossermelli W.[Lyme disease. Report of a case observed in Brazil]. [Article in Portuguese]. Rev Hosp Clin Fac Med Sao Paulo. 1993 Jul-Aug;48(4):170-4.

Yoshinari NH, Steere AC, Cossermelli W. [A review of Lyme disease]. [Article in Portuguese]. AMB Rev Assoc Med Bras. 1989 Jan-Feb;35(1):34-8. Review.

Yoshinari NH, Reinhardt BN, Steere AC. T cell responses to polypeptide fractions of Borrelia burgdorferi in patients with Lyme arthritis. Arthritis Rheum. 1991 Jun;34(6):707-13.

Youn H. Review of zoonotic parasites in medical and veterinary fields in the Republic of Korea. Korean J Parasitol. 2009 Oct;47 Suppl:S133-41. Review.

Younger DS, Orsher S. Lyme Neuroborreliosis: Preliminary Results from an Urban Referral Center Employing Strict CDC Criteria for Case Selection. Neurol Res Int. 2010;2010:525206. Epub 2010 Jun 23.

Youssef D, Shams WE, El Abbassi A, Moorman JP, Al-Abbadi MA. Combining cytomorphology and serology for the diagnosis of cat scratch disease. Diagn Cytopathol. 2011 Mar;39(3):210-3.

Yrjänäinen H, Hytönen J, Hartiala P, Oksi J, Viljanen MK, Persistence of borrelial DNA in the joints of Borrelia burgdorferi-infected mice after ceftriaxone treatment. APMIS, 118(9):665-73.

Yrjänäinen H, Hytönen J, Song XY, Oksi J, Hartiala K, Viljanen MK. Anti-tumor necrosis factor-alpha treatment activates Borrelia burgdorferi spirochetes 4 weeks after ceftriaxone treatment in C3H/He mice. 2007. J Infect Dis, 195(10):1489-96.

Yu DH, Li YH, Yoon JS, Lee JH, Lee MJ, Yu IJ, Chae JS, Park JH. Ehrlichia chaffeensis infection in dogs in South Korea. Vector Borne Zoonotic Dis. 2008 Jun;8(3):355-8.

Yuan C, Zhu C, Wu Y, Pan X, Hua X. Bacteriological and molecular identification of bartonella species in cats from different regions of china. PLoS Negl Trop Dis. 2011 Sep;5(9):e1301. Epub 2011 Sep 6.

Zagorski Z, Biziorek B, Haszcz D. [Ophthalmic manifestations in Lyme borreliosis]. [Article in Polish]. Przegl Epidemiol. 2002;56 Suppl 1:85-90.

Zamponi N, Cardinali C, Tavoni MA, Porfiri L, Rossi R, Manca A. Chronic neuroborreliosis in infancy. Ital J Neurol Sci. 1999 Oct;20(5):303-7.

Zarkovic A, McMurray C, Deva N, Ghosh S, Whitley D, Guest S. Seropositivity rates for Bartonella henselae, Toxocara canis and Toxoplasma gondii in New Zealand blood donors. Clin Experiment Ophthalmol. 2007 Mar;35(2):131-4. Erratum in: Clin Experiment Ophthalmol. 2007 Jul;35(5):500. MacMurray, Catherine [corrected to McMurray, Catherine].

Zarrella TM, Singh A, Bitsaktsis C, Rahman T, Sahay B, Feustel PJ, Gosselin EJ, Sellati TJ, Hazlett KR. Host-Adaptation of Francisella tularensis Alters the Bacterium's Surface-Carbohydrates to Hinder Effectors of Innate and Adaptive Immunity. PLoS One. 2011;6(7):e22335. Published online 2011 July 22.

Zarzycka B, Pieczara A, Skowron-Kobos J, Krzemiński Z. [Prevalence IgG antibodies against Bartonella henselae in children with lymphadenopathy].[Article in Polish]. Przegl Epidemiol. 2008;62(4):759-65.

Zeaiter Z, Fournier PE, Greub G, Raoult D. Diagnosis of Bartonella endocarditis by a real-time nested PCR assay using serum. J Clin Microbiol. 2003 Mar;41(3):919-25.

Zeaiter Z, Fournier PE, Ogata H, Raoult D. Phylogenetic classification of Bartonella species by comparing groEL sequences. Int J Syst Evol Microbiol. 2002 Jan;52(Pt 1):165-71.

Zekraoui Y, Megzari A, El Alloussi T, Berraho A. [Unilateral neuroretinitis revealing cat-scratch disease].[Article in French]. Rev Med Interne. 2011 Apr;32(4):e46-8. Epub 2010 Jun 19.

Zemel L. Lyme disease and pseudotumor. Mayo Clinic Proc. 2000;75(3):315.

Zenz W, Trop M, Kollaritsch H, Reinthaler F. [Congenital malaria due to Plasmodium falciparum and Plasmodium malariae]. Wien Klin Wochenschr. 2000 May 19;112(10):459-61. [Article in German]. Comment in: Wien Klin Wochenschr. 2000 May 19;112(10):421-2.

Zhang L, Shan A, Mathew B, Yin J, Fu X, Zhang J, Lu J, Xu J, Dumler JS. Rickettsial Seroepidemiology among farm workers, Tianjin, People's Republic of China. Emerg Infect Dis. 2008 Jun;14(6):938-40.

Zhang L, Zhang Y, Adusumilli S, Liu L, Narasimhan S, Dai J, Zhao YO, Fikrig E. Molecular interactions that enable movement of the Lyme disease agent from the tick gut into the hemolymph. PLoS Pathog. 2011 Jun;7(6):e1002079. Epub 2011 Jun 9.

Zhang Q, Zhang Y. Lyme disease and modern Chinese medicine. New York, NY:Sino-Med Reseach Institute. 2006;pp.1-5, 34-5, 42-3, 76-82.

Zhao KC, Xuan WY, Zhao Y, Song ZY. The pharmacokinetics of a transdermal preparation of artesunate in mice and rabbits.Yao Xue Xue Bao. 1989;24(11):813-6.

Zhao Z, Fleming R, McCloud B, Klempner MS. CD14 Mediates Cross Talk between Mononuclear Cells and Fibroblasts for Upregulation of Matrix Metalloproteinase 9 by Borrelia burgdorferi. Infect Immun. 2007 Jun;75(6):3062-9. Published online 2007 April 2.

Zhao Y, Love KR, Hall SW, Beardell FV. A fatal case of transfusion-transmitted babesiosis in the State of Delaware. Transfusion. 2009 Dec;49(12):2583-7. Epub 2009 Nov 9.

Zhou X, Miller MR, Motaleb M, Charon NW, He P. Spent Culture Medium from Virulent Borrelia burgdorferi Increases Permeability of Individually Perfused Microvessels of Rat Mesentery. PLoS One. 2008;3(12):e4101. Epub 2008 Dec 31.

Ziemssen F, Bartz-Schmidt KU, Gelisken F. Secondary unilateral glaucoma and neuroretinitis: atypical manifestation of cat-scratch disease. Jpn J Ophthalmol. 2006 Mar-Apr;50(2):177-9.

Ziska MH, Donta ST, Demarest FC. Physician preferences in the diagnosis and treatment of Lyme disease in the United States. Infection. 1996 Mar-Apr;24(2):182-6.

Zivkovic Z, Torina A, Mitra R, Alongi A, Scimeca S, Kocan KM, Galindo RC, Almazán C, Blouin EF, Villar M, Nijhof AM, Mani R, La Barbera G, Caracappa S, Jongejan F, de la Fuente J. Subolesin expression in response to pathogen infection in ticks. BMC Immunol. 2010 Feb 19;11:7. Published online 2010 February 19.

Zobba R, Chessa G, Mastrandrea S, Pinna Parpaglia ML, Patta C, Masala G. Serological and molecular detection of Bartonella spp. in humans, cats and dogs from northern Sardinia, Italy. Clin Microbiol Infect. 2009 Dec;15 Suppl 2:134-5. Epub 2009 May 18.

Zobba R, Parpaglia ML, Spezzigu A, Pittau M, Alberti A. First molecular identification and phylogeny of a Babesia sp. from a symptomatic sow (Sus scrofa Linnaeus 1758). J Clin Microbiol. 2011 Jun;49(6):2321-4. Epub 2011 Apr 13.

Bibliography for Babesia Treatment

Why Publish a Babesia Treatment Bibliography?

Since it may be some time before I publish my updated Babesia treatments textbook, with options that are significantly modified and more effective than what has been in past publications, I offer these preliminary references for anyone interested in suggesting a 2012 approach to Babesia treatment, or any academics interesting in reading in this area of emerging medicine.

Abbas HM, Brenes RA, Ajemian MS, Scholand SJ. Successful conservative treatment of spontaneous splenic rupture secondary to Babesiosis: a case report and literature review. Conn Med. 2011 Mar;75(3):143-6. PMID:21500704

Abdalla HS, Hussein HS, Kreier JP. Babesia rodhaini: passive protection of mice with immune serum. Tropenmed Parasitol. 1978 Sep;29(3):295-306. PMID:726044

AbouLaila M, Sivakumar T, Yokoyama N, Igarashi I. Inhibitory effect of terpene nerolidol on the growth of Babesia parasites. Parasitol Int. 2010 Jun;59(2):278-82. Epub 2010 Feb 21. PMID:20178862

Abrams Y. Complications of coinfection with Babesia and Lyme disease after splenectomy. J Am Board Fam Med. 2008 Jan-Feb;21(1):75-7. PMID:18178707

Adams LG, Todorovic RA. The chemotherapeutic efficacy of imidocarb dihydrochloride on concurrent bovine anaplasmosis and babesiosis. I. The effects of a single treatment. Trop Anim Health Prod. 1974 May;6(2):71-8. PMID:4416121

Adams LG, Todorovic RA. The chemotherapeutic efficacy of imidocarb dihydrochloride on concurrent bovine anaplasmosis and babesiosis. II. The effects of multiple treatments. Trop Anim Health Prod. 1974 May;6(2):79-84. PMID:4416122

Adan GL. Development of malaria control in the Philippines. J Philipp Med Assoc. 1954 Jan;30(1):29-35. PMID:13143503

Adedotun AA, Morenikeji OA, Odaibo AB. Knowledge, attitudes and practices about malaria in an urban community in south-western Nigeria. J Vector Borne Dis. 2010 Sep;47(3):155-9. PMID:20834085

Aderinboye O, Syed SS. Congenital babesiosis in a four-week-old female infant. Pediatr Infect Dis J. 2010 Feb;29(2):188. PMID:20118748

Aeschlimann A, Suter H. [Apropos of "Babesia" rodhaini].[Article in French]. Acta Trop. 1965;22(4):303-20. PMID:4379113

Ahmed OA, Odunukwe NN, Akinwale OP, Raheem TY, Efienemokwu CE, Ogedengbe O, Salako LA. Knowledge and practices of traditional birth attendants in prenatal services in Lagos State, Nigeria. Afr J Med Med Sci. 2005 Mar;34(1):55-8. PMID:15971555

Ahorlu CK, Dunyo SK, Afari EA, Koram KA, Nkrumah FK. Malaria-related beliefs and behaviour in southern Ghana: implications for treatment, prevention and control. Trop Med Int Health. 1997 May;2(5):488-99. PMID:9217705

Aikawa M, Beaudoin RL. Plasmodium fallax: high-resolution autoradiography of exoerythrocytic stages treated with Primaquine in vitro. Exp Parasitol. 1970 Jun;27(3):454-63. PMID:5419455

Aikins MK, Pickering H, Greenwood BM. Attitudes to malaria, traditional practices and bednets (mosquito nets) as vector control measures: a comparative study in five west African countries. J Trop Med Hyg. 1994 Apr;97(2):81-6. PMID:8170007

Ajayi IO, Falade CO, Olley BO, Yusuf B, Gbotosho S, Iyiola T, Olaniyan O, Happi C, Munguti K, Pagnoni F. A qualitative study of the feasibility and community perception on the effectiveness of artemether-lumefantrine use in the context of home management of malaria in south-west Nigeria. BMC Health Serv Res. 2008 Jun 1;8:119. PMID:18513447

Akiba M, Saeki H, Ishii T, Yamamoto S, Ueda K. Immunological changes in Babesia rodhaini infected BALB/c mice after treated with anti-babesial drug; diminazene diaceturate. J Vet Med Sci. 1991 Jun;53(3):371-7. PMID:1832024

Alabay M, Duzgun A, Cerci H, Wright IG, Waltisbuhl DJ, Goodger BV. Ovine babesiosis: induction of a protective immune response with crude extracts of either Babesia bovis or B ovis. Res Vet Sci. 1987 Nov;43(3):401-2. PMID:3444987

Aldighieri J, Blancard A, Boizis N, Dupoux R, Sautet G, Sautet J. [Influence of the environmental temperature on the development of Plasmodium berghei infections in white mice treated with nivaquine].[Article in French]. Bull Soc Pathol Exot Filiales. 1965 May-Jun;58(3):423-8. PMID:5898834

Alekseev AN. [The possibility of the detection of one more tick-borne infection--babesiosis--on the territory of Russia].[Article in Russian]. Zh Mikrobiol Epidemiol Immunobiol. 2003 May-Jun;(3):39-43. PMID:12886630

Alekseev AN, Rudakov NV, Dubinina EV. [Possible types of tick-borne diseases and the predictive role of history data in their diagnosis (parasitological aspects of the problem)].[Article in Russian]. Med Parazitol (Mosk). 2004 Oct-Dec;(4):31-6. PMID:15689134

Alhassan A, Govind Y, Tam NT, Thekisoe OM, Yokoyama N, Inoue N, Igarashi I. Comparative evaluation of the sensitivity of LAMP, PCR and in vitro culture methods for the diagnosis of equine piroplasmosis. Parasitol Res. 2007 Apr;100(5):1165-8. Epub 2007 Jan 11. PMID:17216488

Aliu YO, Odegaard S. Pharmacokinetics of diminazene in sheep. J Pharmacokinet Biopharm. 1985 Apr;13(2):173-84. PMID:4057056

Alkhalil A, Hill DA, Desai SA. Babesia and plasmodia increase host erythrocyte permeability through distinct mechanisms. Cell Microbiol. 2007 Apr;9(4):851-60. Epub 2006 Nov 3. PMID:17087736

Allison AC, Eugui EM. Approaches to vaccines against protozoan parasites of cattle. Adv Exp Med Biol. 1981;137:225-37. PMID:6800224

Almerìa S, Delgado-Neira Y, Adelantado C, Huguet M, Vinent J, Nicolàs A. Mediterranean theileriosis and other tick transmitted piroplasmoses in cattle in Minorca (Balearic Islands, Spain): the effect of tick control on prevalence levels analyzed by reverse line blot (RLB) macroarrays. J Parasitol. 2009 Jun;95(3):598-603. PMID:19086744

Alonso M, Blandino T, Mendoza E, Savon L, Camacho M. Development of a Babesia bovis live attenuated vaccine. Arch Med Res. 1994 Summer;25(2):273-7. PMID:7919825

Alter HJ, Stramer SL, Dodd RY. Emerging infectious diseases that threaten the blood supply. Semin Hematol. 2007 Jan;44(1):32-41. PMID:17198845

Altstatt LB. A clinical view of the biology of Plasmodia. Ann Intern Med. 1969 Jan;70(1):130-4. PMID:4884380

Alvarez JA, Ramos JA, Rojas EE, Mosqueda JJ, Vega CA, Olvera AM, Figueroa JV, Cantó GJ. Field challenge of cattle vaccinated with a combined Babesia bovis and Babesia bigemina frozen immunogen. Ann N Y Acad Sci. 2004 Oct;1026:277-83. PMID:15604506

Alward W, Javaid M, Garner J. Babesiosis in a Connecticut resident. Conn Med. 1990 Aug;54(8):425-7. PMID:2225809

Amer A, Mehlhorn H. Repellency effect of forty-one essential oils against Aedes, Anopheles, and Culex mosquitoes. Parasitol Res. 2006 Sep;99(4):478-90. Epub 2006 Apr 27. PMID:16642384

Anders JC, Chung H, Theoharides AD. Methemoglobin formation resulting from administration of candidate 8-aminoquinoline antiparasitic drugs in the dog. Fundam Appl Toxicol. 1988 Feb;10(2):270-5. PMID:3356313

Anderson AE, Cassaday PB, Healy GR. Babesiosis in man. Sixth documented case. Am J Clin Pathol. 1974 Nov;62(5):612-8. PMID:4412160

Ansari MA, Razdan RK. Relative efficacy of various oils in repelling mosquitoes. Indian J Malariol. 1995 Sep;32(3):104-11. PMID:8936292

Arai S, Tsuji M, Kaiho I, Murayama H, Zamoto A, Wei Q, Okabe N, Kamiyama T, Ishihara C. Retrospective seroepidemiological survey for human babesiosis in an area in Japan where a tick-borne disease is endemic. J Vet Med Sci. 2003 Mar;65(3):335-40. PMID:12679563

Arai S, Tsuji M, Kim SJ, Nakade T, Kanno Y, Ishihara C. Babesia canis infection in canine-red blood cell-substituted SCID mice. Int J Parasitol. 1998 Sep;28(9):1429-35. PMID:9770629

Ardington PC. Bovine fluid therapy. J S Afr Vet Assoc. 1977 Oct;48(3):215-8. PMID:599536

Armstrong PM, Brunet LR, Spielman A, Telford SR 3rd. Risk of Lyme disease: perceptions of residents of a Lone Star tick-infested community. Bull World Health Organ. 2001;79(10):916-25. PMID:11693973

Arnez M, Luznik-Bufon T, Avsic-Zupanc T, Ruzic-Sabljic E, Petrovec M, Lotric-Furlan S, Strle F. Causes of febrile illnesses after a tick bite in Slovenian children. Pediatr Infect Dis J. 2003 Dec;22(12):1078-83. PMID:14688569

Arulogun OS, Gregory AU. Management practices of childhood malaria among caregivers in Ojo Military Cantonment, Lagos, Nigeria: implication for child survival. Afr J Med Med Sci. 2009 Mar;38(1):45-54. PMID:19722428

Asad S, Sweeney J, Mermel LA. Transfusion-transmitted babesiosis in Rhode Island. Transfusion. 2009 Dec;49(12):2564-73. Epub 2009 Sep 16. PMID:19761547

Babu RV, Sharma G. A 57-year-old man with abdominal pain, jaundice, and a history of blood transfusion. Chest. 2007 Jul;132(1):347-50. PMID:17625097

Banerjee DP, Singh B, Gautam OP, Sarup S. Cell-mediated immune response in equine babesiosis. Trop Anim Health Prod. 1977 Aug;9(3):153-8. PMID:910301

Barnard CJ, Collins SA, Daisley JN, Behnke JM. Odour learning and immunity costs in mice. Behav Processes. 2006 Mar;72(1):74-83. Epub 2006 Jan 26. PMID:16442748

Barratt JL, Harkness J, Marriott D, Ellis JT, Stark D. Importance of nonenteric protozoan infections in immunocompromised people. Clin Microbiol Rev. 2010 Oct;23(4):795-836. PMID:20930074

Barré N, Happold J, Delathière JM, Desoutter D, Salery M, de Vos A, Marchal C, Perrot R, Grailles M, Mortelecque A. A campaign to eradicate bovine babesiosis from New Caledonia. Ticks Tick Borne Dis. 2011 Mar;2(1):55-61. Epub 2011 Jan 26. PMID:21771538

Barriga OO. A review on vaccination against protozoa and arthropods of veterinary importance. Vet Parasitol. 1994 Oct;55(1-2):29-55. PMID:7886919

Barry DN. Metabolism of Babesia parasites in vitro. Change in adenylate energy charge and infectivity of Babesia rodhaini-infected erythrocytes. Aust J Exp Biol Med Sci. 1984 Feb;62 (Pt 1):63-71. PMID:6743142

Bartlett MS, Queener SF, Durkin MM, Shaw MA, Smith JW. Inoculated mouse model of Pneumocystis carinii infection. Diagn Microbiol Infect Dis. 1992 Feb;15(2):129-34. PMID:1572137

Basu SK. A health profile of tribal India. Health Millions. 1994 Apr;2(2):12-4. PMID:12287763

Baumann D, Pusterla N, Péter O, Grimm F, Fournier PE, Schär G, Bossart W, Lutz H, Weber R. [Fever after a tick bite: clinical manifestations and diagnosis of acute tick bite-associated infections in northeastern Switzerland]. [Article in German] Dtsch Med Wochenschr. 2003 May 9;128(19):1042-7. PMID:12736854

Baumeister S, Wiesner J, Reichenberg A, Hintz M, Bietz S, Harb OS, Roos DS, Kordes M, Friesen J, Matuschewski K, Lingelbach K, Jomaa H, Seeber F. Fosmidomycin uptake into Plasmodium and Babesia-infected erythrocytes is facilitated by parasite-induced new permeability pathways. PLoS One. 2011 May 4;6(5):e19334. PMID:21573242

Bautista CR, Sandoval A, Aguilar BR. Effect of high- and low-molecular-weight components of Lactobacillus casei on resistance against Babesia microti in NIH mice. Ann N Y Acad Sci. 2008 Dec;1149:152-4. PMID:19120196

Bautista-Garfias CR, Gómez MB, Aguilar BR, Ixta O, Martínez F, Mosqueda J. The treatment of mice with Lactobacillus casei induces protection against Babesia microti infection. Parasitol Res. 2005 Dec;97(6):472-7. Epub 2005 Sep 17. PMID:16170567

Bayés M, Rabasseda X. Gateways to clinical trials. Methods Find Exp Clin Pharmacol. 2008 Jan-Feb;30(1):67-99. PMID:18389098

Bayes M, Rabasseda X, Prous JR. Gateways to clinical trials. Methods Find Exp Clin Pharmacol. 2003 Nov;25(9):747-71. PMID:14685303

Bayés M, Rabasseda X, Prous JR. Gateways to clinical trials. Methods Find Exp Clin Pharmacol. 2005 Jun;27(5):331-72. PMID:16082422

Becker JL. Vector-borne illnesses and the safety of the blood supply. Curr Hematol Rep. 2003 Nov;2(6):511-7. PMID:14561396

Belloli C, Crescenzo G, Lai O, Carofiglio V, Marang O, Ormas P. Pharmacokinetics of imidocarb dipropionate in horses after intramuscular administration. Equine Vet J. 2002 Sep;34(6):625-9. PMID:12358005

Belongia EA, Reed KD, Mitchell PD, Mueller-Rizner N, Vandermause M, Finkel MF, Kazmierczak JJ. Tickborne infections as a cause of nonspecific febrile illness in Wisconsin. Clin Infect Dis. 2001 May 15;32(10):1434-9. Epub 2001 Apr 17. PMID:11317244

Ben Musa N, Dawoud HA. The protective activity of serum and fractionated serum from rats against Babesia divergens. J Egypt Soc Parasitol. 2004 Aug;34(2):407-22. PMID:15287167

Ben Musa N, Phillips RS. The adaptation of three isolates of Babesia divergens to continuous culture in rat erythrocytes. Parasitology. 1991 Oct;103 Pt 2:165-70. PMID:1745544

Benach JL, Habicht GS, Holbrook TW, Cook JA. Glucan as an adjuvant for a murine Babesia microti immunization trial. Infect Immun. 1982 Mar;35(3):947-51. PMID:7068224

Benavides MV, Sacco AM. Differential Bos taurus cattle response to Babesia bovis infection. Vet Parasitol. 2007 Nov 30;150(1-2):54-64. Epub 2007 Oct 24. PMID:17919816

Beniwal RP, Nichani AK, Rakha NK, Sharma RD, Sarup S. An immunisation trial with in vitro produced Babesia bigemina exoantigens. Trop Anim Health Prod. 1997 Nov;29(4 Suppl):124S-126S. PMID:9512758

Berglund J. [Ticks--a medical topic of current interest which sticks].[Article in Swedish]. Lakartidningen. 1998 Jun 3;95(23):2695-700. PMID:9656623

Berkman SA. The spectrum of transfusion reactions. Hosp Pract (Off Ed). 1984 Jun;19(6):205-8, 210-2, 217-9. PMID:6427247

Berkman SA. Infectious complications of blood transfusion. Blood Rev. 1988 Sep;2(3):206-10. PMID:3052666

Beveridge E. Babesicidal effect of basically substituted carbanilides. II. Imidocarb in rats and mice: toxicity and activity against Babesia rodhaini. Res Vet Sci. 1969 Nov;10(6):534-9. PMID:5368455

Bianchi MW, Barré N, Messad S. Factors related to cattle infestation level and resistance to acaricides in Boophilus microplus tick populations in New Caledonia. Vet Parasitol. 2003 Feb 28;112(1-2):75-89. PMID:12581586

Birkenheuer AJ, Levy MG, Breitschwerdt EB. Efficacy of combined atovaquone and azithromycin for therapy of chronic Babesia gibsoni (Asian genotype) infections in dogs. J Vet Intern Med. 2004 Jul-Aug;18(4):494-8. PMID:15320586

Birkenheuer AJ, Whittington J, Neel J, Large E, Barger A, Levy MG, Breitschwerdt

EB. Molecular characterization of a Babesia species identified in a North American raccoon. J Wildl Dis. 2006 Apr;42(2):375-80. PMID:16870860

Birkett MA, Hassanali A, Hoglund S, Pettersson J, Pickett JA. Repellent activity of catmint, Nepeta cataria, and iridoid nepetalactone isomers against Afro-tropical mosquitoes, ixodid ticks and red poultry mites. Phytochemistry. 2011 Jan;72(1):109-14. Epub 2010 Nov 4. PMID:21056438

Bishop JP, Adams LG. Babesia bigemina: immune response of cattle inoculated with irradiated parasites. Exp Parasitol. 1974 Feb;35(1):35-43. PMID:4815017

Bishop JP, Adams LG, Thompson KC, Corrier DE. The isolation, separation and preservation of Babesia bigemina. Trop Anim Health Prod. 1973 Aug;5(3):141-5. PMID:4802625

Blue D, Graves V, McCarthy L, Cruz J, Gregurek S, Smith D. Fatal transfusion-transmitted Babesia microti in the Midwest. Transfusion. 2009 Jan;49(1):8. Epub 2008 Aug 6. PMID:18694463

Bock R, Jackson L, de Vos A, Jorgensen W. Babesiosis of cattle. Parasitology. 2004;129 Suppl:S247-69. PMID:15938514

Bock RE, Blight GW, Kingston TG, de Vos AJ. A survey of cattle producers in the Boophilus microplus endemic area of Queensland to determine attitudes to the control of and vaccination against tick fever. Aust Vet J. 1995 Mar;72(3):88-92. PMID:7611988

Bock RE, de Vos AJ. Immunity following use of Australian tick fever vaccine: a review of the evidence. Aust Vet J. 2001 Dec;79(12):832-9. PMID:11837905

Bock RE, de Vos AJ, Kingston TG, Shiels IA, Dalgliesh RJ. Investigations of breakdowns in protection provided by living Babesia bovis vaccine. Vet Parasitol. 1992 Jun;43(1-2):45-56. PMID:1496802

Bomfim MR, Ko A, Koury MC. Evaluation of the recombinant LipL32 in enzyme-linked immunosorbent assay for the serodiagnosis of bovine leptospirosis. Vet Microbiol. 2005 Aug 10;109(1-2):89-94. PMID:15950404

Bono MF, Mangold AJ, Baravalle ME, Valentini BS, Thompson CS, Wilkowsky SE, Echaide IE, Farber MD, Torioni de Echaide SM. Efficiency of a recombinant MSA-2c-based ELISA to establish the persistence of antibodies in cattle vaccinated with Babesia bovis. Vet Parasitol. 2008 Nov 7;157(3-4):203-10. Epub 2008 Aug 5. PMID:18783887

Bonoan JT, Johnson DH, Cunha BA. Life-threatening babesiosis in an asplenic patient treated with exchange transfusion, azithromycin, and atovaquone. Heart Lung. 1998 Nov-Dec;27(6):424-8. PMID:9835673

Bora U, Sahu A, Saikia AP, Ryakala VK, Goswami P. Medicinal plants used by the people of Northeast India for curing malaria. Phytother Res. 2007 Aug;21(8):800-4. PMID:17533627

Botros BA, Moch RW, Barsoum IS. Some observations on experimentally induced infection of dogs with Babesia gibsoni. Am J Vet Res. 1975 Mar;36(3):293-6. PMID:1115427

Bourdoiseau G. Canine babesiosis in France. Vet Parasitol. 2006 May 31;138(1-2):118-25. Epub 2006 Feb 28. PMID:16507334

Boustani MR, Lepore TJ, Gelfand JA, Lazarus DS. Acute respiratory failure in patients treated for babesiosis. Am J Respir Crit Care Med. 1994 Jun;149(6):1689-91. PMID:8004331

Bown KJ, Lambin X, Telford GR, Ogden NH, Telfer S, Woldehiwet Z, Birtles RJ. Relative importance of Ixodes ricinus and Ixodes trianguliceps as vectors for Anaplasma phagocytophilum and Babesia microti in field vole (Microtus agrestis) populations. Appl Environ Microbiol. 2008 Dec;74(23):7118-25. Epub 2008 Sep 26. PMID:18820068

Boyom FF, Ngouana V, Kemgne EA, Zollo PH, Menut C, Bessiere JM, Gut J, Rosenthal PJ. Antiplasmodial volatile extracts from Cleistopholis patens Engler & Diels and Uvariastrum pierreanum Engl. (Engl. & Diels) (Annonaceae) growing in Cameroon. Parasitol Res. 2011 May;108(5):1211-7. Epub 2010 Nov 25. PMID:21107862

Boyom FF, Ngouana V, Zollo PH, Menut C, Bessiere JM, Gut J, Rosenthal PJ. Composition and anti-plasmodial activities of essential oils from some Cameroonian medicinal plants. Phytochemistry. 2003 Dec;64(7):1269-75. PMID:14599525

Bradbury-Golas K, Washart C. A 56-year-old woman with fever, generalized body aches, and anemia after a tick bite. J Emerg Nurs. 2005 Apr;31(2):137-8. PMID:15856537

Braga W, Venasco J, Willard L, Moro MH. Ultrastructure of Babesia WA1 (Apicomplexa: Piroplasma) during infection of erythrocytes in a hamster model. J Parasitol. 2006 Oct;92(5):1104-7. PMID:17152960

Brasseur P, Gorenflot A. Human babesial infections in Europe. Rocz Akad Med Bialymst. 1996;41(1):117-22. PMID:8673796

Brasseur P, Lecoublet S, Kapel N, Favennec L, Ballet JJ. Quinine in the treatment of Babesia divergens infections in humans. Eur J Clin Microbiol Infect Dis. 1996 Oct;15(10):840-1. PMID:8950568

Breitschwerdt EB, Maggi RG. A confusing case of canine vector-borne disease: clinical signs and progression in a dog co-infected with Ehrlichia canis and Bartonella vinsonii ssp. berkhoffii. Parasit Vectors. 2009 Mar 26;2 Suppl 1:S3. PMID:19426442

Brigden ML. Detection, education and management of the asplenic or hyposplenic patient. Am Fam Physician. 2001 Feb 1;63(3):499-506, 508. PMID:11272299

Brizuela CM, Ortellado CA, Sanabria E, Torres O, Ortigosa D. The safety and efficacy of Australian tick-borne disease vaccine strains in cattle in Paraguay. Vet Parasitol. 1998 Mar 31;76(1-2):27-41. PMID:9653988

Brocklesby DW, Harness E, Sellwood SA. The effect of age on the natural immunity of cattle to Babesia divergens. Res Vet Sci. 1971 Jan;12(1):15-7. PMID:4252543

Brocks DR, Mehvar R. Stereoselectivity in the pharmacodynamics and pharmacokinetics of the chiral antimalarial drugs. Clin Pharmacokinet. 2003;42(15):1359-82. PMID:14674788

Brown KN. Immunity to protozoal infections. Proc R Soc Med. 1969 Mar 3;62(3):301-2. PMID:4181289

Brown WC. Molecular approaches to elucidating innate and acquired immune responses to Babesia bovis, a protozoan parasite that causes persistent infection. Vet Parasitol. 2001 Nov 22;101(3-4):233-48. PMID:11707299

Brown WC, McElwain TF, Hötzel I, Suarez CE, Palmer GH. Helper T-cell epitopes encoded by the Babesia bigemina rap-1 gene family in the constant and variant domains are conserved among parasite strains. Infect Immun. 1998 Apr;66(4):1561-9. PMID:9529082

Brown WC, Zhao S, Logan KS, Grab DJ, Rice-Ficht AC. Identification of candidate vaccine antigens of bovine hemoparasites Theileria parva and Babesia bovis by use of helper T cell clones. Vet Parasitol. 1995 Mar;57(1-3):189-203. PMID:7597783

Bruce-Chwatt LJ. Transfusion associated parasitic infections. Prog Clin Biol Res. 1985;182:101-25. PMID:3929259

Brueckner RP, Coster T, Wesche DL, Shmuklarsky M, Schuster BG. Prophylaxis of Plasmodium falciparum infection in a human challenge model with WR 238605, a new 8-aminoquinoline antimalarial. Antimicrob Agents Chemother. 1998 May;42(5):1293-4. PMID:9593172

Brueckner RP, Fleckenstein L. Simultaneous modeling of the pharmacokinetics and methemoglobin pharmacodynamics of an 8-aminoquinoline candidate antimalarial (WR 238605). Pharm Res. 1991 Dec;8(12):1505-10. PMID:1808614

Brueckner RP, Lasseter KC, Lin ET, Schuster BG. First-time-in-humans safety and pharmacokinetics of WR 238605, a new antimalarial. Am J Trop Med Hyg. 1998 May;58(5):645-9. PMID:9598455

Brumlik MJ, Pandeswara S, Ludwig SM, Murthy K, Curiel TJ. Parasite mitogen-activated protein kinases as drug discovery targets to treat human protozoan pathogens. J Signal Transduct. 2011;2011:971968. Epub 2011 Feb 27. PMID:21637385

Brüning A. Equine piroplasmosis an update on diagnosis, treatment and prevention. Br Vet J. 1996 Mar;152(2):139-51. PMID:8680838

Bryceson AD, Fleming AF, Edington GM. Splenomegaly in Northern Nigeria. Acta Trop. 1976;33(3):185-214. PMID:11654

Bu Jassoum S, Fong IW, Hannach B, Kain KC. Transfusion-transmitted babesiosis in Ontario: first reported case in Canada. [Article in English, French]. Can Commun Dis Rep. 2000 Jan 15;26(2):9-13. PMID:10680253

Buckingham SC. Tick-borne infections in children: epidemiology, clinical manifestations, and optimal management strategies. Paediatr Drugs. 2005;7(3):163-76. PMID:15977962

Buelvas F, Alvis N, Buelvas I, Miranda J, Mattar S. [A high prevalence of antibodies against Bartonella and Babesia microti has been found in villages and urban populations in Cordoba, Colombia].[Article in Spanish]. Rev Salud Publica (Bogota). 2008 Jan-Feb;10(1):168-77. PMID:18368229

Buma AH, van Thiel P. Experiences with malaria chemoprophylaxis in Dutch troops. Med Trop (Mars). 2001;61(1):77-8. PMID:11584661

Bunin KV. [A brief essay on the development of chemotherapy of malaria and recurrent typhus in Russia].[Article in Russian]. Zh Mikrobiol Epidemiol Immunobiol. 1957 Feb;28(2):122-7. PMID:13423825

Burgess RW, Young MD. The development of pyrimethamine resistance by Plasmodium falciparum. Bull World Health Organ. 1959;20(1):37-46. PMID:13638788

Butler CM, van Gils JA, van der Kolk JH. [A literature review of equine piroplasmosis after an episode of acute babesiosis in a Dutch Standardbred foal after a stay in Normandy].[Article in Dutch]. Tijdschr Diergeneeskd. 2005 Dec 1;130(23):726-31. PMID:16363205

Butler T, Warren KS, Mahmoud AA. Algorithms in the diagnosis and management of exotic diseases. XIII. Malaria. J Infect Dis. 1976 Jun;133(6):721-6. PMID:932498

Button C. Fluid therapy in canine babesiosis. J S Afr Vet Assoc. 1976 Dec;47(4):284-7. PMID:1035270

Cable RG, Leiby DA. Risk and prevention of transfusion-transmitted babesiosis and other tick-borne diseases. Curr Opin Hematol. 2003 Nov;10(6):405-11. PMID:14564169

Cacciò S, Cammà C, Onuma M, Severini C. The beta-tubulin gene of Babesia and Theileria parasites is an informative marker for species discrimination. Int J Parasitol. 2000 Oct;30(11):1181-5. PMID:11027785

Cahill KM. Babesiosis: unappreciated even in endemic areas. J Community Health. 1995 Aug;20(4):315-20. PMID:7593737

Cahill KM, Benach JL, Reich LM, Bilmes E, Zins JH, Siegel FP, Hochweis S. Red cell exchange: treatment of babesiosis in a splenectomized patient. Transfusion. 1981 Mar-Apr;21(2):193-8. PMID:7194528

Callow LL. Vaccination against bovine babesiosis. Adv Exp Med Biol. 1977;93:121-49. PMID:596295

Callow LL. Some aspects of the epidemiology and control of bovine babesiosis in Australia. J S Afr Vet Assoc. 1979 Dec;50(4):353-6. PMID:399977

Callow LL, Dalgliesh RJ, de Vos AJ. Development of effective living vaccines against bovine babesiosis--the longest field trial? Int J Parasitol. 1997 Jul;27(7):747-67. PMID:9279577

Callow LL, McGregor W. Vaccination against Babesia argentina infection in cattle during chemoprophylaxis with a quinuronium compound. Aust Vet J. 1969 Sep;45(9):408-10. PMID:5389523

Callow LL, Stewart NP. Immunosuppression by Babesia bovis against its tick vector, Boophilus microplus. Nature. 1978 Apr 27;272(5656):818-9. PMID:643072

Cambournac FJ. [The development of the eradication of malaria. A practical public health lesson].[Article in French]. An Esc Nacl Saude Publica Med Trop (Lisb). 1969 Jan-Dec;3(1):33-46. PMID:5404998

Canfield CJ, Rozman RS. Clinical testing of new antimalarial compounds. Bull World Health Organ. 1974;50(3-4):203-12. PMID: 4613503

Cangelosi JJ, Sarvat B, Sarria JC, Herwaldt BL, Indrikovs AJ. Transmission of Babesia microti by blood transfusion in Texas. Vox Sang. 2008 Nov;95(4):331-4. PMID:19138264

Canto GJ, Figueroa JV, Ramos JA, Rojas EE, Garcia-Tapia D, Alvarez JA, Allred DR, Carson CA. Evaluation of cattle inoculated with Babesia bovis clones adhesive in vitro to bovine brain endothelial cells. Ann N Y Acad Sci. 2006 Oct;1081:397-404. PMID:17135543

Carbrey EA, Avery RJ, Knowles RC, Sash SC. Chemotherapy of equine babesiosis. J Am Vet Med Assoc. 1971 Dec 1;159(11):1538-45. PMID:5005185

Cardoso L, Tuna J, Vieira L, Yisaschar-Mekuzas Y, Baneth G. Molecular detection of Anaplasma platys and Ehrlichia canis in dogs from the North of Portugal. Vet J. 2010 Feb;183(2):232-3. Epub 2008 Dec 3. PMID:19056304

Carlsson T, Bergqvist L, Hellgren U. Homeopathic Resistant Malaria. J Travel Med. 1996 Mar 1;3(1):62. PMID:9815426

Carter WJ, Yan Z, Cassai ND, Sidhu GS. Detection of extracellular forms of babesia in the blood by electron microscopy: a diagnostic method for differentiation from Plasmodium falciparum. Ultrastruct Pathol. 2003 Jul-Aug;27(4):211-6. PMID:12907365

Carvalho L, Luque-Ortega JR, Manzano JI, Castanys S, Rivas L, Gamarro F. Tafenoquine, an antiplasmodial 8-aminoquinoline, targets leishmania respiratory complex III and induces apoptosis. Antimicrob Agents Chemother. 2010 Dec;54(12):5344-51. Epub 2010 Sep 13. PMID:20837758

Centeno-Lima S, do Rosário V, Parreira R, Maia AJ, Freudenthal AM, Nijhof AM, Jongejan F. A fatal case of human babesiosis in Portugal: molecular and phylogenetic analysis. Trop Med Int Health. 2003 Aug;8(8):760-4. PMID:12869099

Chambers JA. Military aviators, special operations forces, and causal malaria prophylaxis. Mil Med. 2003 Dec;168(12):1001-6. PMID:14719625

Chansiri K, Sarataphan N. Molecular phylogenetic study of Theileria sp. (Thung Song) based on the thymidylate synthetase gene. Parasitol Res. 2002 May;88(13 Suppl 1):S33-5. PMID:12051604

Chapman WE, Ward PA. The complement profile in babesiosis. J Immunol. 1976 Sep;117(3):935-8. PMID:956661

Chapman WE, Ward PA. Babesia rodhaini: requirement of complement for penetration of human erythrocytes. Science. 1977 Apr 1;196(4285):67-70. PMID:841340

Chapman WL Jr, Hanson W. Plasmodium berghei infection in neonatallythymectomized hamsters. J Parasitol. 1971 Feb;57(1):24-8. PMID:4101132

Charles BG, Miller AK, Nasveld PE, Reid MG, Harris IE, Edstein MD. Population pharmacokinetics of tafenoquine during malaria prophylaxis in healthy subjects. Antimicrob Agents Chemother. 2007 Aug;51(8):2709-15. Epub 2007 May 21. PMID:17517850

Chatel G, Gulletta M, Matteelli A, Marangoni A, Signorini L, Oladeji O, Caligaris S. Short report: Diagnosis of tick-borne relapsing fever by the quantitative buffy coat fluorescence method. Am J Trop Med Hyg. 1999 May;60(5):738-9. PMID:10344644

Chaudhuri S, Varshney JP. Clinical management of babesiosis in dogs with homeopathic Crotalus horridus 200C. Homeopathy. 2007 Apr;96(2):90-4. PMID:17437935

Chaykovsky M, Rosowsky A, Papathanasopoulos N, Chen KK, Modest EJ, Kisliuk RL, Gaumont Y. Methotrexate analogs. 3. Synthesis and biological properties of some side-chain altered analogs. J Med Chem. 1974 Nov;17(11):1212-6. PMID:4213249

Chema S, Chumo RS, Dolan TT, Gathuma JM, Irvin AD, James AD, Young AS. Clinical trial of halofuginone lactate for the treatment of East Coast fever in Kenya. Vet Rec. 1987 Jun 13;120(24):575-7. PMID:3303642

Chen LH, Keystone JS. New strategies for the prevention of malaria in travelers. Infect Dis Clin North Am. 2005 Mar;19(1):185-210. PMID:15701554

Christensson DA, Morén T. Seroresponse (IgG) after vaccination and natural infection of cattle with Babesia divergens. Acta Vet Scand. 1987;28(3-4):393-402. PMID:3454550

Cichocka A, Skotarczak B. [Babesosis--difficulty of diagnosis]. [Article in Polish]. Wiad Parazytol. 2001;47(3):527-33. PMID:16894770

Clark IA. Resistance to Babesia spp. and Plasmodium sp. in mice pretreated with an extract of Coxiella burnetii. Infect Immun. 1979 May;24(2):319-25. PMID:378850

Clark IA, Allison AC, Cox FE. Protection of mice against Babesia and Plasmodium with BCG. Nature. 1976 Jan 29;259(5541):309-11. PMID:765838

Clark IA, Budd AC, Hsue G, Haymore BR, Joyce AJ, Thorner R, Krause PJ. Absence of erythrocyte sequestration in a case of babesiosis in a splenectomized human patient. Malar J. 2006 Aug 4;5:69. PMID:16887045

Clark IA, Cox FE, Allison AC. Protection of mice against Babesia spp. and Plasmodium spp. with killed Corynebacterium parvum. Parasitology. 1977 Feb;74(1):9-18. PMID:320544

Clyde DF. The problem of drug-resistant malaria. Am J Trop Med Hyg. 1972 Sep;21(5):736-43. PMID:4561521

Clyde DF, McCarthy VC, Rebert CC, Miller RM. Prophylactic activity of a phenanthrene methanol (WR 33063) and a quinoline methanol (WR 30090) in human malaria. Antimicrob Agents Chemother. 1973 Feb;3(2):220-3. PMID:4597716

Clyde DF, Shute GT, McCarthy VC, Sangalang RP. Characterization of a drug resistant strain of Plasmodium falciparum from the Philippines. J Trop Med Hyg. 1971 May;74(5):101-5. PMID:4931686

Cohen S, Butcher GA. Serum antibody in acquired malarial immunity. Trans R Soc Trop Med Hyg. 1971;65(2):125-35. PMID:4934028

Coleman RE. Sporontocidal activity of the antimalarial WR-238605 against Plasmodium berghei ANKA in Anopheles stephensi. Am J Trop Med Hyg. 1990 Mar;42(3):196-205. PMID:2180334

Coleman RE, Clavin AM, Milhous WK. Gametocytocidal and sporontocidal activity of antimalarials against Plasmodium berghei ANKA in ICR Mice and Anopheles stephensi mosquitoes. Am J Trop Med Hyg. 1992 Feb;46(2):169-82. PMID:1539752

Coleman M, Girotto JE, Spielman A. Persistent and relapsing babesiosis in immunocompromised patients. Clin Infect Dis. 2008 Feb 1;46(3):370-6. PMID:18181735

Collins WE, Contacos PG. Immunization of monkeys against Plasmodium cynomolgi by X-irradiated sporozoites. Nat New Biol. 1972 Apr 12;236(67):176-7. PMID:4624244

Collins WE, Contacos PG, Garnham PC, Warren M, Skinner JC. Plasmodium hylobati: a malaria parasite of the gibbon. J Parasitol. 1972 Feb;58(1):123-8. PMID:4335047

Collins WE, Contacos PG, Skinner JC, Chin W, Guinn E. Fluorescent antibody studies on simian malaria. I. Development of antibodies to Plasmodium knowlesi. Am J Trop Med Hyg. 1967 Jan;16(1):1-6. PMID:4960484

Collins WE, Jeffrey GM, Skinner JC. Fluorescent Antibody Studies In Human Malaria. II. Development And Persistence Of Antibodies To Plasmodium Falciparum. Am J Trop Med Hyg. 1964 Mar;13:256-60. PMID:14125876

Collins WE, Skinner JC, Contacos PG, Guinn EG. Fluorescent-antibody studies on simian malaria. II. Development of antibodies to Plasmodium cynomolgi. Am J Trop Med Hyg. 1967 May;16(3):267-72. PMID:4960704

Combrink MP, Troskie PC, Du Plessis F, Latif AA. Serological responses to Babesia bovis vaccination in cattle previously infected with Babesia bigemina. Vet Parasitol. 2010 May 28;170(1-2):30-6. Epub 2010 Feb 18. PMID:20207488

Commins MA, Goodger BV, Wright IG. Proteinases in the lysate of bovine erythrocytes infected with Babesia bovis: initial vaccination studies. Int J Parasitol. 1985 Oct;15(5):491-5. PMID:3905658

Conly GN. The impact of malaria on economic development. A case study. Am J Trop Med Hyg. 1972 Sep;21(5):668-74. PMID:5074689

Conrad PA, Kjemtrup AM, Carreno RA, Thomford J, Wainwright K, Eberhard M, Quick R, Telford SR 3rd, Herwaldt BL. Description of Babesia duncani n.sp. (Apicomplexa: Babesiidae) from humans and its differentiation from other piroplasms. Int J Parasitol. 2006 Jun;36(7):779-89. Epub 2006 May 4. PMID:16725142

Cooke BM, Mohandas N, Coppel RL. The malaria-infected red blood cell: structural and functional changes. Adv Parasitol. 2001;50:1-86. PMID:11757330

Cooper PE, Watson PM. Discontinuation of redwater treatments. Vet Rec. 1989 Jun 17;124(24):643. PMID:2773215

Cooper RD, Milhous WK, Rieckmann KH. The efficacy of WR238605 against the blood stages of a chloroquine resistant strain of Plasmodium vivax. Trans R Soc Trop Med Hyg. 1994 Nov-Dec;88(6):691-2. PMID:7886774

Corash L. Inactivation of viruses, bacteria, protozoa, and leukocytes in platelet concentrates. Vox Sang. 1998;74 Suppl 2:173-6. PMID:9704443

Corash L. Inactivation of viruses, bacteria, protozoa and leukocytes in platelet and red cell concentrates. Vox Sang. 2000;78 Suppl 2:205-10. PMID: 10938954

Corash L. New technologies for the inactivation of infectious pathogens in cellular blood components and the development of platelet substitutes. Baillieres Best Pract Res Clin Haematol. 2000 Dec;13(4):549-63. PMID:11102276

Corash L. Inactivation of infectious pathogens in labile blood components: meeting the challenge. Transfus Clin Biol. 2001 Jun;8(3):138-45. PMID:11499954

Corpelet C, Vacher P, Coudore F, Laurichesse H, Conort N, Souweine B. Role of quinine in life-threatening Babesia divergens infection successfully treated with clindamycin. Eur J Clin Microbiol Infect Dis. 2005 Jan;24(1):74-5. PMID:15616840

Corradetti A. Some remarks on the use of avian malaria parasites in research. Ann Parasitol Hum Comp. 1973 Mar-Apr;48(2):217-9. PMID:4785849

Corrier DE, Vizcaino O, Terry M, Betancourt A, Kuttler KL, Carson CA, Trevino G, Ristic M. Mortality, weight loss and anaemia in Bos taurus calves exposed to Boophilus microplus ticks in the tropics of Colombia. Trop Anim Health Prod. 1979 Nov;11(4):215-21. PMID:552671

Corrier DE, Wagner GG. Comparison of the effect of T-2 toxin with that of dexamethasone or cyclophosphamide on resistance to Babesia microti infection in mice. Am J Vet Res. 1988 Nov;49(11):2000-3. PMID:3247926

Corrier DE, Wagner GG, Kuttler KL. Viability and virulence of Babesia rodhaini eight years after cryogenic preservation with dimethyl sulfoxide. Vet Parasitol. 1985 Jun;18(1):71-3. PMID:4049729

Cottrell BJ, Playfair JH, de Sousa B. Plasmodium yoelii and Plasmodium vinckei: the effects of nonspecific immunostimulation on murine malaria. Exp Parasitol. 1977 Oct;43(1):45-53. PMID:330190

Covell G. A brief review of the history and development of the more important antimalarial drugs. Indian J Malariol. 1947 Jun;1(2):231-41. PMID:18901444

Cox FE. Heterologous immunity between piroplasms and malaria parasites: the simultaneous elimination of Plasmodium vinckei and Babesia microti from the blood of doubly infected mice. Parasitology. 1978 Feb;76(1):55-60. PMID:622306

Cox HW, Saleh SM. Anemia and thrombocytopenia from Corynebacterium parvum-stimulated resistance against malaria, trypanosomiasis, and babesiosis. J Parasitol. 1983 Aug;69(4):654-9. PMID:6355427

Cranwell MP. Efficacy of long-acting oxytetracycline for the prevention of tick-borne fever in calves. Vet Rec. 1990 Apr 7;126(14):334-6. PMID:2339491

Criado-Fornelio A. A review of nucleic-acid-based diagnostic tests for Babesia and Theileria, with emphasis on bovine piroplasms. Parassitologia. 2007 May;49 Suppl 1:39-44. PMID:17691606

Criado-Fornelio A, Martinez-Marcos A, Buling-Saraña A, Barba-Carretero JC. Presence of Mycoplasma haemofelis, Mycoplasma haemominutum and piroplasmids in cats from southern Europe: a molecular study. Vet Microbiol. 2003 Jun 10;93(4):307-17. PMID:12713893

Crockett M, Kain KC. Tafenoquine: a promising new antimalarial agent. Expert Opin Investig Drugs. 2007 May;16(5):705-15. PMID:17461742

Cunha BA, Cohen YZ, McDermott B. Fever of unknown origin (FUO) due to babesiosis in a immunocompetent host. Heart Lung. 2008 Nov-Dec;37(6):481-4. Epub 2008 Sep 30. PMID:18992633

Cunha BA, Nausheen S, Szalda D. Pulmonary complications of babesiosis: case report and literature review. Eur J Clin Microbiol Infect Dis. 2007 Jul;26(7):505-8. PMID:17558489 da Silva RA, Corrêa Fdo N, Botteon Rde C, Botteon Pde T. [Natural infection by hemoparasites in calves submitted to chemoprophylaxis at 30 days of age].[Article in Portuguese]. Rev Bras Parasitol Vet. 2007 Jul-Sep;16(3):163-5. PMID:18078605

Dalgliesh RJ. Field observations on Babesia argentina vaccination in Queensland. Aust Vet J. 1968 Mar;44(3):103-4. PMID:5689432

Dalgliesh RJ. Dimethyl sulphoxide in the low-temperature preservation of Babesia bigemina. Res Vet Sci. 1971 Sep;12(5):469-71. PMID:4999644

Dalgliesh RJ. Effects of low temperature preservation and route of inoculation on infectivity of Babesia bigemina in blood diluted with glycerol. Res Vet Sci. 1972 Nov;13(6):540-5. PMID:4630813

Dalgliesh RJ, Callow LL, Mellors LT, McGregor W. Development of a highly infective Babesia bigemina vaccine of reduced virulence. Aust Vet J. 1981 Jan;57(1):8-11. PMID:7236153

Dalgliesh RJ, Jorgensen WK, de Vos AJ. Australian frozen vaccines for the control of babesiosis and anaplasmosis in cattle--a review. Trop Anim Health Prod. 1990 Feb;22(1):44-52. PMID:2181745

Dalgliesh RJ, Mellors LT. Survival of the parasitic protozoan, Babesia bigemina, in blood cooled at widely different rates to -196 degrees C. Int J Parasitol. 1974 Apr;4(2):169-72. PMID:4822484

Dantas-Torres F, Figueredo LA. Canine babesiosis: a Brazilian perspective. Vet Parasitol. 2006 Nov 5;141(3-4):197-203. Epub 2006 Sep 8. PMID:16962707

Dantrakool A, Somboon P, Hashimoto T, Saito-Ito A. Identification of a new type of Babesia species in wild rats (Bandicota indica) in Chiang Mai Province, Thailand. J Clin Microbiol. 2004 Feb;42(2):850-4. PMID:14766871

Dao AH. Human babesiosis. Compr Ther. 1996 Nov;22(11):713-8. PMID:8978977

Davidson RN, Wall RA. Prevention and management of infections in patients without a spleen. Clin Microbiol Infect. 2001 Dec;7(12):657-60. PMID:11843905

de Almeida RR, Souto RN, Bastos CN, da Silva MH, Maia JG. Chemical variation in Piper aduncum and biological properties of its dillapiole-rich essential oil. Chem Biodivers. 2009 Sep;6(9):1427-34. PMID:19774604

de la Fuente J, Rodríguez M, Montero C, Redondo M, García-García JC, Méndez L, Serrano E, Valdés M, Enríquez A, Canales M, Ramos E, Boué O, Machado H, Lleonart R. Vaccination against ticks (Boophilus spp.): the experience with the Bm86-based vaccine Gavac. Genet Anal. 1999 Nov;15(3-5):143-8. PMID:10596754

de la Fuente J, Rodríguez M, Redondo M, Montero C, García-García JC, Méndez L, Serrano E, Valdés M, Enriquez A, Canales M, Ramos E, Boué O, Machado H, Lleonart R, de Armas CA, Rey S, Rodríguez JL, Artiles M, García L. Field studies and cost-effectiveness analysis of vaccination with Gavac against the cattle tick Boophilus microplus. Vaccine. 1998 Feb;16(4):366-73. PMID:9607057

De Souza CM, Silva ED, Ano Bom AP, Bastos RC, Nascimento HJ, Da Silva Junior JG. Evaluation of an ELISA for canine leishmaniasis immunodiagnostic using recombinant proteins. Parasite Immunol. 2012 Jan;34(1):1-7. PMID:21929686

de-Thé G, Geser A. [Prospective epidemiologic studies and the nature of the association between Epstein-Barr virus (EBV) and Burkitt's lymphoma (BL)].[Article in French]. C R Acad Sci Hebd Seances Acad Sci D. 1976 Apr 5;282(14):1387-90. PMID:181158 de Vos AJ. Epidemiology and control of bovine babesiosis in South Africa. J S Afr Vet Assoc. 1979 Dec;50(4):357-62. PMID:576018

De Vos AJ, Bessenger R, Fourie CG. Virulence and heterologous strain immunity of South African and Australian Babesia bovis strains with reduced pathogenicity. Onderstepoort J Vet Res. 1982 Sep;49(3):133-6. PMID:7177589

De Vos AJ, Bock RE. Vaccination against bovine babesiosis. Ann N Y Acad Sci. 2000;916:540-5. PMID:11193669

de Waal DT, Combrink MP. Live vaccines against bovine babesiosis. Vet Parasitol. 2006 May 31;138(1-2):88-96. Epub 2006 Feb 28. PMID:16504404

Delbecq S, Precigout E, Schetters T, Gorenflot A. Babesia divergens: cloning of a Ran binding protein 1 homologue. Vet Parasitol. 2003 Jul 29;115(3):205-11. PMID:12935735

Della-Giustina D, Laird TW Jr, Smith T. Transfusion-acquired babesiosis in a nonendemic area. Mil Med. 2005 Apr;170(4):295-6. PMID:15916297

Diggs CL, Osler AG. Humoral immunity in rodent malaria. III: Studies on the site of antibody action. J Immunol. 1975 Apr;114(4):1243-7. PMID:1090670

Dimmock CK. Blood group antibody production in cattle by a vaccine against Babesia argentina. Res Vet Sci. 1973 Nov;15(3):305-9. PMID:4792010

Dimmock CK, Bell K. Haemolytic disease of the newborn in calves. Aust Vet J. 1970 Feb;46(2):44-7. PMID:5463721

DoAmaral JR, French FA, Blanz EJ Jr, French DA. Antimalarial activity of guanylhydrazone salts of aromatic ketones. 2. Development of active polyhalo derivatives. J Med Chem. 1971 Sep;14(9):862-6. PMID:5140015

Dobroszycki J, Herwaldt BL, Boctor F, Miller JR, Linden J, Eberhard ML, Yoon JJ, Ali NM, Tanowitz HB, Graham F, Weiss LM, Wittner M. A cluster of transfusion-associated babesiosis cases traced to a single asymptomatic donor. JAMA. 1999 Mar 10;281(10):927-30. PMID:10078490

Dodd JD, Aquino SL, Sharma A. Babesiosis: CT and hematologic findings. J Thorac Imaging. 2007 Aug;22(3):271-3. PMID:17721341

Dodd RY. Transmission of parasites by blood transfusion. Vox Sang. 1998;74 Suppl 2:161-3. PMID:9704440

Dodd RY. Current risk for transfusion transmitted infections. Curr Opin Hematol. 2007 Nov;14(6):671-6. PMID:17898573

Dodd RY. Emerging pathogens in transfusion medicine. Clin Lab Med. 2010 Jun;30(2):499-509. Epub 2010 May 6. PMID:20513567

Dorman SE, Cannon ME, Telford SR 3rd, Frank KM, Churchill WH. Fulminant babesiosis treated with clindamycin, quinine, and whole-blood exchange transfusion. Transfusion. 2000 Mar;40(3):375-80. PMID:10738042

Dow GS, Gettayacamin M, Hansukjariya P, Imerbsin R, Komcharoen S, Sattabongkot J, Kyle D, Milhous W, Cozens S, Kenworthy D, Miller A, Veazey J, Ohrt C. Radical curative efficacy of tafenoquine combination regimens in Plasmodium cynomolgi-infected Rhesus monkeys (Macaca mulatta). Malar J. 2011 Jul 29;10:212. PMID:21801400

Dowsett KF, Dimmock CK, Hill MW. Haemolytic disease in new born calves. Aust Vet J. 1978 Feb;54(2):65-7. PMID:566099

Doyle E, Fowles SE, Summerfield S, White TJ. Rapid determination of tafenoquine in small volume human plasma samples by high-performance liquid chromatography-tandem mass spectrometry. J Chromatogr B Analyt Technol Biomed Life Sci. 2002 Mar 25;769(1):127-32. PMID:11936685

Dreyer K, Fourie LJ, Kok DJ. The efficacy of used engine oil against ticks on cattle. Onderstepoort J Vet Res. 1998 Dec;65(4):275-9. PMID:10192839

Dua VK, Pandey AC, Dash AP. Adulticidal activity of essential oil of Lantana camara leaves against mosquitoes. Indian J Med Res. 2010 Mar;131:434-9. PMID:20418559

Duh D, Jelovsek M, Avsic-Zupanc T. Evaluation of an indirect fluorescence immunoassay for the detection of serum antibodies against Babesia divergens in humans. Parasitology. 2007 Feb;134(Pt 2):179-85. Epub 2006 Oct 11. PMID:17032478

Dunn MA, Quinn TC, Terwedow HA Jr. Pre-erythrocytic rodent malaria, Plasmodium berghei--prevention of development in the ethionine fatty liver. Am J Trop Med Hyg. 1972 May;21(3):288-92. PMID:5025613

Dvoraková HM, Dvoráckova M. [Babesiosis, a little known zoonosis].[Article in Czech]. Epidemiol Mikrobiol Imunol. 2007 Nov;56(4):176-80. PMID:18072299

Dy FJ. Present status of malaria control in Asia. Bull World Health Organ. 1954;11(4-5):725-63. PMID:13209318

East IJ, Zakrzewski H, Gale KR, Leatch G, Dimmock CM, Thomas MB, Waltisbuhl DJ. Vaccination against Babesia bovis: T cells from protected and unprotected animals show different cytokine profiles. Int J Parasitol. 1997 Dec;27(12):1537-45. PMID:9467739

Eberhard ML, Walker EM, Steurer FJ. Survival and infectivity of Babesia in blood maintained at 25 C and 2-4 C. J Parasitol. 1995 Oct;81(5):790-2. PMID:7472878

Echaide IE, de Echaide ST, Guglielmone AA. Live and soluble antigens for cattle protection to Babesia bigemina. Vet Parasitol. 1993 Dec;51(1-2):35-40. PMID:8128585

Eder AF, Dy BA, Barton J, Kennedy JM, Benjamin RJ. The American Red Cross Hemovigilance Program: advancing the safety of blood donation and transfusion. Immunohematology. 2009;25(4):179-85. PMID:20406027

Edstein MD, Kocisko DA, Brewer TG, Walsh DS, Eamsila C, Charles BG. Population pharmacokinetics of the new antimalarial agent tafenoquine in Thai soldiers. Br J Clin Pharmacol. 2001 Dec;52(6):663-70. PMID:11736877

Edstein MD, Kocisko DA, Walsh DS, Eamsila C, Charles BG, Rieckmann KH. Plasma concentrations of tafenoquine, a new long-acting antimalarial agent, in thai soldiers receiving monthly prophylaxis. Clin Infect Dis. 2003 Dec 15;37(12):1654-8. Epub 2003 Nov 20. PMID:14689348

Edstein MD, Nasveld PE, Kocisko DA, Kitchener SJ, Gatton ML, Rieckmann KH. Gender differences in gastrointestinal disturbances and plasma concentrations of tafenoquine in healthy volunteers after tafenoquine administration for post-exposure vivax malaria prophylaxis. Trans R Soc Trop Med Hyg. 2007 Mar;101(3):226-30. Epub 2006 Jun 30. PMID:16814823

Edstein MD, Walsh DS, Eamsila C, Sasiprapha T, Nasveld PE, Kitchener S, Rieckmann KH. Malaria prophylaxis/radical cure: recent experiences of the Australian Defence Force. Med Trop (Mars). 2001;61(1):56-8. PMID:11584657

Egdell HG, Stanfield JP. Paediatric neurology in Africa: a Ugandan report. Br Med J. 1972 Feb 26;1(5799):548-52. PMID:5015052

El-Bahnasawy MM, Morsy TA. Egyptian human babesiosis and general review. J Egypt Soc Parasitol. 2008 Apr;38(1):265-72. PMID:19143136

Elmes NJ, Nasveld PE, Kitchener SJ, Kocisko DA, Edstein MD. The efficacy and tolerability of three different regimens of tafenoquine versus primaquine for post-exposure prophylaxis of Plasmodium vivax malaria in the Southwest Pacific. Trans R Soc Trop Med Hyg. 2008 Nov;102(11):1095-101. Epub 2008 Jun 9. PMID:18541280

Emmerson FR, Knott SG, Callow LL. Vaccination with Babesia argentina in 5 beef herds in south-eastern Queensland. Aust Vet J. 1976 Oct;52(10):451-4. PMID:1016135

Englund L, Pringle J. New diseases and increased risk of diseases in companion animals and horses due to transport. Acta Vet Scand Suppl. 2003-2004;100:19-25. PMID:16429803

Enwere OO. Herbs in orthodox practice: a view by medical students. Afr J Tradit Complement Altern Med. 2009 Mar 7;6(2):203-6. PMID:20209013

Erbsloh JK. Babesiosis in the newborn foal. J Reprod Fertil Suppl. 1975 Oct;(23):725-6. PMID:1060872

Erol E, Kumar N, Carson CA. Immunogenicity of recombinant Babesia microti hsp70 homologue in mice. Int J Parasitol. 1999 Feb;29(2):263-6. PMID:10221626

Erp EE, Smith RD, Ristic M, Osorno BM. Optimization of the suspension culture method for in vitro cultivation of Babesia bovis. Am J Vet Res. 1980 Dec;41(12):2059-62. PMID:7212439

Eskow ES, Krause PJ, Spielman A, Freeman K, Aslanzadeh J. Southern extension of the range of human babesiosis in the eastern United States. J Clin Microbiol. 1999 Jun;37(6):2051-2. PMID:10325378

Evenson DA, Perry E, Kloster B, Hurley R, Stroncek DF. Therapeutic apheresis for babesiosis. J Clin Apher. 1998;13(1):32-6. PMID:9590496

Ezzelarab M, Yeh P, Wagner R, Cooper DK. Babesia as a complication of immunosuppression following pig-to-baboon heart transplantation. Xenotransplantation. 2007 Mar;14(2):162-5. PMID:17381691

Falagas ME, Klempner MS. Babesiosis in patients with AIDS: a chronic infection presenting as fever of unknown origin. Clin Infect Dis. 1996 May;22(5):809-12. PMID:8722936

Farzad E, Cator M, Giulivi A, Zhang J. Physician survey on knowledge and reporting practices of transfusion-transmitted infections in Canada. Can J Public Health. 2004 Nov-Dec;95(6):451-5. PMID:15622796

Fasan PO. The control of malaria in a holoendemic region. Niger Med J. 1973 Jul;3(3):124-7. PMID:16366343

Fawole OI, Akinboye DO, Falade CO, Arulogun OS, Adeniyi JD. Case management of childhood fever by traditional healers in southwest Nigeria: identification of training and collaborative needs. Int Q Community Health Educ. 2007-2008;28(4):319-35. PMID:19193526

Fawole OI, Onadeko MO. Knowledge and home management of malaria fever by mothers and care givers of under five children. West Afr J Med. 2001 Apr-Jun;20(2):152-7. PMID:11768016

Fell E. An update on Lyme disease and other tick-borne illnesses. Nurse Pract. 2000 Oct;25(10):38-40, 43-4, 47-8 passim; quiz 56-7. PMID:11068777

Fernandes Fde F, Freitas Ede P. Analysis of the use of fenthion via epicutaneous in dogs for Rhipicephalus sanguineus control. Rev Soc Bras Med Trop. 2001 Jul-Aug;34(4):339-42. PMID:11562726

Figueroa JV, Alvarez JA, Rojas EE, Ramos JA, Mosqueda JJ, Cantó GJ, Vega CA, Buening GM. Use of a duplex PCR/DNA probe assay to monitor Babesia bovis and Babesia bigemina in cattle during a vaccination trial. Rev Latinoam Microbiol. 1998 Jan-Jun;40(1-2):39-44. PMID:10932733

Filbin MR, Mylonakis EE, Callegari L, Legome E. Babesiosis. J Emerg Med. 2001 Jan;20(1):21-4. PMID:11165832

Finerty JF, Krehl EP. Cyclophosphamide pretreatment and protection against malaria. Infect Immun. 1976 Oct;14(4):1103-5. PMID:791863

Fink E. Assessment of causal prophylactic activity in Plasmodium berghei yoelii and its

value for the development of new antimalarial drugs. Bull World Health Organ. 1974;50(3-4):213-22. PMID: 4155355

Fink E, Dann O. [Further development of the Roehl test for testing antimalarial agents on Plasmodium cathemerium in the canary by intravenous administration].[Article in German]. Z Tropenmed Parasitol. 1967 Dec;18(4):466-74. PMID:5613461

Fish L, Leibovich B, Krigel Y, McElwain T, Shkap V. Vaccination of cattle against B. bovis infection with live attenuated parasites and non-viable immunogens. Vaccine. 2008 Dec 19;26 Suppl 6:G29-33. PMID:19178890

Fish L, Pipano E, Indrakamhang P. Lyophilised bovine serum as a substitute for frozen serum in the cultivation of Babesia bigemina and B bovis. Res Vet Sci. 1992 Jan;52(1):115-6. PMID:1553430

Fleck SL, Robinson BL, Peters W. The chemotherapy of rodent malaria. LIV. Combinations of 'Fenozan B07' (Fenozan-50F), a difluorinated 3,3'-spirocyclopentane 1,2,4-trioxane, with other drugs against drug-sensitive and drug-resistant parasites. Ann Trop Med Parasitol. 1997 Jan;91(1):33-9. PMID:9093427

Fletcher TI, Wigg JL, Rolls PJ, de Vos AJ. Viability assays of intra-erythrocytic organisms using fluorescent dyes. Vet Parasitol. 2009 Jul 7;163(1-2):144-7. Epub 2009 Mar 31. PMID:19380205

Floch H. [Development of the malaria campaign in French Guiana from 1950 to 1954].[Article in French]. Publ Inst Pasteur Guyane Fr Inini. 1954 Nov;15(345):1-8. PMID:14377655

Florescu D, Sordillo PP, Glyptis A, Zlatanic E, Smith B, Polsky B, Sordillo E. Splenic infarction in human babesiosis: two cases and discussion. Clin Infect Dis. 2008 Jan 1;46(1):e8-11. PMID:18171204

Florin-Christensen M, Schnittger L, Dominguez M, Mesplet M, Rodríguez A, Ferreri L, Asenzo G, Wilkowsky S, Farber M, Echaide I, Suarez C. Search for Babesia bovis vaccine candidates. Parassitologia. 2007 May;49 Suppl 1:9-12. PMID:17691600

Foppa IM, Krause PJ, Spielman A, Goethert H, Gern L, Brand B, Telford SR 3rd. Entomologic and serologic evidence of zoonotic transmission of Babesia microti, eastern Switzerland. Emerg Infect Dis. 2002 Jul;8(7):722-6. PMID:12095442

Fowler JL, Ruff MD, Fernau RC, Furusho Y. Babesia gibsoni: chemotherapy in dogs. Am J Vet Res. 1972 Jun;33(6):1109-14. PMID:5022393

Fox LM, Wingerter S, Ahmed A, Arnold A, Chou J, Rhein L, Levy O. Neonatal babesiosis: case report and review of the literature. Pediatr Infect Dis J. 2006 Feb;25(2):169-73. PMID:16462298

Freeman MJ, Kirby BM, Panciera DL, Henik RA, Rosin E, Sullivan LJ. Hypotensive shock syndrome associated with acute Babesia canis infection in a dog. J Am Vet Med Assoc. 1994 Jan 1;204(1):94-6. PMID:8125828

Frerichs WM, Allen PC, Holbrook AA. Equine piroplasmosis (Babesia equi): therapeutic trials of imidocarb dihydrochloride in horses and donkeys. Vet Rec. 1973 Jul 21;93(3):73-5. PMID:4748680

Frerichs WM, Holbrook AA. Treatment of equine piroplasmosis (B caballi) with imidocarb dipropionate. Vet Rec. 1974 Aug 31;95(9):188-9. PMID:4450446

Froberg MK, Dannen D, Bakken JS. Babesiosis and HIV. Lancet. 2004 Feb 28;363(9410):704. PMID:15001329

Froberg MK, Dannen D, Bernier N, Shieh WJ, Guarner J, Zaki S. Case report: spontaneous splenic rupture during acute parasitemia of Babesia microti. Ann Clin Lab Sci. 2008 Autumn;38(4):390-2. PMID:18988934

Frölich S, Entzeroth R, Wallach M. Comparison of protective immune responses to apicomplexan parasites. J Parasitol Res. 2012;2012:852591. Epub 2011 Aug 18. PMID:21876783

Fukumoto S, Tamaki Y, Igarashi I, Suzuki H, Xuan X. Immunogenicity and growth inhibitory efficacy of the prime-boost immunization regime with DNA followed by recombinant vaccinia virus carrying the P29 gene of Babesia gibsoni in dogs. Exp Parasitol. 2009 Dec;123(4):296-301. Epub 2009 Aug 25. PMID:19712674

Fukumoto S, Tamaki Y, Okamura M, Bannai H, Yokoyama N, Suzuki T, Igarashi I, Suzuki H, Xuan X. Prime-boost immunization with DNA followed by a recombinant vaccinia virus expressing P50 induced protective immunity against Babesia gibsoni infection in dogs. Vaccine. 2007 Jan 26;25(7):1334-41. Epub 2006 Oct 10. PMID:17055131

Fukumoto S, Tamaki Y, Shirafuji H, Harakawa S, Suzuki H, Xuan X. Immunization with recombinant surface antigen P50 of Babesia gibsoni expressed in insect cells induced parasite growth inhibition in dogs. Clin Diagn Lab Immunol. 2005 Apr;12(4):557-9. PMID:15817768

Fukumoto S, Xuan X, Igarashi I, Zhang S, Mugisha J, Ogata T, Nagasawa H, Fujisaki K, Suzuki N, Mikami T. Morphological changes of Babesia gibsoni grown in canine red blood cell-substituted severe combined immune deficiency mice. J Parasitol. 2000 Oct;86(5):956-8. PMID:11128518.

Fukumoto S, Xuan X, Kadota K, Igarashi I, Sugimoto C, Fujisaki K, Nagasawa H, Mikami T, Suzuki H. High-level expression of truncated surface antigen P50 of Babesia gibsoni in insect cells by baculovirus and evaluation of its immunogenicity and antigenicity. Clin Diagn Lab Immunol. 2003 Jul;10(4):596-601. PMID:12853391

Fukumoto S, Xuan X, Takabatake N, Igarashi I, Sugimoto C, Fujisaki K, Nagasawa H, Mikami T, Suzuki H. Inhibitory effect of antiserum to surface antigen P50 of Babesia gibsoni on growth of parasites in severe combined immunodeficiency mice given canine red blood cells. Infect Immun. 2004 Mar;72(3):1795-8. PMID:14977989

Galay RL, Maeda H, Aung KM, Umemiya-Shirafuji R, Xuan X, Igarashi I, Tsuji N, Tanaka T, Fujisaki K. Anti-babesial activity of a potent peptide fragment derived from longicin of Haemaphysalis longicornis. Trop Anim Health Prod. 2011 Nov 20. [Epub ahead of print]

PMID:22102016

Gallagher LG, Chau S, Owaisi AS, Konczyk M, Bishop HS, Arguin PM, Trenholme GM. An 84-year-old woman with fever and dark urine. Clin Infect Dis. 2009 Jul 15;49(2):278, 310-1. PMID:19538064

Garnham PC, Warren M, Killick-Kendrick R. The action of 'terramycin' on the primary exoerythrocytic development of Plasmodium vivax and Plasmodium cynomolgi ceylonensis. J Trop Med Hyg. 1971 Feb;74(2):32-5. PMID:4993964

Garrett-Jones C, Gramiccia G. Evidence of the development of resistance to DDT by Anopheles sacharovi in the Levant. Bull World Health Organ. 1954;11(4-5):865-83. PMID:13209325

Gary AT, Webb JA, Hegarty BC, Breitschwerdt EB. The low seroprevalence of tick-transmitted agents of disease in dogs from southern Ontario and Quebec. Can Vet J. 2006 Dec;47(12):1194-200. PMID:17217089

Gear JH. The occurrence and diagnosis of malaria. S Afr Med J. 1974 May 25;48(25):1078-84. PMID:4602110

Gerber MA, Shapiro ED, Krause PJ, Cable RG, Badon SJ, Ryan RW. The risk of acquiring Lyme disease or babesiosis from a blood transfusion. J Infect Dis. 1994 Jul;170(1):231-4. PMID:8014507

Gern L, Lienhard R, Péter O. [Diseases and pathogenic agents transmitted by ticks in Switzerland].[Article in French]. Rev Med Suisse. 2010 Oct 13;6(266):1906-9. PMID:21089555

Gero AM, Wood AM. New nucleoside transport pathways induced in the host erythrocyte membrane of malaria and Babesia infected cells. Adv Exp Med Biol. 1991;309A:169-72. PMID:1789200

Gharoro EP, Igbafe AA. Pattern of drug use amongst antenatal patients in Benin City, Nigeria. Med Sci Monit. 2000 Jan-Feb;6(1):84-7. PMID:11208289

Gill AC, Cowman AF, Stewart NP, Kemp DJ, Timms P. Babesia bovis: molecular and biological characteristics of cloned parasite lines. Exp Parasitol. 1987 Apr;63(2):180-8. PMID:3032666

Gillet J, Herman F. [Development of Plasmodium berghei berghei in mice embryos].[Article in French]. C R Seances Soc Biol Fil. 1971;165(9):2029-31. PMID:4263149

Gleason NN, Wolf RE. Entopolypoides macaci (Babesiidae) in Macaca mulatta. J Parasitol. 1974 Oct;60(5):844-7. PMID:4214908

Gleckman RA, Roth RM. Fever following abdominal surgery. Unusual infectious causes. Postgrad Med. 1986 Feb 1;79(2):287-94. PMID:3945600

Goethert HK, Telford SR 3rd. Enzootic transmission of Babesia divergens among cottontail rabbits on Nantucket Island, Massachusetts. Am J Trop Med Hyg. 2003 Nov;69(5):455-60. PMID:14695079

Goheen MP, Bartlett MS, Shaw MM, Queener SF, Smith JW. Effects of 8-aminoquinolines on the ultrastructural morphology of Pneumocystis carinii. Int J Exp Pathol. 1993 Aug;74(4):379-87. PMID:8398811

Golightly LM, Hirschhorn LR, Weller PF. Fever and headache in a splenectomized woman. Rev Infect Dis. 1989 Jul-Aug;11(4):629-37. PMID:2772469

Gonçalves PM, Passos LM, Ribeiro MF. Detection of IgM antibodies against Babesia bovis in cattle. Vet Parasitol. 1999 Mar 22;82(1):11-7. PMID:10223346

González EF, Todorovic RA, Thompson KC. Immunization against anaplasmosis and babesiosis: Part I. Evaluation of immunization using minimum infective doses under laboratory conditions. Tropenmed Parasitol. 1976 Dec;27(4):427-37. PMID:1006801

Goo YK, Terkawi MA, Jia H, Aboge GO, Ooka H, Nelson B, Kim S, Sunaga F, Namikawa K, Igarashi I, Nishikawa Y, Xuan X. Artesunate, a potential drug for treatment of Babesia infection. Parasitol Int. 2010 Sep;59(3):481-6. Epub 2010 Jun 9. PMID:20541037

Goodger BV, Commins MA, Waltisbuhl DJ, Wright IG, Rode-Bramanis K. Babesia bovis: immunity induced by vaccination with a lipid enriched fraction. Int J Parasitol. 1990 Aug;20(5):685-7. PMID:2228430

Goodger BV, Commins MA, Wright IG, Mirre GB, Waltisbuhl DJ, White M. Babesia bovis: vaccination trial with a dominant immunodiffusion antigen in splenectomised calves. Z Parasitenkd. 1986;72(6):715-22. PMID:3099492

Goodger BV, Commins MA, Wright IG, Waltisbuhl DJ, Mirre GB. Successful homologous vaccination against Babesia bovis using a heparin-binding fraction of infected erythrocytes. Int J Parasitol. 1987 Apr;17(4):935-40. PMID:3583543

Goodger BV, Waltisbuhl DJ, Commins MA, Wright IG. Babesia bovis: dextran sulphate as an adjuvant for and precipitant of protective immunogens. Int J Parasitol. 1992 Jul;22(4):465-9.

PMID:1644521

Goodger BV, Waltisbuhl DJ, Wright IG, Mahoney DF, Commins MA. Babesia bovis--analysis and vaccination trial with the cryoprecipitable immune complex. Vet Immunol Immunopathol. 1987 Jan;14(1):57-65. PMID:3103316

Goodger BV, Waltisbuhl DJ, Wright IG, White M. Babesia bovis: analysis of and preliminary vaccination studies with a defined infected erythrocyte membrane binding antigen. Int J Parasitol. 1992 Jul;22(4):533-5. PMID:1644530

Goodger BV, Wright IG, Mahoney DF. The use of pathophysiological reactions to assess the efficacy of the immune response to Babesia bovis in cattle. Z Parasitenkd. 1981;66(1):41-8. PMID:6172907

Goodger BV, Wright IG, Waltisbuhl DJ. The lysate from bovine erythrocytes infected with Babesia bovis. Analysis of antigens and a report on their immunogenicity when polymerized with glutaraldehyde. Z Parasitenkd. 1983;69(4):473-82. PMID:6414195

Goodger BV, Wright IG, Waltisbuhl DJ, Mirre GB. Babesia bovis: successful vaccination against homologous challenge in splenectomised calves using a fraction of haemagglutinating antigen. Int J Parasitol. 1985 Apr;15(2):175-9. PMID:3997349

Gordon S, Cordon RA, Mazdzer EJ, Valigorsky JM, Blagg NA, Barnes SJ. Adult respiratory distress syndrome in babesiosis. Chest. 1984 Oct;86(4):633-4. PMID:6541117

Gorenflot A, Bazin C, Ambroise-Thomas P. [Human babesiosis. Treatment of severe forms].[Article in French]. Presse Med. 1987 Jun 13;16(22):1099. PMID:2955343

Gorenflot A, Brasseur P, Bonmarchand G, Laneele D, Simonin D. [2 cases of severe human babesiosis treated successfully].[Article in French]. Presse Med. 1990 Feb 24;19(7):335. PMID:2138308

Gorenflot A, Moubri K, Precigout E, Carcy B, Schetters TP. Human babesiosis. Ann Trop Med Parasitol. 1998 Jun;92(4):489-501. PMID:9683900

Gorenflot A, Precigout E, Bissuel G, Lecointre O, Brasseur P, Vidor E, L'Hostis M, Schrevel J. Identification of major Babesia divergens polypeptides that induce protection against homologous challenge in gerbils. Infect Immun. 1990 Dec;58(12):4076-82. PMID:2254031

Gorenflot A, Precigout E, Valentin A, Bissuel G, Carcy B, Brasseur P, Moreau Y, Schrevel J. Babesia divergens vaccine. Mem Inst Oswaldo Cruz. 1992;87 Suppl 3:279-81. PMID:1343703

Grabowski EF, Giardina PJ, Goldberg D, Masur H, Read SE, Hirsch RL, Benach JL. Babesiosis transmitted by a transfusion of frozen-thawed blood. Ann Intern Med. 1982 Apr;96(4):466-7. PMID:7199884

Graham HA, Palczuk NC, Stauber LA. Immunity to exoerythrocytic forms of malaria. II. Passive transfer of immunity to exoerythrocytic forms. Exp Parasitol. 1973 Dec;34(3):372-81. PMID:4773576

Graham HA, Stauber LA, Palczuk NC, Barnes WD. Immunity to exoerythrocytic forms of malaria. I. Course of infection of Plasmodium fallax in turkeys. Exp Parasitol. 1973 Dec;34(3):364-71. PMID:4773575

Gray GD, Phillips RS. Use of sorbitol in the cryopreservation of babesia. Res Vet Sci. 1981 May;30(3):388-9. PMID:7255935

Gray GD, Phillips RS. Suppression of primary and secondary antibody responses and inhibition of antigen priming during Babesia microti infections in mice. Parasite Immunol. 1983 Mar;5(2):123-34. PMID:6844029

Gray JS, Gannon P. Preliminary development of a live drug-controlled vaccine against bovine babesiosis using the Mongolian gerbil, Meriones unguiculatus. Vet Parasitol. 1992 May;42(3-4):179-88. PMID:1496778

Gray JS, Langley RJ, Brophy PO, Gannon P. Vaccination against bovine babesiosis with drug-controlled live parasites. Vet Rec. 1989 Sep 30;125(14):369-72. PMID:2683338

Gray JS, Pudney M. Activity of atovaquone against Babesia microti in the Mongolian gerbil, Meriones unguiculatus. J Parasitol. 1999 Aug;85(4):723-8. PMID:10461956

Gregory KG, Peters W. The chemotherapy of rodent malaria. IX. Causal prophylaxis. I. A method for demonstrating drug action on exo-erythrocytic stages. Ann Trop Med Parasitol. 1970 Mar;64(1):15-24. PMID:5485706

Grellier P, Benach J, Labaied M, Charneau S, Gil H, Monsalve G, Alfonso R, Sawyer L, Lin L, Steiert M, Dupuis K. Photochemical inactivation with amotosalen and long-wavelength ultraviolet light of Plasmodium and Babesia in platelet and plasma components. Transfusion. 2008 Aug;48(8):1676-84. Epub 2008 May 22. PMID:18503613

Grellier P, Santus R, Mouray E, Agmon V, Mazière JC, Rigomier D, Dagan A, Gatt S, Schrével J. Photosensitized inactivation of Plasmodium falciparum- and Babesia divergens-infected erythrocytes in whole blood by lipophilic pheophorbide derivatives. Vox Sang. 1997;72(4):211-20. PMID:9228710

Grima KM. Therapeutic apheresis in hematological and oncological diseases. J Clin Apher. 2000;15(1-2):28-52. PMID:10767050

Grimble RF, Tappia PS. Modulation of pro-inflammatory cytokine biology by unsaturated fatty acids. Z Ernahrungswiss. 1998;37 Suppl 1:57-65. PMID:9558730

Guan G, Chauvin A, Luo J, Inoue N, Moreau E, Liu Z, Gao J, Thekisoe OM, Ma M, Liu A, Dang Z, Liu J, Ren Q, Jin Y, Sugimoto C, Yin H. The development and evaluation of a loop-mediated isothermal amplification (LAMP) method for detection of Babesia spp. infective to sheep and goats in China. Exp Parasitol. 2008 Sep;120(1):39-44. Epub 2008 Apr 18. PMID:18504039

Guan G, Chauvin A, Yin H, Luo J, Moreau E. Course of infection by Babesia sp. BQ1 (Lintan) and B. divergens in sheep depends on the production of IFNgamma and IL10. Parasite Immunol. 2010 Feb;32(2):143-52. PMID:20070828

Gubernot DM, Lucey CT, Lee KC, Conley GB, Holness LG, Wise RP. Babesia infection through blood transfusions: reports received by the US Food and Drug Administration, 1997-2007. Clin Infect Dis. 2009 Jan 1;48(1):25-30. PMID:19035776

Gubernot DM, Nakhasi HL, Mied PA, Asher DM, Epstein JS, Kumar S. Transfusion-transmitted babesiosis in the United States: summary of a workshop. Transfusion. 2009 Dec;49(12):2759-71. Epub 2009 Oct 10. PMID:19821952

Guerrero FD, Miller RJ, Rousseau ME, Sunkara S, Quackenbush J, Lee Y, Nene V. BmiGI: a database of cDNAs expressed in Boophilus microplus, the tropical/southern cattle tick. Insect Biochem Mol Biol. 2005 Jun;35(6):585-95. Epub 2005 Mar 27. PMID:15857764

Guglielmone AA, Lugaresi CI, Volpogni MM, Anziani OS, Vanzini VR. Babesial antibody dynamics after cattle immunisation with live vaccines, measured

with an indirect immunofluorescence test. Vet Parasitol. 1997 Jun;70(1-3):33-9. PMID:9195707

Gummow B, Swan GE, Du Preez JL. A bioequivalence and pharmacokinetic evaluation of two commercial diminazene aceturate formulations administered intramuscularly to cattle. Onderstepoort J Vet Res. 1994 Dec;61(4):317-26. PMID:7501363

Gupta P, Hurley RW, Helseth PH, Goodman JL, Hammerschmidt DE. Pancytopenia due to hemophagocytic syndrome as the presenting manifestation of babesiosis. Am J Hematol. 1995 Sep;50(1):60-2. PMID:7668227

Gutman JD, Kotton CN, Kratz A. Case records of the Massachusetts General Hospital. Weekly clinicopathological exercises. Case 29-2003. A 60-year-old man with fever, rigors, and sweats. N Engl J Med. 2003 Sep 18;349(12):1168-75. PMID:13679532

Gutteridge WE. Antimalarial drugs currently in development. J R Soc Med. 1989;82 Suppl 17:63-6; discussion 66-8. PMID:2693729

Gwadz RW. Successful immunization against the sexual stages of Plasmodium gallinaceum. Science. 1976 Sep 17;193(4258):1150-1. PMID:959832

Hagimori I, Machida H, Goi R, Mencke N. Efficacy of imidacloprid/permethrin and fipronil/(S)-methoprene combinations against Haemaphysalis longicornis ticks evaluated under in vitro and in vivo conditions. Parasitol Res. 2005 Oct;97 Suppl 1:S120-6. PMID:16228268

Hale BR, Owusu-Agyei S, Fryauff DJ, Koram KA, Adjuik M, Oduro AR, Prescott WR, Baird JK, Nkrumah F, Ritchie TL, Franke ED, Binka FN, Horton J, Hoffman SL. A randomized, double-blind, placebo-controlled, dose-ranging trial of tafenoquine for weekly prophylaxis against Plasmodium falciparum. Clin Infect Dis. 2003 Mar 1;36(5):541-9. Epub 2003 Feb 14. PMID:12594633

Hamer SA, Tsao JI, Walker ED, Mansfield LS, Foster ES, Hickling GJ. Use of tick surveys and serosurveys to evaluate pet dogs as a sentinel species for emerging Lyme disease. Am J Vet Res. 2009 Jan;70(1):49-56. PMID:19119948

Han JI, Lee SJ, Jang HJ, Na KJ. Asymptomatic Babesia microti-like parasite infection in wild raccoon dogs (Nyctereutes procyonoides) in South Korea. J Wildl Dis. 2010 Apr;46(2):632-5. PMID:20688664

Hanafusa Y, Onuma M, Kamiyama T. Partial protection of severe combined immunodeficient mice against infection with Babesia microti by in vitro-generated CD4+ T cell clones. J Vet Med Sci. 1998 Apr;60(4):401-4. PMID:9592710

Hansford CF. The use of antimalarial drugs. S Afr Med J. 1974 Jun 22;48(30):1314-6. PMID:4605355

Harrison KA, Ibeziako PA. Maternal anaemia and fetal birthweight. J Obstet Gynaecol Br Commonw. 1973 Sep;80(9):798-804. PMID:4743068

Harvey WT, Martz D. Motor neuron disease recovery associated with IV ceftriaxone and anti-Babesia therapy. Acta Neurol Scand. 2007 Feb;115(2):129-31. PMID:17212618

Harwin RM. Gametocytes, sporozoites and liver schizonts. S Afr Med J. 1974 Jun 1;48(26):1123-4. PMID:4135674

Häselbarth K, Kurz M, Hunfeld KP, Krieger G. [Babesiosis in an immunocompromised German patient].[Article in German]. Med Klin (Munich). 2008 Feb 15;103(2):104-7. PMID:18270666

Häselbarth K, Tenter AM, Brade V, Krieger G, Hunfeld KP. First case of human babesiosis in Germany - Clinical presentation and molecular characterisation of the pathogen. Int J Med Microbiol. 2007 Jun;297(3):197-204. Epub 2007 Mar 12. PMID:17350888

Hashemi-Fesharki R. Ovine and caprine babesiosis in Iran: treatment with imidocarb. Vet Rec. 1991 Oct 26;129(17):383-4. PMID:1746117

Hatcher JC, Greenberg PD, Antique J, Jimenez-Lucho VE. Severe babesiosis in Long Island: review of 34 cases and their complications. Clin Infect Dis. 2001 Apr 15;32(8):1117-25. Epub 2001 Mar 26. PMID:11283800

Hemmer RM, Wozniak EJ, Lowenstine LJ, Plopper CG, Wong V, Conrad PA. Endothelial cell changes are associated with pulmonary edema and respiratory distress in mice infected with the WA1 human Babesia parasite. J Parasitol. 1999 Jun;85(3):479-89. PMID:10386441

Hentrich B, Böse R. Cryopreservation of Babesia divergens from jirds as a live vaccine for cattle. Int J Parasitol. 1993 Sep;23(6):771-6. PMID:8300287

Hentrich B, Böse R, Doherr M. Cryopreservation of Babesia caballi cultures. Int J Parasitol. 1994 Apr;24(2):253-4. PMID:8026902

Herman JH, Ayache S, Olkowska D. Autoimmunity in transfusion babesiosis: a spectrum of clinical presentations. J Clin Apher. 2010;25(6):358-61. Epub 2010 Sep 7. PMID:20824620

Herman R, Shiroishi T. Plasmodium gallinaceum: selective immunosuppression by cyclophosphamide in preerythrocytic malaria. Exp Parasitol. 1973 Oct;34(2):295-305. PMID:4583057

Herman R, Shiroishi T, Buckler CE. Viral interference with exoerythrocytic forms of malaria (Plasmodium gallinaceum) in ovo. J Infect Dis. 1973 Aug;128(2):148-55. PMID:4353044

Hermanowska-Szpakowicz T, Skotarczak B, Kondrusik M, Rymaszewska A, Sawczuk M, Maciejewska A, Adamska M, Pancewicz S, Zajkowska J. Detecting DNAs of Anaplasma phagocytophilum and Babesia in the blood of patients suspected of Lyme disease. Ann Agric Environ Med. 2004;11(2):351-4. PMID:15627349

Herod E, Clark IA, Allison AC. Protection of mice against haemoprotozoan Babesia microti with Brucella abortus strain 19. Clin Exp Immunol. 1978 Mar;31(3):518-23. PMID:95914

Herwaldt BL, Cacciò S, Gherlinzoni F, Aspöck H, Slemenda SB, Piccaluga P, Martinelli G, Edelhofer R, Hollenstein U, Poletti G, Pampiglione S, Löschenberger , Tura S, Pieniazek NJ. Molecular characterization of a non-Babesia divergens organism causing zoonotic babesiosis in Europe. Emerg Infect Dis. 2003 Aug;9(8):942-8. PMID:12967491

Herwaldt BL, Kjemtrup AM, Conrad PA, Barnes RC, Wilson M, McCarthy MG, Sayers MH, Eberhard ML. Transfusion-transmitted babesiosis in Washington State: first reported case caused by a WA1-type parasite. J Infect Dis. 1997 May;175(5):1259-62. PMID:9129100

Herwaldt BL, Linden JV, Bosserman E, Young C, Olkowska D, Wilson M. Transfusion-associated babesiosis in the United States: a description of cases. Ann Intern Med. 2011 Oct 18;155(8):509-19. Epub 2011 Sep 5. PMID:21893613

Herwaldt BL, McGovern PC, Gerwel MP, Easton RM, MacGregor RR. Endemic babesiosis in another eastern state: New Jersey. Emerg Infect Dis. 2003 Feb;9(2):184-8. PMID:12603988

Herwaldt BL, Neitzel DF, Gorlin JB, Jensen KA, Perry EH, Peglow WR, Slemenda SB,

Won KY, Nace EK, Pieniazek NJ, Wilson M. Transmission of Babesia microti in Minnesota through four blood donations from the same donor over a 6-month period. Transfusion. 2002 Sep;42(9):1154-8. PMID:12430672

Herwaldt BL, Springs FE, Roberts PP, Eberhard ML, Case K, Persing DH, Agger WA. Babesiosis in Wisconsin: a potentially fatal disease. Am J Trop Med Hyg. 1995 Aug;53(2):146-51. PMID:7677215

Heyman P, Cochez C, Hofhuis A, van der Giessen J, Sprong H, Porter SR, Losson B, Saegerman C, Donoso-Mantke O, Niedrig M, Papa A. A clear and present danger: tick-borne diseases in Europe. Expert Rev Anti Infect Ther. 2010 Jan;8(1):33-50. PMID:20014900

Hildebrandt A, Hunfeld KP, Baier M, Krumbholz A, Sachse S, Lorenzen T, Kiehntopf M, Fricke HJ, Straube E. First confirmed autochthonous case of human Babesia microti infection in Europe. Eur J Clin Microbiol Infect Dis. 2007 Aug;26(8):595-601. PMID:17587072

Hilton E, DeVoti J, Benach JL, Halluska ML, White DJ, Paxton H, Dumler JS. Seroprevalence and seroconversion for tick-borne diseases in a high-risk population in the northeast United States. Am J Med. 1999 Apr;106(4):404-9. PMID:10225242

Hinaidy HK. [Bovine babesiasis in Austria. IV. Studies with killed vaccines].[Article in German]. Berl Munch Tierarztl Wochenschr. 1981 Apr 1;94(7):121-5. PMID:7247917

Hines SA, Palmer GH, Jasmer DP, Goff WL, McElwain TF. Immunization of cattle with recombinant Babesia bovis merozoite surface antigen-1. Infect Immun. 1995 Jan;63(1):349-52. PMID:7806376

Hjelm K, Mufunda E. Zimbabwean diabetics' beliefs about health and illness: an interview study. BMC Int Health Hum Rights. 2010 May 12;10:7. PMID:20462425

Hohenschild S. [Babesiosis--a dangerous infection for splenectomized children and adults].[Article in German]. Klin Padiatr. 1999 May-Jun;211(3):137-40. PMID:10412122

Hollenberg D, Zakus D, Cook T, Xu XW. Re-positioning the role of traditional, complementary and alternative medicine as essential health knowledge in global health: do they still have a role to play? World Health Popul. 2008;10(4):62-75. PMID:19550163

Holman PJ, Frerichs WM, Chieves L, Wagner GG. Culture confirmation of the carrier status of Babesia caballi-infected horses. J Clin Microbiol. 1993 Mar;31(3):698-701. PMID:8458966

Holman PJ, Petrini K, Rhyan J, Wagner GG. In vitro isolation and cultivation of a Babesia from an American woodland caribou (Rangifer tarandus caribou). J Wildl Dis. 1994 Apr;30(2):195-200. PMID:7913142

Holman PJ, Spencer AM, Droleskey RE, Goethert HK, Telford SR 3rd. In vitro cultivation of a zoonotic Babesia sp. isolated from eastern cottontail rabbits (Sylvilagus floridanus) on Nantucket Island, Massachusetts. J Clin Microbiol. 2005 Aug;43(8):3995-4001. PMID:16081941

Holman PJ, Spencer AM, Telford SR 3rd, Goethert HK, Allen AJ, Knowles DP, Goff WL. Comparative infectivity of Babesia divergens and a zoonotic Babesia divergens-like parasite in cattle. Am J Trop Med Hyg. 2005 Nov;73(5):865-70. PMID:16282295

Holman PJ, Waldrup KA, Droleskey RE, Corrier DE, Wagner GG. In vitro growth of Babesia bovis in white-tailed deer (Odocoileus virginianus) erythrocytes. J Parasitol. 1993 Apr;79(2):233-7. PMID:8459334

Holman PJ, Waldrup KA, Wagner GG. In vitro cultivation of a Babesia isolated from a white-tailed deer (Odocoileus virginianus). J Parasitol. 1988 Feb;74(1):111-5. PMID:3357095

Homer MJ, Aguilar-Delfin I, Telford SR 3rd, Krause PJ, Persing DH. Babesiosis. Clin Microbiol Rev. 2000 Jul;13(3):451-69. PMID:10885987

Homer MJ, Lodes MJ, Reynolds LD, Zhang Y, Douglass JF, McNeill PD, Houghton RL, Persing DH. Identification and characterization of putative secreted antigens from Babesia microti. J Clin Microbiol. 2003 Feb;41(2):723-9. PMID:12574273

Horowitz ML, Coletta F, Fein AM. Delayed onset adult respiratory distress syndrome in babesiosis. Chest. 1994 Oct;106(4):1299-301. PMID:7924525

Houghton RL, Homer MJ, Reynolds LD, Sleath PR, Lodes MJ, Berardi V, Leiby DA, Persing DH. Identification of Babesia microti-specific immunodominant epitopes and development of a peptide EIA for detection of antibodies in serum. Transfusion. 2002 Nov;42(11):1488-96. PMID:12421223

Huang X, Xuan X, Yokoyama N, Katayama Y, Anzai T, Igarashi I. Evaluation of enzyme-linked immunosorbent assays with recombinant antigens for the serodiagnosis of equine Babesia infections. Vet Parasitol. 2006 Aug 31;140(1-2):158-61. Epub 2006 Apr 18. PMID:16621293

Hughes CC, Hunter JM. Disease and "development" in Africa. Soc Sci Med. 1970 Apr;3(4):443-93. PMID:5483543

Hughes WT, Oz HS. Successful prevention and treatment of babesiosis with atovaquone. J Infect Dis. 1995 Oct;172(4):1042-6. PMID:7561178

Hugoson G. Studies on lymphocytosis in regions with high and low incidences of bovine leukosis and babesiosis. Bibl Haematol. 1970;(36):537-43. PMID:5538363.

Hugoson G, Vennström R, Henriksson K. The occurrence of bovine leukosis following the introduction of babesiosis vaccination. Bibl Haematol. 1968;30:157-61. PMID:5695478

Hunfeld KP, Allwinn R, Peters S, Kraiczy P, Brade V. Serologic evidence for tick-borne pathogens other than Borrelia burgdorferi (TOBB) in Lyme borreliosis patients from midwestern Germany. Wien Klin Wochenschr. 1998 Dec 23;110(24):901-8. PMID:10048174

Hunfeld KP, Brade V. Zoonotic Babesia: possibly emerging pathogens to be considered for tick-infested humans in Central Europe. Int J Med Microbiol. 2004 Apr;293 Suppl 37:93-103. PMID:15146990

Hunfeld KP, Hildebrandt A, Gray JS. Babesiosis: recent insights into an ancient disease. Int J Parasitol. 2008 Sep;38(11):1219-37. Epub 2008 Mar 20. PMID:18440005

Hunfeld KP, Lambert A, Kampen H, Albert S, Epe C, Brade V, Tenter AM. Seroprevalence of Babesia infections in humans exposed to ticks in Midwestern Germany. J Clin Microbiol. 2002 Jul;40(7):2431-6. PMID:12089258

Hutchings CL, Li A, Fernandez KM, Fletcher T, Jackson LA, Molloy JB, Jorgensen WK, Lim CT, Cooke BM. New insights into the altered adhesive and mechanical properties of red blood cells parasitized by Babesia bovis. Mol Microbiol. 2007 Aug;65(4):1092-105. Epub 2007 Jul 19. PMID:17640278

Huwer M, Schwarzmaier A, Hamel HD, Will R. [The occurrence of Babesia divergens in the Freiburg i. Br. district and piroplasmosis prevention trials in cattle].[Article in German]. Berl Munch Tierarztl Wochenschr. 1994 Jun;107(6):198-202. PMID:8067991

Ibidapo CA. Perception of causes of malaria and treatment-seeking behaviour of nursing mothers in a rural community. Aust J Rural Health. 2005 Aug;13(4):214-8. PMID:16048462

Idowu ET, Mafe MA, Otubanjo OA, Adeneye AK. Herbal remedy in the treatment of malaria: cross sectional survey of residents of Lagos State, Nigeria. Afr J Med Med Sci. 2006 Jun;35(2):149-53. PMID:17209310

Idowu OR, Peggins JO, Brewer TG, Kelley C. Metabolism of a candidate 8-aminoquinoline antimalarial agent, WR 238605, by rat liver microsomes. Drug Metab Dispos. 1995 Jan;23(1):1-17. PMID:7720510

Igarashi I, Suzuki R, Waki S, Tagawa Y, Seng S, Tum S, Omata Y, Saito A, Nagasawa H, Iwakura Y, Suzuki N, Mikami T, Toyoda Y. Roles of CD4(+) T cells and gamma interferon in protective immunity against Babesia microti infection in mice. Infect Immun. 1999 Aug;67(8):4143-8. PMID:10417185

Ijarotimi SO, Agbedahunsi JM, Onyeji CO, Adewunmi CO. Chemotherapeutic interaction between Khaya grandifoliola (WELW) CDC stem bark extract and two anti-malarial drugs in mice. Afr J Tradit Complement Altern Med. 2010;7(4):370-6. Epub 2010 Jul 3. PMID:21731168

Ilchmann G. [New findings on the immunology of protozoan blood parasitoses in domestic animals].[Article in German]. Beitr Trop Landwirtsch Veterinarmed. 1978;16(3):305-12. PMID:373747

Innocent E, Joseph CC, Gikonyo NK, Nkunya MH, Hassanali A. Constituents of the essential oil of Suregada zanzibariensis leaves are repellent to the mosquito, Anopheles gambiae s.s. J Insect Sci. 2010;10:57. PMID:20569134

Irvin AD. Control of tick-borne diseases. Int J Parasitol. 1987 Feb;17(2):649-57. PMID:3294675

Israili ZH, Lyoussi B. Ethnopharmacology of the plants of genus Ajuga. Pak J Pharm Sci. 2009 Oct;22(4):425-62. PMID:19783524

Ittarat I, Webster HK, Yuthavong Y. High-performance liquid chromatographic determination of dihydroorotate dehydrogenase of Plasmodium falciparum and effects of antimalarials on enzyme activity. J Chromatogr. 1992 Nov 6;582(1-2):57-64. PMID:1491058

Jack RM, Ward PA. Babesia rodhaini interactions with complement: relationship to parasitic entry into red cells. J Immunol. 1980 Apr;124(4):1566-73. PMID:6767771

Jackson LA, Waldron SJ, Weier HM, Nicoll CL, Cooke BM. Babesia bovis: culture of laboratory-adapted parasite lines and clinical isolates in a chemically defined medium. Exp Parasitol. 2001 Nov;99(3):168-74. PMID:11846527

Jacobs RL, Koontz LC. Plasmodium berghei: development of resistance to clindamycin and minocycline in mice. Exp Parasitol. 1976 Aug;40(1):116-23. PMID:780118

Jacoby GA, Hunt JV, Kosinski KS, Demirjian ZN, Huggins C, Etkind P, Marcus LC, Spielman A. Treatment of transfusion-transmitted babesiosis by exchange transfusion. N Engl J Med. 1980 Nov 6;303(19):1098-100. PMID:7191475

Jahangir A, Kolbert C, Edwards W, Mitchell P, Dumler JS, Persing DH. Fatal pancarditis associated with human granulocytic Ehrlichiosis in a 44-year-old man. Clin Infect Dis. 1998 Dec;27(6):1424-7. PMID:9868655

Jahiel RI, Nussenzweig RS, Vanderberg J, Vilcek J. Anti-malarial effect of interferon inducers at different stages of development of Plasmodium berghei in the mouse. Nature. 1968 Nov 16;220(5168):710-1. PMID:5688147

Jahiel RI, Vilcek J, Nussenzweig R, Vanderberg J. Interferon inducers protect mice against plasmodium berghei malaria. Science. 1968 Aug 23;161(3843):802-4. PMID:5663811

James B. Control of malaria cycle. Lancet. 1968 Apr 6;1(7545):758. PMID:4170998

James MA. Antibody levels during bovine hemoparasitic diseases: trypanosomiasis, anaplasmosis, and babesiosis. Acta Cient Venez. 1983;34(3-4):185-90. PMID:6399967

James MA, Kuttler KL, Levy MG, Ristic M. Antibody kinetics in response to vaccination against Babesia bovis. Am J Vet Res. 1981 Nov;42(11):1999-2001. PMID:7337297

Jayaseelan C, Rahuman AA, Rajakumar G, Vishnu Kirthi A, Santhoshkumar T, Marimuthu S, Bagavan A, Kamaraj C, Zahir AA, Elango G. Synthesis of pediculocidal and larvicidal silver nanoparticles by leaf extract from heartleaf moonseed plant, Tinospora cordifolia Miers. Parasitol Res. 2011 Jul;109(1):185-94. Epub 2011 Jan 7. PMID:21212979

Jeffery GM, McWilson W, Collins WE, Lobel H. Application of the indirect fluorescent antibody method in a study of malaria endemicity in Mato Grosso, Brazil. Am J Trop Med Hyg. 1975 May;24(3):402-11. PMID:1098491

Jeffrey HC. Morphological changes in lasmodium vivax in patients under treatment with chloroquine. Trans R Soc Trop Med Hyg. 1968;62(1):47-50. PMID:4170613

Jeneby MM, Ngeiywa M, Yole DS, Mwenda JM, Suleman MA, Carlson HE. Enzootic simian piroplasm (Entopolypoides macaci) in wild-caught Kenyan non-human primates. J Med Primatol. 2008 Dec;37(6):329-36. Epub 2008 May 27. PMID:18507704

Jenkins MC. Advances and prospects for subunit vaccines against protozoa of veterinary importance. Vet Parasitol. 2001 Nov 22;101(3-4):291-310. PMID:11707303

Jittapalapong S, Jansawan W, Barriga OO, Stich RW. Reduced incidence of Babesia bigemina infection in cattle immunized against the cattle tick, Boophilus microplus. Ann N Y Acad Sci. 2004 Oct;1026:312-8. PMID:15604511

Johnson ST, Cable RG, Tonnetti L, Spencer B, Rios J, Leiby DA. Seroprevalence of Babesia microti in blood donors from Babesia-endemic areas of the northeastern United States: 2000 through 2007. Transfusion. 2009 Dec;49(12):2574-82. Epub 2009 Oct 10. PMID:19821951

Jorgensen WK, de Vos AJ, Dalgliesh RJ. Infectivity of cryopreserved Babesia bovis, Babesia bigemina and Anaplasma centrale for cattle after thawing, dilution and incubation at 30 degrees C. Vet Parasitol. 1989 Jun;31(3-4):243-51. PMID:2763444

Jorgensen WK, De Vos AJ, Dalgliesh RJ. Comparison of immunogenicity and virulence between Babesia bigemina parasites from continuous culture and from a splenectomised calf. Aust Vet J. 1989 Nov;66(11):371-2. PMID:2619652

Joseph JT, Roy SS, Shams N, Visintainer P, Nadelman RB, Hosur S, Nelson J, Wormser GP. Babesiosis in Lower Hudson Valley, New York, USA. Emerg Infect Dis. 2011 May;17(5):843-7. PMID:21529393

Joubert KE, Kettner F, Lobetti RG, Miller DM. The effects of diminazene aceturate on systemic blood pressure in clinically healthy adult dogs. J S Afr Vet Assoc. 2003 Sep;74(3):69-71. PMID:15029949

Kachani M, Oliver RA, Brown CG, Ouhelli H, Spooner RL. Common and stage-specific antigens of Theileria annulata. Vet Immunol Immunopathol. 1992 Nov;34(3-4):221-34. PMID:1280878

Kain KC, Jassoum SB, Fong IW, Hannach B. Transfusion-transmitted babesiosis in Ontario: first reported case in Canada. CMAJ. 2001 Jun 12;164(12):1721-3. PMID:11450217

Kain KC, Shanks GD, Keystone JS. Malaria chemoprophylaxis in the age of drug resistance. I. Currently recommended drug regimens. Clin Infect Dis. 2001 Jul 15;33(2):226-34. Epub 2001 Jun 14. PMID:11418883

Kania SA, Allred DR, Barbet AF. Babesia bigemina: host factors affecting the invasion of erythrocytes. Exp Parasitol. 1995 Feb;80(1):76-84. PMID:7821413

Kareru PG, Kenji GM, Gachanja AN, Keriko JM, Mungai G. Traditional medicines among the Embu and Mbeere peoples of Kenya. Afr J Tradit Complement Altern Med. 2006 Aug 28;4(1):75-86. PMID:20162075

Karle JM, Olmeda R. Rapid and sensitive quantitative analysis of the new antimalarial N4-[2,6-dimethoxy-4-methyl-5-[(3-trifluoromethyl)phenoxy]-8-quinolinyl]-1,4-pentanediamine in plasma by liquid chromatography and electrochemical detection. J Chromatogr. 1988 Feb 26;424(2):347-56. PMID:3372627

Karle JM, Olmeda R, Freeman SG, Schroeder AC. Quantification of the individual enantiomer plasma concentrations of the candidate antimalarial agent N4-[2,6-dimethoxy-4-methyl-5-[(3-trifluoromethyl)phenoxy]-8-quinolinyl] -1,4-pentanediamine (WR 238,605). J Chromatogr B Biomed Appl. 1995 Aug 18;670(2):251-7. PMID:8548015

Kasahara K, Nomura S, Subeki, Matsuura H, Yamasaki M, Yamato O, Maede Y, Katakura K, Suzuki M, Trimurningsih, Chairul, Yoshihara T. Anti-babesial compounds from Curcuma zedoaria. Planta Med. 2005 May;71(5):482-4. PMID:15977324

Katz TM, Miller JH, Hebert AA. Insect repellents: historical perspectives and new developments. J Am Acad Dermatol. 2008 May;58(5):865-71. Epub 2008 Feb 13. PMID:18272250

Kayode J. Conservation of indigenous medicinal botanicals in Ekiti State, Nigeria. J Zhejiang Univ Sci B. 2006 Sep;7(9):713-8. PMID:16909472

Kengeya-Kayondo JF, Seeley JA, Kajura-Bajenja E, Kabunga E, Mubiru E, Sembajja F, Mulder DW. Recognition, treatment seeking behaviour and perception of cause of malaria among rural women in Uganda. Acta Trop. 1994 Dec;58(3-4):267-73. PMID:7709865

Khai PN, Van NT, Lua TT, Huu VT, Dang DT, Huong PT, Salazar N, Sukthana Y, Singhasivanon P. The situation of malaria along the Vietnam-Lao PDR border and some related factors. Southeast Asian J Trop Med Public Health. 2000;31 Suppl 1:99-105. PMID:11414469

Khalacheva M. [Immunological studies of Babesia ovis strains isolated from various regions of Bulgaria].[Article in Bulgarian]. Vet Med Nauki. 1974;11(8):103-8. PMID:4446350

Kim CM, Blanco LB, Alhassan A, Iseki H, Yokoyama N, Xuan X, Igarashi I. Development of a rapid immunochromatographic test for simultaneous serodiagnosis of bovine babesioses caused by Babesia bovis and Babesia bigemina. Am J Trop Med Hyg. 2008 Jan;78(1):117-21. PMID:18187794

Kim JY, Cho SH, Joo HN, Tsuji M, Cho SR, Park IJ, Chung GT, Ju JW, Cheun HI, Lee

HW, Lee YH, Kim TS. First case of human babesiosis in Korea: detection and characterization of a novel type of Babesia sp. (KO1) similar to ovine babesia. J Clin Microbiol. 2007 Jun;45(6):2084-7. Epub 2007 Mar 28. PMID:17392446

Kimbi HK, Fagbenro-Beyioku AF, Oyibo WA. Antimalarial herbs against chloroquine-resistant P. yoelii nigeriensis in mice. Indian J Malariol. 1998 Mar;35(1):35-8. PMID:10212890

King AC. Regression of mouse sarcoma M(52)B treated with bovine fascia lata extract from animals previously inoculated with Babesia bovis and B. bigemina. S Afr Med J. 1980 Aug 2;58(5):191-3. PMID:7404219

Kinnamon KE, Rothe WE. Biological screening in the U.S. Army antimalarial drug development program. Am J Trop Med Hyg. 1975 Mar;24(2):174-8. PMID:804264

Kinung'hi SM, Mashauri F, Mwanga JR, Nnko SE, Kaatano GM, Malima R, Kishamawe C, Magesa S, Mboera LE. Knowledge, attitudes and practices about malaria among communities: comparing epidemic and non-epidemic prone communities of Muleba district, North-western Tanzania. BMC Public Health. 2010 Jul 5;10:395. PMID:20602778

Kirira PG, Rukunga GM, Wanyonyi AW, Muregi FM, Gathirwa JW, Muthaura CN, Omar SA, Tolo F, Mungai GM, Ndiege IO. Anti-plasmodial activity and toxicity of extracts of plants used in traditional malaria therapy in Meru and Kilifi Districts of Kenya. J Ethnopharmacol. 2006 Jul 19;106(3):403-7. Epub 2006 Mar 13. PMID:16530996

Kitchener S, Nasveld P, Edstein MD. Tafenoquine for the treatment of recurrent Plasmodium vivax malaria. Am J Trop Med Hyg. 2007 Mar;76(3):494-6. PMID:17360873

Kiurtov N. [Trial of a live vaccine against babesiasis in sheep]. [Article in Bulgarian]. Vet Med Nauki. 1977;14(4):25-30. PMID:929961

Kiurtov N. [Deep freezing of Babesia ovis in liquid nitrogen]. [Article in Bulgarian]. Vet Med Nauki. 1977;14(6):11-5. PMID:595370

Kiurtov N. [Soluble Babesia ovis antigen].[Article in Bulgarian]. Vet Med Nauki. 1979;16(3):15-22. PMID:93342

Kiurtov N. [Production of a Babesia ovis extract and its testing for antigenic properties].[Article in Bulgarian]. Vet Med Nauki. 1979;16(4):84-90. PMID:532096

Kivaria FM, Ruheta MR, Mkonyi PA, Malamsha PC. Epidemiological aspects and economic impact of bovine theileriosis (East Coast fever) and its control: a preliminary assessment with special reference to Kibaha district, Tanzania. Vet J. 2007 Mar;173(2):384-90. Epub 2005 Oct 5. PMID:16169755

Kjemtrup AM, Conrad PA. A review of the small canine piroplasms from California: Babesia conradae in the literature. Vet Parasitol. 2006 May 31;138(1-2):112-7. Epub 2006 Mar 7. PMID:16522352

Kjemtrup AM, Lee B, Fritz CL, Evans C, Chervenak M, Conrad PA. Investigation of transfusion transmission of a WA1-type babesial parasite to a premature infant in California. Transfusion. 2002 Nov;42(11):1482-7. PMID:12421222

Kjemtrup AM, Wainwright K, Miller M, Penzhorn BL, Carreno RA. Babesia conradae, sp. Nov., a small canine Babesia identified in California. Vet Parasitol. 2006 May 31;138(1-2):103-11. Epub 2006 Mar 9. PMID:16524663

Knight DJ. Babesia rodhaini and Plasmodium berghei. A highly active series of chlorophenoxyalkoxy-substituted diamino-dihydrotriazines against experimental infections in mice. Ann Trop Med Parasitol. 1981 Feb;75(1):1-6. PMID:7023398

Knowles JH. Editorial: American medicine and world health 1976. Ann Intern Med. 1976 Apr;84(4):483-5. PMID:1259295

Koch HT, Kambeva L, Ocama JG, Munatswa FC, Franssen FF, Uilenberg G, Dolan TT, Norval RA. Immunization of cattle against Theileria parva bovis and their exposure to natural challenge. Vet Parasitol. 1990 Nov;37(3-4):185-96. PMID:2125158

Kocisko DA, Walsh DS, Eamsila C, Edstein MD. Measurement of tafenoquine (WR 238605) in human plasma and venous and capillary blood by high-pressure liquid chromatography. Ther Drug Monit. 2000 Apr;22(2):184-9. PMID:10774631

Kok LD, Wong CK, Leung KN, Tsang SF, Fung KP, Choy YM. Activation of the anti-tumor effector cells by Radix bupleuri. Immunopharmacology. 1995 Jun;30(1):79-87. PMID:7591716

Kolabskiĭ NA, Gaĭdukov AKh, Vorob'ev VV, Sivak DA, Voevoda NI. [Combined chemoprophylaxis of babesiasis in cattle].[Article in Russian]. Veterinariia. 1973 Feb;3:71-3. PMID:4770054

Kolören Z, Avşar C, Şekeroğlu ZA. [Diagnosis of protozoa by loop-mediated isothermal amplification: (LAMP)].[Article in Turkish]. Turkiye Parazitol Derg. 2010;34(4):207-11. PMID:21391196

Kosower NS, Kosower EM. Molecular basis for selective advantage of glucose-6-phosphate-dehydrogenase-deficient individuals exposed to malaria. Lancet. 1970 Dec 26;2(7687):1343-4. PMID:4098912

Köster LS, Van Schoor M, Goddard A, Thompson PN, Matjila PT, Kjelgaard-Hansen M. C-reactive protein in canine babesiosis caused by Babesia rossi and its association with outcome. J S Afr Vet Assoc. 2009 Jun;80(2):87-91. PMID:19831269

Krause PJ. Babesiosis. Med Clin North Am. 2002 Mar;86(2):361-73. PMID:11982307

Krause PJ. Babesiosis diagnosis and treatment. Vector Borne Zoonotic Dis. 2003 Spring;3(1):45-51. PMID:12804380

Krause PJ, Gewurz BE, Hill D, Marty FM, Vannier E, Foppa IM, Furman RR, Neuhaus E, Skowron G, Gupta S, McCalla C, Pesanti EL, Young M, Heiman D, Hsue G, Gelfand JA, Wormser GP, Dickason J, Bia FJ, Hartman B, Telford SR 3rd, Christianson D, Dardick K, Coleman M, Girotto JE, Spielman A. Persistent and relapsing babesiosis in immunocompromised patients. Clin Infect Dis. 2008 Feb 1;46(3):370-6. PMID:18181735

Krause PJ, Gewurz BE, Hill D, Marty FM, Vannier E, Foppa IM, Furman RR, Neuhaus E, Skowron G, Gupta S, McCalla C, Pesanti EL, Young M, Heiman D, Hsue G, Gelfand JA, Wormser GP, Dickason J, Bia FJ, Hartman B, Telford SR 3rd, Christianson D, Dardick K, da Silva RA, Corrêa Fdo N, Botteon Rde C, Botteon Pde T. [Natural infection by hemoparasites in calves submitted to chemoprophylaxis at 30 days of age].[Article in Portuguese]. Rev Bras Parasitol Vet. 2007 Jul-Sep;16(3):163-5. PMID:18078605

Krause PJ, Lepore T, Sikand VK, Gadbaw J Jr, Burke G, Telford SR 3rd, Brassard P, Pearl D, Azlanzadeh J, Christianson D, McGrath D, Spielman A. Atovaquone and azithromycin for the treatment of babesiosis. N Engl J Med. 2000 Nov 16;343(20):1454-8. PMID:11078770

Krause PJ, Spielman A, Telford SR 3rd, Sikand VK, McKay K, Christianson D, Pollack RJ, Brassard P, Magera J, Ryan R, Persing DH. Persistent parasitemia after acute babesiosis. N Engl J Med. 1998 Jul 16;339(3):160-5. PMID:9664092

Kremsner P. [New preventive antimalaria drug. 3 tables, 2 months of protection. Interview by Petra Eiden].[Article in German]. MMW Fortschr Med. 2000 Sep 21;142(38):13. PMID:11050883

Krishnan S, Krishnan AD, Mustafa AS, Talwar GP, Ramalingaswami V. Effect of vitamin A and undernutrition on the susceptibility of rodents to a malarial parasite Plasmodium berghei. J Nutr. 1976 Jun;106(6):784-91.

PMID: 818347.

Kuhner A. The impact of public health programs on economic development. Report of a study of malaria in Thailand. Int J Health Serv. 1971 Aug;1(3):285-92. PMID:5136231

Kumar S, Gupta AK, Pal Y, Dwivedi SK. In-vivo therapeutic efficacy trial with artemisinin derivative, buparvaquone and imidocarb dipropionate against Babesia equi infection in donkeys. J Vet Med Sci. 2003 Nov;65(11):1171-7. PMID:14665744

Kumar S, Kumar R, Sugimoto C. A perspective on Theileria equi infections in donkeys. Jpn J Vet Res. 2009 Feb;56(4):171-80. PMID:19358444

Kumar S, Malhotra DV, Dhar S, Nichani AK. Vaccination of donkeys against Babesia equi using killed merozoite immunogen. Vet Parasitol. 2002 May 30;106(1):19-33. PMID:11992708

Kumar S, Malhotra DV, Nichani AK. Identification of immunoreactive polypeptides of Babesia equi parasite during immunization. Vet Parasitol. 2002 Aug 22;107(4):295-301. PMID:12163241

Kung'u MW, Goodger BV, Bushell GR, Wright IG, Waltisbuhl DJ. Vaccination of cattle with dextran sulphate-binding Babesia bigemina antigens. Int J Parasitol. 1992 Aug;22(5):621-5. PMID:1399246

Kuttler KL. The effect of Imidocarb treatment on Babesia in the bovine and the tick (Boophilus microplus). Res Vet Sci. 1975 Mar;18(2):198-200. PMID:1129539

Kuttler KL, Johnson LW. Immunization of cattle with a Babesia bigemina antigen in Freund's complete adjuvant. Am J Vet Res. 1980 Apr;41(4):536-8. PMID:7406273

Kuttler KL, Levy MG, James MA, Ristic M. Efficacy of a nonviable culture-derived Babesia bovis vaccine. Am J Vet Res. 1982 Feb;43(2):281-4. PMID:7046534

Kuttler KL, Levy MG, Ristic M. Cell culture-derived Babesia bovis vaccine: sequential challenge exposure of protective immunity during a 6-month postvaccination period. Am J Vet Res. 1983 Aug;44(8):1456-9. PMID:6354014

Kuttler KL, Zaugg JL, Gipson CA. Imidocarb and parvaquone in the treatment of piroplasmosis (Babesia equi) in equids. Am J Vet Res. 1987 Nov;48(11):1613-6. PMID:3434908

Kuttler KL, Zaugg JL, Yunker CE. The pathogenicity and immunologic relationship of a virulent and a tissue-culture-adapted Babesia bovis. Vet Parasitol. 1988 Mar;27(3-4):239-44. PMID:3285573

Kuwayama DP, Briones RJ. Spontaneous splenic rupture caused by Babesia microti infection. Clin Infect Dis. 2008 May 1;46(9):e92-5. PMID:18419430

Kweka EJ, Mosha F, Lowassa A, Mahande AM, Kitau J, Matowo J, Mahande MJ, Massenga CP, Tenu F, Feston E, Lyatuu EE, Mboya MA, Mndeme R, Chuwa G, Temu EA. Ethnobotanical study of some of mosquito repellent plants in north-eastern Tanzania. Malar J. 2008 Aug 7;7:152. PMID:18687119

Kweka EJ, Mosha FW, Lowassa A, Mahande AM, Mahande MJ, Massenga CP, Tenu F, Lyatuu EE, Mboya MA, Temu EA. Longitudinal evaluation of Ocimum and other plants effects on the feeding behavioral response of mosquitoes (Diptera: Culicidae) in the field in Tanzania. Parasit Vectors. 2008 Oct 22;1(1):42. PMID:18945343

Kweka EJ, Nyindo M, Mosha F, Silva AG. Insecticidal activity of the essential oil from fruits and seeds of Schinus terebinthifolia Raddi against African malaria vectors. Parasit Vectors. 2011 Jul 5;4:129. PMID:21729280

Labarthe NV, Remião JO, Sacco AM, Maia LC. Cross-reaction of tick salivary antigens in the Boophilus microplus-cattle system. Vet Parasitol. 1985 Mar;17(3):259-63. PMID:3992881

Labbé AC, Loutfy MR, Kain KC. Recent Advances in the Prophylaxis and Treatment of Malaria. Curr Infect Dis Rep. 2001 Feb;3(1):68-76. PMID:11177733

Laing AB. Studies on the chemotherapy of malaria. II. Pyrimethamine resistance in The Gambia. Trans R Soc Trop Med Hyg. 1970;64(4):569-80. PMID:4922133

Lantos PM, Krause PJ. Babesiosis: similar to malaria but different. Pediatr Ann. 2002 Mar;31(3):192-7. PMID:11905293

Lau AO. An overview of the Babesia, Plasmodium and Theileria genomes: a comparative perspective. Mol Biochem Parasitol. 2009 Mar;164(1):1-8. Epub 2008 Dec 6. PMID:19110007

Lawrence JA. Conventional vaccines for tick-borne haemoparasitic diseases of sheep and goats. Parassitologia. 1997 Jun;39(2):119-21. PMID:9530695

Lawrence JA, de Vos AJ. Methods currently used for the control of anaplasmosis and babesiosis: their validity and proposals for future control strategies. Parassitologia. 1990 Apr;32(1):63-71. PMID:2284136

Lawrence JA, Malika J, Whiteland AP, Kafuwa P. Efficacy of an Australian Babesia bovis vaccine strain in Malawi. Vet Rec. 1993 Mar 20;132(12):295-6. PMID:8470344

Lawrence JA, Musisi FL, Mfitilodze MW, Tjornehoj K, Whiteland AP, Kafuwa PT, Chamambala KE. Integrated tick and tick-borne disease control trials in crossbred dairy cattle in Malawi. Trop Anim Health Prod. 1996 Nov;28(4):280-8. PMID:8983132

Lawrence JA, Whiteland AP, Malika J, Kafuwa P, Jongejan F. Use of serological response to evaluate heartwater immunization of cattle. Rev Elev Med Vet Pays Trop. 1993;46(1-2):211-5. PMID:8134634

Leary KJ, Riel MA, Roy MJ, Cantilena LR, Bi D, Brater DC, van de Pol C, Pruett K, Kerr C, Veazey JM Jr, Beboso R, Ohrt C. A randomized, double-blind, safety and tolerability study to assess the ophthalmic and renal effects of tafenoquine 200 mg weekly versus placebo for 6 months in healthy volunteers. Am J Trop Med Hyg. 2009 Aug;81(2):356-62. PMID:19635898

Lee BP. Apnea, bradycardia and thrombocytopenia in a premature infant. Pediatr Infect Dis J. 2001 Aug;20(8):816, 820-2. PMID:11734753

Lee S, Carson K, Rice-Ficht A, Good T. Small heat shock proteins differentially affect Abeta aggregation and toxicity. Biochem Biophys Res Commun. 2006 Aug 25;347(2):527-33. Epub 2006 Jun 30. PMID:16828710

Leiby DA. Threats to blood safety posed by emerging protozoan pathogens. Vox Sang. 2004 Jul;87 Suppl 2:120-2. PMID:15209895

Leiby DA. Babesiosis and blood transfusion: flying under the radar. Vox Sang. 2006 Apr;90(3):157-65. PMID:16507014

Leiby DA. Transfusion-transmitted Babesia spp.: bull's-eye on Babesia microti. Clin Microbiol Rev. 2011 Jan;24(1):14-28. PMID:21233506

Leiby DA. Transfusion-associated babesiosis: shouldn't we be ticked off? Ann Intern Med. 2011 Oct 18;155(8):556-7. Epub 2011 Sep 5. PMID:21893616

Leiby DA, Chung AP, Cable RG, Trouern-Trend J, McCullough J, Homer MJ, Reynolds LD, Houghton RL, Lodes MJ, Persing DH. Relationship between tick bites and the seroprevalence of Babesia microti and Anaplasma phagocytophila (previously Ehrlichia sp.) in blood donors. Transfusion. 2002 Dec;42(12):1585-91. PMID:12473139

Leiby DA, Chung AP, Gill JE, Houghton RL, Persing DH, Badon S, Cable RG. Demonstrable parasitemia among Connecticut blood donors with antibodies to Babesia microti. Transfusion. 2005 Nov;45(11):1804-10. PMID:16271108

Leiby DA, Gill JE. Transfusion-transmitted tick-borne infections: a cornucopia of threats. Transfus Med Rev. 2004 Oct;18(4):293-306. PMID:15497129

Leisewitz AL, Guthrie AJ, Berry WL. Evaluation of the effect of whole-blood transfusion on the oxygen status and acid-base balance of Babesia canis infected dogs using the oxygen status algorithm. J S Afr Vet Assoc. 1996 Mar;67(1):20-6. PMID:8786612

Leisewitz AL, Jacobson LS, de Morais HS, Reyers F. The mixed acid-base disturbances of severe canine babesiosis. J Vet Intern Med. 2001 Sep-Oct;15(5):445-52. PMID:11596731

Lell B, Faucher JF, Missinou MA, Borrmann S, Dangelmaier O, Horton J, Kremsner PG. Malaria chemoprophylaxis with tafenoquine: a randomised study. Lancet. 2000 Jun 10;355(9220):2041-5. PMID:10885356

Lepes T. Research related to malaria. A review of achievements and further needs. Am J Trop Med Hyg. 1972 Sep;21(5):640-7. PMID:4627544

Lewis BD, Penzhorn BL, Volkmann DH. Could treatment of pregnant mares prevent abortions due to equine piroplasmosis? J S Afr Vet Assoc. 1999 Jun;70(2):90-1. PMID:10855828

Lewis RL. Blood transfusion in a case of bovine piroplasmosis. Vet Rec. 1946 Nov 30;58(48):568. PMID:20279641

L'Hostis M. Epidemiology and vaccination strategy: Babesia divergens bovine babesiosis example. Vet Res. 1995;26(3):240-3. PMID:7795691

Li J, Zhu JD, Appiah A, McCutchan TF, Long GW, Milhous WK, Hollingdale MR. Plasmodium berghei: quantitation of in vitro effects of antimalarial drugs on exoerythrocytic development by a ribosomal RNA probe. Exp Parasitol. 1991 May;72(4):450-8. PMID:2026219

Li PN, Khitenkova LP. [Imidocarb, a highly effective preparation in animal piroplasmosis (a survey of the foreign literature)]. [Article in Russian]. Veterinariia. 1973 Jan;49(1):117-9. PMID:4756636

Lin MY, Huang HP. Use of a doxycycline-enrofloxacin-metronidazole combination with/without diminazene diaceturate to treat naturally occurring canine babesiosis caused by Babesia gibsoni. Acta Vet Scand. 2010 Apr 24;52:27. PMID:20416095

Linden JV, Wong SJ, Chu FK, Schmidt GB, Bianco C. Transfusion-associated transmission of babesiosis in New York State. Transfusion. 2000 Mar;40(3):285-9. PMID:10738027

Lindholm PF, Annen K, Ramsey G. Approaches to minimize infection risk in blood banking and transfusion practice. Infect Disord Drug Targets. 2011 Feb;11(1):45-56. PMID:21303341

Littman MP. Canine borreliosis. Vet Clin North Am Small Anim Pract. 2003 Jul;33(4):827-62. PMID:12910746

Liu AR, Yu ZY, Lu LL, Sui ZY. [The synergistic action of guanghuoxiang volatile oil and sodium artesunate against Plasmodium berghei and reversal of SA-resistant Plasmodium berghei].[Article in Chinese]. Zhongguo Ji Sheng Chong Xue Yu Ji Sheng Chong Bing Za Zhi. 2000;18(2):76-8. PMID:12567719

Loa CC, Adelson ME, Mordechai E, Raphaelli I, Tilton RC. Serological diagnosis of human babesiosis by IgG enzyme-linked immunosorbent assay. Curr Microbiol. 2004 Dec;49(6):385-9. PMID:15696612

Lobetti RG, Reyers F, Nesbit JW. The comparative role of haemoglobinaemia and hypoxia in the development of canine babesial nephropathy. J S Afr Vet Assoc. 1996 Dec;67(4):188-98. PMID:9284030

Lodes MJ, Dillon DC, Houghton RL, Skeiky YA. Expression cloning. Methods Mol Med. 2004;94:91-106. PMID:14959824

Lodes MJ, Houghton RL, Bruinsma ES, Mohamath R, Reynolds LD, Benson DR, Krause PJ, Reed SG, Persing DH. Serological expression cloning of novel immunoreactive antigens of Babesia microti. Infect Immun. 2000 May;68(5):2783-90. PMID:10768973

Löhr KF. [Immunization against babesiasis and anaplasmosis in 40 Charollais cattle imported to Kenya and report the incidence of photosensitization].[Article in German]. Zentralbl Veterinarmed B. 1969 Feb;16(1):40-6. PMID:5389131

Löhr KF. [Contribution to the problem of the natural resistance of calves to Babesia bigemina].[Article in German]. Zentralbl Veterinarmed B. 1969 Mar;16(2):158-63. PMID:5814189

Looareesuwan S, Phillips RE, Karbwang J, White NJ, Flegg PJ, Warrell DA. Plasmodium falciparum hyperparasitaemia: use of exchange transfusion in seven patients and a review of the literature. Q J Med. 1990 May;75(277):471-81. PMID:2201995

Lopes NP, Kato MJ, Andrade EH, Maia JG, Yoshida M, Planchart AR, Katzin AM. Antimalarial use of volatile oil from leaves of Virola surinamensis (Rol.) Warb. by Waiãpi Amazon Indians. J Ethnopharmacol. 1999 Nov 30;67(3):313-9. PMID:10617066

Losos GJ, Crockett E. Toxicity of beril in the dog. Vet Rec. 1969 Aug 16;85(7):196. PMID:5816642

Losson B, Patz R. [Babesia divergens: activity of long-acting oxytetracycline in the gerbil, Meriones unguiculatus].[Article in French]. Ann Rech Vet. 1989;20(4):501-7. PMID:2619208

Lubin AS, Snydman DR, Miller KB. Persistent babesiosis in a stem cell transplant recipient. Leuk Res. 2011 Jun;35(6):e77-8. Epub 2010 Dec 24. PMID:21185598

Luo Y, Jia H, Terkawi MA, Goo YK, Kawano S, Ooka H, Li Y, Yu L, Cao S, Yamagishi J, Fujisaki K, Nishikawa Y, Saito-Ito A, Igarashi I, Xuan X. Identification and characterization of a novel secreted antigen 1 of Babesia microti and evaluation of its potential use in enzyme-linked immunosorbent assay and immunochromatographic test. Parasitol Int. 2011 Jun;60(2):119-25. Epub 2010 Nov 8. PMID:21070864

Lux JZ, Weiss D, Linden JV, Kessler D, Herwaldt BL, Wong SJ, Keithly J, Della-Latta P, Scully BE. Transfusion-associated babesiosis after heart transplant. Emerg Infect Dis. 2003 Jan;9(1):116-9. PMID:12533293

Lykins JD, Ristic M, Weisiger RM. Babesia microti: pathogenesis of parasite of human origin in the hamster. Exp Parasitol. 1975 Jun;37(3):388-97. PMID:805058

Ma C, Wang H, Lu X, Li H, Liu B, Xu G. Analysis of Artemisia annua L. volatile oil by comprehensive two-dimensional gas chromatography time-of-flight mass spectrometry. J Chromatogr A. 2007 May 25;1150(1-2):50-3. Epub 2006 Oct 12. PMID:17045598

Ma X, Zheng C, Hu C, Rahman K, Qin L. The genus Desmodium (Fabaceae)-traditional uses in Chinese medicine, phytochemistry and pharmacology. J Ethnopharmacol. 2011 Nov 18;138(2):314-32. Epub 2011 Oct 17. PMID:22004895

Macgregor JD, Avery JG. Malaria transmission and fetal growth. Br Med J. 1974 Aug 17;3(5928):433-6. PMID:4606777

Machado RZ, McElwain TF, Pancracio HP, Freschi CR, Palmer GH. Babesia bigemina: immunization with purified rhoptries induces protection against acute parasitemia. Exp Parasitol. 1999 Oct;93(2):105-8. PMID:10502474

Machtinger L, Telford SR 3rd, Inducil C, Klapper E, Pepkowitz SH, Goldfinger D. Treatment of babesiosis by red blood cell exchange in an HIV-positive, splenectomized patient. J Clin Apher. 1993;8(2):78-81. PMID:8226709

Mahoney DF, Goodger BV. Babesia argentina: immunogenicity of plasma from infected animals. Exp Parasitol. 1972 Aug;32(1):71-85. PMID:4626125

Mahoney DF, Kerr JD, Goodger BV, Wright IG. The immune response of cattle to Babesia bovis (syn. B. argentina). Studies on the nature and specificity of protection. Int J Parasitol. 1979 Aug;9(4):297-306. PMID:489236

Mahoney DF, Mirre GB. Babesia argentina: the infection of splenectomized calves with extracts of larval ticks (Boophilus microplus). Res Vet Sci. 1974 Jan;16(1):112-4. PMID:4819982

Mahoney DF, Wright IG, Goodger BV. Immunity in cattle to Babesia bovis after single infections with parasites of various origin. Aust Vet J. 1979 Jan;55(1):10-2. PMID:435202

Mahoney DF, Wright IG, Goodger BV. Changes in the haemolytic activity of serum complement during acute Babesia bovis infection in cattle. Z Parasitenkd. 1980;62(1):39-45. PMID:7395306

Mahoney DF, Wright IG, Goodger BV. Bovine babesiosis: the immunization of cattle with fractions of erythrocytes infected with Babesia bovis (syn B. argentina). Vet Immunol Immunopathol. 1981 Apr;2(2):145-56. PMID:7344266

Mahoney DF, Wright IG, Goodger BV, Mirre GB, Sutherst RW, Utech KB. The transmission of Babesia bovis in herds of European and Zebu x European cattle infested with the tick, Boophilus microplus. Aust Vet J. 1981 Oct;57(10):461-9. PMID:7337597

Mahoney DF, Wright IG, Ketterer PJ. Babesia argentina: the infectivity and immunogenicity of irradiated blood parasites for splenectomized calves. Int J Parasitol. 1973 Mar;3(2):209-17. PMID:4196318

Malagon F, Tapia JL. Experimental transmission of Babesia microti infection by the oral route. Parasitol Res. 1994;80(8):645-8. PMID:7886033

Malik EM, Hanafi K, Ali SH, Ahmed ES, Mohamed KA. Treatment-seeking behaviour for malaria in children under five years of age: implication for home management in rural areas with high seasonal transmission in Sudan. Malar J. 2006 Jul 22;5:60. PMID:16859565

Malimbo M, Mugisha E, Kato F, Karamagi C, Talisuna AO. Caregivers' perceived treatment failure in home-based management of fever among Ugandan children aged less than five years. Malar J. 2006 Dec 15;5:124. PMID:17173675

Mangold AJ, Aguirre DH, Cafrune MM, de Echaide ST, Guglielmone AA. Evaluation of the infectivity of a vaccinal and a pathogenic Babesia bovis strain from Argentina to Boophilus microplus. Vet Parasitol. 1993 Dec;51(1-2):143-8. PMID:8128578

Mangold AJ, Aguirre DH, Guglielmone AA. Post-thawing viability of vaccines for bovine babesiosis and anaplasmosis cryopreserved with glycerol. Vet Parasitol. 1990 Nov;37(3-4):301-6. PMID:2267730

Mangold AJ, Vanzini VR, Echaide IE, de Echaide ST, Volpogni MM, Guglielmone AA. Viability after thawing and dilution of simultaneously cryopreserved vaccinal Babesia bovis and Babesia bigemina strains cultured in vitro. Vet Parasitol. 1996 Feb;61(3-4):345-8. PMID:8720572

Manzano JI, Carvalho L, García-Hernández R, Poveda JA, Ferragut JA, Castanys S, Gamarro F. Uptake of the antileishmania drug tafenoquine follows a sterol-dependent diffusion process in Leishmania. J Antimicrob Chemother. 2011 Nov;66(11):2562-5. Epub 2011 Aug 16. PMID:21846675

Manzano JI, Carvalho L, Pérez-Victoria JM, Castanys S, Gamarro F. Increased glycolytic ATP synthesis is associated with tafenoquine resistance in Leishmania major. Antimicrob Agents Chemother. 2011 Mar;55(3):1045-52. Epub 2011 Jan 3. PMID:21199921

Marathe A, Tripathi J, Handa V, Date V. Human babesiosis--a case report. Indian J Med Microbiol. 2005 Oct;23(4):267-9. PMID:16327127

Marco I, Velarde R, Castellà J, Ferrer D, Lavín S. Presumptive Babesia ovis infection in a spanish ibex (Capra pyrenaica). Vet Parasitol. 2000 Jan;87(2-3):217-21. PMID:10622613

Marcotty T, Berkvens D, Besa RK, Losson B, Dolan TT, Madder M, Chaka G, Van den Bossche P, Brandt J. Lyophilisation and resuscitation of sporozoites of Theileria parva: preliminary experiments. Vaccine. 2003 Dec 12;22(2):213-6. PMID:14615148

Marcu CB, Caracciolo E, Libertin C, Donohue T. Fulminant babesiosis manifested soon after coronary bypass surgery. Conn Med. 2005 Feb;69(2):67-8. PMID:15779600

Marcus LC, Mabray CJ, Sturgis GH. Babesia microti infection in the hamster: failure of quinine and pyrimethamine in chemotherapeutic trials. Am J Trop Med Hyg. 1984 Jan;33(1):21-3. PMID:6696180

Marcus LC, Valigorsky JM, Fanning WL, Joseph T, Glick B. A case report of transfusion-induced babesiosis. JAMA. 1982 Jul 23;248(4):465-7. PMID:7201036

Marley SE, Eberhard ML, Steurer FJ, Ellis WL, McGreevy PB, Ruebush TK 2nd. Evaluation of selected antiprotozoal drugs in the Babesia microti-hamster model. Antimicrob Agents Chemother. 1997 Jan;41(1):91-4. PMID:8980761

Marshall CL. Health, nutrition, and the roots of world population growth. Int J Health Serv. 1974 Fall;4(4):677-90. PMID:4463173

Martinot M, Zadeh MM, Hansmann Y, Grawey I, Christmann D, Aguillon S, Jouglin M, Chauvin A, De Briel D. Babesiosis in immunocompetent patients, Europe. Emerg Infect Dis. 2011 Jan;17(1):114-6. PMID:21192869

Máthé A, Vörös K, Németh T, Biksi I, Hetyey C, Manczur F, Tekes L. Clinicopathological changes and effect of imidocarb therapy in dogs experimentally infected with Babesia canis. Acta Vet Hung. 2006 Mar;54(1):19-33. PMID:16613023

Matjila PT, Penzhorn BL, Leisewitz AL, Bhoora R, Barker R. Molecular characterisation of Babesia gibsoni infection from a pit-bull terrier pup recently imported into South Africa. J S Afr Vet Assoc. 2007 Mar;78(1):2-5. PMID:17665757

Matsui T, Inoue R, Kajimoto K, Tamekane A, Okamura A, Katayama Y, Shimoyama M, Chihara K, Saito-Ito A, Tsuji M. [First documentation of transfusion-associated babesiosis in Japan].[Article in Japanese]. Rinsho Ketsueki. 2000 Aug;41(8):628-34. PMID:11020989

Matsuu A, Koshida Y, Kawahara M, Inoue K, Ikadai H, Hikasa Y, Okano S, Higuchi S. Efficacy of atovaquone against Babesia gibsoni in vivo and in vitro. Vet Parasitol. 2004 Sep 20;124(1-2):9-18. PMID:15350657

Matthews J, Rattigan E, Yee H. Case 29-2003: a 60-year-old man with fever, rigors, and sweats. N Engl J Med. 2003 Dec 18;349(25):2467; author reply 2467. PMID:14681519

Mattioli RC, Dampha K, Bah M, Verhulst A, Pandey VS. Effect of controlling natural field-tick infestation on the growth of N'Dama and Gobra zebu cattle in the Gambia. Prev Vet Med. 1998 Feb 27;34(2-3):137-46. PMID:9604263

Mbati PA, Hlatshwayo M, Mtshali MS, Mogaswane KR, De Waal TD, Dipeolu OO. Ticks and tick-borne diseases of livestock belonging to resource-poor farmers in the eastern Free State of South Africa. Exp Appl Acarol. 2002;28(1-4):217-24. PMID:14570134

Mbonye AK, Neema S, Magnussen P. Treatment-seeking practices for malaria in pregnancy among rural women in Mukono district, Uganda. J Biosoc Sci. 2006 Mar;38(2):221-37. PMID:16490155

Mbonye AK, Neema S, Magnussen P. Malaria in pregnancy, risk perceptions and care seeking practices among adolescents in Mukono district Uganda. Int J Adolesc Med Health. 2006 Oct-Dec;18(4):561-73. PMID:17340848

McCarthy VC, Clyde DF. Influence of sulfalene upon gametocytogenesis of Plasmodium falciparum and subsequent infection patterns in Anopheles stephensi. Exp Parasitol. 1973 Feb;33(1):73-8. PMID:4570982

McElroy B, Wiseman V, Matovu F, Mwengee W. Malaria prevention in north-eastern Tanzania: patterns of expenditure and determinants of demand at the household level. Malar J. 2009 May 7;8:95. PMID:19422704

McElwain TF, Perryman LE, Musoke AJ, McGuire TC. Molecular characterization and immunogenicity of neutralization-sensitive Babesia bigemina merozoite surface proteins. Mol Biochem Parasitol. 1991 Aug;47(2):213-22. PMID:1944418

McGregor IA. Immunity to plasmodial infections; consideration of factors relevant to malaria in man. Int Rev Trop Med. 1971;4:1-52. PMID:4944095

McHardy N. Immunization of rats against Babesia (Nuttalia) rodhaini. Nature. 1967 May 20;214(5090):805. PMID:4963880

McHardy N. Protective effect of haemolytic serum on mice infected with Babesia rodhaini. Ann Trop Med Parasitol. 1972 Mar;66(1):1-5. PMID:5021569

McHardy N. Effects of stimulating erythropoiesis in mice infected with Babesia rodhaini. Ann Trop Med Parasitol. 1973 Sep;67(3):301-6. PMID:4761938

McHardy N, Simpson RM. Imidocarb dipropionate therapy in Kenyan anaplasmosis and babesiosis. Trop Anim Health Prod. 1974 May;6(2):63-70. PMID:4413774

McLaughlin GL, Montenegro-James S, Vodkin MH, Howe D, Toro M, Leon E, Armijos R, Kakoma I, Greenwood BM, Hassan-King M, et al. Molecular approaches to malaria and babesiosis diagnosis. Mem Inst Oswaldo Cruz. 1992;87 Suppl 3:57-68. PMID:1343727

McQuiston JH, Childs JE, Chamberland ME, Tabor E. Transmission of tick-borne agents of disease by blood transfusion: a review of known and potential risks in the United States. Transfusion. 2000 Mar;40(3):274-84. PMID:10738026

Meer-Scherrer L, Adelson M, Mordechai E, Lottaz B, Tilton R. Babesia microti infection in Europe. Curr Microbiol. 2004 Jun;48(6):435-7. PMID:15170239

Meeusen E, Lloyd S, Soulsby EJ. Babesia microti in mice. Adoptive transfer of immunity with serum and cells. Aust J Exp Biol Med Sci. 1984 Oct;62 (Pt 5):551-66. PMID:6335965

Meeusen E, Lloyd S, Soulsby EJ. Babesia microti in mice. Subpopulations of cells involved in the adoptive transfer of immunity with immune spleen cells. Aust J Exp Biol Med Sci. 1984 Oct;62 (Pt 5):567-75. PMID:6442859

Meeusen E, Lloyd S, Soulsby EJ. Antibody levels in adoptively immunized mice after infection with Babesia microti or injection with antigen fractions. Aust J Exp Biol Med Sci. 1985 Jun;63 (Pt 3):261-72. PMID:2415100

Meister J. Human babesiosis: a case study. Clin Excell Nurse Pract. 1999 Jul;3(4):214-6. PMID:10711060

Mellors LT, Dalgliesh RJ, Timms P, Rodwell BJ, Callow LL. Preparation and laboratory testing of a frozen vaccine containing Babesia bovis, Babesia bigemina and Anaplasma centrale. Res Vet Sci. 1982 Mar;32(2):194-7. PMID:7079601

Mesfin F, Demissew S, Teklehaymanot T. An ethnobotanical study of medicinal plants in Wonago Woreda, SNNPR, Ethiopia. J Ethnobiol Ethnomed. 2009 Oct 12;5:28. PMID:19821994

Metcalf ES. The role of international transport of equine semen on disease transmission. Anim Reprod Sci. 2001 Dec 3;68(3-4):229-37. PMID:11744267

Meyer C, Guthrie AJ, Stevens KB. Clinical and clinicopathological changes in 6 healthy ponies following intramuscular administration of multiple doses of imidocarb dipropionate. J S Afr Vet Assoc. 2005 Mar;76(1):26-32. PMID:15900897

Miguel CA, Manderson L, Lansang MA. Patterns of treatment for malaria in Tayabas, The Philippines: implications for control. Trop Med Int Health. 1998 May;3(5):413-21. PMID:9623948

Miguel CA, Tallo VL, Manderson L, Lansang MA. Local knowledge and treatment of malaria in Agusan del Sur, The Philippines. Soc Sci Med. 1999 Mar;48(5):607-18. PMID:10080362

Milhous W. Development of new drugs for chemoprophylaxis of malaria. Bull Soc Pathol Exot. 2001 Jul;94(2 Pt 2):149-51. PMID:16579068

Minodier P, Noël G, Blanc P, Tsaregorodtseva N, Retornaz K, Garnier JM. [Malaria chemoprophylaxis in traveling children]. [Article in French]. Arch Pediatr. 2005 Jan;12(1):53-8. PMID:15653056

Mintz ED, Anderson JF, Cable RG, Hadler JL. Transfusion-transmitted babesiosis: a case report from a new endemic area. Transfusion. 1991 May;31(4):365-8. PMID:2021001

Mitchell GH, Butcher GA, Cohen S. A merozoite vaccine effective against Plasmodium knowlesi malaria. Nature. 1974 Nov 22;252(5481):311-3. PMID:4431452

Mitchell GF, Handman E, Howard RJ. Protection of mice against plasmodium and babesia infections: attempts to raise host-protective sera. Aust J Exp Biol Med Sci. 1978 Oct;56(5):553-9. PMID:375903

Mitrović S, Kranjcić-Zec I, Arsić-Arsenijević V, Dzamić A, Radonjić I. [Human babesiosis--recent discoveries]. [Article in Serbian]. Med Pregl. 2004 Jul-Aug;57(7-8):349-53. PMID:15626291

Molinar E, James MA, Kakoma I, Holland C, Ristic M. Antigenic and immunogenic studies on cell culture-derived Babesia canis. Vet Parasitol. 1982 Mar;10(1):29-40. PMID:6179286

Molloy JB, Bock RE, Templeton JM, Bruyeres AG, Bowles PM, Blight GW, Jorgensen WK. Identification of antigenic differences that discriminate between cattle vaccinated with Anaplasma centrale and cattle naturally infected with Anaplasma marginale. Int J Parasitol. 2001 Feb;31(2):179-86. PMID:11239938

Montenegro-James S. Immunoprophylactic control of bovine babesiosis: role of exoantigens of Babesia. Trans R Soc Trop Med Hyg. 1989;83 Suppl:85-94. PMID:2696166

Montenegro-James S. Prevalence and control of babesiosis in the Americas. Mem Inst Oswaldo Cruz. 1992;87 Suppl 3:27-36. PMID:1343700

Montenegro-James S, Ristic M, Toro Benitez M, Leon E, Lopez R. Heterologous strain immunity in bovine babesiosis using a culture-derived soluble Babesia bovis immunogen. Vet Parasitol. 1985 Dec;18(4):321-37.PMID:4090242

Montenegro-James S, Toro Benitez M, Leon E, Lopez R, Ristic M. Bovine babesiosis: induction of protective immunity with culture-derived Babesia bovis and Babesia bigemina immunogens. Parasitol Res. 1987;74(2):142-50. PMID:3325981

Montenegro-James S, Toro M, Leon E, Guillen AT. Field evaluation of an exoantigen-containing Babesia vaccine in Venezuela. Mem Inst Oswaldo Cruz. 1992;87 Suppl 3:283-8. PMID:1343704

Montenegro-James S, Toro M, Leon E, Guillen AT, Lopez R, Lopez W. Immunization of cattle with an inactivated polyvalent vaccine against anaplasmosis and babesiosis. Ann N Y Acad Sci. 1992 Jun 16;653:112-21. PMID:1626861

Montero E, Rodriguez M, Oksov Y, Lobo CA. Babesia divergens apical membrane antigen 1 and its interaction with the human red blood cell. Infect Immun. 2009 Nov;77(11):4783-93. Epub 2009 Aug 31. PMID:19720759

Moore DJ. Therapeutic implications of Babesia canis infection in dogs. J S Afr Vet Assoc. 1979 Dec;50(4):346-52. PMID:553976

Moore SJ, Hill N, Ruiz C, Cameron MM. Field evaluation of traditionally used plant-based insect repellents and fumigants against the malaria vector Anopheles darlingi in Riberalta, Bolivian Amazon. J Med Entomol. 2007 Jul;44(4):624-30. PMID:17695017

Moore SJ, Lenglet A, Hill N. Field evaluation of three plant-based insect repellents against malaria vectors in Vaca Diez Province, the Bolivian Amazon. J Am Mosq Control Assoc. 2002 Jun;18(2):107-10. PMID:12083351

Moreau Y, Vidor E, Bissuel G, Dubreuil N. Vaccination against canine babesiosis: an overview of field observations. Trans R Soc Trop Med Hyg. 1989;83 Suppl:95-6. PMID:2623757

Moreno Giménez JC, Jiménez Puya R, Galán Gutiérrez M, Ortega Salas R, Dueñas Jurado JM. Erythema figuratum in septic babesiosis. J Eur Acad Dermatol Venereol. 2006 Jul;20(6):726-8. PMID:16836504

Morita T, Saeki H, Imai S, Ishii T. Reactivity of anti-erythrocyte antibody induced by Babesia gibsoni infection against aged erythrocytes. Vet Parasitol. 1995 Jul;58(4):291-9. PMID:8533268

Morzaria SP, Brocklesby DW, Harradine DL, Barnett SF. Babesia major in Britain: infectivity of suspensions derived from ground-up Haemaphysalis punct at a nymphs. Int J Parasitol. 1974 Aug;4(4):437-8. PMID:4448585

Morzaria SP, Brocklesby DW, Harradine DL, Luther PD. Babesia major in Britain: infectivity for cattle of cryopreserved parasites derived from Haemaphysalis punctata nymphs. Res Vet Sci. 1977 Mar;22(2):190-3. PMID:860093

Morzaria SP, Young AS, Hudson EB. Babesia bigemina in Kenya: experimental transmission by Boophilus decoloratus and the production of tick-derived stabilates. Parasitology. 1977 Jun;74(3):291-8. PMID:876684

Moshkovskiĭ ShD, Tareev EM, Dukhanina NN, Stavrovskaia VI, Ozeretskovskaia NN, Rabinovich SA. [Development of the main trends of malariology in the USSR].[Article in Russian]. Med Parazitol (Mosk). 1967 Nov-Dec;36(6):643-63. PMID:4887958

Mosqueda J, Figueroa JV, Alvarez A, Bautista R, Falcon A, Ramos A, Canto G, Vega CA. Advances in the development of molecular tools for the control of bovine babesiosis in Mexico. Parassitologia. 2007 May;49 Suppl 1:19-22. PMID:17691602

Motabar M, Tabibzadeh I, Manouchehri AV. Malaria and its control in Iran. Trop Geogr Med. 1975 Mar;27(1):71-8. PMID:1094644

Mott GA, Wilson R, Fernando A, Robinson A, MacGregor P, Kennedy D, Schaap D, Matthews JB, Matthews KR. Targeting cattle-borne zoonoses and cattle pathogens using a novel trypanosomatid-based delivery system. PLoS Pathog. 2011 Oct;7(10):e1002340. Epub 2011 Oct 27. PMID:22046137

Mubyazi G, Bloch P, Kamugisha M, Kitua A, Ijumba J. Intermittent preventive treatment of malaria during pregnancy: a qualitative study of knowledge, attitudes and practices of district health managers, antenatal care staff and pregnant women in Korogwe District, North-Eastern Tanzania. Malar J. 2005 Jul 20;4:31. PMID:16033639

Munro JB, Silva JC. Ribonucleotide Reductase as a Target to Control Apicomplexan Diseases. Curr Issues Mol Biol. 2011 Jul 26;14(1):9-26. [Epub ahead of print]. PMID:21791713

Murnigsih T, Subeki, Matsuura H, Takahashi K, Yamasaki M, Yamato O, Maede Y, Katakura K, Suzuki M, Kobayashi S, Chairul, Yoshihara T. Evaluation of the inhibitory activities of the extracts of Indonesian traditional medicinal plants against Plasmodium falciparum and Babesia gibsoni. J Vet Med Sci. 2005 Aug;67(8):829-31. PMID:16141673

Mustofa, Sholikhah EN, Wahyuono S. In vitro and in vivo antiplasmodial activity and cytotoxicity of extracts of Phyllanthus niruri L. herbs traditionally used to treat malaria in Indonesia. Southeast Asian J Trop Med Public Health. 2007 Jul;38(4):609-15. PMID:17882995

Muthee JK, Gakuya DW, Mbaria JM, Kareru PG, Mulei CM, Njonge FK. Ethnobotanical study of anthelmintic and other medicinal plants traditionally used in Loitoktok district of Kenya. J Ethnopharmacol. 2011 Apr 26;135(1):15-21. Epub 2011 Feb 22. PMID:21349318

Mylonakis E. When to suspect and how to monitor babesiosis. Am Fam Physician. 2001 May 15;63(10):1969-74. PMID:11388711

Nadembega P, Boussim JI, Nikiema JB, Poli F, Antognoni F. Medicinal plants in Baskoure, Kourittenga Province, Burkina Faso: an ethnobotanical study. J Ethnopharmacol. 2011 Jan 27;133(2):378-95. Epub 2010 Oct 13. PMID:20950680

Nagao E, Arie T, Dorward DW, Fairhurst RM, Dvorak JA. The avian malaria parasite Plasmodium gallinaceum causes marked structural changes on the surface of its host erythrocyte. J Struct Biol. 2008 Jun;162(3):460-7. Epub 2008 Mar 21. PMID:18442920

Naidoo V, Mulders MS, Swan GE. The intravenous pharmacokinetics of diminazene in healthy dogs. J S Afr Vet Assoc. 2009 Dec;80(4):215-9. PMID:20458860

Naidoo V, Zweygarth E, Eloff JN, Swan GE. Identification of anti-babesial activity for four ethnoveterinary plants in vitro. Vet Parasitol. 2005 Jun 10;130(1-2):9-13. Epub 2005 Apr 12. PMID:15893064

Naing C, Aung K, Win DK, Wah MJ. Efficacy and safety of chloroquine for treatment in patients with uncomplicated Plasmodium vivax infections in endemic countries. Trans R Soc Trop Med Hyg. 2010 Nov;104(11):695-705. Epub 2010 Sep 20. PMID:20850161

Nakamura Y, Tsuji M, Arai S, Ishihara C. A method for rapid and complete substitution of the circulating erythrocytes in SCID mice with bovine erythrocytes and use of the substituted mice for bovine hemoprotozoa infections. J Immunol Methods. 1995 Dec 27;188(2):247-54. PMID:8551053

Nakao R, Mizukami C, Kawamura Y, Subeki, Bawm S, Yamasaki M, Maede Y, Matsuura H, Nabeta K, Nonaka N, Oku Y, Katakura K. Evaluation of efficacy of bruceine A, a natural quassinoid compound extracted from a medicinal plant, Brucea javanica, for canine babesiosis. J Vet Med Sci. 2009 Jan;71(1):33-41. PMID:19194074

Namangala B, Inoue N, Sugimoto C. Preliminary studies on the effects of orally-administered Transforming Growth Factor-beta on protozoan diseases in mice. Jpn J Vet Res. 2009 Aug;57(2):101-8. PMID:19827745

Narasimhan S, Montgomery RR, DePonte K, Tschudi C, Marcantonio N, Anderson JF, Sauer JR, Cappello M, Kantor FS, Fikrig E. Disruption of Ixodes scapularis anticoagulation by using RNA interference. Proc Natl Acad Sci U S A. 2004 Feb 3;101(5):1141-6. Epub 2004 Jan 26. PMID:14745044

Nari A. Strategies for the control of one-host ticks and relationship with tick-borne diseases in South America. Vet Parasitol. 1995 Mar;57(1-3):153-65. PMID:7597780

Nasveld P, Kitchener S. Treatment of acute vivax malaria with tafenoquine. Trans R Soc Trop Med Hyg. 2005 Jan;99(1):2-5. PMID:15550254

Nasveld P, Kitchener S, Edstein M, Rieckmann K. Comparison of tafenoquine (WR238605) and primaquine in the post-exposure (terminal) prophylaxis of vivax malaria in Australian Defence Force personnel. Trans R Soc Trop Med Hyg. 2002 Nov-Dec;96(6):683-4. PMID:12625150

Nasveld PE, Edstein MD, Reid M, Brennan L, Harris IE, Kitchener SJ, Leggat PA, Pickford P, Kerr C, Ohrt C, Prescott W; Tafenoquine Study Team. Randomized, double-blind study of the safety, tolerability, and efficacy of tafenoquine versus mefloquine for malaria prophylaxis in nonimmune subjects. Antimicrob Agents Chemother. 2010 Feb;54(2):792-8. Epub 2009 Dec 7. PMID:19995933

Neal RA, Garnham PC, Cohen S. Immunization against protozoal diseases. Br Med Bull. 1969 May;25(2):194-201. PMID:4918534

Neal RA, Garnham PC, Cohen S. [Immunization against protozoal diseases].[Article in Spanish]. Bol Oficina Sanit Panam. 1973 Oct;75(4):337-53. PMID:4272727

Németh K, Tárkányi G, Varga E, Imre T, Mizsei R, Iványi R, Visy J, Szemán J, Jicsinszky L, Szente L, Simonyi M. Enantiomeric separation of antimalarial drugs by capillary electrophoresis using neutral and negatively charged cyclodextrins. J Pharm Biomed Anal. 2011 Feb 20;54(3):475-81. Epub 2010 Sep 19. PMID:20943339

Ngo V, Civen R. Babesiosis acquired through blood transfusion, California, USA. Emerg Infect Dis. 2009 May;15(5):785-7. PMID:19402969

Nicholson GT, Walsh CA, Madan RP. Transfusion-associated babesiosis in a 7-month-old infant after bidirectional Glenn procedure. Congenit Heart Dis. 2010 Nov-Dec;5(6):607-13. PMID:21106022

Nicolas X, Granier H, Laborde JP, Talarmin F, Klotz F. [Plasmodium vivax: therapy update].[Article in French]. Presse Med. 2001 Apr 21;30(15):767-71. PMID:11360746

Nishisaka M, Yokoyama N, Xuan X, Inoue N, Nagasawa H, Fujisaki K, Mikami T, Igarashi I. Characterisation of the gene encoding a protective antigen from Babesia microti identified it as eta subunit of chaperonin containing T-complex protein 1. Int J Parasitol. 2001 Dec;31(14):1673-9. PMID:11730795

[No authors listed]. DEVELOPMENT of the antimalarial paludrine. Am Prof Pharm. 1946 Apr;12:352-4. PMID:21027189

[No authors listed]. DEVELOPMENT of the antimalarial paludrine. Am Prof Pharm. 1946 Apr;12:352-4. PMID:21027189

[No authors listed]. Malaria and economic development in Papua New Guinea. Med J Aust. 1972 Dec 30;2(27):1473-4. PMID:4655125

[No authors listed]. Timing antimalarial prophylaxis: when to start and how long to go on. Drug Ther Bull. 1974 Aug 16;12(17):65-7. PMID:4457297

[No authors listed] Developments in malaria immunology. Report of a WHO scientific group. World Health Organ Tech Rep Ser. 1975;(579):1-68. PMID:813400

[No authors listed]. Vaccines against malaria and babesiosis. Lancet. 1983 Nov 26;2(8361):1232-3. PMID:6139575

[No authors listed]. Research needs on internal parasites of horses. Am J Vet Res. 1984 Aug;45(8):1614-8. PMID:6383147

[No authors listed]. OSHA's bloodborne pathogens standard: analysis and recommendations. Health Devices. 1993 Feb;22(2):35-92. PMID:8444629

[No authors listed]. Molecule of the month. Tafenoquine succinate. Drug News Perspect. 2003 May;16(4):238. PMID:12942153

Nohýnková E, Kubek J, Měst'ánková O, Chalupa P, Hubálek Z. [A case of Babesia microti imported into the Czech Republic from the USA].[Article in Czech]. Cas Lek Cesk. 2003;142(6):377-81. PMID:12924039

Nonaka D, Vongseththa K, Kobayashi J, Bounyadeth S, Kano S, Phompida S, Jimba M. Public and private sector treatment of malaria in Lao PDR. Acta Trop. 2009 Dec;112(3):283-7. Epub 2009 Aug 14. PMID:19683502

Norimine J, Mosqueda J, Palmer GH, Lewin HA, Brown WC. Conservation of Babesia bovis small heat shock protein (Hsp20) among strains and definition of T helper cell epitopes recognized by cattle with diverse major histocompatibility complex class II haplotypes. Infect Immun. 2004 Feb;72(2):1096-106. PMID:14742557

Nussenzweig RS, Vanderberg J, Spitalny GL, Rivera CI, Orton C, Most H. Sporozoite-induced immunity in mammalian malaria. A review. Am J Trop Med Hyg. 1972 Sep;21(5):722-8. PMID:4561520

Obaldia N 3rd, Rossan RN, Cooper RD, Kyle DE, Nuzum EO, Rieckmann KH, Shanks GD. WR 238605, chloroquine, and their combinations as blood schizonticides against a chloroquine-resistant strain of Plasmodium vivax in Aotus monkeys. Am J Trop Med Hyg. 1997 May;56(5):508-10. PMID:9180599

Oehme R, Hartelt K, Backe H, Brockmann S, Kimmig P. Foci of tick-borne diseases in southwest Germany. Int J Med Microbiol. 2002 Jun;291 Suppl 33:22-9. PMID:12141751

Ohgitani T, Okabe T, Sasaki N. [Studies on immunity to Babesia gibsoni in dogs immunostimulation by Bordetella bronchiseptica]. [Article in Japanese]. Nihon Saikingaku Zasshi. 1990 Jul;45(4):785-95. PMID:2232161

Ohrt C, Willingmyre GD, Lee P, Knirsch C, Milhous W. Assessment of azithromycin in combination with other antimalarial drugs against Plasmodium falciparum in vitro. Antimicrob Agents Chemother. 2002 Aug;46(8):2518-24. PMID:12121927

Okamura M, Yokoyama N, Takabatake N, Okubo K, Ikehara Y, Igarashi I. Modification of host erythrocyte membranes by trypsin and chymotrypsin treatments and effects on the in vitro growth of bovine and equine Babesia parasites. J Parasitol. 2007 Feb;93(1):208-11. PMID:17436968

Okpako LC, Ajaiyeoba EO. In vitro and in vivo antimalarial studies of Striga hermonthica and Tapinanthus sessilifolius extracts. Afr J Med Med Sci. 2004 Mar;33(1):73-5. PMID:15490799

Oladosu LA. Effects of intravenous corticosteroid on the pathogenicity of Babesia equi infection of donkeys (Equus asinus). Zentralbl Veterinarmed B. 1988 Aug;35(7):509-14. PMID:3188726

Oladosu LA, Olufemi BE. Haematology of experimental babesiosis and ehrlichiosis in steroid immunosuppressed horses. Zentralbl Veterinarmed B. 1992 Jul;39(5):345-52. PMID:1519411

Oleson CV, Sivalingam JJ, O'Neill BJ, Staas WE Jr. Transverse myelitis secondary to coexistent Lyme disease and babesiosis. J Spinal Cord Med. 2003 Summer;26(2):168-71. PMID:12828297

Oliveira TM, Furuta PI, de Carvalho D, Machado RZ. A study of cross-reactivity in serum samples from dogs positive for Leishmania sp., Babesia canis and Ehrlichia canis in enzyme-linked immunosorbent assay and indirect fluorescent antibody test. Rev Bras Parasitol Vet. 2008 Jan-Mar;17(1):7-11. PMID:18554433

Omar MS, Collins WE. Studies on the antimalarial effects of RC-12 and WR 14,997 on the development of Plasmodium cynomolgi in mosquitoes and Rhesus monkeys. Am J Trop Med Hyg. 1974 May;23(3):339-49. PMID:4207342

Omar MS, Collins WE, Contacos PG. Gametocytocidal and sporontocidal effects of antimalarial drugs on malaria parasites. I. Effect of single and multiple doses of primaquine on Plasmodium cynomolgi. Exp Parasitol. 1973 Oct;34(2):229-41. PMID:4200769

Omar MS, Gwadz RW, Miller LH. Incorporation of nucleic acid precursors by Plasmodium cynomolgi in Anopheles balabacensis. Tropenmed Parasitol. 1975 Sep;26(3):303-6. PMID:1189024

Ong KR, Stavropoulos C, Inada Y. Babesiosis, asplenia, and AIDS. Lancet. 1990 Jul 14;336(8707):112. PMID:1975291

Ooka H, Terkawi MA, Goo YK, Luo Y, Li Y, Yamagishi J, Nishikawa Y, Igarashi I, Xuan X. Babesia microti: molecular and antigenic characterizations of a novel 94-kDa protein (BmP94). Exp Parasitol. 2011 Jan;127(1):287-93. Epub 2010 Jun 25. PMID:20599995

Orinda GO, Gale KR, Wright IG, Parrodi F. Bovine babesiosis: failure to induce interferon gamma production in response to Babesia bovis antigens in cattle. Int J Parasitol. 1992 May;22(3):395-8. PMID:1639576

Orinda GO, Waltisbuhl DJ, Young AS, Wright IG. Low doses of natural human interferon alpha inhibit the development of Babesia microti infection in BALB/c mice. Vet Parasitol. 1994 May;53(1-2):53-8. PMID:8091618

Overdulve JP, Antonisse HW. Measurement of the effect of low temperature on protozoa by titration. II. Titration of Babesia rodhaini, using prepatent period and survival time, before and after storage at minus 76 degree C. Exp Parasitol. 1970 Apr;27(2):323-41. PMID:5446635

Oz HS, Hughes WT. Acute fulminating babesiosis in hamsters infected with Babesia microti. Int J Parasitol. 1996 Jun;26(6):667-70. PMID:8875313

Palacios Fraire S. Analysis of the principal problems impeding normal development of malaria eradication programs. Bull Pan Am Health Organ. 1975;9(4):283-94. PMID:1240013

Palmer DA, Buening GM, Carson CA. Cryopreservation of Babesia bovis for in vitro cultivation. Parasitology. 1982 Jun;84(Pt 3):567-72. PMID:7099713

Pancewicz S, Moniuszko A, Bieniarz E, Puciło K, Grygorczuk S, Zajkowska J, Czupryna P, Kondrusik M, Swierzbińska-Pijanowska R. Anti-Babesia microti antibodies in foresters highly exposed to tick bites in Poland. Scand J Infect Dis. 2011 Mar;43(3):197-201. Epub 2010 Dec 9. PMID:21142620

Pantanowitz L, Aufranc S 3rd, Monahan-Earley R, Dvorak A, Telford SR 3rd. Transfusion medicine illustrated. Morphologic hallmarks of Babesia. Transfusion. 2002 Nov;42(11):1389. PMID:12421208

Pantanowitz L, Telford SR 3rd, Cannon ME. The impact of babesiosis on transfusion medicine. Transfus Med Rev. 2002 Apr;16(2):131-43. PMID:11941575

Pasvol G, Weatherall DJ, Wilson RJ, Smith DH, Gilles HM. Fetal haemoglobin and malaria. Lancet. 1976 Jun 12;1(7972):1269-72. PMID:73695

Patarroyo JH, Prates AA, Tavares CA, Mafra CL, Vargas MI. Exoantigens of an attenuated strain of Babesia bovis used as a vaccine against bovine babesiosis. Vet Parasitol. 1995 Oct;59(3-4):189-99. PMID:8533277

Pates HV, Line JD, Keto AJ, Miller JE. Personal protection against mosquitoes in Dar es Salaam, Tanzania, by using a kerosene oil lamp to vaporize transfluthrin. Med Vet Entomol. 2002 Sep;16(3):277-84. PMID:12243228

Paul JH, Seaforth CE, Tikasingh T. Eryngium foetidum L.: a review. Fitoterapia. 2011 Apr;82(3):302-8. Epub 2010 Nov 6. PMID:21062639

Payne RC. Cryopreservation of bovine blood infected with Babesia major for use in the indirect fluorescent antibody test. Res Vet Sci. 1978 May;24(3):375. PMID:353926

Payne RC, Osorio O, Ybañez A. Tick-borne diseases of cattle in Paraguay. II. Immunisation against anaplasmosis and babesiosis. Trop Anim Health Prod. 1990 May;22(2):101-8. PMID:2196724

Pearce GW, Gooden EL, Johnson DR. Specifications of the International Cooperation Administration for DDT water-dispersible powder for use in malaria control programmes. Bull World Health Organ. 1959;20:913-20. PMID:14431217

Pearson CD, McLean SA, Tetley K, Phillips RS. Induction of secondary antibody responses to Plasmodium chabaudi in vitro. Clin Exp Immunol. 1983 Apr;52(1):121-8. PMID:6861369

Peirce MA, Norton CC, Donnelly J. The preservation of Cytoecetes phagocytophila in liquid nitrogen. Res Vet Sci. 1974 May;16(3):393-4. PMID:4855005

Pendse S, Bilyk JR, Lee MS. The ticking time bomb. Surv Ophthalmol. 2006 May-Jun;51(3):274-9. PMID:16644367

Penzhorn BL, Lewis BD, de Waal DT, López Rebollar LM. Sterilisation of Babesia canis infections by imidocarb alone or in combination with diminazene. J S Afr Vet Assoc. 1995 Sep;66(3):157-9. PMID:8596187

Perdrizet GA, Olson NH, Krause PJ, Banever GT, Spielman A, Cable RG. Babesiosis in a renal transplant recipient acquired through blood transfusion. Transplantation. 2000 Jul 15;70(1):205-8. PMID:10919602

Peregrine AS. Chemotherapy and delivery systems: haemoparasites. Vet Parasitol. 1994 Aug;54(1-3):223-48. PMID:7846852

Perkins HA, Busch MP. Transfusion-associated infections: 50 years of relentless challenges and remarkable progress. Transfusion. 2010 Oct;50(10):2080-99. PMID:20738828

Permin A, Yelifari L, Bloch P, Steenhard N, Hansen NP, Nansen P. Parasites in cross-bred pigs in the Upper East region of Ghana. Vet Parasitol. 1999 Nov;87(1):63-71. PMID:10628701

Peters W. The evolution of tafenoquine--antimalarial for a new millennium? J R Soc Med. 1999 Jul;92(7):345-52. PMID:10615272

Peters W. The chemotherapy of rodent malaria. II. Host-parasite relationships. 2. The relationship between chloroquine sensitivity and the age of the host cell. Ann Trop Med Parasitol. 1968 Jun;62(2):246-61. PMID:5751426

Peters W. Partial inhibition by mepacrine of the development of sulphonamide resistance in Plasmodium berghei. Nature. 1969 Aug 23;223(5208):858-9. PMID:5799037

Peters W. The chemotherapy of rodent malaria. X. Dynamics of drug resistance. II. Acquisition and loss of chloroquine resistance in Plasmodium berghei observed by continuous bioassay. Ann Trop Med Parasitol. 1970 Mar;64(1):25-40. PMID:5485708

Peters W. The chemotherapy of rodent malaria. XVII. Dynamics of drug resistance. 3. Influence of drug combinations on the development of resistance to chloroquine in P. berghei. Ann Trop Med Parasitol. 1973 Jun;67(2):143-54. PMID:4578935

Peters W. Prevention of drug resistance in rodent malaria by the use of drug mixtures. Bull World Health Organ. 1974;51(4):379-83. PMID:4619060

Peters W. Recent advances in antimalarial chemotherapy and drug resistance. Adv Parasitol. 1974;12:69-114. PMID:4217563

Peters W, Bafort J, Ramkaran AE. The chemotherapy of rodent malaria. XI. Cyclically transmitted, chloroquine-resistant variants of the Keyberg 173 strain of Plasmodium berghei. Ann Trop Med Parasitol. 1970 Mar;64(1):41-51. PMID:5485709

Peters W, Porter M. The chemotherapy of rodent malaria, XXVI. The potential value of WR 122,455 (a 9-phenanthrenemethanol) against drug-resistant malaria parasites. Ann Trop Med Parasitol. 1976 Sep;70(3):271-81. PMID:788658

Peters W, Robinson BL, Milhous WK. The chemotherapy of rodent malaria. LI. Studies on a new 8-aminoquinoline, WR 238,605. Ann Trop Med Parasitol. 1993 Dec;87(6):547-52. PMID:8122915

Peters W, Stewart LB, Robinson BL. The chemotherapy of rodent malaria. LXI. Drug combinations to impede the selection of drug resistance, part 4: the potential role of 8-aminoquinolines. Ann Trop Med Parasitol. 2003 Apr;97(3):221-36. PMID:12803854

Petersen E. Malaria chemoprophylaxis: when should we use it and what are the options? Expert Rev Anti Infect Ther. 2004 Feb;2(1):119-32. PMID:15482177

Phillips RS. Resistance of mice and rats to Babesia rodhaini challenge after inoculation with irradiated B. rodhaini infected red cells. Trans R Soc Trop Med Hyg. 1970;64(4):470. PMID:4991940

Phillips RS. Resistance of mice and rats to challenge by Babesia rodhaini after inoculation with irradiated red cells infected with B. rodhaini. Nature. 1970 Sep 19;227(5264):1255. PMID:4989140

Phillips RS. Immunity of rats and mice following injection with 60Co irradiated Babesia rodhaini infected red cells. Parasitology. 1971 Apr;62(2):221-31. PMID:4995421

Phillips RS. Evidence that piroplasms can undergo antigenic variation. Nature. 1971 Jun 4;231(5301):323. PMID:4930987

Phillips RS. Antigenic variation in Babesia rodhaini demonstrated by immunization with irradiated parasites. Parasitology. 1971 Oct;63(2):315-22. PMID:5002030

Phillips RS, Wakelin D. Trichuris muris: effect of concurrent infections with rodent piroplasms on immune expulsion from mice. Exp Parasitol. 1976 Feb;39(1):95-100. PMID:1253888

Pipano E. Immunization against intracellular blood protozoans of cattle. Prog Clin Biol Res. 1980;47:301-14. PMID:6782586

Pipano E, Alekceev E, Galker F, Fish L, Samish M, Shkap V. Immunity against Boophilus annulatus induced by the Bm86 (Tick-GARD) vaccine. Exp Appl Acarol. 2003;29(1-2):141-9. PMID:14580066

Pipano E, Jeruham I, Frank M. Pentamidine in chemoimmunisation of cattle against Babesia bigemina infection. Trop Anim Health Prod. 1979 Feb;11(1):13-6. PMID:442205

Pipano E, Krigel Y, Markovics A, Rubinstein E, Frank M. Mitigation of the response of Friesian calves to live Babesia bovis vaccine by treatment with long acting oxytetracycline. Vet Rec. 1985 Oct 19;117(16):413-4. PMID:4071930

Pipano E, Markovics A, Kriegel Y, Frank M, Fish L. Use of long-acting oxytetracycline in the immunisation of cattle against Babesia bovis and B bigemina. Res Vet Sci. 1987 Jul;43(1):64-6. PMID:3628985

Pipano E, Shkap V, Kriegel Y, Leibovitz B, Savitsky I, Fish L. Babesia bovis and B. bigemina: Persistence of infection in friesian cows following vaccination with live antibabesial vaccines. Vet J. 2002 Jul;164(1):64-8. PMID:12359486

Pitasawat B, Champakaew D, Choochote W, Jitpakdi A, Chaithong U, Kanjanapothi D, Rattanachanpichai E, Tippawangkosol P, Riyong D, Tuetun B, Chaiyasit D.

Aromatic plant-derived essential oil: an alternative larvicide for mosquito control. Fitoterapia. 2007 Apr;78(3):205-10. Epub 2007 Feb 6. PMID:17337133

Ploemen IH, Prudêncio M, Douradinha BG, Ramesar J, Fonager J, van Gemert GJ, Luty AJ, Hermsen CC, Sauerwein RW, Baptista FG, Mota MM, Waters AP, Que I, Lowik CW, Khan SM, Janse CJ, Franke-Fayard BM. Visualisation and quantitative analysis of the rodent malaria liver stage by real time imaging. PLoS One. 2009 Nov 18;4(11):e7881. PMID:19924309

Pohlit AM, Lopes NP, Gama RA, Tadei WP, Neto VF. Patent literature on mosquito repellent inventions which contain plant essential oils--a review. Planta Med. 2011 Apr;77(6):598-617. Epub 2011 Feb 15. PMID:21328177

Pohlit AM, Rezende AR, Lopes Baldin EL, Lopes NP, Neto VF. Plant extracts, isolated phytochemicals, and plant-derived agents which are lethal to arthropod vectors of human tropical diseases--a review. Planta Med. 2011 Apr;77(6):618-30. Epub 2011 Mar 22. PMID:21432748

Ponsa N, Sattabongkot J, Kittayapong P, Eikarat N, Coleman RE. Transmission-blocking activity of tafenoquine (WR-238605) and artelinic acid against naturally circulating strains of Plasmodium vivax in Thailand. Am J Trop Med Hyg. 2003 Nov;69(5):542-7. PMID:14695093

Popovsky MA. Transfusion-transmitted babesiosis. Transfusion. 1991 May;31(4):296-8. PMID:2020992

Popovsky MA, Lindberg LE, Syrek AL, Page PL. Prevalence of Babesia antibody in a selected blood donor population. Transfusion. 1988 Jan-Feb;28(1):59-61. PMID:3341068

Posnett ES, Fehrsen J, De Waal DT, Ambrosio RE. Detection of Babesia equi in infected horses and carrier animals using a DNA probe. Vet Parasitol. 1991 Jul;39(1-2):19-32. PMID:1897117

Posnett ES, Metaferia E, Wiliamson S, Brown CG, Canning EU. In vitro cultivation of an African strain of Babesia bigemina, its characterisation and infectivity in cattle. Parasitol Res. 1998;84(4):302-9. PMID:9569096

Potgieter FT. Chemotherapy of Babesia felis infection: efficacy of certain drugs. J S Afr Vet Assoc. 1981 Dec;52(4):289-93. PMID:7341778

Potgieter FT, Van Vuuren AS. The transmission of Babesia bovis using frozen infective material obtained from Boophilus microplus larvae. Onderstepoort J Vet Res. 1974 Jun;41(2):79-80. PMID:4449642

Powell RD. Development of new antimalarial drugs. Am J Trop Med Hyg. 1972 Sep;21(5):744-8. PMID:4561522

Powell RD, Berglund EM. Effects of chloroquine upon the maturation of asexual erythrocytic forms of Plasmodium vivax in vitro. Am J Trop Med Hyg. 1974 Nov;23(6):1007-14. PMID:4611251

Powell VI, Grima K. Exchange transfusion for malaria and Babesia infection. Transfus Med Rev. 2002 Jul;16(3):239-50. PMID:12075561

Pradines B, Mamfoumbi MM, Tall A, Sokhna C, Koeck JL, Fusai T, Mosnier J, Czarnecki E, Spiegel A, Trape JF, Kombila M, Rogier C. In vitro activity of tafenoquine against the asexual blood stages of Plasmodium falciparum isolates from Gabon, Senegal, and Djibouti. Antimicrob Agents Chemother. 2006 Sep;50(9):3225-6. PMID:16940138

Pradines B, Mamfoumbi MM, Tall A, Sokhna C, Koeck JL, Fusai T, Mosnier J, Czarnecki E, Spiegel A, Trape JF, Kombila M, Rogier C. In vitro activity of tafenoquine against the asexual blood stages of Plasmodium falciparum isolates from Gabon, Senegal, and Djibouti. Antimicrob Agents Chemother. 2006 Sep;50(9):3225-6. PMID:16940138

Precigout E, Delbecq S, Vallet A, Carcy B, Camillieri S, Hadj-Kaddour K, Kleuskens J, Schetters T, Gorenflot A. Association between sequence polymorphism in an epitope of Babesia divergens Bd37 exoantigen and protection induced by passive transfer. Int J Parasitol. 2004 Apr;34(5):585-93. PMID:15064123

Precigout E, Gorenflot A, Valentin A, Bissuel G, Carcy B, Brasseur P, Moreau Y, Schrevel J. Analysis of immune responses of different hosts to Babesia divergens isolates from different geographic areas and capacity of culture-derived exoantigens to induce efficient cross-protection. Infect Immun. 1991 Aug;59(8):2799-805. PMID:1713201

Price JE, Dolan TT. A comparison of the efficacy of imidocarb dipropionate and tetracycline hydrochloride in the treatment of canine ehrlichiosis. Vet Rec. 1980 Sep 20;107(12):275-7. PMID:7210420

Priest JW, Kwon JP, Montgomery JM, Bern C, Moss DM, Freeman AR, Jones CC, Arrowood MJ, Won KY, Lammie PJ, Gilman RH, Mead JR. Cloning and characterization of the acidic ribosomal protein P2 of Cryptosporidium parvum, a new 17-kilodalton antigen. Clin Vaccine Immunol. 2010 Jun;17(6):954-65. Epub 2010 Apr 21. PMID:20410328

Prince HE, Lapé-Nixon M, Patel H, Yeh C. Comparison of the Babesia duncani (WA1) IgG detection rates among clinical sera submitted to a reference laboratory for WA1 IgG testing and blood donor specimens from diverse geographic areas of the United States. Clin Vaccine Immunol. 2010 Nov;17(11):1729-33. Epub 2010 Sep 22. PMID:20861326

Przyjemski CJ. Was babesiosis transmitted by transfusion? N Engl J Med. 1981 Mar 19;304(12):733. PMID:7193287

Purfield AE, Tidwell RR, Meshnick SR. Interactions of DB75, a novel antimalarial agent, with other antimalarial drugs in vitro. Antimicrob Agents Chemother. 2008 Jun;52(6):2253-5. Epub 2008 Mar 24. PMID:18362196

Puri SK, Dutta GP. Blood schizontocidal activity of WR 238605 (Tafenoquine) against Plasmodium cynomolgi and Plasmodium fragile infections in rhesus monkeys. Acta Trop. 2003 Apr;86(1):35-40. PMID:12711101

Purnell RE, Brocklesby DW. Babesia divergens in splenectomised calves: immunogenicity of lyophilised plasma from an infected animal. Res Vet Sci. 1977 Sep;23(2):255-6. PMID:928989

Purnell RE, Gunter TD, Schroder J. Development of a prophylactic regime using long-acting tetracycline for the control of redwater and heartwater in susceptible cattle moved into an endemic area. Trop Anim Health Prod. 1989 Feb;21(1):11-9. PMID:2711456

Purnell RE, Lewis D, Brocklesby DW, Taylor SM. Bovine babesiosis: steps towards an irradiated vaccine. J S Afr Vet Assoc. 1979 Dec;50(4):339-44. PMID:553975

Purnell RE, Lewis D, Young ER. Investigations on the prophylactic effect of treatment with imidocarb diproprionate on Babesia divergens infections in splenectomized calves. Br Vet J. 1980 Sep-Oct;136(5):452-6. PMID:7225772

Purvis AC. Immunodepression in Babesia microti infections. Parasitology. 1977 Oct;75(2):197-205. PMID:337221

Qi C, Zhou D, Liu J, Cheng Z, Zhang L, Wang L, Wang Z, Yang D, Wang S, Chai T. Detection of Babesia divergens using molecular methods in anemic patients in Shandong Province, China. Parasitol Res. 2011 Jul;109(1):241-5. Epub 2011 Apr 19. PMID:21503639

Queener SF, Dean RA, Bartlett MS, Milhous WK, Berman JD, Ellis WY, Smith JW. Efficacy of intermittent dosage of 8-aminoquinolines for therapy or prophylaxis of Pneumocystis pneumonia in rats. J Infect Dis. 1992 Apr;165(4):764-8. PMID:1532406

Quintão-Silva MG, Melo MN, Ribeiro MF. Comparison of duplex PCR and microscopic techniques for the identification of Babesia bigemina and Babesia bovis in engorged female ticks of Boophilus microplus. Zoonoses Public Health. 2007;54(3-4):147-51. PMID:17456146

Rabinovich SA. [Experimental investigation of the antimalarial drug haloquine. 3. Investigation of the possibility to restrain the development of chemoresistance to chloridine (daraprim) by combined administration of chloridine with haloquine].[Article in Russian]. Med Parazitol (Mosk). 1965 Jul-Aug;34(4):434-9. PMID:5871367

Radford AJ, Van Leeuwen H, Christian SH. Social aspects in the changing epidemiology of malaria in the highlands of New Guinea. Ann Trop Med Parasitol. 1976 Mar;70(1):11-23. PMID:1267506

Raether W, Seidenath H. Survival of Aegyptianella pullorum, Anaplasma marginale and various parasitic protozoa following prolonged storage in liquid nitrogen. Z Parasitenkd. 1977 Aug 25;53(1):41-6. PMID:919686

Rajgor DD, Gogtay NJ, Kadam VS, Kamtekar KD, Dalvi SS, Chogle AR, Aigal U, Bichile LS, Kain KC, Kshirsagar NA. Efficacy of a 14-day primaquine regimen in preventing relapses in patients with Plasmodium vivax malaria in Mumbai, India. Trans R Soc Trop Med Hyg. 2003 Jul-Aug;97(4):438-40. PMID:15259476

Raju M, Salazar JC, Leopold H, Krause PJ. Atovaquone and azithromycin treatment for babesiosis in an infant. Pediatr Infect Dis J. 2007 Feb;26(2):181-3. PMID:17259886

Ramazani A, Sardari S, Zakeri S, Vaziri B. In vitro antiplasmodial and phytochemical study of five Artemisia species from Iran and in vivo activity of two species. Parasitol Res. 2010 Aug;107(3):593-9. Epub 2010 May 18. PMID:20480374

Ramharter M, Noedl H, Thimasarn K, Wiedermann G, Wernsdorfer G, Wernsdorfer WH. In vitro activity of tafenoquine alone and in combination with artemisinin against Plasmodium falciparum. Am J Trop Med Hyg. 2002 Jul;67(1):39-43. PMID:12363062

Ramharter M, Walochnik J, Lagler H, Winkler S, Wernsdorfer WH, Stoiser B, Graninger W. Clinical and molecular characterization of a near fatal case of human babesiosis in Austria. J Travel Med. 2010 Nov-Dec;17(6):416-8. PMID:21050324

Ranatunga P, Wanduragala L. Reactions and haematology in imported Jersey cattle premunized in Ceylon. Br Vet J. 1972 Jan;128(1):9-18. PMID:5062160

Rank RG, Weidanz WP, Bondi A. Nonsterilizing immunity in avian malaria: an antibody-independent phenomenon. Proc Soc Exp Biol Med. 1976 Feb;151(2):257-9. PMID:1082596

Ranque S. The treatment of babesiosis. N Engl J Med. 2001 Mar 8;344(10):773-4. PMID:11236790

Raoult D, Soulayrol L, Toga B, Dumon H, Casanova P. Babesiosis, pentamidine, and cotrimoxazole. Ann Intern Med. 1987 Dec;107(6):944. PMID:3500663

Rashina MG, Sarikian SIa. [On the development of a network of special institutions for the control of malaria and other parasitic diseases in the USSR].[Article in Russian]. Med Parazitol (Mosk). 1970 Mar-Apr;39(2):132-8. PMID:5473684

Rech A, Bittar CM, de Castro CG, Azevedo KR, dos Santos RP, Machado AR, Schwartsmann G, Goldani L, Brunetto AL. Asymptomatic babesiosis in a child with hepatoblastoma. J Pediatr Hematol Oncol. 2004 Mar;26(3):213. PMID:15125618

Reesink HW. European strategies against the parasite transfusion risk. Transfus Clin Biol. 2005 Feb;12(1):1-4. PMID:15814284

Regassa A, Penzhorn BL, Bryson NR. Progression towards endemic stability to bovine babesiosis in cattle introduced onto a game ranch. Onderstepoort J Vet Res. 2004 Dec;71(4):333-6. PMID:15732461

Reine NJ. Infection and blood transfusion: a guide to donor screening. Clin Tech Small Anim Pract. 2004 May;19(2):68-74. PMID:15179926

Reis C, Cote M, Paul RE, Bonnet S. Questing ticks in suburban forest are infected by at least six tick-borne pathogens. Vector Borne Zoonotic Dis. 2011 Jul;11(7):907-16. Epub 2010 Dec 15. PMID:21158500

Reis RC, Melo DR, Perinotto WM, Bittencourt VR. [In vitro pathogenicity of fungic formulation on nymphs and adults of Rhipicephalus sanguineus (Latreile, 1806) (Acari:Ixodidae)]. [Article in Portuguese]. Rev Bras Parasitol Vet. 2005 Jul-Sep;14(3):101-5. PMID:16229753

Reis SP, Maddineni S, Rozenblit G, Allen D. Spontaneous splenic rupture secondary to Babesia microti infection: treatment with splenic artery embolization. J Vasc Interv Radiol. 2011 May;22(5):732-4. PMID:21514529

Rieckmann KH, Trenholme GM, Williams RL, Carson PE, Frischer H, Desjardins RE. Prophylactic activity of mefloquine hydrochloride (WR 142490) in drug-resistant malaria. Bull World Health Organ. 1974;51(4):375-7. PMID:4619059

Ríos L, Alvarez G, Blair S. Serological and parasitological study and report of the first case of human babesiosis in Colombia. Rev Soc Bras Med Trop. 2003 Jul-Aug;36(4):493-8. Epub 2003 Aug 13. PMID:12937727

Roberts JA. Some quantitative aspects of the adoptive transfer of immunity to Plasmodium berghei with immune spleen cells. J Protozool. 1971 Aug;18(3):437-40. PMID:5132318

Roberts JA, Tracey-Patte PD. Babesia rodhaini: a study of the effects of immune serum. Int J Parasitol. 1975 Dec;5(6):577-81. PMID:1201890

Roberts MC, Groenendyk S. Splenectomy in the horse. Aust Vet J. 1978 Apr;54(4):196-7. PMID:687278

Rodriguez RI, Trees AJ. In vitro responsiveness of Babesia bovis to imidocarb dipropionate and the selection of a drug-adapted line. Vet Parasitol. 1996 Mar;62(1-2):35-41. PMID:8638391

Rodríguez SD, Palmer GH, McElwain TF, McGuire TC, Ruef BJ, Chitko-McKown MG, Brown WC. CD4+ T-helper lymphocyte responses against Babesia bigemina rhoptry-associated protein I. Infect Immun. 1996 Jun;64(6):2079-87. PMID:8675310

Rodríguez-Vivas RI, Quiñones-Avila FJ, Ramírez-Cruz GT, Cruz D, Wagner G. [Isolation of a field strain of Babesia bigemina (Piroplasma: Babesiidae) and establishment of in vitro culture for antigen production].[Article in Spanish]. Rev Biol Trop. 2007 Mar;55(1):127-33. PMID:18457120

Rogers RJ. The acquired resistance to Babesia argentina of cattle exposed to light infestation with cattle tick (Boophilus microplus). Aust Vet J. 1971 Jun;47(6):237-41. PMID:5106905

Rogers RJ. Serum opsonins and the passive transfer of protection in Babesia rodhaini infections of rats. Int J Parasitol. 1974 Apr;4(2):197-201. PMID:4822486

Rojas C, Figueroa JV, Alvarado A, Mejia P, Mosqueda JJ, Falcon A, Vega CA, Alvarez A. Bovine babesiosis live vaccine production: use of gamma irradiation on the substrate. Ann N Y Acad Sci. 2006 Oct;1081:405-16. PMID:17135544

Rollo IM. Antiplasmodial efficacy of 2,4--diaminopyrimidine0sylfonamide combinations, especially against chloroquine-resistant malaria. Can Med Assoc J. 1975 Jun 14;112(13 Spec No):50-3. PMID:805650

Römsing S, Lindegardh N, Bergqvist Y. Determination of tafenoquine in dried blood spots and plasma using LC and fluorescence detection. Bioanalysis. 2011 Aug;3(16):1847-53. PMID:21877894

Rosenblatt JE. Antiparasitic agents. Mayo Clin Proc. 1999 Nov;74(11):1161-75. PMID:10560606

Rosa FW. International aspects of perinatal mortality. Clin Obstet Gynecol. 1970 Mar;13(1):57-78. PMID:5430770

Rosenblatt JE. Laboratory diagnosis of infections due to blood and tissue parasites. Clin Infect Dis. 2009 Oct 1;49(7):1103-8. PMID:19691431

Rosner F, Zarrabi MH, Benach JL, Habicht GS. Babesiosis in splenectomized adults. Review of 22 reported cases. Am J Med. 1984 Apr;76(4):696-701. PMID:6424470

Rosowsky A, Huang PC, Papathanasopoulos N, Modest EJ. Quinazolines. 12. 1,3-Diaminobenzo(f)quinazolines containing long-chain alkyl or chloro substituents on the central ring. Synthesis and biological evaluation as candidate antifolate and antimalarial agents. J Med Chem. 1974 Nov;17(11):1217-22. PMID:4606974

Rousset JJ, Couzineau P, Baufine-Ducrocq H. [Plasmodium ovale (Stephens 1922)].[Article in French]. Ann Parasitol Hum Comp. 1969 May-Jun;44(3):273-328. PMID:4905936

Rowin KS, Tanowitz HB, Wittner M. Therapy of experimental babesiosis. Ann Intern Med. 1982 Oct;97(4):556-8. PMID:7125412

Ruebush MJ, Hanson WL. Transfer of immunity to Babesia microti of human origin using T lymphocytes in mice. Cell Immunol. 1980 Jul 1;52(2):255-65. PMID:6969120

Ruebush MJ, Steel LK, Kennedy DA. Prostaglandin-mediated suppression of delayed-type hypersensitivity to infected erythrocytes during Babesia microti infection in mice. Cell Immunol. 1986 Apr 1;98(2):300-10. PMID:2944617

Ruebush MJ, Troutman EH, Kennedy DA. Delayed-type hypersensitivity to Babesia microti-infected erythrocytes in mice. Cell Immunol. 1986 Apr 1;98(2):289-99. PMID:3757050

Ruef BJ, Tuo W, Rodriguez SD, Roussel AJ, Chitko-McKown CG, Palmer GH, McElwain TF, Canals A, Zarlenga DS, Gasbarre LC, Brown WC. Immunization with Babesia bigemina rhoptry-associated protein 1 induces a type 1 cytokine response. J Interferon Cytokine Res. 1997 Jan;17(1):45-54. PMID:9041471

Ruff MD, Fowler JL, Fernau RC, Matsuda K. Action of certain antiprotozoal compounds against Babesia gibsoni in dogs. Am J Vet Res. 1973 May;34(5):641-5. PMID:4703508

Russell BM, Udomsangpetch R, Rieckmann KH, Kotecka BM, Coleman RE, Sattabongkot J. Simple in vitro assay for determining the sensitivity of Plasmodium vivax isolates from fresh human blood to antimalarials in areas where P. vivax is endemic. Antimicrob Agents Chemother. 2003 Jan;47(1):170-3. PMID:12499187.

Ryan R, Krause PJ, Radolf J, Freeman K, Spielman A, Lenz R, Levin A. Diagnosis of babesiosis using an immunoblot serologic test. Clin Diagn Lab Immunol. 2001 Nov;8(6):1177-80. PMID:11687460

Saeki H, Ishii T. Studies on route of immunization with a mixture of killed parasites and adjuvants against Babesia rodhaini infection in mice. Nihon Juigaku Zasshi. 1989 Dec;51(6):1173-8. PMID:2601229

Saeki H, Ishii T. Effect of silica treatment on resistance to Babesia rodhaini infection in immunized mice. Vet Parasitol. 1996 Feb;61(3-4):201-10. PMID:8720558

Saito-Ito A, Dantrakool A, Kawai A, Yano Y, Takada N. [Babesiosis].[Article in Japanese]. Nihon Rinsho. 2003 Feb;61 Suppl 2:623-8. PMID:12722292

Saito-Ito A, Tsuji M, Wei Q, He S, Matsui T, Kohsaki M, Arai S, Kamiyama T, Hioki K, Ishihara C. Transfusion-acquired, autochthonous human babesiosis in Japan: isolation of Babesia microti-like parasites with hu-RBC-SCID mice. J Clin Microbiol. 2000 Dec;38(12):4511-6. PMID:11101588

Saitoito A, Rai SK, He S, Kohsaki M, Tsuji M, Ishihara C. [First demonstration of Babesia parasitizing in human in Japan]. [Article in Japanese]. Kansenshogaku Zasshi. 1999 Nov;73(11):1163-4. PMID:10624098

Salem GH, Liu X, Johnsrude JD, Dame JB, Roman Reddy G. Development and evaluation of an extra chromosomal DNA-based PCR test for diagnosing bovine babesiosis. Mol Cell Probes. 1999 Apr;13(2):107-13. PMID:10208801

Salih DA, Ali AM, Liu Z, Bakheit MA, Taha KM, El Imam AH, Kullmann B, El Hussein AM, Ahmed JS, Seitzer U. Development of a loop-mediated isothermal amplification method for detection of Theileria lestoquardi. Parasitol Res. 2011 Jul 9. [Epub ahead of print]. PMID:21744022

Sambri V, Marangoni A, Storni E, Cavrini F, Moroni A, Sparacino M, Cevenini R. [Tick borne zoonosis: selected clinical and diagnostic aspects].[Article in Italian]. Parassitologia. 2004 Jun;46(1-2):109-13. PMID:15305697

Sam-Wobo SO, Akinboroye T, Anosike JC, Adewale B. Knowledge and practices on malaria treatment measures among pregnant women in Abeokuta, Nigeria. Tanzan J Health Res. 2008 Oct;10(4):226-31. PMID:19402584

Sandler SG, Yu H, Rassai N. Risks of blood transfusion and their prevention. Clin Adv Hematol Oncol. 2003 May;1(5):307-13. PMID:16224428

Sannusi A, Aliu YO. Field observations on adult zebu bulls immunised against anaplasmosis by infection and treatment plus integrated tick control. Trop Anim Health Prod. 1986 Feb;18(1):13-20. PMID:3705174

Santoro F, Bernal J, Capron A. Complement activation by parasites. A review. Acta Trop. 1979 Mar;36(1):5-14. PMID:35934

Sato M, Hori Z, Hirose T, Suzuki N. Immune effect of toxoplasma lysate antigen (TLA) on cattle against Theileria sergenti infection. Nihon Juigaku Zasshi. 1985 Dec;47(6):921-9. PMID:4094277

Sato M, Igarashi I, Saito A, Hirose T, Suzuki N. Protection against Babesia infection in beagles immunized with Toxoplasma lysate antigen. Nihon Juigaku Zasshi. 1990 Feb;52(1):155-8. PMID:2179608

Schaller JL, Burkland GA, Langhoff PJ. Are various Babesia species a missed cause for hypereosinophilia? A follow-up on the first reported case of imatinib mesylate for idiopathic hypereosinophilia. MedGenMed. 2007 Feb 27;9(1):38. PMID:17435644

Scharf BA, Fricke RF, Baskin SI. Comparison of methemoglobin formers in protection against the toxic effects of cyanide. Gen Pharmacol. 1992 Jan;23(1):19-25. PMID:1592224

Schetters T. Vaccination against canine babesiosis. Trends Parasitol. 2005 Apr;21(4):179-84. PMID:15780840

Schetters TH, Kleuskens J, Scholtes N, Bos HJ. Strain variation limits protective activity of vaccines based on soluble Babesia canis antigens. Parasite Immunol. 1995 Apr;17(4):215-8. PMID:7542765

Schetters TP, Eling WM. Can Babesia infections be used as a model for cerebral malaria? Parasitol Today. 1999 Dec;15(12):492-7. PMID:10557150

Schetters TP, Kleuskens J, Carcy B, Gorenflot A, Vermeulen A. Vaccination against large Babesia species from dogs. Parassitologia. 2007 May;49 Suppl 1:13-7. PMID:17691601

Schetters TP, Kleuskens J, Scholtes N, Bos HJ. Vaccination of dogs against Babesia canis infection using parasite antigens from in vitro culture. Parasite Immunol. 1992 May;14(3):295-305. PMID:1625906

Schetters TP, Kleuskens J, Scholtes N, Gorenflot A. Parasite localization and dissemination in the Babesia-infected host. Ann Trop Med Parasitol. 1998 Jun;92(4):513-9.

PMID:9683902

Schetters TP, Kleuskens JA, Scholtes NC, Gorenflot A, Moubri K, Vermeulen AN. Vaccination of dogs against heterologous Babesia canis infection using antigens from culture supernatants. Vet Parasitol. 2001 Sep 12;100(1-2):75-86. PMID:11522408

Schetters TP, Kleuskens JA, Scholtes NC, Pasman JW, Bos HJ. Vaccination of dogs against Babesia canis infection using antigens from culture supernatants with emphasis on clinical babesiosis. Vet Parasitol. 1994 Apr;52(3-4):219-33. PMID:8073606

Schetters TP, Moubri K, Cooke BM. Comparison of Babesia rossi and Babesia canis isolates with emphasis on effects of vaccination with soluble parasite antigens: a review. J S Afr Vet Assoc. 2009 Jun;80(2):75-8. PMID:19831266

Schetters TP, Scholtes NC, Kleuskens JA, Bos HJ. Not peripheral parasitaemia but the level of soluble parasite antigen in plasma correlates with vaccine efficacy against Babesia canis. Parasite Immunol. 1996 Jan;18(1):1-6. PMID:9223150

Schetters TP, Strydom T, Crafford D, Kleuskens JA, van de Crommert J, Vermeulen AN. Immunity against Babesia rossi infection in dogs vaccinated with antigens from culture supernatants. Vet Parasitol. 2007 Mar 15;144(1-2):10-9. Epub 2006 Oct 23. PMID:17056181

Schindler R, Wokatsch R, Schröder G. [Immunity and serological reactions against Babesia canis in dogs after infection with living parasites and after immunization with a soluble antigen].[Article in German]. Z Tropenmed Parasitol. 1966 Jul;17(2):226-40. PMID:4969377

Schoeler GB, Manweiler SA, Wikel SK. Ixodes scapularis: effects of repeated infestations with pathogen-free nymphs on macrophage and T lymphocyte cytokine responses of BALB/c and C3H/HeN mice. Exp Parasitol. 1999 Aug;92(4):239-48. PMID:10425152

Schoeman JP. Canine babesiosis. Onderstepoort J Vet Res. 2009 Mar;76(1):59-66. PMID:19967929

Schoeman JP, Herrtage ME. Adrenal response to the low dose ACTH stimulation test and the cortisol-to-adrenocorticotrophic hormone ratio in canine babesiosis. Vet Parasitol. 2008 Jul 4;154(3-4):205-13. Epub 2008 Apr 7. PMID:18468798

Semel ME, Tavakkolizadeh A, Gates JD. Babesiosis in the immediate postoperative period after splenectomy for trauma. Surg Infect (Larchmt). 2009 Dec;10(6):553-6. PMID:19622029

Senthil Nathan S. The use of Eucalyptus tereticornis Sm. (Myrtaceae) oil (leaf extract) as a natural larvicidal agent against the malaria vector Anopheles stephensi Liston (Diptera: Culicidae). Bioresour Technol. 2007 Jul;98(9):1856-60. Epub 2006 Sep 25. PMID:16997545

Sethi S, Alcid D, Kesarwala H, Tolan RW Jr. Probable congenital babesiosis in infant, new jersey, USA. Emerg Infect Dis. 2009 May;15(5):788-91. PMID:19402971

Setty S, Khalil Z, Schori P, Azar M, Ferrieri P. Babesiosis. Two atypical cases from Minnesota and a review. Am J Clin Pathol. 2003 Oct;120(4):554-9. PMID:14560566

Shaio MF, Yang KD. Response of babesiosis to a combined regimen of quinine and azithromycin. Trans R Soc Trop Med Hyg. 1997 Mar-Apr;91(2):214-5. PMID:9196774

Shanks GD, Edstein MD. Modern malaria chemoprophylaxis. Drugs. 2005;65(15):2091-110. PMID:16225366

Shanks GD, Kain KC, Keystone JS. Malaria chemoprophylaxis in the age of drug resistance. II. Drugs that may be available in the future. Clin Infect Dis. 2001 Aug 1;33(3):381-5. Epub 2001 Jul 5. PMID:11438908

Shanks GD, Oloo AJ, Aleman GM, Ohrt C, Klotz FW, Braitman D, Horton J, Brueckner R. A new primaquine analogue, tafenoquine (WR 238605), for prophylaxis against Plasmodium falciparum malaria. Clin Infect Dis. 2001 Dec 15;33(12):1968-74. Epub 2001 Nov 7. PMID:11700577

Sharma SK, Jalees S, Kumar K, Rahman SJ. Knowledge, attitude and beliefs about malaria in a tribal area of Bastar district (Madhya Pradesh). Indian J Public Health. 1993 Oct-Dec;37(4):129-32. PMID:8077001

Sharma SP, Bansal GC. Chemoprophylaxis with diminazene aceturate in experimental Babesia bigemina infection in cattle. Res Vet Sci. 1984 Jul;37(1):126-7. PMID:6473911

Shepard CC, Walker LL, Van Landingham M, Redus MA. Kinetic testing of drugs against Mycobacterium leprae in mice. Activity of cephaloridine, rifampin, streptovaricin, vadrine, and viomycin. Am J Trop Med Hyg. 1971 Jul;20(4):616-20. PMID:4398128

Sherr VT. Human babesiosis--an unrecorded reality. Absence of formal registry undermines its detection, diagnosis and treatment, suggesting need for immediate mandatory reporting. Med Hypotheses. 2004;63(4):609-15. PMID:15325004

Shih CM, Wang CC. Ability of azithromycin in combination with quinine for the elimination of babesial infection in humans. Am J Trop Med Hyg. 1998 Oct;59(4):509-12. PMID:9790419

Shimada T, Shikano S, Hashiguchi R, Matsuki N, Ono K. Effects of depletion of T cell subpopulations on the course of infection and anti-parasite delayed type hypersensitivity response in mice infected with Babesia microti and Babesia rodhaini. J Vet Med Sci. 1996 Apr;58(4):343-7. PMID:8741267

Shipitcina NK. [Main results of the study of malaria vectors and development of control measures for them in the Soviet Union for the past 50 years].[Article in Russian]. Med Parazitol (Mosk). 1967 Sep-Oct;36(5):525-32. PMID:4886730

Shiraki H, Kozar MP, Melendez V, Hudson TH, Ohrt C, Magill AJ, Lin AJ. Antimalarial activity of novel 5-aryl-8-aminoquinoline derivatives. J Med Chem. 2011 Jan 13;54(1):131-42. Epub 2010 Dec 8. PMID:21141892

Shkap V, Leibovitz B, Krigel Y, Hammerschlag J, Marcovics A, Fish L, Molad T, Savitsky I, Mazuz M. Vaccination of older Bos taurus bulls against bovine babesiosis. Vet Parasitol. 2005 May 15;129(3-4):235-42. PMID:15845278

Shkap V, Pipano E, McElwain TF, Herzberg U, Krigel Y, Fish L, Palmer GH. Cross-protective immunity induced by Babesia bovis clones with antigenically unrelated variable merozoite surface antigens. Vet Immunol Immunopathol. 1994 Jun;41(3-4):367-74. PMID:7941314

Shkap V, Rasulov I, Abdurasulov S, Fish L, Leibovitz B, Krigel Y, Molad T, Mazuz ML, Savitsky I. Babesia bigemina: attenuation of an Uzbek isolate for immunization of cattle with live calf- or culture-derived parasites. Vet Parasitol. 2007 May 31;146(3-4):221-6. Epub 2007 Mar 26. PMID:17368728

Shoemaker JP. Plasmodium berghei: possible role of thyroxine in growth and metabolism. Exp Parasitol. 1974 Oct;36(2):261-4. PMID:4606914

Shoemaker JP, McAllister RG Jr, Selby JB, Hoffman RV Jr. Effect of hypothyroidism on parasitemia and survival in rodent malaria. Am J Med Sci. 1974 Nov;268(5):281-5. PMID:4617503

Shoemaker RC, Hudnell HK, House DE, Van Kempen A, Pakes GE; COL40155 Study Team. Atovaquone plus cholestyramine in patients coinfected with Babesia microti and Borrelia burgdorferi refractory to other treatment. Adv Ther. 2006 Jan-Feb;23(1):1-11. PMID:16644602

Shulman IA. Parasitic infections and their impact on blood donor selection and testing. Arch Pathol Lab Med. 1994 Apr;118(4):366-70. PMID:8166586

Shulman IA, Appleman MD. Transmission of parasitic and bacterial infections through blood transfusion within the U.S. Crit Rev Clin Lab Sci. 1991;28(5-6):447-59. PMID:1772589

Shute PG, Maryon M. Some observations on true latency and long-term relapses in P. vivax malaria. Arch Roum Pathol Exp Microbiol. 1968 Dec;27(4):893-8. PMID:4393171

Sibinovic KH, Milar R, Ristic M, Cox HW. In vivo and in vitro effects of serum antigens of babesial infection and their antibodies on parasitized and normal erythrocytes. Ann Trop Med Parasitol. 1969 Sep;63(3):327-36. PMID:4906995

Sibinovic KH, Sibinovic S, Ristic M, Cox HW. Immunogenic properties of babesial serum antigens. J Parasitol. 1967 Dec;53(6):1121-9. PMID:4169599

Simonsen KA, Harwell JI, Lainwala S. Clinical presentation and treatment of transfusion-associated babesiosis in premature infants. Pediatrics. 2011 Oct;128(4):e1019-24. Epub 2011 Sep 2. PMID:21890833

Siński E, Welc-Faleciak R, Pogłód R. Babesia spp. infections transmitted through blood transfusion. Wiad Parazytol. 2011;57(2):77-81. PMID:21682090

Sipos W, Schmoll F, Bagó Z, Hobbiger A, Wodak E. [Isoimmune haemolytic icterus in neonatal calves as a consequence of vaccination against piroplasmosis].[Article in German]. Berl Munch Tierarztl Wochenschr. 2002 May-Jun;115(5-6):167-72. PMID:12058589

Skotarczak B. [Babesiosis of human and domestic dog; ethiology, pathogenesis, diagnostics].[Article in Polish]. Wiad Parazytol. 2007;53(4):271-80. PMID:18441872

Skotarczak B, Cichocka A. Isolation and amplification by polymerase chain reaction DNA of Babesia microti and Babesia divergens in ticks in Poland. Ann Agric Environ Med. 2001;8(2):187-9. PMID:11748876

Skotarczak B, Sawczuk M. [Occurrence of Babesia microti in ticks Ixodes ricinus on selected areas of western Pomerania].[Article in Polish]. Wiad Parazytol. 2003;49(3):273-80. PMID:16889031

Slovut DP, Benedetti E, Matas AJ. Babesiosis and hemophagocytic syndrome in an asplenic renal transplant recipient. Transplantation. 1996 Aug 27;62(4):537-9. PMID:8781622

Smith LA, Wright-Kanuth MS. Transfusion-transmitted parasites. Clin Lab Sci. 2003 Fall;16(4):239-45, 251. PMID:14626442

Smith RD, Carpenter J, Cabrera A, Gravely SM, Erp EE, Osorno M, Ristic M. Bovine babesiosis: vaccination against tick-borne challenge exposure with culture-derived Babesia bovis immunogens. Am J Vet Res. 1979 Dec;40(12):1678-82. PMID:230765

Smith RD, James MA, Ristic M, Aikawa M, Vega y Murguia CA. Bovine babesiosis: protection of cattle with culture-derived soluble Babesia bovis antigen. Science. 1981 Apr 17;212(4492):335-8. PMID:7209532

Smith RP, Evans AT, Popovsky M, Mills L, Spielman A. Transfusion-acquired babesiosis and failure of antibiotic treatment. JAMA. 1986 Nov 21;256(19):2726-7. PMID:3773183

Snow M. Babesiosis: another tick-borne disease. Nursing. 2009 Jun;39(6):55. PMID:19474614

Snyder EL, Dodd RY. Reducing the risk of blood transfusion. Hematology Am Soc Hematol Educ Program. 2001:433-42. PMID:11722997

Snyman HW. Malaria symposium--opening address. S Afr Med J. 1974 May 25;48(25):1075-7. PMID:4602109

Sodeman TM, Contacos PG, Collins WE, Smith CS, Jumper JR. Studies on the prophylactic and radical curative activity of RC-12 against Plasmodium cynomolgi in Macaca mulatta. Bull World Health Organ. 1972;47(3):425-8. PMID:4631044

Soerono M, Badawi AS, Muir DA, Soedono A, Siran M. Observations on doubly resistant Anopheles aconitus Dönitz in Java, Indonesia, and on its amenability to treatment with malathion. Bull World Health Organ. 1965;33(4):453-9. PMID:5294991

Solari MA, Nari A, Cardozo H. Impact of Babesia bovis and Babesia bigemina on the production of beef cattle in Uruguay. Mem Inst Oswaldo Cruz. 1992;87 Suppl 3:143-9. PMID:1343684

Soltys MA. A review of studies on immunization against protozoan diseases of animals. Z Tropenmed Parasitol. 1973 Sep;24(3):309-22. PMID:4598206

Spaete J, Patrozou E, Rich JD, Sweeney JD. Red cell exchange transfusion for babesiosis in Rhode Island. J Clin Apher. 2009;24(3):97-105. PMID:19291782

Specos MM, García JJ, Tornesello J, Marino P, Vecchia MD, Tesoriero MV, Hermida LG. Microencapsulated citronella oil for mosquito repellent finishing of cotton textiles. Trans R Soc Trop Med Hyg. 2010 Oct;104(10):653-8. Epub 2010 Jul 31. PMID:20673937

Squires JM, Ferreira JF, Lindsay DS, Zajac AM. Effects of artemisinin and Artemisia extracts on Haemonchus contortus in gerbils (Meriones unguiculatus). Vet Parasitol. 2011 Jan 10;175(1-2):103-8. Epub 2010 Sep 16. PMID:20943323

Sréter T, Sréterné Lancz Z, Széll Z, Egyed L. [Rickettsia helvetica: an emerging tick-borne pathogen in Hungary and Europe]. [Article in Hungarian]. Orv Hetil. 2005 Dec 11;146(50):2547-52. PMID:16440500

Sréter T, Kálmán D, Sréterné Lancz Z, Széll Z, Egyed L. [Babesia microti and Anaplasma phagocytophilum: two emerging zoonotic pathogens in Europe and Hungary].[Article in Hungarian]. Orv Hetil. 2005 Mar 27;146(13):595-600. PMID:15856623

Sserugga JN, Jonsson NN, Bock RE, More SJ. Serological evidence of exposure to tick fever organisms in young cattle on Queensland dairy farms. Aust Vet J. 2003 Mar;81(3):147-52. PMID:15080428

Stańczak J, Myjak P, Bajer A, Siński E, Wedrychowicz H, Majewska AC, Gołab E, Budak A. [Usefulness of the molecular techniques for detecting and/or identifing of parasites and fungi in humans and animals or pathogens transmitted by ticks. Part III].[Article in Polish]. Wiad Parazytol. 2001;47(3):465-75. PMID:16894762

Standfast NF, Bock RE, Wiecek MM, deVos AJ, Jorgensen WK, Kingston TG. Overcoming constraints to meeting increased demand for Babesia bigemina vaccine in Australia. Vet Parasitol. 2003 Jul 29;115(3):213-22. PMID:12935736

Standfast NF, Jorgensen WK. Comparison of the infectivity of Babesia bovis, Babesia bigemina and Anaplasma centrale for cattle after cryopreservation in either dimethylsulphoxide (DMSO) or polyvinylpyrrolidone (PVP). Aust Vet J. 1997 Jan;75(1):62-3. PMID:9034504

Steele JH. Veterinary public health in the United States, 1776 to 1976. J Am Vet Med Assoc. 1976 Jul 1;169(1):74-82. PMID:776913

Stegeman JR, Birkenheuer AJ, Kruger JM, Breitschwerdt EB. Transfusion-associated Babesia gibsoni infection in a dog. J Am Vet Med Assoc. 2003 Apr 1;222(7):959-63, 952. PMID:12685786

Steinhaus RK, Baskin SI, Clark JH, Kirby SD. Formation of methemoglobin and metmyoglobin using 8-aminoquinoline derivatives or sodium nitrite and subsequent reaction with cyanide. J Appl Toxicol. 1990 Oct;10(5):345-51. PMID:2254586

Stewart NP, de Vos AJ, Shiels I. Elimination of Theileria buffeli infections from cattle by concurrent treatment with primaquine phosphate and halofuginone lactate. Trop Anim Health Prod. 1990 May;22(2):109-15. PMID:2115212

Stowell CP, Gelfand JA, Shepard JA, Kratz A. Case records of the Massachusetts General Hospital. Case 17-2007. A 25-year-old woman with relapsing fevers and recent onset of dyspnea. N Engl J Med. 2007 May 31;356(22):2313-9. PMID:17538091

Stramer SL, Hollinger FB, Katz LM, Kleinman S, Metzel PS, Gregory KR, Dodd RY. Emerging infectious disease agents and their potential threat to transfusion safety. Transfusion. 2009 Aug;49 Suppl 2:1S-29S. PMID:19686562

Stricker RB. Counterpoint: long-term antibiotic therapy improves persistent symptoms associated with lyme disease. Clin Infect Dis. 2007 Jul 15;45(2):149-57. Epub 2007 Jun 5. PMID:17578772

Stricker RB, Lautin A, Burrascano JJ. Lyme disease: point/ counterpoint. Expert Rev Anti Infect Ther. 2005 Apr;3(2):155-65. PMID:15918774

Stricker RB, Lautin A, Burrascano JJ. Lyme disease: the quest for magic bullets. Chemotherapy. 2006;52(2):53-9. Epub 2006 Feb 22. PMID:16498239.

Suarez CE, McElwain TF. Transfection systems for Babesia bovis: a review of methods for the transient and stable expression of exogenous genes. Vet Parasitol. 2010 Feb 10;167(2-4):205-15. Epub 2009 Sep 19. PMID:19819628

Suarez CE, Noh S. Emerging perspectives in the research of bovine babesiosis and anaplasmosis. Vet Parasitol. 2011 Aug 4;180(1-2):109-25. Epub 2011 May 27. PMID:21684084

Subeki, Matsuura H, Yamasaki M, Yamato O, Maede Y, Katakura K, Suzuki M, Trimurningsih, Chairul, Yoshihara T. Effects of Central Kalimantan plant extracts on intraerythrocytic Babesia gibsoni in culture. J Vet Med Sci. 2004 Jul;66(7):871-4. PMID:15297762

Subeki, Nomura S, Matsuura H, Yamasaki M, Yamato O, Maede Y, Katakura K, Suzuki M, Trimurningsih, Chairul, Yoshihara T. Anti-babesial activity of some central kalimantan plant extracts and active oligostilbenoids from Shorea balangeran. Planta Med. 2005 May;71(5):420-3. PMID:15931579

Sun T, Tenenbaum MJ, Greenspan J, Teichberg S, Wang RT, Degnan T, Kaplan MH. Morphologic and clinical observations in human infection with Babesia microti. J Infect Dis. 1983 Aug;148(2):239-48. PMID:6684141

Suzuki K, Wakabayashi H, Takahashi M, Fukushima K, Yabuki A, Endo Y. A Possible treatment strategy and clinical factors to estimate the treatment response in Bebesia gibsoni infection. J Vet Med Sci. 2007 May;69(5):563-8. PMID:17551236

Taiwo B, Lee C, Venkat D, Tambar S, Sutton SH. Can tumor necrosis factor alpha blockade predispose to severe babesiosis? Arthritis Rheum. 2007 Feb 15;57(1):179-81. PMID:17266091

Tajima T, Zhi N, Lin Q, Rikihisa Y, Horowitz HW, Ralfalli J, Wormser GP, Hechemy KE. Comparison of two recombinant major outer membrane proteins of the human granulocytic ehrlichiosis agent for use in an enzyme-linked immunosorbent assay. Clin Diagn Lab Immunol. 2000 Jul;7(4):652-7. PMID:10882667

Takabatake N, Okamura M, Yokoyama N, Okubo K, Ikehara Y, Igarashi I. Involvement of a host erythrocyte sialic acid content in Babesia bovis infection. J Vet Med Sci. 2007 Oct;69(10):999-1004. PMID:17984585

Takahashi M, Omata Y, Oikawa H, Claveria F, Igarashi I, Saito A, Suzuki N. Protective immune response of Isospora felis-infected mice against Babesia microti infection. J Vet Med Sci. 1993 Aug;55(4):587-90. PMID:8399737

Talour K, Karam A, Dreux N, Lemasson G, Gilbert D, Abasq C, Misery L. Incipiens linear IgA disease with IgA antibodies directed against 200-kDa epidermal antigens. Eur J Dermatol. 2011 May-Jun;21(3):411-2. PMID:21515442

Tammemagi L. Iron-dextran in the treatment of anaemia associated with bovine babesiosis. Aust Vet J. 1966 Jul;42(7):260-1. PMID:4961184

Taraskina LA. [The development of public health in the Democratic Republic of Vietnam].[Article in Russian]. Sov Zdravookhr. 1968;27(3):80-2. PMID:5675744

Tarello W. Cutaneous lesions in dogs with Dirofilaria (Nochtiella) repens infestation and concurrent tick-borne transmitted diseases. Vet Dermatol. 2002 Oct;13(5):267-74. PMID:12358611

Tarello W. Dermatitis associated with Dirofilaria (Nochtiella) repens microfilariae in dogs from central Italy. Acta Vet Hung. 2002;50(1):63-78. PMID:12061238

Tarello W. Dermatitis associated with Dirofilaria repens microfilariae in three dogs in Saudi Arabia. J Small Anim Pract. 2003 Mar;44(3):132-4. PMID:12653329

Taylor RJ, McHardy N. Preliminary observations on the combined use of imidocarb and Babesia blood vaccine in cattle. J S Afr Vet Assoc. 1979 Dec;50(4):326-9. PMID:553972

Taylor SM, Elliott CT, Kenny J. Babesia divergens: sequential exposure to heterologous tick-borne challenge of cattle immunized with a fraction of parasitized erythrocytes. J Comp Pathol. 1986 Jan;96(1):101-7. PMID:3944282

Taylor SM, Elliott CT, Kenny J. Isolation of antigenic proteins from erythrocytes parasitised with Babesia divergens and a comparison of their immunising potential. Vet Parasitol. 1986 Jun;21(2):99-105. PMID:3739209

Taylor SM, Kenny J, Mallon T. The effect of route of administration of a Babesia divergens inactivated vaccine on protection against homologous challenge. J Comp Pathol. 1983 Jul;93(3):423-8. PMID:6886086

Taylor SM, Kenny J, Mallon T, Elliott CT. The immunization of cattle against Babesia divergens with fractions of parasitized erythrocytes. Vet Parasitol. 1984 Nov;16(3-4):235-42. PMID:6542721

Taylor SM, Kenny J, Purnell RE, Lewis D. Exposure of cattle immunised against redwater to tick challenge in the field: challenge by a homologous strain of B divergens. Vet Rec. 1980 Feb 23;106(8):167-70. PMID:7361409

Taylor SM, Kenny J, Purnell RE, Lewis D. Exposure of cattle immunised against redwater to tick-induced challenge in the field: challenge by a heterologous strain of Babesia divergens. Vet Rec. 1980 Apr 26;106(17):385-7. PMID:7434497

Taylor WM, Simpson CF, Martin FG. Certain aspects of toxicity of an amicarbalide formulation to ponies. Am J Vet Res. 1972 Mar;33(3):533-41. PMID:5014461

Tchoumbougnang F, Zollo PH, Dagne E, Mekonnen Y. In vivo antimalarial activity of essential oils from Cymbopogon citratus and Ocimum gratissimum on mice infected with Plasmodium berghei. Planta Med. 2005 Jan;71(1):20-3. PMID:15678368

Tekwani BL, Walker LA. 8-Aminoquinolines: future role as antiprotozoal drugs. Curr Opin Infect Dis. 2006 Dec;19(6):623-31. PMID:17075340

Terkawi MA, Jia H, Zhou J, Lee EG, Igarashi I, Fujisaki K, Nishikawa Y, Xuan X. Babesia gibsoni ribosomal phosphoprotein P0 induces cross-protective immunity against B. microti infection in mice. Vaccine. 2007 Mar 1;25(11):2027-35. Epub 2006 Dec 8. PMID:17229504

Terkawi MA, Zhang G, Jia H, Aboge G, Goo YK, Nishikawa Y, Yokoyama N, Igarashi I, Kawazu SI, Fujisaki K, Xuan X. C3 contributes to the cross-protective immunity induced by Babesia gibsoni phosphoriboprotein P0 against a lethal B. rodhaini infection. Parasite Immunol. 2008 Jun-Jul;30(6-7):365-70. PMID:18533933

Terzian LA, Stahler N, Dawkins AT Jr. The sporogonous of Plasmodium vivax in Anopheles mosquitoes as a system for evaluating the prophylactic and curative capabilities of potential antimalarial compounds. Exp Parasitol. 1968 Aug;23(1):56-66. PMID:4876903

Tetzlaff CL, Rice-Ficht AC, Woods VM, Brown WC. Induction of proliferative responses of T cells from Babesia bovis-immune cattle with a recombinant 77-kilodalton merozoite protein (Bb-1). Infect Immun. 1992 Feb;60(2):644-52. PMID:1730498

Thomford JW, Conrad PA, Boyce WM, Holman PJ, Jessup DA. Isolation and in vitro cultivation of Babesia parasites from free-ranging desert bighorn sheep (Ovis canadensis nelsoni) and mule deer (Odocoileus hemionus) in California. J Parasitol. 1993 Feb;79(1):77-84. PMID:8437062

Thompson C, Spielman A, Krause PJ. Coinfecting deer-associated zoonoses: Lyme disease, babesiosis, and ehrlichiosis. Clin Infect Dis. 2001 Sep 1;33(5):676-85. Epub 2001 Aug 6. PMID:11486290

Thompson JH. Gametocytemia in falciparum malaria. JAMA. 1971 Jun 14;216(11):1866. PMID:4931429

Thompson KC, Todorovic RA, Mateus G, Adams LG. Methods to improve the health of cattle in the tropics: immunisation and chemoprophylaxis against haemoparasitic infections. Trop Anim Health Prod. 1978 May;10(2):75-81. PMID:664017

Thoongsuwan S, Cox HW. Antigenic variants of the haemosporidian parasite, Babesia rodhaini, selected by in vitro treatment with immune globulin. Ann Trop Med Parasitol. 1973 Dec;67(4):373-85. PMID:4132544

Thoongsuwan S, Cox HW, Patrick RA. Serologic specificity of immunoconglutinin associated with infectious anemia of rats and its role in nonspecific acquired resistance. J Parasitol. 1978 Dec;64(6):1060-6. PMID:739300

Timms P, Barry DN, Gill AC, Sharp PJ, de Vos AJ. Failure of a recombinant Babesia bovis antigen to protect cattle against heterologous strain challenge. Res Vet Sci. 1988 Sep;45(2):267-9. PMID:3194602

Timms P, Dalgliesh RJ, Barry DN, Dimmock CK, Rodwell BJ. Babesia bovis: comparison of culture-derived parasites, non-living antigen and conventional vaccine in the protection of cattle against heterologous challenge. Aust Vet J. 1983 Mar;60(3):75-7. PMID:6347164

Timms P, Stewart NP. Growth of Babesia bovis parasites in stationary and suspension cultures and their use in experimental vaccination of cattle. Res Vet Sci. 1989 Nov;47(3):309-14. PMID:2595088

Timms P, Stewart NP, Dalgliesh RJ. Comparison of tick and blood challenge for assessing immunity to Babesia bovis. Aust Vet J. 1983 Aug;60(8):257-9. PMID:6639533

Timofeev BA, Bolotin IM, Stepanova LP, Bogdanov AA Jr, Georgiu K, Malyshev SN, Petrovsky VV, Klibanov AL, Torchilin VP. Liposomal diamidine (imidocarb): preparation and animal studies. J Microencapsul. 1994 Nov-Dec;11(6):627-32. PMID:7884627

Timofeev BA, Bolotin IM, Stepanova LP, Bogdanov AA, Georgiu Kh, Malyshev SN, Petrovskiĭ, Klibanov AL, Torchilin VP. [A liposomal form of diamidine: reduced toxicity]. [Article in Russian]. Antibiot Khimioter. 1991 Sep;36(9):34-6. PMID:1781710

Titanji VP, Zofou D, Ngemenya MN. The antimalarial potential of medicinal plants used for the treatment of malaria in Cameroonian folk medicine. Afr J Tradit Complement Altern Med. 2008 Apr 10;5(3):302-21. PMID:20161952

Tjornehoj K, Lawrence JA, Whiteland AP, Kafuwa PT. Field observations on the duration of immunity in cattle after vaccination against Anaplasma and Babesia species. Onderstepoort J Vet Res. 1996 Mar;63(1):1-5. PMID:8848296

Todorovic R, Gonzalez E, Lopez G. Immunization against anaplasmosis and babesiosis. Part II. Evaluation of cryo-preserved vaccines using different doses and routes of inoculation. Tropenmed Parasitol. 1978 Jun;29(2):210-4. PMID:675843

Todorovic RA. Bovine babesiasis: its diagnosis and control. Am J Vet Res. 1974 Aug;35(8):1045-52. PMID:4850812

Todorovic RA, Gonzalez EF, Adams LG. Bovine babesiosis: sterile immunity to Babesia bigemina and Babesia argentina infections. Trop Anim Health Prod. 1973 Nov;5(4):234-45. PMID:4807692

Todorovic RA, Gonzalez EF, Adams LG. Babesia bigemina, Babesia argentina, and Anaplasma marginale: Coinfectious immunity in bovines. Exp Parasitol. 1975 Apr;37(2):179-92. PMID:1123013

Todorovic RA, Gonzalez EF, Garcia O. Immunization against anaplasmosis and babesiosis. Part III. Evaluation of immunization under field conditions in the Cauca River Valley. Tropenmed Parasitol. 1979 Mar;30(1):43-52. PMID:442200.

Todorovic RA, Vizcaino OG, Gonzalez EF, Adams LG. Chemoprophylaxis (Imidocarb) against Babesia bigemina and Babesia argentina infections. Am J Vet Res. 1973 Sep;34(9):1153-61. PMID:4747036

Tomillero A, Moral MA. Gateways to clinical trials. Methods Find Exp Clin Pharmacol. 2010 Jun;32(5):331-88. PMID:20664824

Tonnetti L, Eder AF, Dy B, Kennedy J, Pisciotto P, Benjamin RJ, Leiby DA. Transfusion-transmitted Babesia microti identified through hemovigilance. Transfusion. 2009 Dec;49(12):2557-63. Epub 2009 Jul 16. PMID:19624607

Tonnetti L, Proctor MC, Reddy HL, Goodrich RP, Leiby DA. Evaluation of the Mirasol pathogen [corrected] reduction technology system against Babesia microti in apheresis platelets and plasma. Transfusion. 2010 May;50(5):1019-27. Epub 2009 Dec 18. PMID:20030791

Topolovec J, Puntarić D, Antolović-Pozgain A, Vuković D, Topolovec Z, Milas J, Drusko-Barisić V, Venus M. Serologically detected "new" tick-borne zoonoses in eastern Croatia. Croat Med J. 2003 Oct;44(5):626-9. PMID:14515426

Torina A, Caracappa S. Anaplasmosis in cattle in Italy. Vet Res Commun. 2007 Aug;31 Suppl 1:73-8. PMID:17682850

Torina A, Vicente J, Alongi A, Scimeca S, Turlá R, Nicosia S, Di Marco V, Caracappa S, de la Fuente J. Observed prevalence of tick-borne pathogens in domestic animals in Sicily, Italy during 2003-2005. Zoonoses Public Health. 2007;54(1):8-15. PMID:17359441

Torres-Vélez FJ, Nace EK, Won KY, Bartlett J, Eberhard M, Guarner J. Development of an immunohistochemical assay for the detection of babesiosis in formalin-fixed, paraffin-embedded tissue samples. Am J Clin Pathol. 2003 Dec;120(6):833-8. PMID:14671971

Trigg PI. Parasite cultivation in relation to research on the chemotherapy of malaria. Bull World Health Organ. 1976;53(4):399-406. PMID:1086733

Trigg PI. Drug use and design in the nineties. Acta Leiden. 1991;60(1):147-56. PMID:1820704

Trigg PI, Gutteridge WE, Williamson J. The effects of cordycepin on malaria parasites. Trans R Soc Trop Med Hyg. 1971;65(4):514-20. PMID:4999656

Tripathi AK, Prajapati V, Ahmad A, Aggarwal KK, Khanuja SP. Piperitenone oxide as toxic, repellent, and reproduction retardant toward malarial vector Anopheles stephensi (Diptera: Anophelinae). J Med Entomol. 2004 Jul;41(4):691-8. PMID:15311462

Trongtokit Y, Rongsriyam Y, Komalamisra N, Krisadaphong P, Apiwathnasorn C. Laboratory and field trial of developing medicinal local Thai plant products against four species of mosquito vectors. Southeast Asian J Trop Med Public Health. 2004 Jun;35(2):325-33. PMID:15691131

Tsuji M, Terada Y, Arai S, Okada H, Ishihara C. Use of the Bo-RBC-SCID mouse model for isolation of a Babesia parasite from grazing calves in Japan. Exp Parasitol. 1995 Dec;81(4):512-8. PMID:8542992

Tsuji N, Miyoshi T, Battsetseg B, Matsuo T, Xuan X, Fujisaki K. A cysteine protease is critical for Babesia spp. transmission in Haemaphysalis ticks. PLoS Pathog. 2008 May 16;4(5):e1000062. PMID:18483546

Tuliaganov KS. [Status and perspectives of development of therapeutic services in Uzbekistan].[Article in Russian]. Ter Arkh. 1974;46(6):98-101. PMID:4279462

Tuo W, Estes DM, Brown WC. Comparative effects of interleukin-12 and interleukin-4 on cytokine responses by antigen-stimulated memory CD4+ T cells of cattle: IL-12 enhances IFN-gamma production, whereas IL-4 has marginal effects on cytokine expression. J Interferon Cytokine Res. 1999 Jul;19(7):741-9. PMID:10454344

Uguen C, Girard L, Brasseur P, Leblay R. .[Human babesiosis in 1997].[Article in French]. Rev Med Interne. 1997;18(12):945-51. PMID:9499998

Uhnoo I, Cars O, Christensson D, Nyström-Rosander C. First documented case of human babesiosis in Sweden. Scand J Infect Dis. 1992;24(4):541-7. PMID:1411322

Uilenberg G. [Notes on bovine babesiosis and anaplasmosis in Madagascar. VI. Artificial premunization].[Article in French]. Rev Elev Med Vet Pays Trop. 1971;24(1):23-35. PMID:5106007

Uilenberg G. [Studies in the field of tick-borne blood parasites].[Article in Dutch]. Tijdschr Diergeneeskd. 1987 Oct 15;112(20):1163-71. PMID:3672475

Uilenberg G, Franssen FF, Perié NM, Spanjer AA. Three groups of Babesia canis distinguished and a proposal for nomenclature. Vet Q. 1989 Jan;11(1):33-40. PMID:2655263

Uilenberg G, Schreuder BE, Silayo RS, Mpangala C. Studies on Theileriidae (Sporozoa) in Tanzania. IV. A field trial on immunization against East Coast fever (Theileria parva infection of cattle). Tropenmed Parasitol. 1976 Sep;27(3):329-36. PMID:982549

Uilenberg G, Verdiesen PA, Zwart D. Imidocarb: a chemoprophylactic experiment with Babesia canis. Vet Q. 1981 Jul;3(3):118-23. PMID:7268745

Ukaga CN, Nwoke BE, Onyeka PI, Anosike JC, Udujih OS, Udujih OG, Obilor RC, Nwachukwu MI. The use of herbs in malaria treatment in parts of Imo State, Nigeria. Tanzan Health Res Bull. 2006 Sep;8(3):183-5. PMID:18254512

Ungar-Waron H, Paz R, Shkap V, Bin H, Pipano E. IgM rheumatoid factor in cattle immunized against babesiosis. Zentralbl Veterinarmed B. 1991 Sep;38(7):492-6. PMID:1776376

Ushe TC, Palmer GH, Sotomayor L, Figueroa JV, Buening GM, Perryman LE, McElwain TF. Antibody response to a Babesia bigemina rhoptry-associated protein 1 surface-exposed and neutralization-sensitive epitope in immune cattle. Infect Immun. 1994 Dec;62(12):5698-701. PMID:7525490

Valbonesi M, Bruni R. Clinical application of therapeutic erythrocytapheresis (TEA). Transfus Sci. 2000 Jun;22(3):183-94. PMID:10831921

Vale N, Moreira R, Gomes P. Primaquine revisited six decades after its discovery. Eur J Med Chem. 2009 Mar;44(3):937-53. Epub 2008 Sep 11. PMID:18930565

Valentin A, Precigout E, L'Hostis M, Carcy B, Gorenflot A, Schrevel J. Cellular and humoral immune responses induced in cattle by vaccination with Babesia divergens culture-derived exoantigens correlate with protection. Infect Immun. 1993 Feb;61(2):734-41. PMID:8423099

Van den Bossche P, Mudenge D. The effect of short-interval deltamethrin applications to control tsetse on the seroprevalence of babesiosis in cattle. Trop Anim Health Prod. 1999 Aug;31(4):215-22. PMID:10504101 van Duivenvoorde LM, Voorberg-van der Wel A, van der Werff NM, Braskamp G, Remarque EJ, Kondova I, Kocken CH, Thomas AW. Suppression of Plasmodium cynomolgi in rhesus macaques by coinfection with Babesia microti. Infect Immun. 2010 Mar;78(3):1032-9. Epub 2010 Jan 4. PMID:20048045

Vanderberg JP. Inactivity of rodent malaria anti-sporozoite antibodies against exoerythrocytic forms. Am J Trop Med Hyg. 1973 Sep;22(5):573-7. PMID:4580967

Vane JR. The fight against rheumatism: from willow bark to COX-1 sparing drugs. J Physiol Pharmacol. 2000 Dec;51(4 Pt 1):573-86. PMID:11192932

van Heerden J. Diamidine poisoning in a dog. J S Afr Vet Assoc. 1981 Dec;52(4):338-9. PMID:7341787

Van Niekerk CJ, Zweygarth E. In vitro cultivation of Babesia occultans. Onderstepoort J Vet Res. 1996 Sep;63(3):259-61. PMID:8917864

Van Solingen RM, Evans J. Lyme disease. Curr Opin Rheumatol. 2001 Jul;13(4):293-9. PMID:11555731

Vannier E, Gewurz BE, Krause PJ. Human babesiosis. Infect Dis Clin North Am. 2008 Sep;22(3):469-88, viii-ix. PMID:18755385

Vannier E, Krause PJ. Update on babesiosis. Interdiscip Perspect Infect Dis. 2009;2009:984568. Epub 2009 Aug 27. PMID:19727410

Vega CA, Buening GM, Rodriguez SD, Carson CA, McLaughlin K. Cryopreservation of Babesia bigemina for in vitro cultivation. Am J Vet Res. 1985 Feb;46(2):421-3. PMID:3922260

Vercammen F, De Deken R, Maes L. Prophylactic activity of imidocarb against experimental infection with Babesia canis. Vet Parasitol. 1996 Jun;63(3-4):195-8. PMID:8966987

Vial HJ, Gorenflot A. Chemotherapy against babesiosis. Vet Parasitol. 2006 May 31;138(1-2):147-60. Epub 2006 Feb 28. PMID:16504402

Vincke IH. The effects of pyrimethamine and sulphormethoxine on the pre-erythrocytic and sporogonous cycle of Plasmodium berghei berghei. Ann Soc Belges Med Trop Parasitol Mycol. 1970;50(3):339-58. PMID:5514572

Vivas L, Rattray L, Stewart LB, Robinson BL, Fugmann B, Haynes RK, Peters W, Croft SL. Antimalarial efficacy and drug interactions of the novel semi-synthetic endoperoxide artemisone in vitro and in vivo. J Antimicrob Chemother. 2007 Apr;59(4):658-65. Epub 2007 Mar 2. PMID:17337512

Vizcaino O, Corrier DE, Terry MK, Carson CA, Lee AJ, Kuttler KL, Ristic M, Treviño GS. Comparison of three methods of immunization against bovine anaplasmosis: evaluation of protection afforded against field challenge exposure. Am J Vet Res. 1980 Jul;41(7):1066-8. PMID:7436100

Vollnberg A, Prajakwong S, Sirichaisinthop J, Wiedermann G, Wernsdorfer G, Wernsdorfer WH. In-vitro interaction of tafenoquine and chloroquine in Plasmodium falciparum from northwestern Thailand. Wien Klin Wochenschr. 2003;115 Suppl 3:28-32. PMID:15508777

Vreden SG, van den Broek MF, Oettinger MC, Verhave JP, Meuwissen JH, Sauerwein RW. Cytokines inhibit the development of liver schizonts of the malaria parasite Plasmodium berghei in vivo. Eur J Immunol. 1992 Sep;22(9):2271-5. PMID:1516619

Vulchovski Ia. [Comparative test of the efficacy of babesicidal agents].[Article in Bulgarian]. Vet Med Nauki. 1977;14(3):79-87. PMID:906312

Vyas JM, Telford SR, Robbins GK. Treatment of refractory Babesia microti infection with atovaquone-proguanil in an HIV-infected patient: case report. Clin Infect Dis. 2007 Dec 15;45(12):1588-90. PMID:18190320

Waki S, Suzuki M. Development and decline of antiplasmodial indirect fluorescent antibodies in mice infected with Plasmodium berghei (NK65) and treated with drugs. Bull World Health Organ. 1974;50(6):521-6. PMID: 4617640.

Waldron SJ, Jorgensen WK. Transmission of Babesia spp by the cattle tick (Boophilus microplus) to cattle treated with injectable or pour-on formulations of ivermectin and moxidectin. Aust Vet J. 1999 Oct;77(10):657-9. PMID:10590793

Wallce AL, Harris A, Allen JP. Reiter treponeme. A review of the literature. Bull World Health Organ. 1967;36 Suppl:1-103. PMID:4865377

Walsh DS, Eamsila C, Sasiprapha T, Sangkharomya S, Khaewsathien P, Supakalin P, Tang DB, Jarasrumgsichol P, Cherdchu C, Edstein MD, Rieckmann KH, Brewer TG. Efficacy of monthly tafenoquine for prophylaxis of Plasmodium vivax and multidrug-resistant P. falciparum malaria. J Infect Dis. 2004 Oct 15;190(8):1456-63. Epub 2004 Sep 20. PMID:15378438

Walsh DS, Looareesuwan S, Wilairatana P, Heppner DG Jr, Tang DB, Brewer TG, Chokejindachai W, Viriyavejakul P, Kyle DE, Milhous WK, Schuster BG, Horton J, Braitman DJ, Brueckner RP. Randomized dose-ranging study of the safety and efficacy of WR 238605 (Tafenoquine) in the prevention of relapse of Plasmodium vivax malaria in Thailand. J Infect Dis. 1999 Oct;180(4):1282-7. PMID:10479159

Walsh DS, Wilairatana P, Tang DB, Heppner DG Jr, Brewer TG, Krudsood S, Silachamroon U, Phumratanaprapin W, Siriyanonda D, Looareesuwan S. Randomized trial of 3-dose regimens of tafenoquine (WR238605) versus low-dose primaquine for preventing Plasmodium vivax malaria relapse. Clin Infect Dis. 2004 Oct 15;39(8):1095-103. Epub 2004 Sep 24. PMID:15486831

Waltisbuhl DJ, Goodger BV, Wright IG, Mirre GB, Commins MA. Babesia bovis: vaccination studies with three groups of high molecular weight antigens from lysate of infected erythrocytes. Parasitol Res. 1987;73(4):319-23. PMID:3303020

Wang TJ, Liang MH, Sangha O, Phillips CB, Lew RA, Wright EA, Berardi V, Fossel AH, Shadick NA. Coexposure to Borrelia burgdorferi and Babesia microti does not worsen the long-term outcome of lyme disease. Clin Infect Dis. 2000 Nov;31(5):1149-54. Epub 2000 Nov 6. PMID:11073744

Wanjohi JM, Ngeranwa JN, Rumberia RM, Muraguri GR, Mbogo SK. Immunization of cattle against East Coast fever using Theileria parva (Marikebuni) and relaxation of tick control in North Rift, Kenya. Onderstepoort J Vet Res. 2001 Sep;68(3):217-23. PMID:11769354

Ward RA. The influence of Ronald Ropss upon the early development of malaria vector control procedures in the United States Army. J Trop Med Hyg. 1973 Aug;76(8):207-9. PMID:4582106

Warhurst DC, Folwell RO. Measurement of the growth rate of the erythrocytic stages of Plasmodium berghei and comparisons of the potency of inocula after various treatments. Ann Trop Med Parasitol. 1968 Sep;62(3):349-60. PMID:5714962

Webert KE, Cserti CM, Hannon J, Lin Y, Pavenski K, Pendergrast JM, Blajchman MA. Proceedings of a Consensus Conference: pathogen inactivation-making decisions about new technologies. Transfus Med Rev. 2008 Jan;22(1):1-34. PMID:18063190

Wei Q, Tsuji M, Zamoto A, Kohsaki M, Matsui T, Shiota T, Telford SR 3rd, Ishihara C. Human babesiosis in Japan: isolation of Babesia microti-like parasites from an asymptomatic transfusion donor and from a rodent from an area where babesiosis is endemic. J Clin Microbiol. 2001 Jun;39(6):2178-83. PMID:11376054

Weilgama DJ, Jorgensen WK, Dalgliesh RJ, Navaratne M, Weerasinghe C. Comparison between Sri Lankan and Australian strains of Babesia bovis in the vaccination of imported cattle in Sri Lanka. Trop Anim Health Prod. 1989 May;21(2):141-5. PMID:2665254

Weinberg GA. Laboratory diagnosis of ehrlichiosis and babesiosis. Pediatr Infect Dis J. 2001 Apr;20(4):435-7. PMID:11332670

Weiss LM. Babesiosis in humans: a treatment review. Expert Opin Pharmacother. 2002 Aug;3(8):1109-15. PMID:12150690

Weiss LM, Wittner M, Tanowitz HB. The treatment of babesiosis. N Engl J Med. 2001 Mar 8;344(10):773. PMID:11236789

Weiss LM, Wittner M, Wasserman S, Oz HS, Retsema J, Tanowitz HB. Efficacy of azithromycin for treating Babesia microti infection in the hamster model. J Infect Dis. 1993 Nov;168(5):1289-92. PMID:8228366

Weld ED, Eimer KM, Saharia K, Orenstein A, Hess JR. Transfusion medicine illustrated. The expanding range and severity of babesiosis. Transfusion. 2010 Feb;50(2):290-1. PMID:20233358

Wen W. China: a new medicine born of tradition. UNESCO Cour. 1979 Jul;7:25-7. PMID:12309932

Wendel Neto S. Current concepts on the transmission of bacteria and parasites by blood components. Sao Paulo Med J. 1995 Nov-Dec;113(6):1036-52. PMID:8731290

Wendel S. Current concepts on transmission of bacteria and parasites by blood components. Vox Sang. 1994;67 Suppl 3:161-74. PMID:7975485

Wendel S, Leiby DA. Parasitic infections in the blood supply: assessing and countering the threat. Dev Biol (Basel). 2007;127:17-41. PMID:17486879

White DJ, Talarico J, Chang HG, Birkhead GS, Heimberger T, Morse DL. Human babesiosis in New York State: Review of 139 hospitalized cases and analysis of prognostic factors. Arch Intern Med. 1998 Oct 26;158(19):2149-54. PMID:9801183

Wiesner J, Ortmann R, Jomaa H, Schlitzer M. New antimalarial drugs. Angew Chem Int Ed Engl. 2003 Nov 10;42(43):5274-93. PMID:14613157

Wiesner J, Reichenberg A, Heinrich S, Schlitzer M, Jomaa H. The plastid-like organelle of apicomplexan parasites as drug target. Curr Pharm Des. 2008;14(9):855-71. PMID:18473835

Wijaya A, Wulansari R, Ano H, Inokuma H, Makimura S. Therapeutic effect of clindamycin and tetracycline on Babesia rodhaini infection in mouse model. J Vet Med Sci. 2000 Aug;62(8):835-9. PMID:10993180

Willadsen P. Vaccines, genetics and chemicals in tick control: the Australian experience. Trop Anim Health Prod. 1997 Nov;29(4 Suppl):91S-94S. PMID:9512752

Willadsen P, Kemp DH. Novel vaccination for control of the Babesia vector, Boophilus microplus. Trans R Soc Trop Med Hyg. 1989;83 Suppl:107. PMID:2623756

Willadsen P, Kemp DH, Cobon GS, Wright IG. Successful vaccination against Boophilus microplus and Babesia bovis using recombinant antigens. Mem Inst Oswaldo Cruz. 1992;87 Suppl 3:289-94. PMID:1343705

Willerson D Jr, Rieckmann KH, Carson PE, Frischer H. Effects of minocycline against chloroquine-resistant falciparum malaria. Am J Trop Med Hyg. 1972 Nov;21(6):857-62. PMID:4564446

Winger CM, Canning EU, Culverhouse JD. A strain of Babesia divergens, attenuated after long term culture. Res Vet Sci. 1989 Jan;46(1):110-3. PMID:2922498

Winger CM, Canning EU, Culverhouse JD. Induction of protective immunity to Babesia divergens in Mongolian gerbils, Meriones unguiculatus, using culture-derived immunogens. Vet Parasitol. 1987 Dec;26(1-2):43-53. PMID:3439004

Winger CM, Canning EU, Culverhouse JD. A strain of Babesia divergens, attenuated after long term culture. Res Vet Sci. 1989 Jan;46(1):110-3. PMID:2922498

Winger CM, Canning EU, Culverhouse JD. A monoclonal antibody-derived antigen of Babesia divergens: characterization and investigation of its ability to protect gerbils against virulent homologous challenge. Parasitology. 1989 Dec;99 Pt 3:341-8. PMID:2608311

Winterburn TJ, Phylip LH, Bur D, Wyatt DM, Berry C, Kay J. N-terminal extension of the yeast IA3 aspartic proteinase inhibitor relaxes the strict intrinsic selectivity. FEBS J. 2007 Jul;274(14):3685-94. Epub 2007 Jul 2. PMID:17608726

Wiseman V, McElroy B, Conteh L, Stevens W. Malaria prevention in The Gambia: patterns of expenditure and determinants of demand at the household level. Trop Med Int Health. 2006 Apr;11(4):419-31. PMID:16553925

Wittner M, Lederman J, Tanowitz HB, Rosenbaum GS, Weiss LM. Atovaquone in the treatment of Babesia microti infections in hamsters. Am J Trop Med Hyg. 1996 Aug;55(2):219-22. PMID:8780464

Wittner M, Rowin KS, Tanowitz HB, Hobbs JF, Saltzman S, Wenz B, Hirsch R, Chisholm E, Healy GR. Successful chemotherapy of transfusion babesiosis. Ann Intern Med. 1982 May;96(5):601-4. PMID:7200341

Wójcik-Fatla A, Cisak E, Chmielewska-Badora J, Zwoliński J, Buczek A, Dutkiewicz

J. Prevalence of Babesia microti in Ixodes ricinus ticks from Lublin region (eastern Poland). Ann Agric Environ Med. 2006;13(2):319-22. PMID:17196008

Wong WS, Chung JY, Wong KF. Images in haematology. Human babesiosis. Br J Haematol. 2008 Feb;140(4):364. Epub 2007 Nov 27. PMID:18042268

Wood PR, Clark IA. Genetic control of Propionibacterium acnes-induced protection of mice against Babesia microti. Infect Immun. 1982 Jan;35(1):52-7. PMID:7054129

Wormser GP, Lombardo G, Silverblatt F, El Khoury MY, Prasad A, Yelon JA, Sanda A, Karim S, Coku L, Savino JA. Babesiosis as a cause of fever in patients undergoing a splenectomy. Am Surg. 2011 Mar;77(3):345-7. PMID:21375849

Wormser GP, Prasad A, Neuhaus E, Joshi S, Nowakowski J, Nelson J, Mittleman A, Aguero-Rosenfeld M, Topal J, Krause PJ. Emergence of resistance to azithromycin-atovaquone in immunocompromised patients with Babesia microti infection. Clin Infect Dis. 2010 Feb 1;50(3):381-6. PMID:20047477

Wright IG, Casu R, Commins MA, Dalrymple BP, Gale KR, Goodger BV, Riddles PW, Waltisbuhl DJ, Abetz I, Berrie DA, et al. The development of a recombinant Babesia vaccine. Vet Parasitol. 1992 Sep;44(1-2):3-13. PMID:1441189

Wright IG, Goodger BV, Leatch G, Aylward JH, Rode-Bramanis K, Waltisbuhl DJ. Protection of Babesia bigemina-immune animals against subsequent challenge with virulent Babesia bovis. Infect Immun. 1987 Feb;55(2):364-8. PMID:3542832

Wright IG, Goodger BV, Rode-Bramanis K, Mattick JS, Mahoney DF, Waltisbuhl DJ. The characterisation of an esterase derived from Babesia bovis and its use as a vaccine. Z Parasitenkd. 1983;69(6):703-14. PMID:6419487

Wright IG, Mirre GB, Rode-Bramanis K, Chamberlain M, Goodger BV, Waltisbuhl DJ. Protective vaccination against virulent Babesia bovis with a low-molecular-weight antigen. Infect Immun. 1985 Apr;48(1):109-13. PMID:3980077

Wright IG, White M, Tracey-Patte PD, Donaldson RA, Goodger BV, Waltisbuhl DJ, Mahoney DF. Babesia bovis: isolation of a protective antigen by using monoclonal antibodies. Infect Immun. 1983 Jul;41(1):244-50. PMID:6345394

Wudhikarn K, Perry EH, Kemperman M, Jensen KA, Kline SE. Transfusion-transmitted babesiosis in an immunocompromised patient: a case report and review. Am J Med. 2011 Sep;124(9):800-5. Epub 2011 Jun 16. PMID:21683324

Xue RD. Introduction to symposium on mosquitoes and plants. J Am Mosq Control Assoc. 2008 Mar;24(1):134-7. PMID:18437828

Yabsley MJ, Davidson WR, Stallknecht DE, Varela AS, Swift PK, Devos JC Jr, Dubay SA. Evidence of tick-borne organisms in mule deer (Odocoileus hemionus) from the western United States. Vector Borne Zoonotic Dis. 2005 Winter;5(4):351-62. PMID:16417431

Yabsley MJ, Romines J, Nettles VF. Detection of Babesia and Anaplasma species in rabbits from Texas and Georgia, USA. Vector Borne Zoonotic Dis. 2006 Spring;6(1):7-13. PMID:16584322

Yadav S, Mittal PK, Saxena PN, Singh RK. Effect of synergist piperonyl butoxide (PBO) on the toxicity of some essential oils against mosquito larvae. J Commun Dis. 2009 Mar;41(1):33-8. PMID:19886173

Yadav S, Mittal PK, Saxena PN, Singh RK. Effect of synergist piperonyl butoxide (PBO) on the toxicity of some essential oils against mosquito larvae. J Commun Dis. 2008 Dec;40(4):263-8. PMID:19579718

Yamasaki M, Tajima M, Yamato O, Hwang SJ, Ohta H, Maede Y. Heat shock response of Babesia gibsoni heat shock protein 70. J Parasitol. 2008 Feb;94(1):119-24. PMID:18372630

Yao B, Zhao J, Ma L, Liu Z. Studies on the pathogenicity of Babesia bovis in water buffaloes after cryopreservation and resuscitation. Trop Anim Health Prod. 1997 Nov;29(4 Suppl):40S-42S. PMID:9512744

Yardley V, Gamarro F, Croft SL. Antileishmanial and antitrypanosomal activities of the 8-aminoquinoline tafenoquine. Antimicrob Agents Chemother. 2010 Dec;54(12):5356-8. Epub 2010 Sep 13. PMID:20837750

Yoeli M. [The development of malaria research before and since Ronald Ross].[Article in German]. Munch Med Wochenschr. 1973 Feb 2;115(5):151-8. PMID:4633457

Yoeli M. Landmarks in malaria research (a review). Acta Trop. 1974;31(4):321-8. PMID:4141222

Yoeli M, Most H. Sporozoite-induced infections of Plasmodium berghei administered by the oral route. Science. 1971 Sep 10;173(4001):1031-2. PMID:5098964

Yoshinari NH, Abrão MG, Bonoldi VL, Soares CO, Madruga CR, Scofield A, Massard CL, da Fonseca AH. Coexistence of antibodies to tick-borne agents of babesiosis and Lyme borreliosis in patients from Cotia county, State of São Paulo, Brazil. Mem Inst Oswaldo Cruz. 2003 Apr;98(3):311-8. Epub 2003 Jul 18. PMID:12886408

Young AS, Cox FE. The effect of betamethasone on Babesia microti and B. rodhaini infections in rodents. Parasitology. 1971 Dec;63(3):447-53. PMID:4945066

Young AS, Groocock CM, Kariuki DP. Integrated control of ticks and tick-borne diseases of cattle in Africa. Parasitology. 1988 Apr;96 (Pt 2):403-32. PMID:3287285

Young AS, Mutugi JJ, Kariuki DP, Lampard D, Maritim AC, Ngumi PN, Linyonyi A, Leitch BL, Ndungu SG, Lesan AC, et al. Immunisation of cattle against theileriosis in Nakuru District of Kenya by infection and treatment and the introduction of unconventional tick control. Vet Parasitol. 1992 May;42(3-4):225-40. PMID: 1496782

Young C, Krause PJ. The problem of transfusion-transmitted babesiosis. Transfusion. 2009 Dec;49(12):2548-50. PMID:20163687

Yu DH, Li YH, Yoon JS, Lee JH, Lee MJ, Yu IJ, Chae JS, Park JH. Ehrlichia chaffeensis infection in dogs in South Korea. Vector Borne Zoonotic Dis. 2008 Jun;8(3):355-8. PMID:18399775

Yunker CE, Kuttler KL, Johnson LW. Attenuation of Babesia bovis by in vitro cultivation. Vet Parasitol. 1987 Apr;24(1-2):7-13. PMID:3590611

Zambelli AB, Leisewitz AL. A prospective, randomized comparison of Oxyglobin (HB-200) and packed red blood cell transfusion for canine babesiosis. J Vet Emerg Crit Care (San Antonio). 2009 Feb;19(1):102-12. PMID:19691591

Zamoto A, Tsuji M, Kawabuchi T, Wei Q, Asakawa M, Ishihara C. U.S.-type Babesia microti isolated from small wild mammals in Eastern Hokkaido, Japan. J Vet Med Sci. 2004 Aug;66(8):919-26. PMID:15353841

Zamoto A, Tsuji M, Wei Q, Cho SH, Shin EH, Kim TS, Leonova GN, Hagiwara K, Asakawa M, Kariwa H, Takashima I, Ishihara C. Epizootiologic survey for Babesia microti among small wild mammals in northeastern Eurasia and a geographic diversity in the beta-tubulin gene sequences. J Vet Med Sci. 2004 Jul;66(7):785-92. PMID:15297749

Zaugg JL, Lane VM. Efficacy of buparvaquone as a therapeutic and clearing agent of Babesia equi of European origin in horses. Am J Vet Res. 1992 Aug;53(8):1396-9. PMID:1510317

Zhang L, Sathunuru R, Caridha D, Pybus B, O'Neil MT, Kozar MP, Lin AJ. Antimalarial activities of new guanidylimidazole and guanidylimidazoline derivatives. J Med Chem. 2011 Oct 13;54(19):6634-46. Epub 2011 Sep 2. PMID:21848332

Zhao JL, Liu ZL, Yao BA, Ma LH. Culture-derived Babesia orientalis exoantigens used as a vaccine against buffalo babesiosis. Parasitol Res. 2002 May;88(13 Suppl 1):S38-40. PMID:12051606

Zhao Y, Love KR, Hall SW, Beardell FV. A fatal case of transfusion-transmitted babesiosis in the State of Delaware. Transfusion. 2009 Dec;49(12):2583-7. Epub 2009 Nov 9. PMID:19906041

Zhu J, Lin S. [Investigation on folk medicine and health care of She ethnic group in Zhejiang province].[Article in Chinese]. Zhonghua Yi Shi Za Zhi. 2002 Oct;32(4):195-9. PMID:12639431

Zhu L, Tian Y. Chemical composition and larvicidal activity of Blumea densiflora essential oils against Anopheles anthropophagus: a malarial vector mosquito. Parasitol Res. 2011 Nov;109(5):1417-22. Epub 2011 May 10. PMID:21556689

Zhu L, Tian YJ. Chemical composition and larvicidal effects of essential oil of Blumea martiniana against Anopheles anthropophagus. Asian Pac J Trop Med. 2011 May;4(5):371-4. Epub 2011 Jun 22. PMID:2177167

Zintl A, Skerrett HE, Gray JS, Brophy PO, Mulcahy G. Babesia divergens (Phylum Apicomplexa) in vitro growth in the presence of calf serum. Vet Parasitol. 2004 Jun 21;122(2):127-30. PMID:15177717

Zivkovic D, Seinen W, Kuil H, Albers-van Bemmel CM, Speksnijder JE. Immunity to Babesia in mice. I. Adoptive transfer of immunity to Babesia rodhaini with immune spleen cells and the effect of irradiation on the protection of immune mice. Vet Immunol Immunopathol. 1984 Mar;5(4):343-57. PMID:6730310

Zivkovic D, Speksnijder JE, Kuil H, Seinen W. Immunity to Babesia in mice. II. Cross protection between various Babesia and Plasmodium species and its relevance to the nature of Babesia immunity. Vet Immunol Immunopathol. 1984 Mar;5(4):359-68. PMID:6730311

Zivkovic Z, Torina A, Mitra R, Alongi A, Scimeca S, Kocan KM, Galindo RC, Almazán C, Blouin EF, Villar M, Nijhof AM, Mani R, La Barbera G, Caracappa S, Jongejan F, de la Fuente J. Subolesin expression in response to pathogen infection in ticks. BMC Immunol. 2010 Feb 19;11:7. PMID:20170494

Zobba R, Parpaglia ML, Spezzigu A, Pittau M, Alberti A. First molecular identification and phylogeny of a Babesia sp. from a symptomatic sow (Sus scrofa Linnaeus 1758). J Clin Microbiol. 2011 Jun;49(6):2321-4. Epub 2011 Apr 13. PMID:21490184

Zsila F, Visy J, Mády G, Fitos I. Selective plasma protein binding of antimalarial drugs to alpha1-acid glycoprotein. Bioorg Med Chem. 2008 Apr 1;16(7):3759-72. Epub 2008 Feb 2. PMID:18289858

Zweygarth E, Just MC, de Waal DT. Continuous in vitro cultivation of erythrocytic stages of Babesia equi. Parasitol Res. 1995;81(4):355-8. PMID:7624296

Zweygarth E, Van Niekerk C, Just MC, De Waal DT. In vitro cultivation of a Babesia sp. from cattle in South Africa. Onderstepoort J Vet Res. 1995 Jun;62(2):139-42. PMID:8600438

Dr. Schaller has been published in:

Journal of the American Medical Association

Journal of Clinical Neuroscience

Medscape (Academic Journal of WebMD)

Journal of the American Society of Child and Adolescent
Psychiatry

American Journal of Psychiatry

European Journal of Child and Adolescent Psychiatry

Compounding Pharmaceuticals: Triad

Fleming Revell Press (Four Languages)

Internal Medicine News

Family Practice News

Spire Mass Market Books

Internet Journal of Family Medicine

Greenwood Press

Child and Adolescent Psychiatry Drug Alerts

Hope Academic Press

Clinical Psychiatry News

Psychiatric Drug Alerts

Townsend Journal

OB/GYN News

AMA News

Currents

A Sample of Other Books by Dr. Schaller

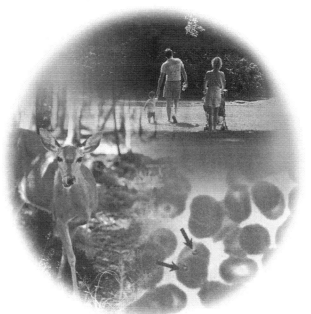

JAMES SCHALLER, M.D.

The Diagnosis and Treatment of

Babesia

Lyme's Cruel Cousin: the OTHER Tick-borne Infection

This large textbook is clear and easy to read. It is really three books. While some points are partially outdated since 2006, much would be considered new to most readers.

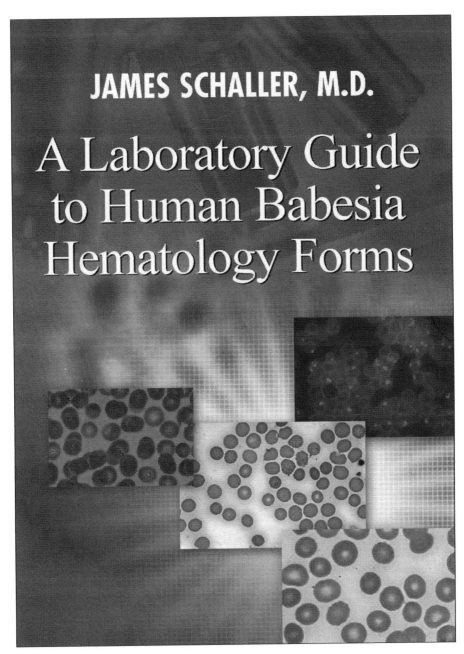

The only hematology book exclusively dedicated to Babesia.

Artemisinin, Artesunate, Artemisinic Acid and Other Derivatives of Artemisia Used for Malaria, Babesia and Cancer

A Health Care Practitioner's Guide to Dosage, Side Effects, Effectiveness, Toxicity and Interactions. A Review of the Research on the Most Common Clinical Artemisia Medications.

JAMES SCHALLER, M.D.

The most up-to-date academic and patient-centered book on practical Artemisia Babesia issues.

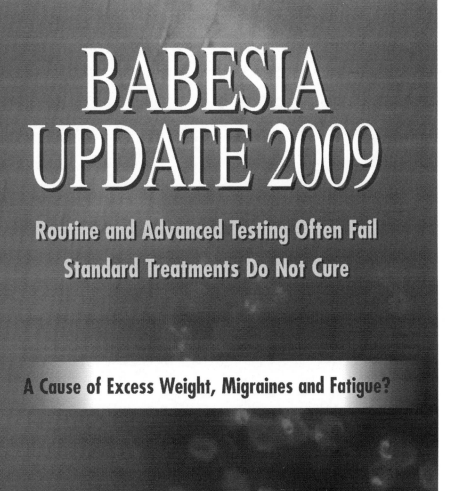

A book with advanced research based information, that moves Babesia medicine into a new decade. It presents highly practical information on ways to detect Babesia that are not mere IgM/G titer tests. Learn how to detect new species being discovered routinely and which seriously undermine function. This text also discusses why some individuals do not experience the easy and fast cure promised in other writings.

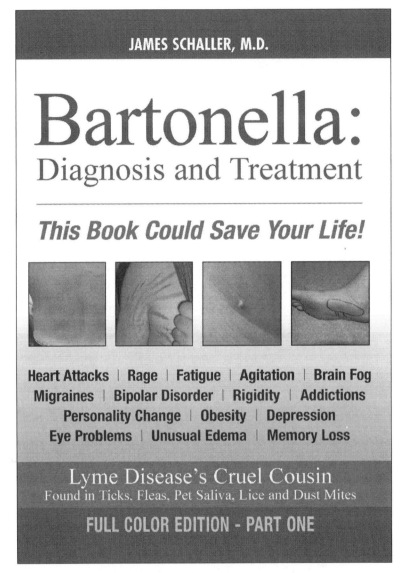

JAMES SCHALLER, M.D.

Bartonella:
Diagnosis and Treatment

This Book Could Save Your Life!

**Heart Attacks | Rage | Fatigue | Agitation | Brain Fog
Migraines | Bipolar Disorder | Rigidity | Addictions
Personality Change | Obesity | Depression
Eye Problems | Unusual Edema | Memory Loss**

Lyme Disease's Cruel Cousin
Found in Ticks, Fleas, Pet Saliva, Lice and Dust Mites

FULL COLOR EDITION - PART ONE

Bartonella diagnosis is very complex. This current text creatively used a new set of tools to assist in diagnosis based on solid research of blood vessel and skin augmentation chemicals created by Bartonella. It literally creates a new Bartonella physical exam. This book helps with limited basic lab testing, and **prevents the use of routinely relapsing or poor treatments promoted in both traditional and integrative medicine.** No other book on this topic is based on over a thousand top research articles, and no one has published anything remotely close to replacing this work in over five years.

When Traditional Medicine Fails...

YOUR GUIDE TO
MOLD TOXINS

Gary Rosen, Ph.D. & James Schaller, M.D.

- **WHAT THEY ARE**
- **WHO THEY HURT**
- **AND WHAT YOU CAN
  DO TO RECLAIM YOUR CHILD'S HEALTH,
  LEARNING AND BEHAVIOR**

Includes Home Detox Program

Dr. Schaller is a Certified Mold Investigator
and a Certified Mold Remediator. Here is a practical
and readable mold mycotoxin book.

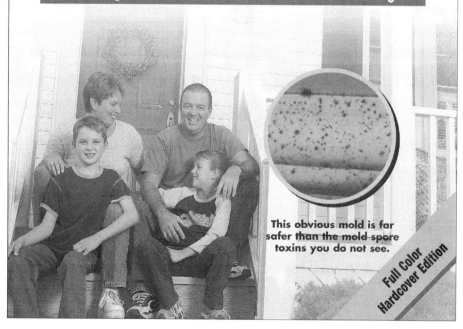

This book is helpful for people who are ill, or have trouble thinking and reading science materials. This is very practical and shows the clean-up errors made by 95% of experienced and expensive licensed mold remediators and renovation workers. Just reading ten pages from this book has shown people why they are not getting better. And this text helps you spot a poor remediators after simply reading 40 easy comics. Most remediations fail and most building hygiene actions are flawed. See why fast. The six best mycotoxin binders **cannot cure you if you are *still* in a "sick" home or moldy work location.**

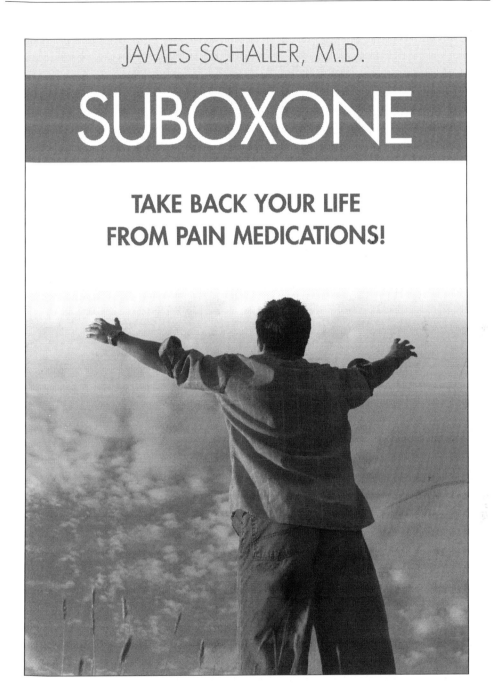

JAMES SCHALLER, M.D.

SUBOXONE

TAKE BACK YOUR LIFE
FROM PAIN MEDICATIONS!

The only current, practical and advanced
clinical book on this revolutionary treatment for
opioid addiction and modest pain.

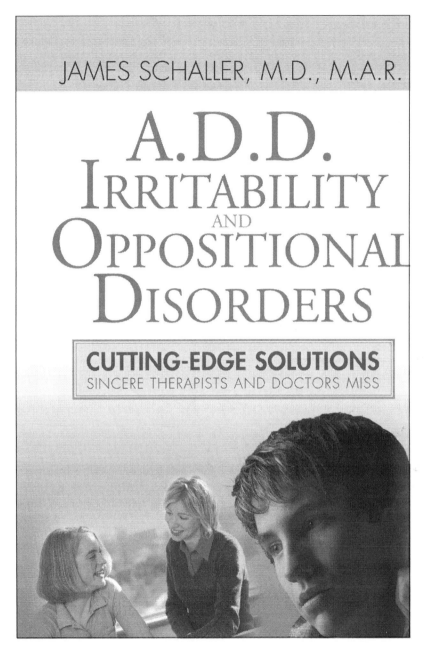

The many missed **medical and neurological** causes of poor focus and bad behaviors can no longer be ignored. This unique text advances medicine and shows how much in youth psychiatry has medical roots that are ignored or unknown even in solid child and adolescent psychiatry practices.

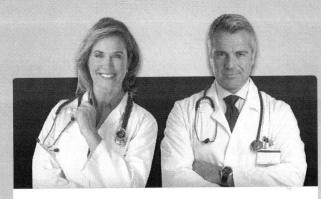

CHECKLISTS FOR BARTONELLA, BABESIA, AND LYME DISEASE
2012 EDITION

A "BEST DOCTOR", "PEOPLE'S CHOICE PHYSICIAN" AND "TOP DOCTOR"
OFFERS HIGHLY RESEARCHED, ADVANCED DIAGNOSTIC CHECKLISTS
FOR DANGEROUS EMERGING INFECTIONS

Which Physician is Going to do a Proper Exam of a
Person With Bartonella, Babesia, and Lyme Disease?

The right physician is the one who is going to take
the time for a very comprehensive evaluation

JAMES SCHALLER, MD, MAR & KIMBERLY MOUNTJOY, MS

The only tick and flea-borne infection diagnostic checklist book
based on over 6,000 references related to Bartonella, Babesia and
Lyme disease. It seeks to prevent false negative diagnosis, meaning,
the advanced and expanded criteria are set to catch these three infections. This book is available from www.personalconsult.com under
"free books" or from Amazon.com.

Disclaimer

Dr. Schaller is not a specialist in infectious disease medicine. He is also not a pathologist. Both of these specialties have over 2,000 diseases to treat and study. Dr. Schaller is only interested in four infections and has read and published on only these four. The medical ideas, health thoughts, health comments, products and any claims made about specific illnesses, diseases, and causes of health problems in this book are purely speculative, hypothetical, and are not meant to be authoritative in any setting. No comment or image has been evaluated by the FDA, CDC, NIH, IDSA or the AMA. Never assume any United States medical body, society, or the majority of American physicians endorse any comment in this book. No comment in this book is approved by any government agency, medical body or medical society. Nothing in this book is to be used to diagnose, treat, cure or prevent disease. The information provided in this book is for educational purposes only. It is not intended as a substitute for the advice from your physician or other health care professionals. This book is not intended to replace or adjust any information contained on, or in, any product label or packaging.

No patient should use the information in this book for the diagnosis or treatment of any health problem, or for prescription of any medication or other treatment. You should consult with a health care professional before deciding on any diagnosis, or initiating any treatment plan of any kind. Dr. Schaller does not claim to be an expert in any illness, disease or treatment. In this book, he is merely sharing one of his interests. Please do not start any diet, exercise or supplementation program, or take any type of nutrient, herb, or medication, without clear consultation with your licensed health care provider.

Babesia or Bartonella diagnosis or treatment comments and reports of possible positive or negative treatment outcomes are hypothetical. No treatment should be rejected or embraced by anyone, based on the preliminary research and study in this book.

In this book, Dr. Schaller makes no authoritative or proven claim about any diagnosis, lab testing or treatment. Dr. Schaller only offers hypothetical ideas. Dr. Schaller makes no authoritative claims about medications, nutrients, herbs or various types of alternative medicine. The ideas in this book will need to be submitted to your local expert in allopathic, osteopathic or progressive medicine, or to other licensed health care practitioners. This book is not meant to be an informal or formal guideline book that presumes to control 800,000 physicians, or the 300 million patients they serve. You are asked to let the wisdom of your health care practitioners, and your own study, be a starting point to guide treatment tailored specifically to your body. Again, Dr. Schaller makes no claim to be an expert in any aspect of medicine. He makes no claim to know more than other physicians.

Additionally, Dr. Schaller makes no claim that any statement in this book is correct.

Since this appears to be the first book exclusively dedicated to advanced modern cutting-edge tick and flea infection expanded diagnosis criteria, it is very likely to contain errors This is common with books that are the first on such sensitive topics. Every reasonable effort has been made not to try to overstate findings. Further, it is important to realize that any single lab finding or treatment outcome can have multiple causes, and not all of these may be known to this author, or to other health practitioners. Therefore, all health care practitioners should look for other confirmations outside this book before beginning on any treatment plan, if possible.

Contacting Dr. Schaller

Should you wish to talk to Dr. Schaller he offers individualized education consults, which can be arranged by calling 239-263-0133. Please leave all your phone numbers, a working email and a fax number. These consults are typically in 15 minute units and can last as long as you wish. All that is required is the completion of a short informed consent form.

If you would like a full diagnostic consult or to see Dr. Schaller as a patient, know he treats patients from all over the USA and from outside the country. He meets with you first and then does follow-up care with you by phone.

If you would like to fly in to see Dr. Schaller, his staff are very familiar with all the closest airports, and we have special hotel discounts.

I wish you the very best health!

Warm Regards,
Rona C. MBA
Office Manager